AF714101

Plastic and Reconstructive Surgery of the Face and Neck

Proceedings of the Second International Symposium

Plastic and Reconstructive Surgery of the Face and Neck

Proceedings of the Second International Symposium

Volume 2: Rehabilitative Surgery

Edited by
George A. Sisson, M.D.
M. Eugene Tardy, Jr., M.D.

GRUNE & STRATTON

A Subsidiary of Harcourt Brace Jovanovich, Publishers

New York San Francisco London

Library of Congress Cataloging in Publication Data

International Symposium on Plastic and Reconstructive
Surgery of the Face and Neck, 2d, Chicago, 1975.
Plastic and reconstructive surgery of the face and neck.

Sponsored by the American Academy of Facial Plastic and Reconstructive Surgery.
Includes bibliographical references and indexes.
CONTENTS: v. 1. Aesthetic surgery—v. 2. Rehabilitative surgery.
1. Surgery, Plastic—Congresses. 2. Face—Surgery—Congresses.
3. Neck—Surgery—Congresses. I. Sisson, George A.
II. Tardy, Medney Eugene, 1934– III. American Academy
of Facial Plastic and Reconstructive Surgery. IV. Title.
[DNLM: 1. Neck—Surgery—Congresses. 2. Face—Congresses.
3. Surgery, Plastic—Congresses. WE705 P713]
RD118.A1I6 1975 617′.52 76-57989
ISBN 0-8089-0941-X (v. 1)
ISBN 0-8089-0956-8 (v. 2)

© 1977 by Grune & Stratton, Inc.

All rights reserved. No part of this publication may be reproduced or transmitted in any form or by any means, electronic or mechanical, including photocopy, recording, or any information storage and retrieval system, without permission in writing from the publisher.

Grune & Stratton, Inc.
111 Fifth Avenue
New York, New York 10003

Distributed in the United Kingdom by
Academic Press, Inc. (London) Ltd.
24/28 Oval Road, London NW 1

Library of Congress Catalog Number 76-57989
International Standard Book Number 0-8089-0956-8

Printed in the United States of America

Table of Contents

Preface

"Medicine is the only world wide profession, following everywhere the same methods, actuated by the same ambitions, and pursuing the same ends. This homogeneity, its most characteristic feature, is not shared by the law, and not by the church, certainly not in the same degree. While in antiquity the law rivals medicine, there is not in it that extraordinary solidarity which makes the physician at home in any country, any place where two or three sons of men are gathered together . . . . A powerful stimulus in promoting this wide organic unity is our great international gatherings . . . . "I may say to you that one of the distressing bewilderments of the layman who only desires the working out of a broad plan is the extraordinary bitterness of professional jealousy between not only schoolmen and nonschoolmen but between schoolmen themselves, and the reflections which are cast on one another as belonging to that clique, which makes it exceedingly difficult for the layman to understand what way there is out of these squabbles."

Sir William Osler
Unity, Peace, and Concord
in Aequanimitas, 1905

In his farewell address to the medical profession seventy years ago, Sir William Osler outlined several truths still inherent in the practice of medicine. Perhaps now, more than ever before, these precepts should be reiterated and recognized as important strengths, since presently our profession is subjected to the greatest scrutiny ever by both the consumer and the lawmaker. Today, it is imperative that the various disciplines of medicine be united. We must not be drawn into jurisdictional disputes which would blur our public image and weaken our position in any political action. Cooperation becomes essential for a favorable future base. The free interchange of information and ideas and the sharing of experiences will help to better gird all specialities so medicine's obligation to the consumer can be well met and its responsibilities to the legislative process intelligently fulfilled.

It was our hope that the Second International Symposium on Plastic and Reconstructive Surgery of the Face and Neck would provide a forum whereby its members, in consortium with its many friends in general surgery, oral surgery, and general plastic surgery could hold a meeting in the continued search for excellence in the teaching and practice of their surgical art.

The Symposium was more than a success. It was gratifying to see the various disciplines sit down for one week and share new concepts, techniques and philosophies without rancor or built-in prejudices.

The multidisiplinary attendance was apparent as was the international flavor, with over twenty countries represented. Approximately 100 papers, 15 panels, 45 instructional courses, and 40 cine-clinics were presented. The true interchange of philosophies and information continued late into the evening social functions.

The mixed background of the 1000 attendees provided a built-in flexibility rather than the traditional rigidities often prominent in the smaller and "select" society meetings. Those in attendance were well aware of the difficulties encountered in gaining new information in this most exacting and complex region. No one man nor one medical specialty can expect to be expert in all the new techniques rapidly developing in the region of the head and neck.

It was apparent early that the American Academy of Facial Plastic and Reconstructive Surgery, host of the Second International Symposium, was obligated to publish these scientific proceedings. A natural division of the presentations into aesthetic and reparative attitudes makes possible the publication of these two volumes. This work should provide ready reference for the attendees as well as make possible further dissemination of this information for those unable to attend. As these volumes take their place in the continuum of medicine, only history can judge their true value.

Today, we can say this international meeting, conceived for the continuing search for excellence, reflected well on the medical profession by demonstrating "unity, peace, and concord."

George A. Sisson, M.D.
General Chairman
and
M. Eugene Tardy, Jr. M.D.
Program Chairman

Second International Symposium
on Plastic and Reconstructive
Surgery of the Face and Neck

Contributors

William A. Alonso, M.D. St. Louis, Missouri

Agustin Arbulu, M.D. Detroit, Michigan

Mohamed A. Arramany, M.D. Pittsburgh, Pennsylvania

R. Baumann, M.D. Wurzburg, W. Germany

David Bernstein, M.D. New York, New York

Dennis Brady, M.D. Minneapolis, Minnesota

Robert W. Cantrell, M.D. San Diego, California

A. D. Cheesman, M.D. London, England

Thomas Christiansen, M.D. Minneapolis, Minnesota

John Conley, M.D. New York, New York

Robin T. Cotton, M.D. Cincinnati, Ohio

Douglas D. Dedo, M.D. St. Louis, Missouri

Bruce K. Defiebre, M.D. San Diego, California

Lawrence W. DeSanto, M.D. Rochester, Minnesota

Ralph L. Dicker, M.D. New York, New York

Blair Fearon, M.D. Cincinnati, Ohio

Stephen C. Ferguson, M.D. Evansville, Indiana

Howard K. Gelman, M.D. Chicago, Illinois

Jerome C. Goldstein, M.D. Albany, New York

Richard L. Goode, M.D. Stanford, California

Malcolm D. Graham, M.D. Los Angeles, California

James A. Grant, M.D. Memphis, Tennessee

Ronald C. Hamaker, M.D. Indianapolis, Indiana

Henry J. Heimlich, M.D. Cincinnati, Ohio

Nobuhiko Isshiki, M.D. Kyoto, Japan

Burton F. Jaffe, M.D. Boston, Massachusetts

Frank M. Kamer, M.D. Los Angeles, California

John Kelly, M.D. Boston, Massachusetts

U. K. Kesselring, M.D. Lausanne, Switzerland

Eugene B. Kern, M.D. Rochester, Minnesota

Charles J. Krause, M.D. Iowa City, Iowa

Marvin L. Kwitko, M.D. Montreal, Canada

Donald Laub, M.D. Stanford, California

James R. Leonard, M.D. Atlanta, Georgia

Ward B. Litton, M.D. Iowa City, Iowa

Richard A. Martin, M.D. Omaha, Nebraska

Robert H. Mathog, M.D. Minneapolis, Minnesota

Ronald S. Matsunaga, M.D. Great Lakes, Illinois

E. Gaylon McCollough, M.D. Birmingham, Alabama

Michael L. Merrin, M.D. Los Angeles, California

Rodolphe Meyer, M.D. Lausanne, Switzerland

William L. Meyerhoff, M.D. Minneapolis, Minnesota

John W. Miles, M.D. Great Lakes, Illinois

Eugene N. Myers, M.D. Pittsburgh, Pennsylvania

Felix Nagel, M.D. Meinz, W. Germany

Alvin J. Novack, M.D. Seattle, Washington

Joseph H. Ogura, M.D. St. Louis, Missouri

Morey L. Parkes, M.D. Los Angeles, California

Deborah Pollak, M.D. Minneapolis, Minnesota

Lionello Ponti, M.D. Rome, Italy

Stephen D. Proffitt, M.D. Pomona, California

Allen M. Putterman, M.D. Chicago, Illinois

F. Mark Rafaty, M.D. Palo Alto, California

W. Richter, M.D. Wurzburg, W. Germany

Eugene Rontal, M.D. Farmington, Missouri

Albert L. Roper, M.D. Charleston, South Carolina

William R. Simpson, M.D. Great Lakes, Illinois

Emanuel M. Skolnick, M.D. Chicago, Illinois

Allen Small, M.D. Washington, D.C.

Raymond O. Smith, Jr., M.D. Oklahoma City, Oklahoma

G. Gordon Snyder, III, M.D. Hartford, Connecticut

Robert H. Sorosky, M.D. Pomona, California

Gershon J. Spector, M.D. St. Louis, Missouri

Samuel J. Stegman, M.D. San Francisco, California

Ronald W. Strahan, M.D. Los Angeles, California

Gordon W. Summers, M.D. Portland, Oregon

Leonard T. Swanson, M.D. Boston, Massachusetts

Victor R. Syracuse, M.D. New York, New York

Stanley E. Thawley, M.D. St. Louis, Missouri

Norman W. Thoms, M.D. Detroit, Michigan

Paul H. Toffel, M.D. Great Lakes, Illinois

James M. Toomey, M.D. Hartford, Connecticut

Theodore Tromovitch, M.D. San Francisco, California

Harvey M. Tucker, M.D. Syracuse, New York

Charles Z. Weingarten, M.D. Evanston, Illinois

Kent Wilson, M.D. Minneapolis, Minnesota

H. L. Wullstein, M.D. Wurzburg, W. Germany

Leonard H. Wurman, M.D. Minneapolis, Minnesota

C. Thomas Yarington, M.D. Omaha, Nebraska

Anthony J. Yonkers, M.D. Omaha, Nebraska

Siegfried Zehm, M.D. Hamburg, W. Germany

Plastic and Reconstructive Surgery of the Face and Neck

Proceedings of the Second International Symposium

Nose

Reconstructive Surgery of the Nose and Orbit

R. Meyer and U.K. Kesselring, Lausanne, Switzerland

Nose Reconstruction

At the first International Symposium four years ago we presented techniques for total and subtotal nasal reconstruction. Now we want to show procedures for partial repair of the nose after tumor ablation and trauma. For partial loss concerning tip, ala and columella the three-stage procedure with fronto-temporal flap is in our hands still the most secure and aesthetically best one. We modified this excellent tiny flap which was advocated by Schmid and adapted it to many types of defects in the fine framework of the nose.[1,7,8]

Our technique consists of prefabricating at the temporal end of the flap a composite construction that is made to measure for the defect which has to be covered (Fig. 1). The components needed are autogenous ear cartilage and split skin grafts. The carrier bridge flap, cut directly above the eyebrow, has bevelled sides which allows to give to a rather narrow strip of skin a considerable amount of subcutaneous tissue. This tissue is covered with an envelope of split skin, the wound above the eyebrow closed primarily. The procedure requires three sessions but has the advantage of being very versatile and of leaving inconspicuous scars.

We not only use this method for the reconstruction of postoperative defects after tumor ablation but also in cases of fresh trauma of the face (Fig. 2). In these cases the fronto-temporal flap is

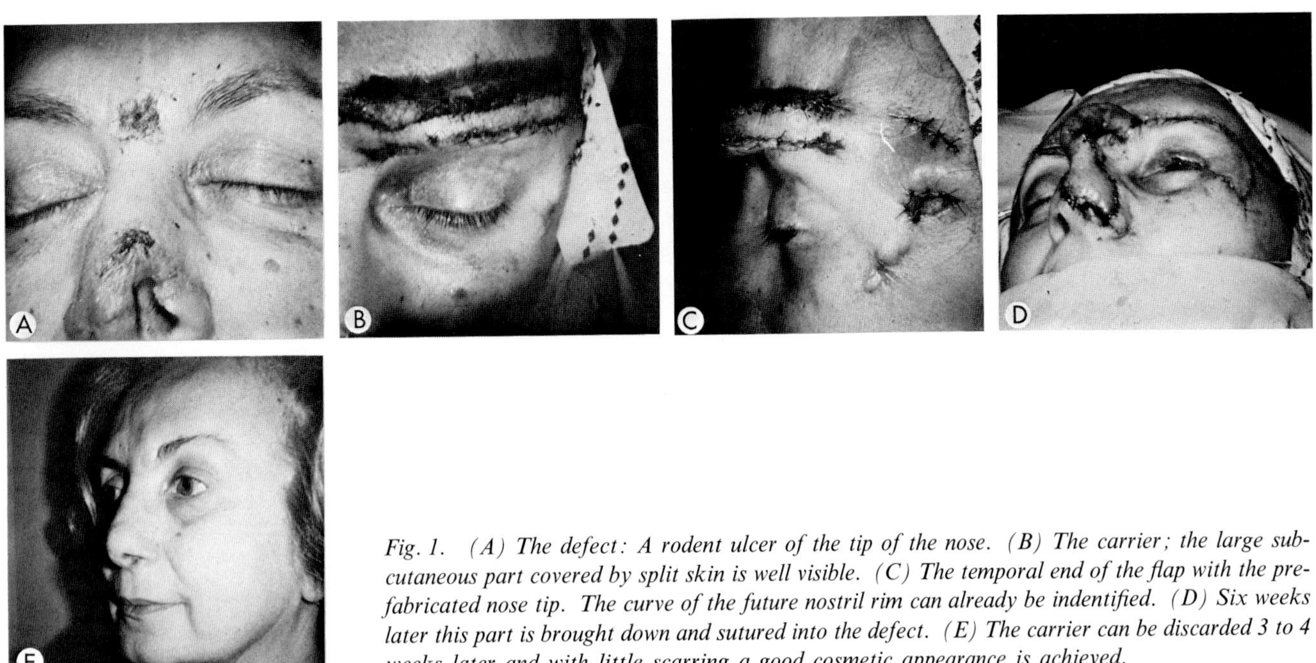

Fig. 1. (A) The defect: A rodent ulcer of the tip of the nose. (B) The carrier; the large subcutaneous part covered by split skin is well visible. (C) The temporal end of the flap with the prefabricated nose tip. The curve of the future nostril rim can already be indentified. (D) Six weeks later this part is brought down and sutured into the defect. (E) The carrier can be discarded 3 to 4 weeks later and with little scarring a good cosmetic appearance is achieved.

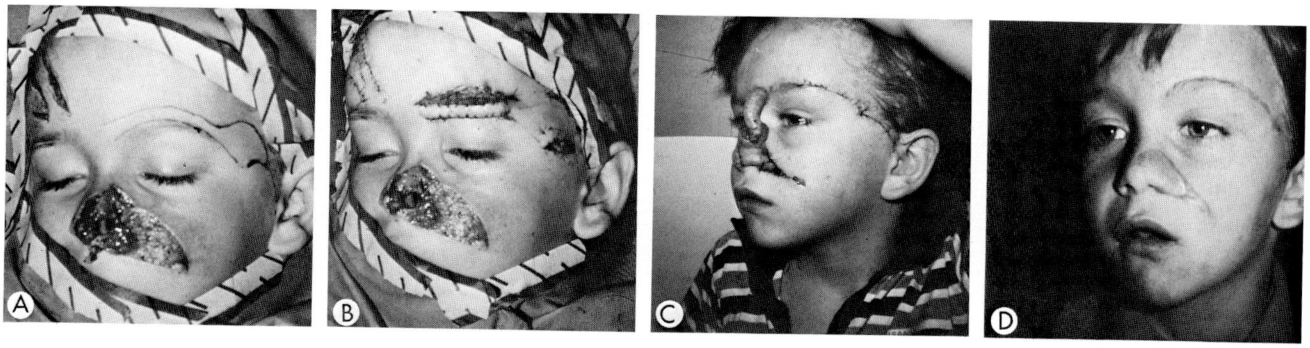

Fig. 2. *(A,B) These dog-bite wounds are cleaned and debrided under general anesthesia and in the same session a fronto-temporal flap is prepared. (C) The flap is brought into the recipient site. (D) The pedicle is discarded; some scar revision will be necessary on the cheek.*

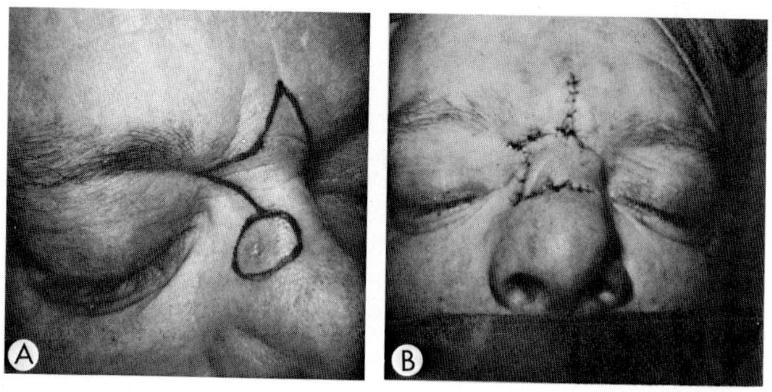

Fig. 3. *(A) A bilobed flap marked out in the glabellar region is intended to cover the defect after basalioma excision. (B) The sutures at the end of the operation. Scarring should be minimal and inconspicuous.*

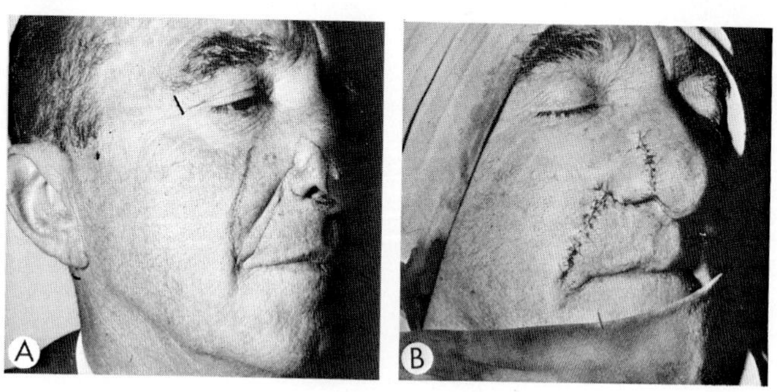

Fig. 4. *A finger flap from the nasolabial fold can be used for non-perforating alar defects.*

already prepared in the first session when the wound is debrided.

For nonperforating defects we use island flaps (which we will not discuss in detail here) and bi- and trilobed flaps (Figs. 3 and 4). Composite grafts are adopted only in rare selected cases (Fig. 5). In certain nostril rim defects for instance we like to use a composite graft from the crus helicis which often offers exactly the arch needed for the reconstruction of a harmoniously curved nostril. The resulting defect is easily covered by advancing the helix in the same manner as we described for the correction of too large auricles.

In the elderly patient with less aesthetic exigence, we limit our reconstructive work to a two-stage procedure. We repair for instance an extensive loss of the lower soft tissue (tip and ala) by combination of two flaps from the nasolabial folds (Fig. 6). Extensive alar defects are covered in two stages by an oblique forehead flap based at the upper border of the eyebrow and containing partially the supraorbital vessels. It can be folded at the extremity in order to provide the alar border (Fig. 7).

Quite obviously these two-stage procedures do not provide the same perfect reconstruction obtained with a composite element as in the cases with fronto-temporal flap repair. They should however be considered whenever any additional anesthesia is a risk since already the second stage can very well be done under local.

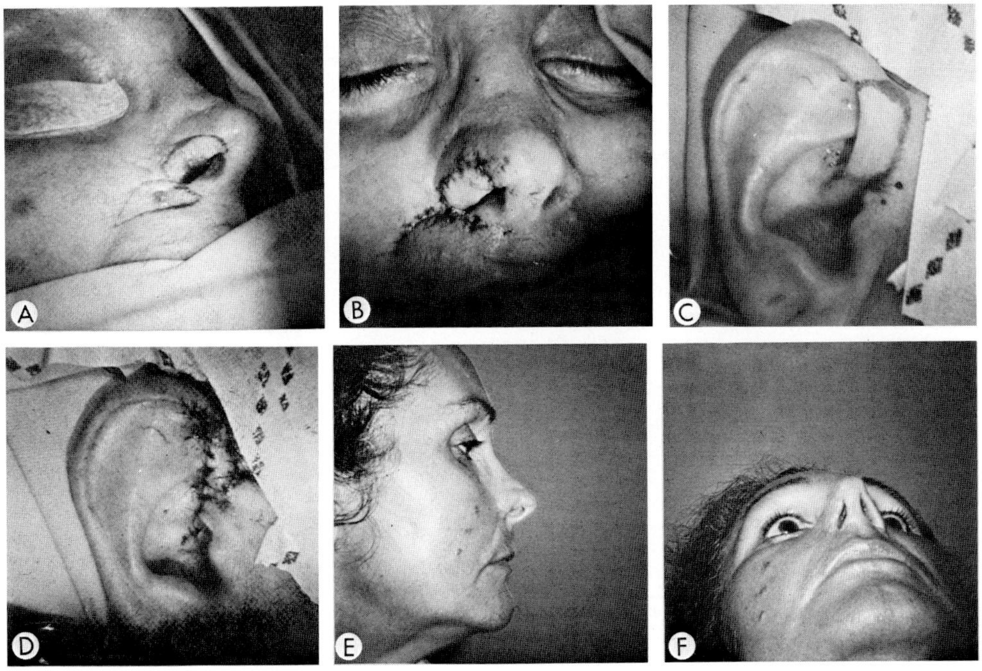

Fig. 5. *(A,B) While one defect after excision of this twin-tumor could be closed primarily, the one on the nose needed a composite graft. (C) The crus helicis provided the desired archiform graft. (D) The secondary defect was easily closed by rotating the helix forward. (E,F) Postoperative result.*

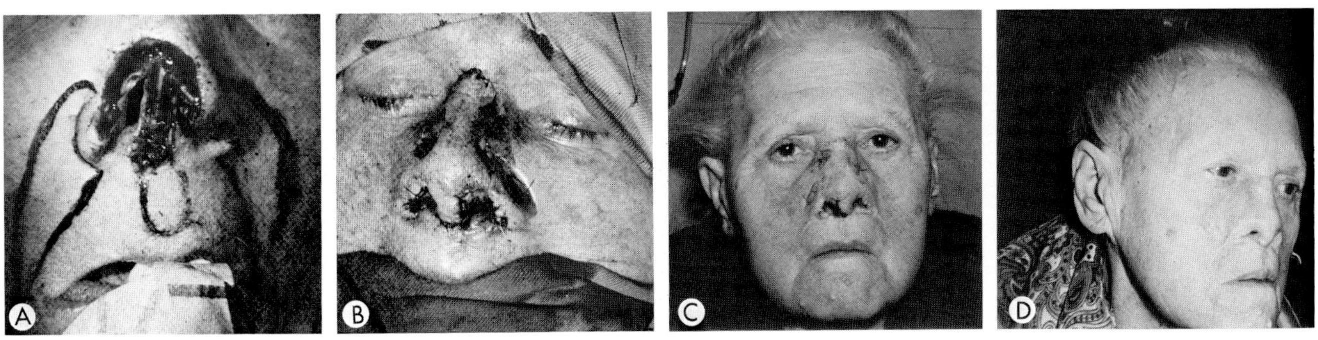

Fig. 6. *The tip of this nose including the columella are reconstructed with two local island flaps from either the nasolabial fold, respectively, from the philtrum.*

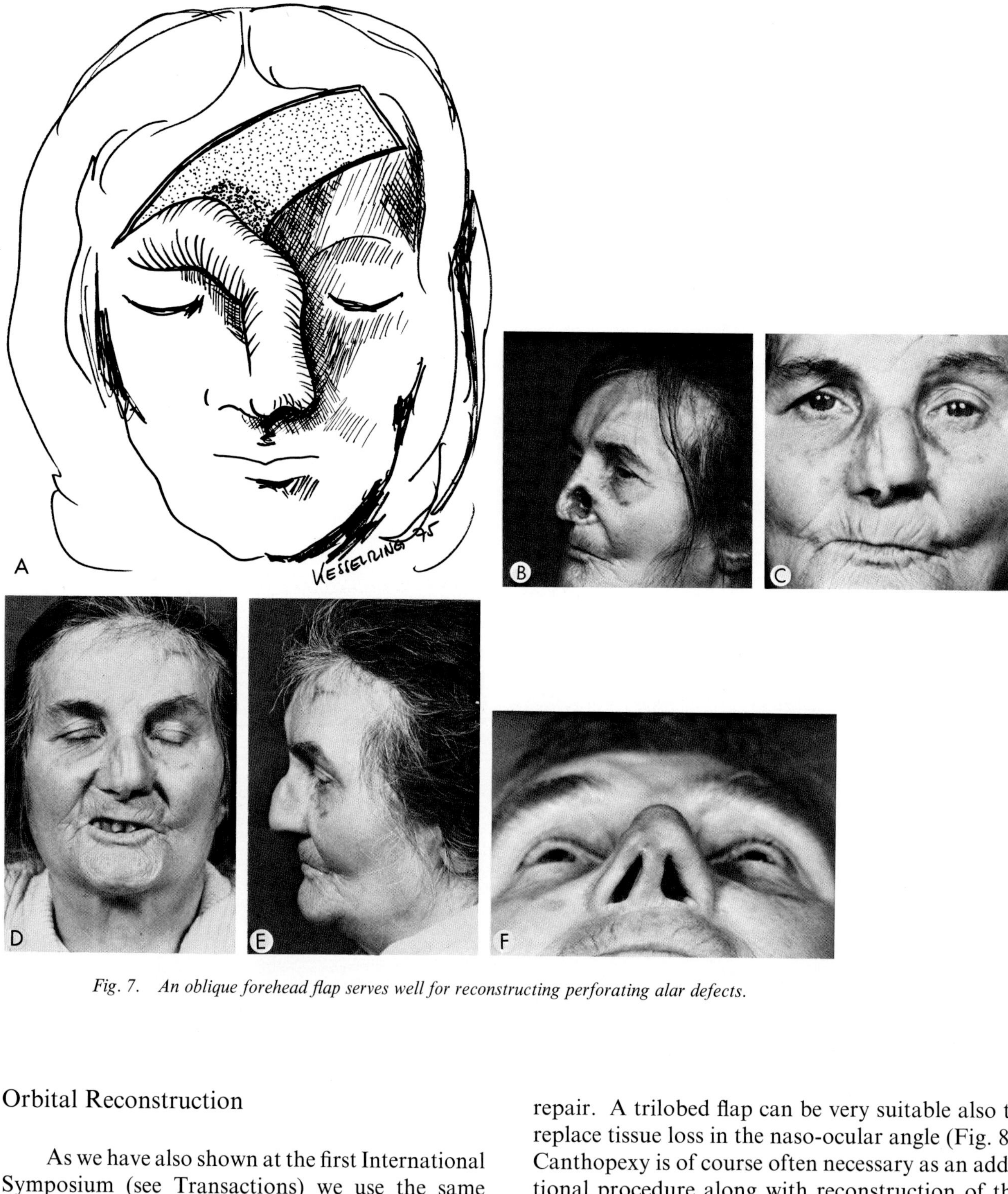

Fig. 7. An oblique forehead flap serves well for reconstructing perforating alar defects.

Orbital Reconstruction

As we have also shown at the first International Symposium (see Transactions) we use the same fronto-temporal flap for the reconstruction of the eyelids.[1,9] Besides this very useful and aesthetically satisfactory flap, we combine external flaps with mucosal flaps and grafts as well as composite flaps and grafts for the partial full thickness lid repair. A trilobed flap can be very suitable also to replace tissue loss in the naso-ocular angle (Fig. 8). Canthopexy is of course often necessary as an additional procedure along with reconstruction of the orbital floor, silicone block implantation, etc. (Fig. 9). To create some bulk and mobility in partially reconstructed eyelids after traumatic exenteration, temporal muscle fascia strips have given satisfactory results in our hands (Fig. 10).

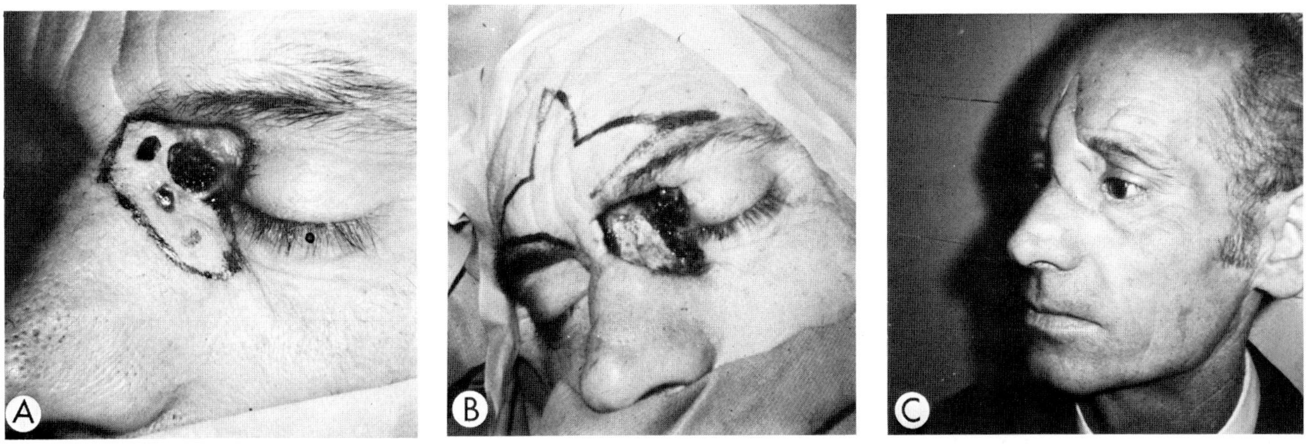

Fig. 8. *The trilobed flap permits one-stage coverage of larger defects. Here employed in a case with multifocal basalioma in the nasoocular angle.*

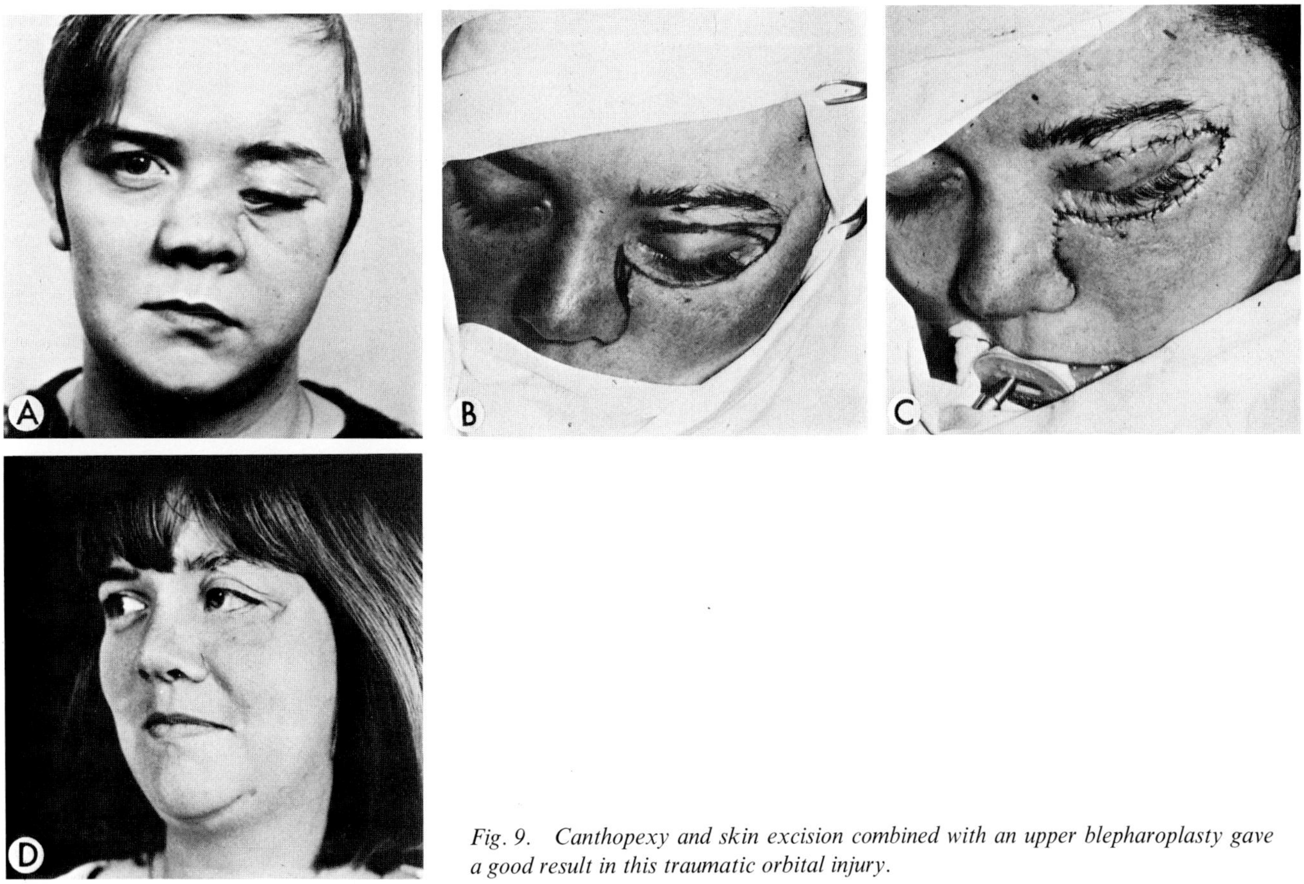

Fig. 9. *Canthopexy and skin excision combined with an upper blepharoplasty gave a good result in this traumatic orbital injury.*

For single-stage total and subtotal reconstruction of the lower lid the wide cheek rotation flap of Mustarde[3] can be combined with Millard's[4] septal mucosal graft which serves well for the eyelid lining (Fig. 11). The graft is sutured into the defect in three layers, using a pull-out suture for the mucosal side.

When the loss of palpebral conjunctiva and tarsal plate is less important its reconstruction may be provided by a free composite graft of the upper

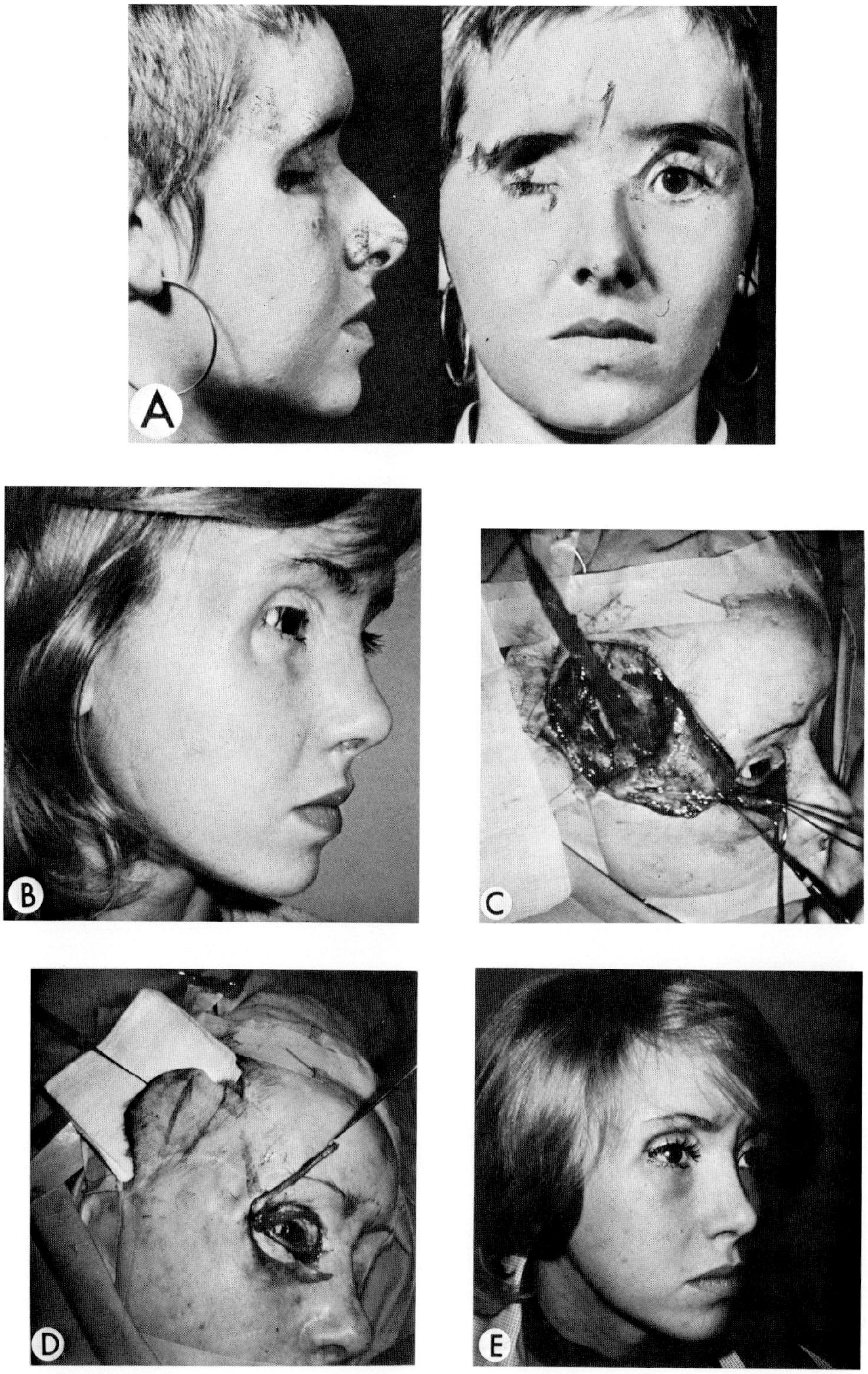

Fig. 10. (A,B) Silicone implants helped to fill up this orbit after traumatic bulb perforation. (C–E) Strips of temporal muscle and fascia are pulled through upper and lower lid and sutured to the medial canthus. Thus, some mobility and some additional bulk helped a great deal to ameliorate the girl's appearance.

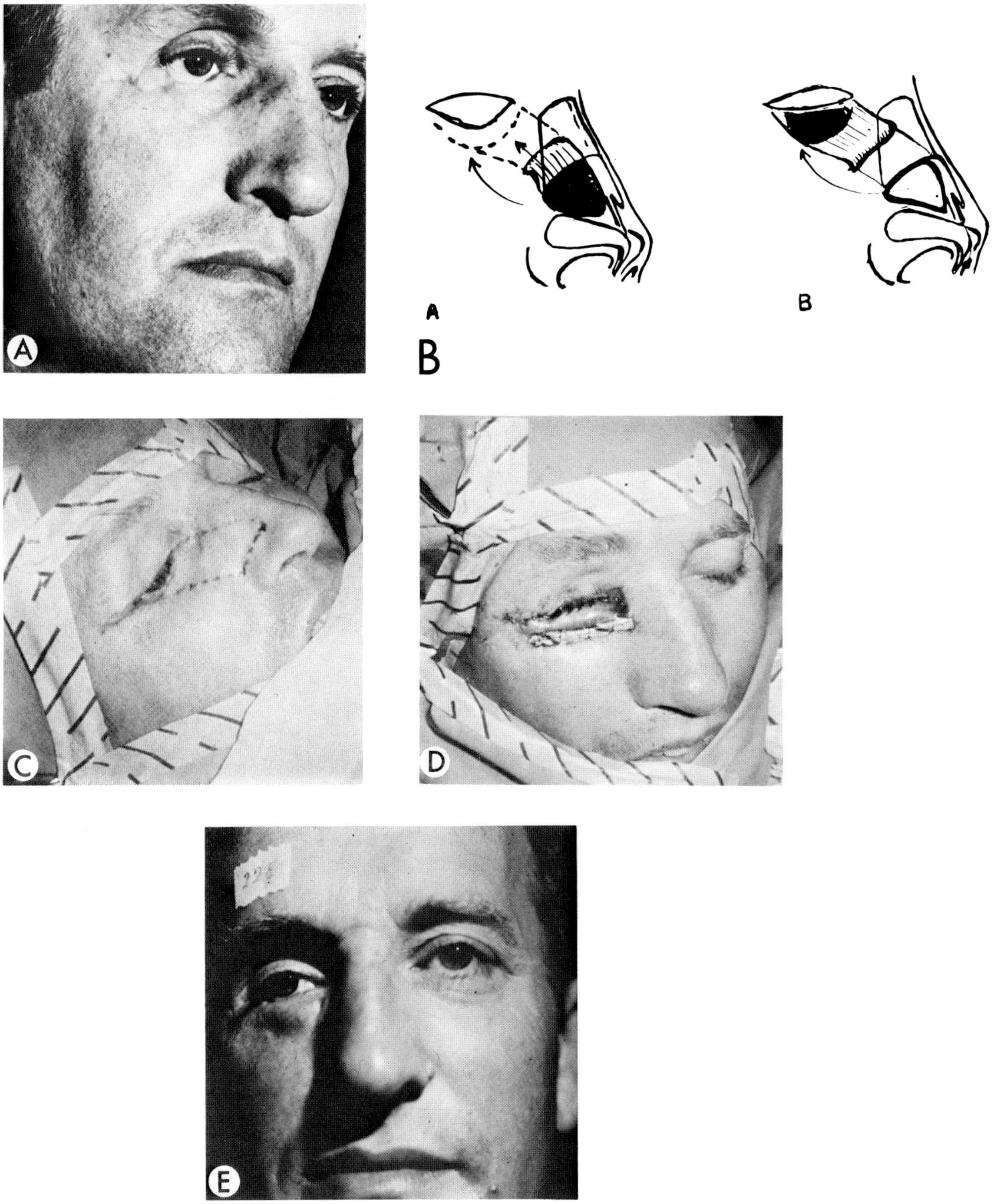

Fig. 11. Full thickness lower lid loss calls for a reconstruction of all planes. A composite graft (cartilage and mucosa) of the upper lateral cartilage can be moved as an island flap to the site of the defect.

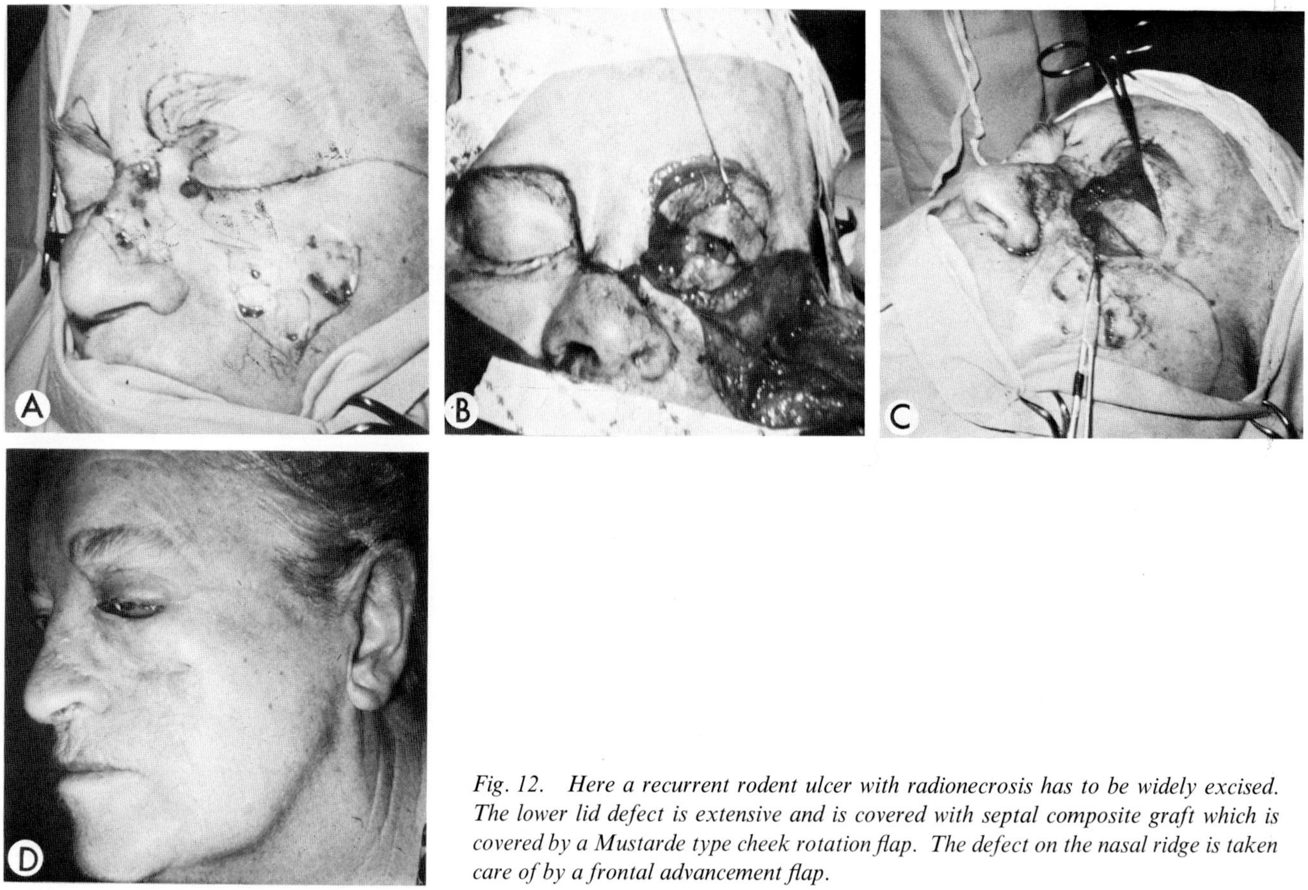

Fig. 12. Here a recurrent rodent ulcer with radionecrosis has to be widely excised. The lower lid defect is extensive and is covered with septal composite graft which is covered by a Mustarde type cheek rotation flap. The defect on the nasal ridge is taken care of by a frontal advancement flap.

lateral nasal cartilage as described by Tessier[5] and by Lipschutz[6] or by transferring this cartilage as an island flap from the homolateral side of the nose with the attached mucosa and with a musculo-subcutaneous pedicle onto the eyelid defect (Fig. 12). We reported this modification at the first International Symposium of Plastic and Reconstructive Surgery of the Face and Neck in New York[1] and have since then extended this island flap technique for wider reconstruction of the tarsal plate and conjunctiva in cases in which the upper lateral cartilage of the nose is too small to fulfill the criteria for repair. This island flap then includes the antero-superior part of the septal cartilage and the upper lateral cartilage leaving its insertion at the mucoperichondrium vault intact. In subtotal loss of the eyelid we transfer the lateral remnant of the lid border to the internal canthus, suturing it to the medial edge of the composite island flap (Fig. 13).

Summary

The modified Schmid[2] fronto-temporal flap is recommended for the repair of partial loss of tip, ala and columella. At its temporal end our flap is shaped, reinforced by autogenous ear cartilage and lined with a split-thickness skin graft in order to obtain a prefabricated part of the nose which fits exactly to the amount and shape of the nasal defect.

The fronto-temporal flap can very well be used for lid reconstruction also. For single-stage lower lid reconstruction the cheek rotation flap of Mustarde[3] combined with Millard's[4] septal mucosal graft serves well. For the reconstruction of wide defects of the tarsal plate and conjunctiva a composite island flap including the antero-superior part of the septal cartilage and the upper lateral cartilage on a musculo-subcutaneous pedicle is advocated.

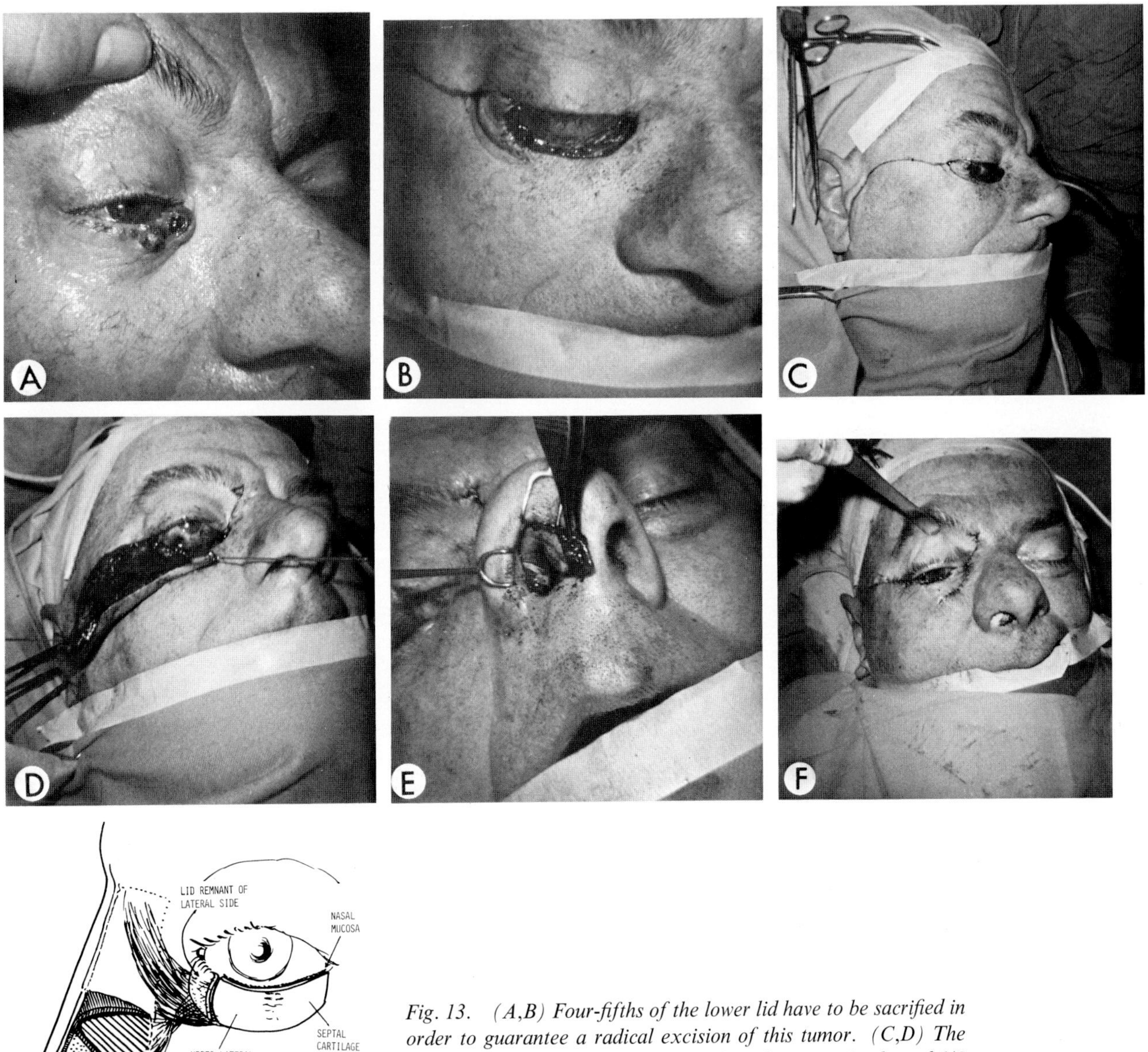

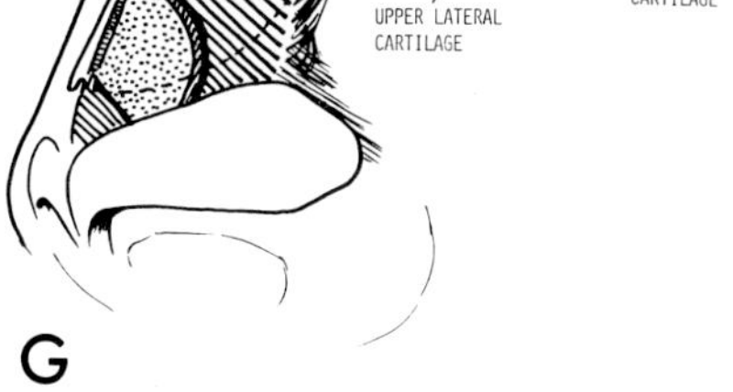

Fig. 13. (A,B) Four-fifths of the lower lid have to be sacrified in order to guarantee a radical excision of this tumor. (C,D) The cheek rotation flap is outlined, including the remaining lateral 1/5 of the lid which is carried to the nasal side. (E,F) The upper lateral cartilage and part of the septal cartilage are freed from their surrounding tissues but the mucoperichondrial vault is left intact. The whole plate is brought to the eye as an island flap and sutured into the defect, the mucosa facing the eye. (G) Diagram of the operation

References

1. Meyer R: Reconstruction of the eyelids. Plastic and Reconstructive Surgery of the Face and Neck, Vol. 2, 285–289, J Conley, JT Dickinson, Thieme Stuttgart 1972
2. Schmid E: Reconstruction of the orbit and lids. Trans the Intern. Society Plastic Surgeons, London 1959, E. & S. Livingstone Ltd. Edinburgh, London, 405–420, 1960
3. Mustarde J: Repair and reconstruction in the orbital region. Churchill Livingstone, Edinburgh, London, 1971
4. Millard R: Eyelid repairs with chondromucosal graft. Journal of Plastic and Reconstructive Surgery 30:267–272, 1962
5. Tessier P: Personal communication
6. Lipschutz, H: Experiences with upper lateral cartilage in reconstruction of the lower eyelid. Amer Ophtalmol 73: 592–594, 1973
7. Meyer R: Reconstructions orbito-palpébrales par lambeau frontotemporal. Ophtalmologica 154:328–333, 1967
8. Meyer R: Plastische Chirurgie bei Verstümmelungen an Kopf und Hals. Helv Chirurgica Acta 37:296–317, 1970
9. Meyer R, Zaoli G: Chirurgia ricostruttiva della regione orbitaria dopo exenteratio. Ed. Minerva medica Bologna 1971

Severe Trauma of the Nose

Lionello Ponti, Rome, Italy

The present brief essay shall treat the fractures of nasal bones accompanied by serious injuries to the skin, to the mucous membrane and to the cartilages forming the nasal pyramid.

These cases, for the most part, concern traumatic emergencies with severe hemorrhage and shock.

The surgical technique obviously varies from case to case, but we will suggest some considerations we find useful to solve some problems.

The first rule for the surgeon is to conserve tissues (skin, mucous membrane, cartilage, and bones) as much as possible.

Once the patient undergoes anesthesia by endotracheal intubation it becomes easier to carefully explore the lesion and to verify the damage suffered to the tissues.

If it is possible to avoid new incisions, the normal anatomy can be reconstructed by reducing first the bony fracture, then the septum and mucosal layers, and finally esthethically repairing the skin.

In these cases it is important to ensure that the bony and cartilaginous septum are on the median line again and support the nasal pyramid.

If reparative surgery is not properly performed a respiratory insufficiency and a nasal deformity may appear after a short time, due to the formation of secondary fibrosis. For this reason it is advisable to suture, where possible, the lacerated mucoperichondrium and "mattressed" orthopaedic stitches can stabilize the dislocated septal cartilage.

In our practice we observed a case of total traumatic extirpation of the bony and cartilagenous nasal septum which after having been washed in "saline solution" was newly grafted and sutured between the upper lateral cartilages with great success.

Occasionally serious traumas, by crushing, present a fracture of the bony-cartilaginous septum with loss of substance: in these cases the support of the nose is lacking and the pyramid presents a large saddleback and a "countersink." In these cases it is necessary to support the nasal pyramid deprived of its principal supporting element, that is a part of the septum.

In one of our previous papers we specify the stages of such operation. In short, primarily we provide for reducing the bony fracture: then we analyze the status of the cartilaginous septum (the saddle depression forms in fact, at this level). By septo-columellar complete transfixion, we unglue the mucoperichondrium from both sides of the septal cartilage attempting to retain every bit of mucosa.

Then we try to reset the cartilaginous structure and we rebuild the frame of the septum on the median line by applying again the muco-perichondrial membranes to the restructured cartilage and attaching them by means of two mattresse sutures. If, notwithstanding these measures, there is a notable saddle on the nasal dorsum provided that there is a certain preservation of the proper bones, we proceed by elevating the skin above the saddle, we divide the upper lateral cartilages and suture them together over the septum by means of one mattressed stitch so that we fill the space caused by the saddle depression.

If the filling thus obtained is not sufficient to obtain a good profile we can insert a free graft of cartilage residual from the previous operation or the septum from a cartilage bank.

The nasal packing and external dressings remain in situ eight days.

In regard to delayed serious nasal pyramid fractures, one must still solve the same problems of the previous fractures made worse by the bony and fibrous cicatrization and by the reabsorption phenomena. The bony structure appears for the most part curved or hollow. The cartilaginous septum, variously deformed and curved, may cause respiratory stenosis.

Almost always at least one part of the septum has been displaced because of its sliding from the vomerine groove causing respiratory obstruction and deformity of the pyramid.

In these cases it is necessary to mobilize all nasal structures following the stages of a normal rhinoplastic operation; however, it is more important to restructure the septum, to correct the eventual curvature and to fill the saddle deformity.

As to the plastic operation of the septum we follow the principles of I. B. Goldman, as previously described. Unlike the operation performed in the case of recent traumas, in this case it is necessary to extirpate bony and cartilaginous fragments to free the nasal fossae from curvatures or slidings.

Once the osteo-cartilaginous septum has been reconstructed on the median line, we go on with the osteotomies to complete the mobilization of the pyramid. The upper lateral cartilages have to be separated from the septum and in case of considerable curvature or saddle they have to be respectively sutured to the septum or between them by means of a mattressed absorbable suture. Assymetries of the upper lateral cartilages associated with a bony pyramid deviation can be corrected by proper trimming and suturing of the septum.

In presence of a saddle, the suture has to be put between the upper lateral cartilages above the septum. The nasal bones, naturally fastened to the upper lateral cartilages follow the traction and become elevated giving an improved projection to the nasal dorsum.

The operation shall be completed by remodeling the tip of the nose and by the usual packing and external dressing.

When the bony and supporting structures of the nasal pyramid (nasal bones and bony septum) are markedly flattened, the above mentioned procedures may not be sufficient: we must then resort to transplantation.

According to our experience the graft of spongy bone drawn from the iliac crest is preferable to heterogeneous transplantations (silicone, etc.) which are subject to rejection.

Transplanting technique is simple and familiar to most rhinoplastic surgeons.

Summary

The general topic of acute nasal trauma including severe fractures of the nasal bones and septal cartilages is discussed. A systematic method is described for correcting the traumatic deviated nose and septum including plastic repair of the covering skin.

An Approach to Repair of Septal Perforations

E. Gaylon McCollough, Birmingham, Alabama

Introduction

The perforated nasal septum remains one of the most difficult management problems in nasal surgery. Patients present to the physicians office complaining of nasal crusting, whistling, bleeding, sinusitis, post nasal drainage, and headache. The size of the perforation and severity of symptoms are directly proportional therefore patients with this defect may be asymptomatic or may have a combination of the previously mentioned complaints. To the physician at first glance it appears that the perforation could be easily repaired and the literature contains many different methods of correcting septal perforations, but the long term results frequently leave much to be desired. The size of the perforation is one of the most important factors in the success of closure regardless of the surgical technique employed.

Since March 1974, we have approached the problem with a transposition flap composed of the entire cartilaginous septum caudal to the perforation, closing the resulting donor defect with a composite graft taken from the auricle of the ear.

Although our experience has been limited, the results are promising. The approach which we will describe seems to be most helpful in anterior or caudal perforations measuring less than 2 cm in diameter.

Methods

Anesthesia

This procedure can be performed utilizing local anesthesia (one percent lidocaine and 1:100,000 epinephrine), but it is helpful to supplement the anesthesia with intravenous sedatives.

Surgical Technique

In order to obtain adequate surgical exposure it may be necessary to perform a modified lateral rhinotomy incision around the alar-facial crease especially when the perforation is greater than 1.5 cm in diameter and more than 1 cm posterior to the caudal end of the septum. The edges of the perforation should be denuded circumferentially on both sides of the nasal septum to produce a raw surface for healing (Fig. 1). An incision is then made through the floor of the perforation down to the maxillary crest. This incision penetrates both sides of the mucoperichondrium and the cartilaginous septum inferior to the perforation.

A complete transfixion incision is carried from the superior septal angle inferiorly to the area of the nasal spine. This transfixion incision is then connected to the incision previously made through the floor of the perforation by a through and through incision at the bony-cartilaginous junction along the floor of the septum.

When all these incisions have been connected the entire caudal end of the septum with its mucosa on both sides may be transposed posteriorly into the perforation. If necessary the mucopericondrium may be elevated on one side of the septum superiorly and anteriorly to the perforation toward the superior septal angle and a triangular portion of cartilage may be removed from the septum to allow easier transposition of the flap (Fig. 2). In some cases it may be necessary to sever the upper lateral cartilages at their caudal attachment to the septum to release any further tension on the flap.

When transposed into the perforation defect the flap is secured with through and through mattress sutures of 4-0 clear Prolene or Neurlon. This maneuver leaves a triangular defect posterior to the columella (Fig. 3) which may be repaired with a triangular composite graft taken from the auricle of the ear (Fig. 4). The composite graft is taken in a stairstep fashion and this defect is closed primarily. We have found it helpful to use a permanent suture of 4-0 or 5-0 clear Prolene or Neurlon buried into the cartilage and perichondrium of the ear to diminish the tension in the closure. The skin closure is accomplished with a running-locking 6-0 chromic catgut suture (Davis, Geck).

The triangular composite graft previously removed from the ear is fashioned to fit into the defect at the caudal end of the septum (Fig. 5). The helical portion of the composite graft is usually discarded and the graft is sutured in place with 6-0 chromic catgut sutures but only six to eight sutures are needed on each side (Fig. 6). These sutures should penetrate only the superficial layer of the skin of the composite graft and the mucosa of the caudal

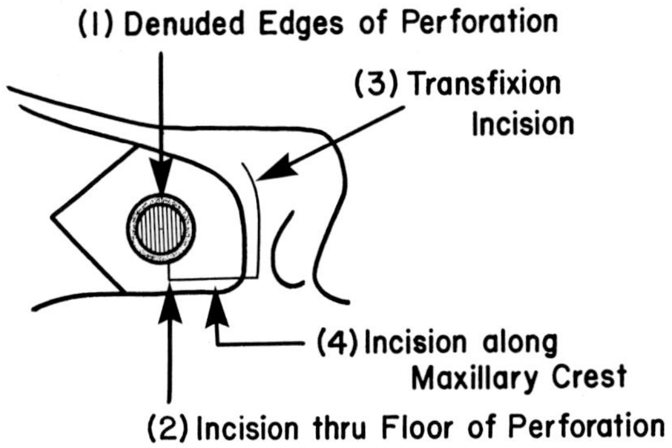

Figure 1.

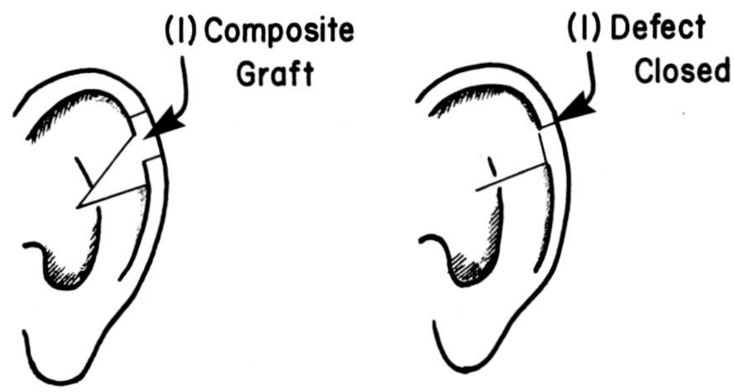

Figure 4.

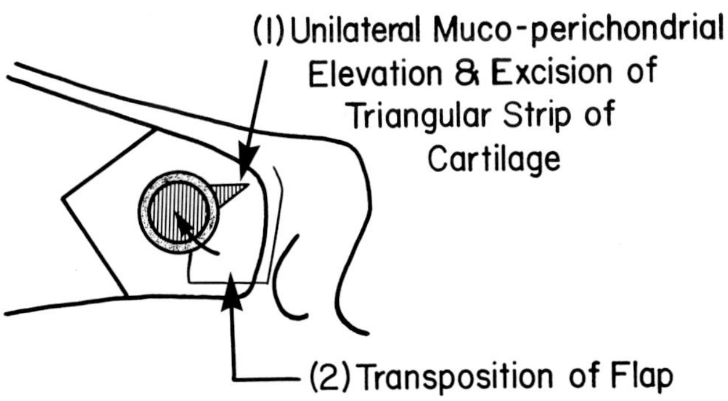

Figure 2.

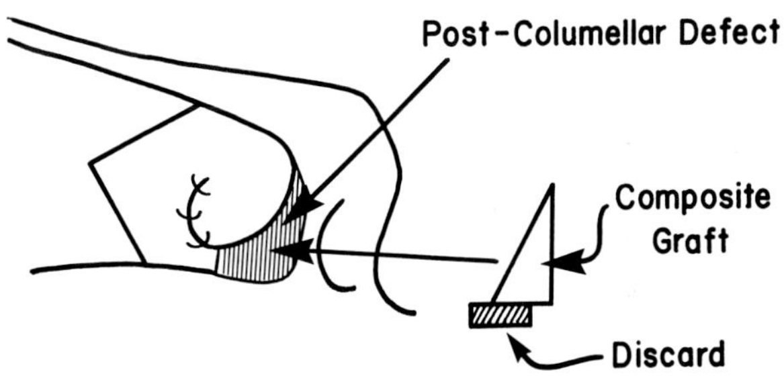

Figure 5.

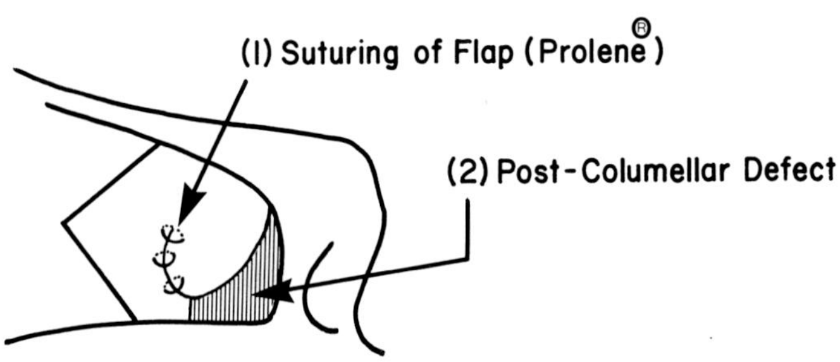

Figure 3.

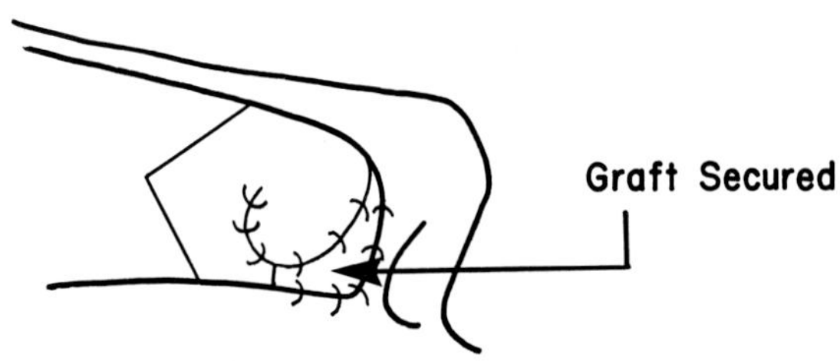

Figure 6.

end of the septum since excessive suturing will impair revascularization of the graft.

A layer of antibiotic ointment is placed on either side of the graft and the transposed septum to prevent crusting and a nasal drip pad is placed for any subsequent nasal draining but no nasal packing is used. The patient is discharged from the hospital the following morning and postoperative care is provided on an outpatient basis.

Comment

At this point in time we have utilized this approach in only four cases. The septal perforations have ranged in size from 1.5 to 2.0 cm in diameter. In two cases the perforation was successfully closed. In another the perforation was reduced in size from 2 cm to 2 mm and the patient became asymptomatic. In the fourth case, failure of closure resulted from a technical error of not denuding enough mucosa from around the superior extent of the perforation to produce a raw surface prior to transposing the flap. All composite grafts have survived and there have been no other appreciable complications.

This technique may appear somewhat more complicated but we offer it for consideration for the following reasons. The septal transposition flap is healthy tissue composed of the three components of nasal septum (cartilage and mucosa on either side) with an additional advantage that it brings its own blood supply into the area. The triangular defect created by swinging the septal transposition flap posteriorly can be closed with a composite graft again containing all three elements of the septum (lining on both sides and the central cartilagenous component). It is placed in a rich vascular bed from the posterior aspect of the columella, caudal end of the septum, and the floor of the nose and the triangular shape of the composite graft increases its likelihood of survival. Finally, the stair-step wedge resection of cartilage and skin from the auricle of the ear provides an acceptable cosmetic result.

Because of the curvature of the composite graft from the ear minimal deviation of the "new" caudal nasal septum may ensue but this is not proved to be a significant factor.

Summary

A technique for repairing perforations of the nasal septum has been described and presented for consideration. With the passage of time and the opportunity to evaluate it in more cases, its effectiveness can be determined.

Negroid Nose Reconstruction

Victor R. Syracuse and Ralph L. Dicker, New York, N.Y.

Introduction

In the black, brown, Asiatic, and Caucasian races it is not uncommon to find all degrees and variations (Fig. 1) of wide and flat noses. Some black patients with these characteristics present themselves to the plastic surgeon with a desire to achieve, as far as possible, the universal conception of the ideal nose. Reports of rhinoplasty in the black race are surprisingly scarce[1–5] while the demand for the surgery is increasing. At this time, we are considering correction of the wide, low profile, bulbous negroid nose.

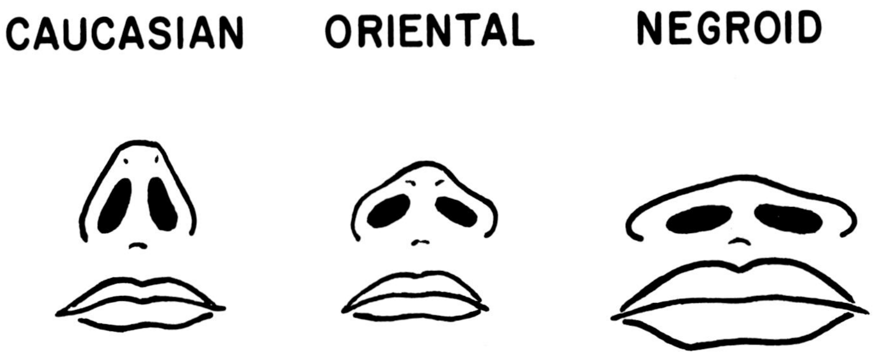

Fig. 1. Appearance of the shape and position of the nostrils in the three major racial groups.

Characteristics of the Negroid Nose

1. Nasal skin: Thick, relatively inelastic with thick subcutaneous tissue.
2. Disproportion between bony cartilaginous dorsum and lobule (Fig. 2).
3. Bridge: Frontal flatness of nasal pyramid[6] (Fig. 3).
4. Nasal tip: Bulbous, drooping, depressed, poorly supported.
5. Alae: Large, flattened, flaring (Fig. 4).
6. Nostrils: Large and round or horizontally ovoid (Fig. 4).
7. Columella: Shortened, wide-based, hidden in profile (Fig. 4).

The characteristics here described dictate the following:

Surgical Goals

1. Lengthening the columella to project the tip.
2. Reducing the size and thickness of the alae.
3. Reducing the size and spring of the lower lateral cartilages.

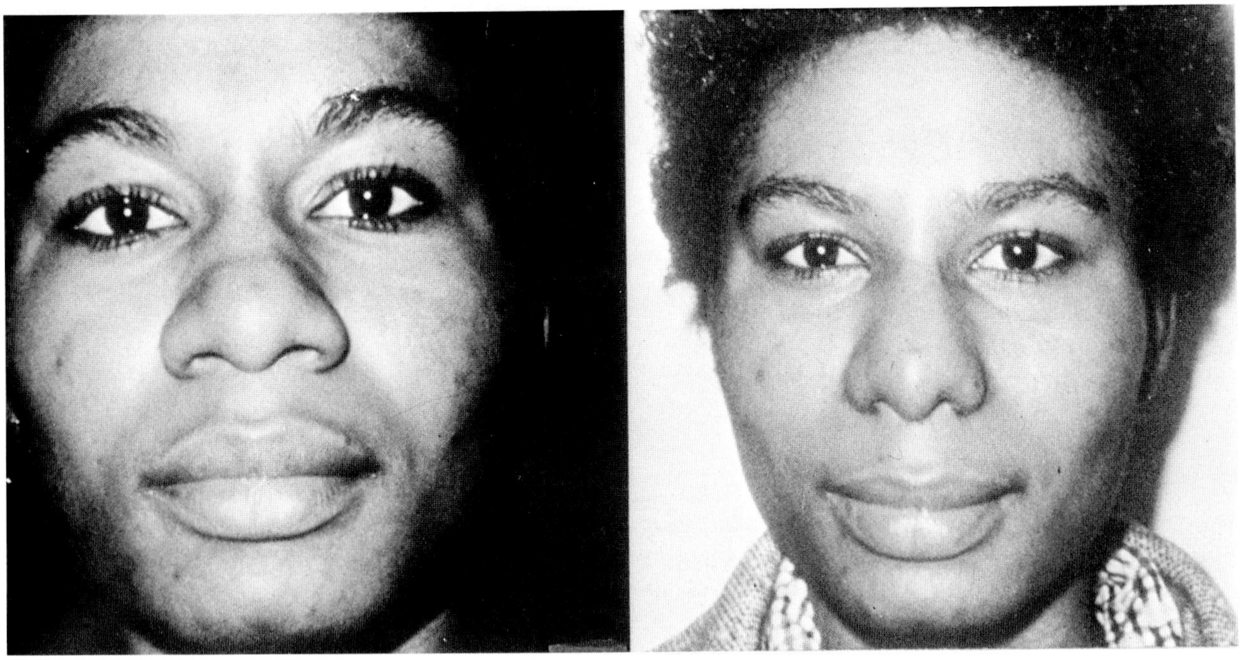

Fig. 2. On this patient the nostrils were narrowed and the tip projected. (Left) Pre-op. (Right) Post-op.

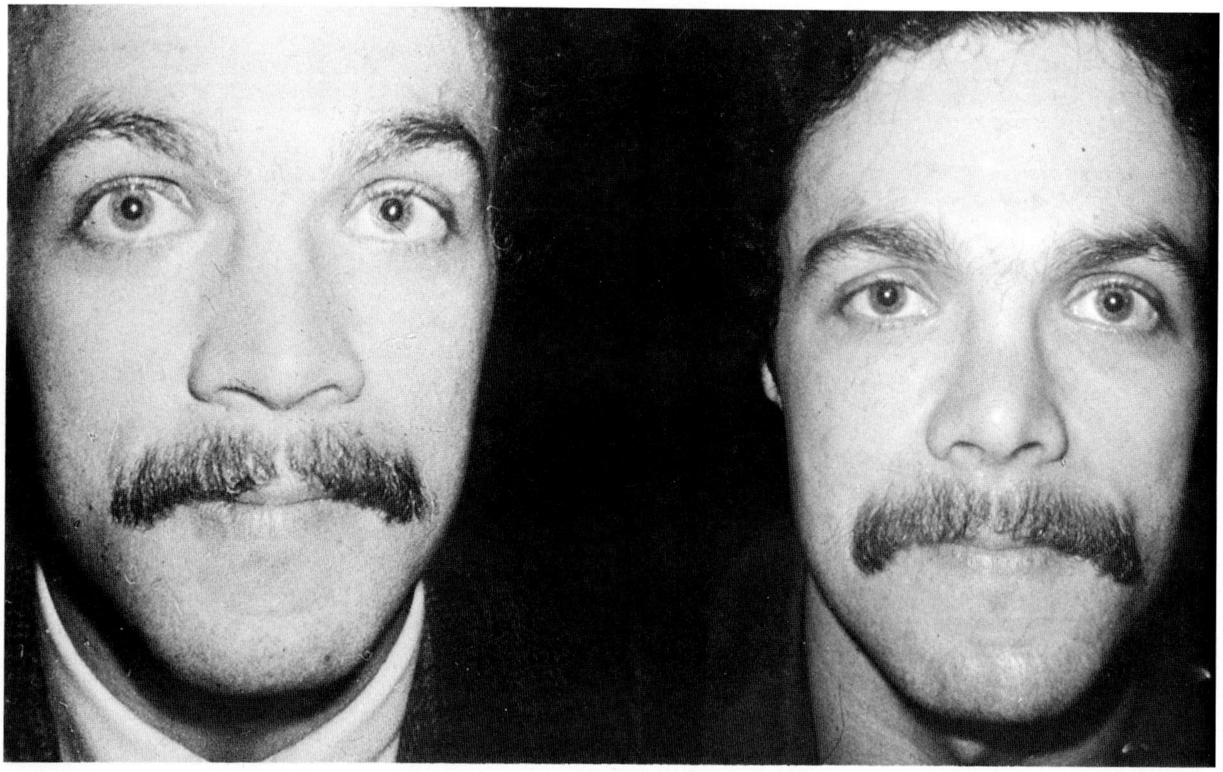

Fig. 3. Example of a dark-skinned Caucasian with a negroid nose who desired a narrowing of the base of the nose. Using the Weir-type wedge excision of the alae to narrow the base of the nose and elevate the tip. (Left) Pre-op. (Right) Post-Op.

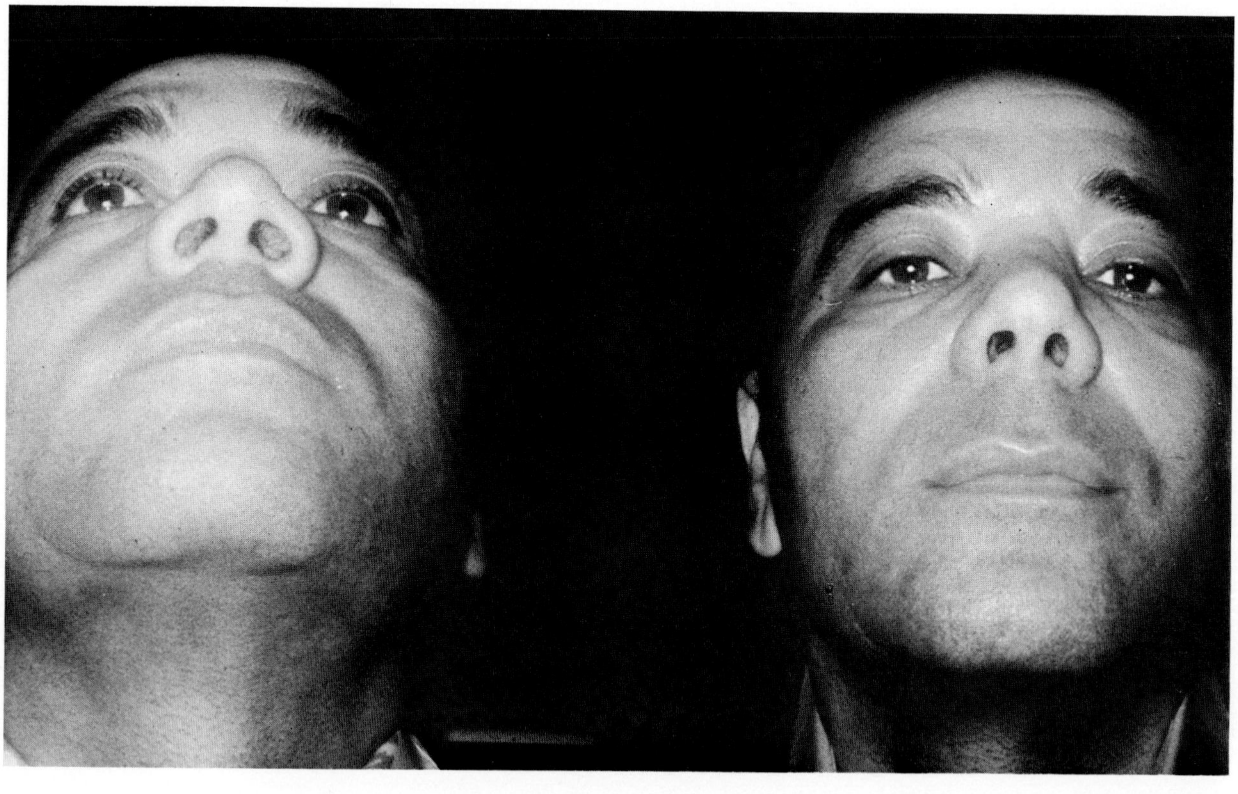

Fig. 4. Looking at same subject as Fig. 2 from below to show the narrowing of the base of the nose and the elevation of the tip. Incidentally, this improves breathing. (Left) Pre-op. (Right) Post-Op.

4. Narrowing the floor of the nostrils.
5. Elevating or projecting the dorsum of the nose.[7–9]

Preoperative Preparation

Frank discussion of possible complications is initiated with the patient, particularly of possible hypertrophied or keloidal scars in the line of projected external incisions.[10,11] Previous body scars are looked for and evaluated in the light of their origin and family history. It is explained that there is no sure way of predicting their occurrence and that if they occur they must be treated with triamcinolone injections.[12] Operating consent and informed consent are obtained with properly executed forms signed by the patient and witnessed.

Hematological studies are important to exclude particularly sickle cell traits, sickle cell anemia, thalassemia, and the thalassemia syndromes where transfusions are usually contraindicated.

Operative Procedures

Remodeling of the nasal tip[2,14] is of the greatest importance to achieve consistently satisfying results. The usual initial vestibular limen or intercartilaginous incisions are made with a No. 11 Bard-Parker knife and extended downward and through the membranous septum to the nasal spine thus detaching the columella and isolating the entire lobule.

The lower laterals are delivered through the usual vestibular incision and separated by dividing them at the angle just lateral to it into separate medial and lateral crura.[7]

The cut ends of the medial crura are now examined (Fig. 5) and, if separated by intervening tissue, this is excised before they are brought together with a surgical absorbable suture. This helps in narrowing and projecting the lobule.[15,16]

Further projection of the tip is obtained by narrowing the width of the columella at its base by various devices[7] (Figs. 6,7): The excess width of the columella may be due to a redundancy of intermediate soft tissue separating the medial crura or to a terminal lateral flare of the feet of the medial crura or to both elements. The detached columella is now retracted with a hook for good visibility, for steadiness and easy access to the raw area. Operating through the newly cut raw area of the columella, the connective tissue is split longitudinally several millimeters in depth and this trough is then deepened with blunt scissors, the flaring medial crura are freed and the excess connective tissue and cartilage are picked up with a Graefe forceps and excised.

The base of the columella is then separated from the maxilla by wide undermining of the adjacent lip with a blunt scissors (Fig. 8).

With a straight needle, a 4-0 chromicized catgut suture is placed horizontally through the very base of the columella sweeping the adjacent soft tissues into a new columellar base. Thus by narrowing the columella at the expense of its width we are helping to project the lobule.

The divided lateral crura, covered medially by vestibular skin, are partly detached from contact with the ala and are redelivered. The connective tissue on its raw surface is picked up, separated, and excised, revealing the underlying cartilage. The latter is partly resected of its upper half or crosshatched or a central oval of cartilage is shaved off its center with a No. 15 Bard-Parker knife held on

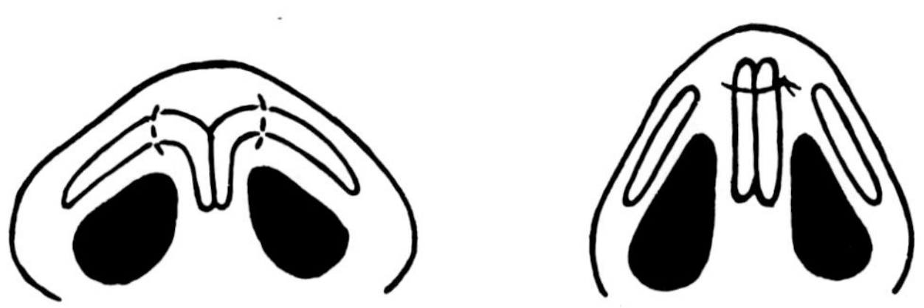

Fig. 5. Narrowing and projecting tip by uniting the cut ends of the medial crura.

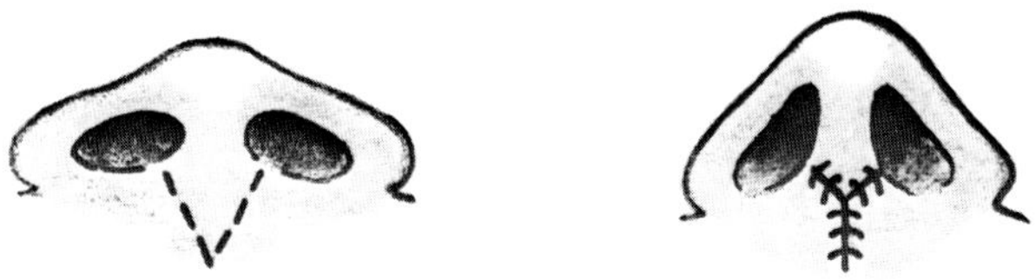

Fig. 6. "V" shaped incision sutured as a "Y."

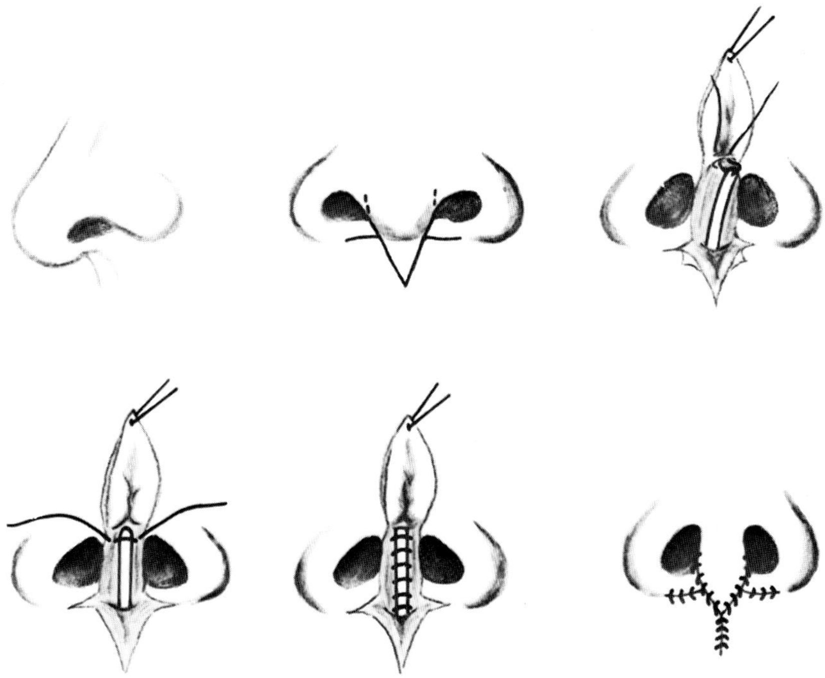

Fig. 7. Correction of short columella and drooping tip using external V incision for introduction of cartilage batten.

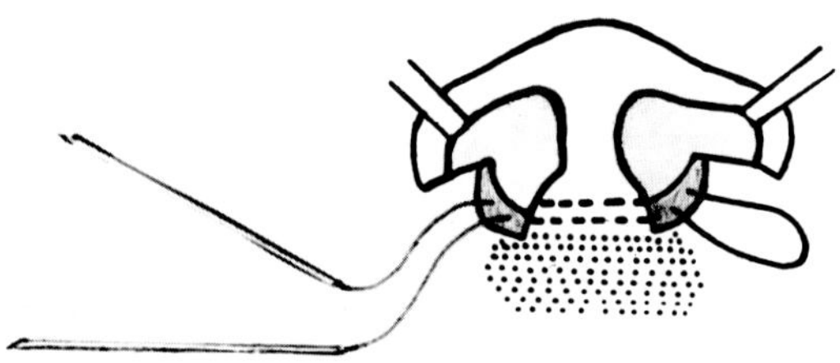

Fig. 8. Lengthening short columella, thus projecting tip. (1) Alae is separated from naso-facial grooves. (2) The base of the columella is separated from the maxilla by wide undermining. (3) Using 3-0 polydec suture with two straight needles, right and left side of base of columella are approximated.

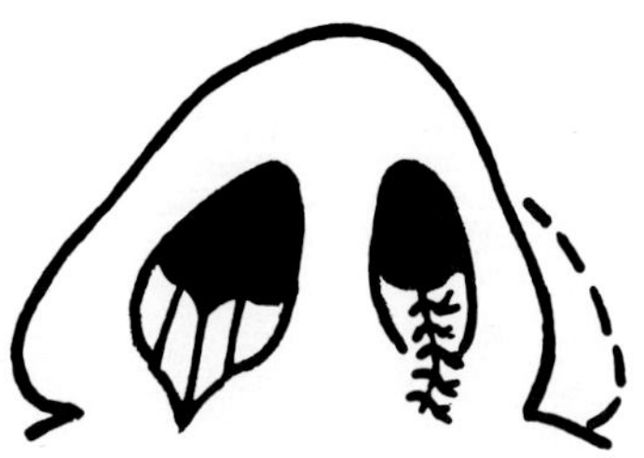

Fig. 9. Weir type wedge excision to narrow floor of nostril.

the flat[7]—thus the spring of this cartilage is greatly reduced or abolished. This structure is then restored to its bed.

Where the standard Weir-type wedge resection (Fig. 9) of the floor of the nostril[17] is inadequate to reduce the large flaring alae, they are separated along the alar facial groove (Fig. 10) with a No. 11 Bard-Parker knife or a special suitably curved and sharp scissors (Figs. 11,12).

If the alae are thick, the cut edge shows a definitely demarcated fatty pad between the vestibular and external skin. With a hook, a No. 11 Bard-Parker blade and a Graefe forceps, a wedge of this fatty pad is excised and the skin surfaces are brought together with a temporary through and through silk suture through a single opening and tied in the vestibule to eliminate possible surface scarring.[7] This procedure effectively thins a thick ala. The undue length and convexity of the ala is corrected (Fig. 12) by removing a wedge from the separated alar flap and suturing the shortened ala at the newly positioned alar facial groove and corresponding vestibule.[7]

Introducing a dorsal implant is the last step in this rhinoplasty.[1,15,18] After all surgical corrective measures have been completed, in the patient who

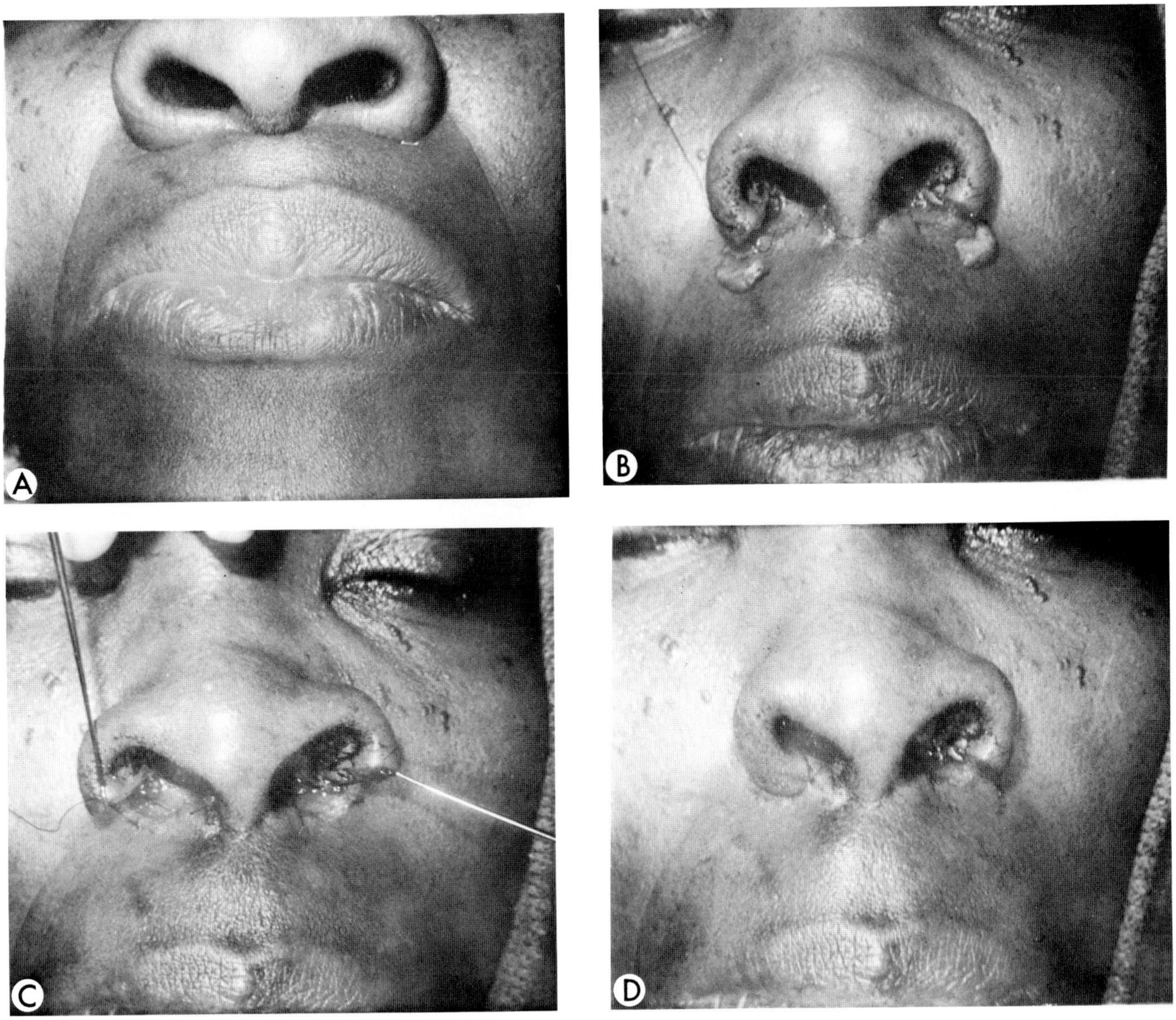

Fig. 10. (A–D) Steps in the reduction of large alae.

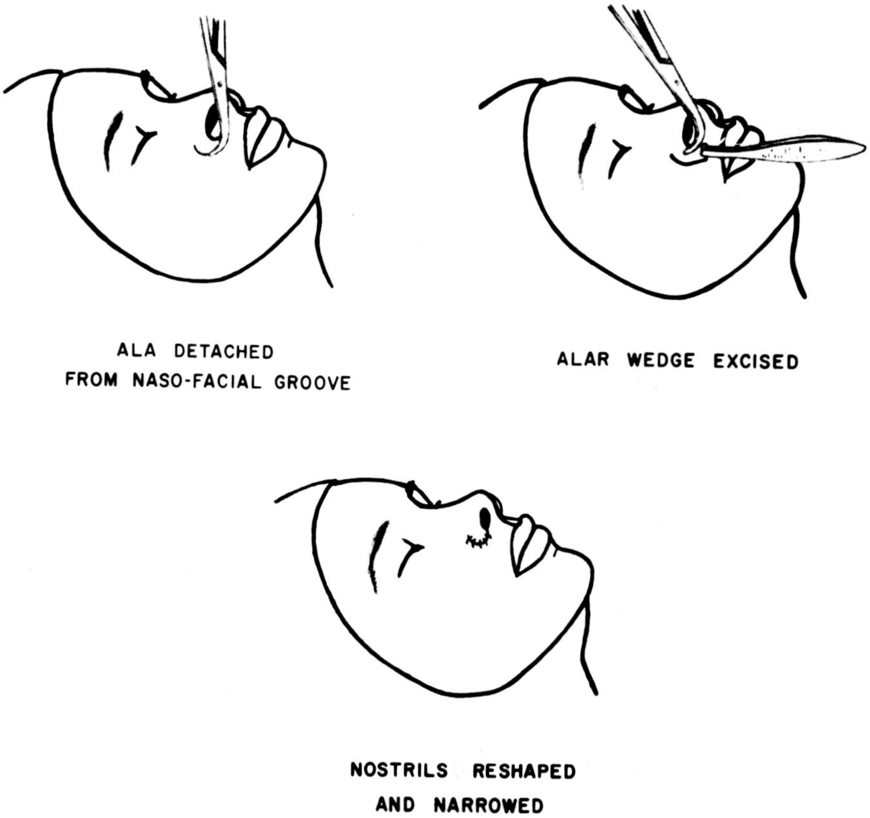

Fig. 11. Use of the No. 11 Bard-Parker knife or a special suitably curved scissor to separate the large alae.

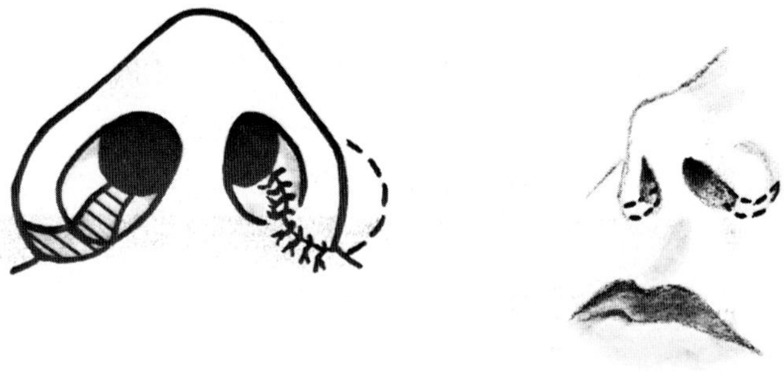

Fig. 12. Wedge shaped excision from detached margin of Ala.

has a significant degree of flattening of the dorsum, or a false saddle nose, a solid medical grade silicone rubber implant to increase projection is used and modeled to fit. The latter is not subject to absorption and rarely extrudes. The elevation of skin and soft tissue directly over the dorsum is carried out with a blunt pointed scissors. The pocket created must be suited to admit and hold the implant snugly in place. Excess tension at the lower end of the implant is to be avoided or the implant will not stay in place. The columella is now sutured to the caudal edge of the septum by through and through 3-0 black silk sutures. These are supplemented by a series of closer interrupted 4-0 black silk sutures. The customary external immobilizing and suspensory dressings and nasal packings are then placed.

Routine postoperative photographs should record the course of healing.

These procedures are well-tolerated under local infiltration and topical anesthesia. We cannot report any hypertrophic or keloidal reactions to sutures thus far, in several routine cases of negroid rhinoplasty. Nor has the literature reported keloids occurring in scars of the vestibules or alar-facial groves. Our results appear good to excellent.

Conclusion

When considering the negroid nose for reconstruction, we must realize that deviations from the ideal nose are either extreme or of varying degree. Accordingly, a plan must be devised that is suitable for the individual nose. There is no one way to deal with the inherent variations. From his own experience and from his repertoire of techniques, the resourceful rhinologic surgeon combines those procedures that will solve the particular problems. Perfection is not always attainable. In the extreme variations only an improvement can be promised.

Summary

The surgical and aesthetic goals discussed here for reconstruction of the negroid nose are to increase the overall projection of the bony cartilaginous dorsum and tip, and to narrow the nostrils to achieve a less bulbous tip.

References

1. Falces et al: Cosmetic surgery of the non-caucasian nose. PRS 45:317, 1970
2. Millard DR: Problem cases in rhinoplasty. Symposium on Aesthetic Surgery of the Nose, Ears Archives, Vol 6, p 45 (C.V. Mosby Co.), 1973
3. Pitanguy I: The negroid nose. PRS of the face and neck. Proceedings of the First International Symposium. Vol I, Aesthetic Surgery, New York, Grune and Stratton, pp 136–138, 1972
4. Rees TD: Nasal plastic surgery in the negro. PRS 43:13, 1969
5. Snyder GB: Rhinoplasty in the negro. PRS 47:572, 1971
6. Schaeffer JP: The nose and olfactory organ, New York, McGraw, pp 64–66, 1920
7. Fomon et al: Rhinoplastic problems in the lower cartilaginous vault. AMA Arch Otolaryng 79:512–521, 1964
8. Holmes EM: Correction of nasal skeletal defects. PRS 29:319, 1962
9. Uchida JA: A design for a prosthesis in augmentation rhinoplasty: The projection method. PRS 33:485, 1964
10. Alhady SMA, Kandian S: Keloids in various races. PRS 44:564, 1969
11. Crockett DJ: Colour, cancer and keloids in the sudan. Brit J Plast Surg 15:408, 1962
12. Griffith BH, Monroe CW, McKinney P: Follow-up study on treatment of keloids with triamcinolone acetonide. PRS 46:145, 1970
13. Rapaport SI: Introduction to hematology, New York, Harper & Row, pp 73–78, 1971
14. Schultz LW: Deformities of the nasal tip. PRS 23:294, 1959
15. Foman S, Schattner A, Bell JW: Narrowing of the wide nose. Arch Otolaryng AMA Arch Otolaryng 59:299, 1954
16. Loeb R: Narrowing of the nasal bases. PRS 36:134, 1965
17. Weir RF: On restoring sunken noses without scarring the face (Classic Reprint) PRS 45:382, 1970
18. Boo-Chai K: A Augmentation rhinoplasty in orientals. PRS 34:81, 42, 1964

Homologous Nasal Hump Implant: Follow-up Studies

David Bernstein, New York, N.Y.

The use of homologous nasal hump implants to reconstruct saddle noses was first reported in 1973.[1] At that time, in an excellent discussion, Howard W. Smith[2] indicated an interest in follow-up results among other pertinent considerations. At this time it is possible to describe experiences with a total of forty-four patients the longest observed for four years compared to twenty patients and two years in the prior report.

Materials and Methods

Basically, with certain exceptions, the method remains unchanged. Nasal humps removed during rhinoplasty are preserved in 1:1000 tincture of merthiolate and are utilized only after six changes of the supernatant fluid over a period of six months. Excised humps remain firm, clean in appearance and supple even after as long as three years. Since removal of perichondrium, endochondrium, periosteum, endosteum, and mucosa would compromise the integrity of the hump no attempt is made to eliminate the tissue over the cartilage and bone. Appropriate trimming is done to remove irregularities and projecting fragments. Persistently negative cultures have been a prime consideration and the material is stored at 4°C. Prior to implantation the donor tissue is rinsed at least six times in sterile Ringer's solution or normal saline. Preparation of the recipient site follows the customary well known rhinoplastic principles.

Good visibility is of paramount importance for proper placement and incisions and lighting must be considered with this in mind. Sharp projections should be avoided in the caudal portion of the implant which will be close to the incised points of entry. The graft is kept as wide as possible in this area consistent with appropriate aesthetic considerations. A one week period of splinting and packing is sufficient for most purposes.

Anatomic Considerations

A typical hump consists of nasal bones above, upper lateral cartilages below and septum in between extending vertically. Wherever possible it would appear preferable to keep like tissues in contact. For this reason most humps with few exceptions have been placed in their natural position rather than being turned around or upside down. No problems of dead space have been encountered and it is always possible to choose a hump or reshape one or combine two in order to correct the existing defect.

Results

There has been no instance of rejection or infection. In one patient mechanical extrusion occurred on the second day postoperatively following violent blowing, sneezing, and continued manipulation resulting in removal of the packing despite sedation and repeated proper instructions. There was no surrounding tissue reaction other than the customary changes seen at this time. Another factor was an unusually scarred skin overlying the nasal bridge the result of many traumatic lacerations. Other than this instance takes have been firm and thus far no resorption has been observed. Mobility sometimes noted following iliac crest grafts has not occurred and there has been no curling or warping as may happen with rib implants. Sharp edges and distortion produced by septal cartilage have been obviated.

In one patient with osteogenesis imperfecta an iliac crest graft had slowly absorbed. A double homologous hump implant was subsequently utilized and has thus far survived in excess of eighteen months. The double hump implant has been placed in eight of the forty-four patients with satisfactory results.

Figure 1A shows one of the earlier patients preoperatively. The saddle has been corrected by a homologous hump implant with the result demonstrated in Figure 1B. His x-ray in Figure 1C shows the preserved hump in place ten months later. Almost three years later there is no clinical evidence of resorption as illustrated in the photograph in Figure 1D and his x-ray in Figure 1E taken at the same time compared with his x-ray in Figure 1C indicates a well calcified implant with a bridge of bone to the recipient site. In Figure 2A, there is an x-ray of a double hump in situ and the patient is shown pre and post operatively in Figures 2B and 2C, respectively. The saddle has been amply corrected. Figure 3A is included because of the very large saddle which required a correspondingly substantial implant. This was supplied by a double hump and the correction is evident in Figure 3B.

A particularly useful application of the homologous hump implant is in instances where during operation a defect becomes apparent following hump removal, lateral osteotomies, upper lateral cartilage resection and tip reconstruction. This is well illustrated in Figure 4A. Autogenous septal cartilage may not be available or suitable and reliance on time or healing is usually illusory. A

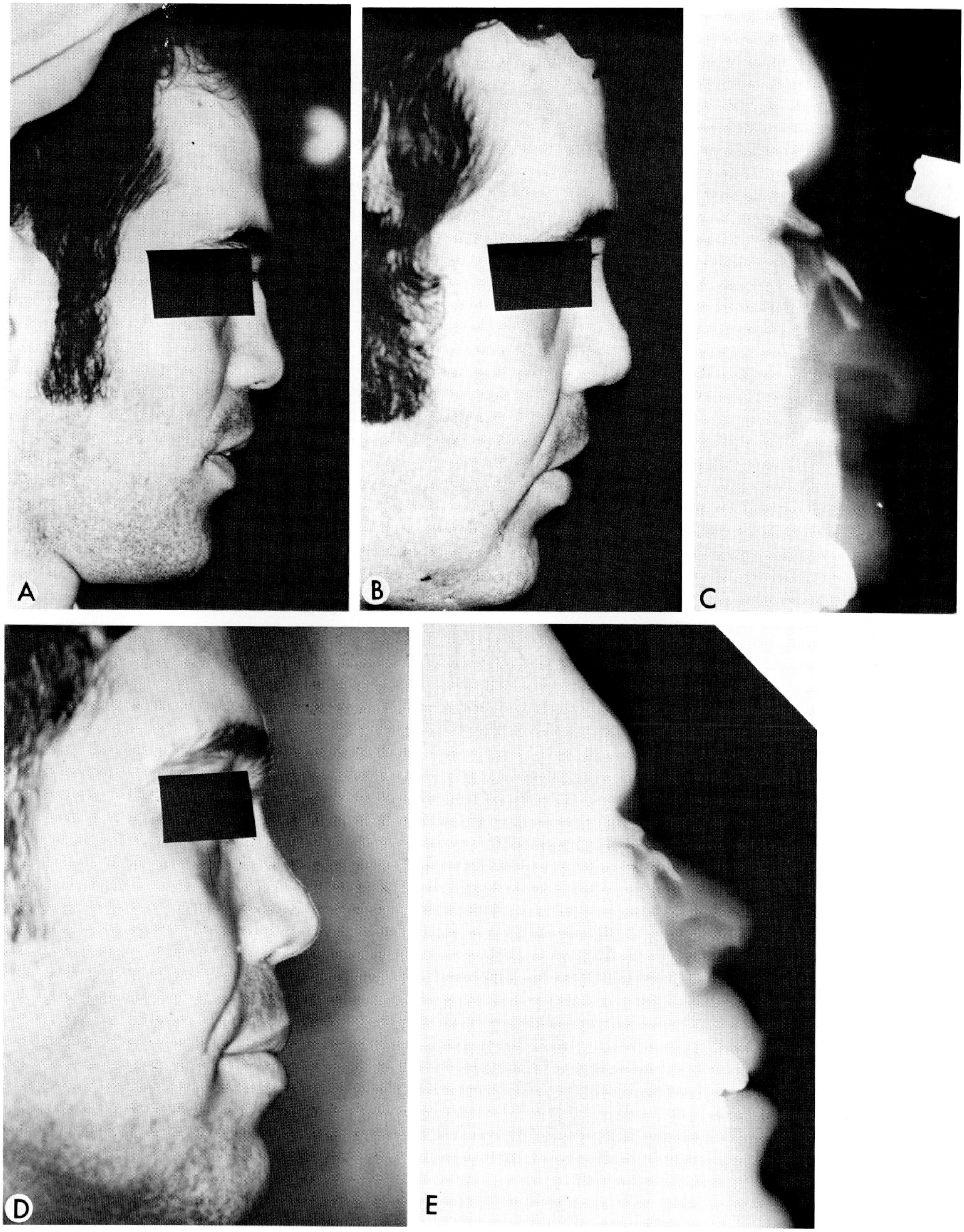

Fig. 1. (A) Preoperative hump-saddle deformity. (B) Defect shown in Figure 1A corrected by homologous nasal implant. (C) X-ray of the same patient demonstrating the preserved hump in situ ten months later. (D) There is no clinical evidence of resorption in this patient, shown in Figure 1, three years later. (E) An x-ray taken at the same time as the photograph in Figure 1C indicates a well-calcified implant with a bridge of bone to the recipient site.

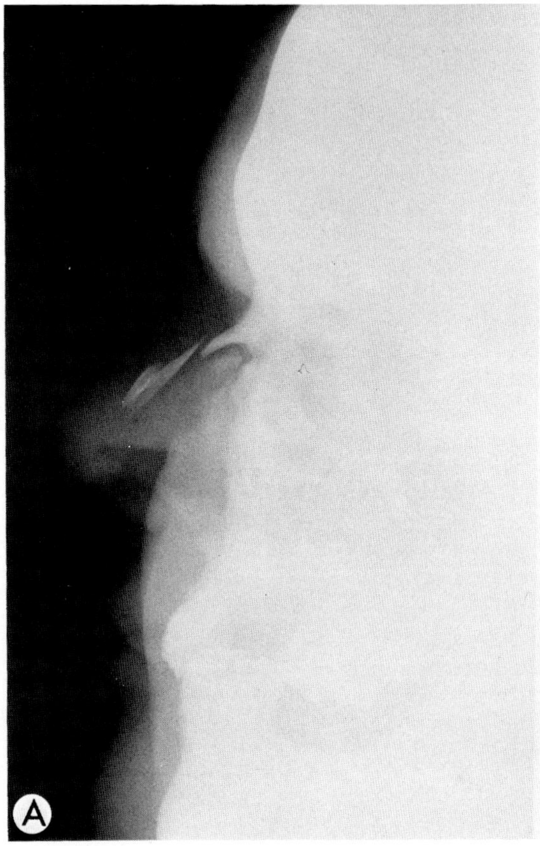

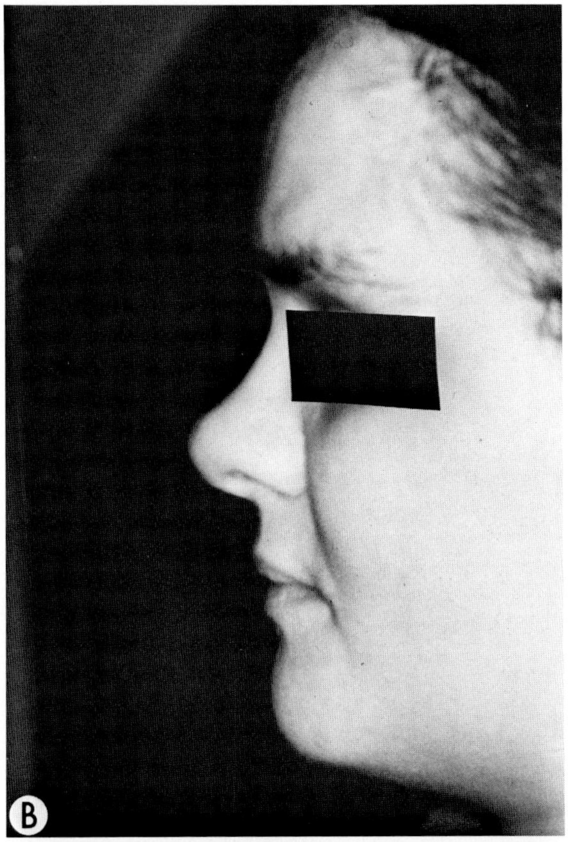

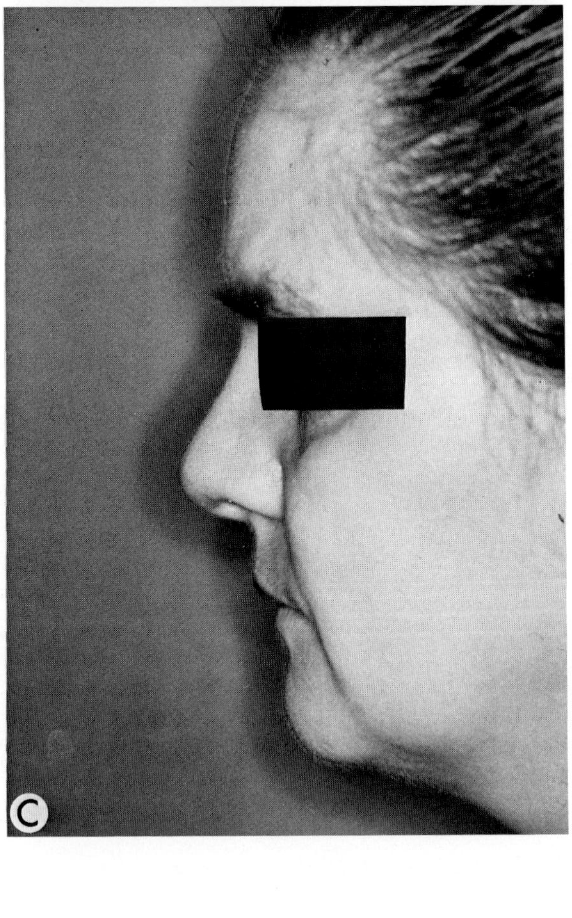

Fig. 2. (A) X-ray of a double hump implant. (B) This patient with a saddle nose deformity is illustrated preoperatively. (C) The saddle has been corrected by a double hump implant.

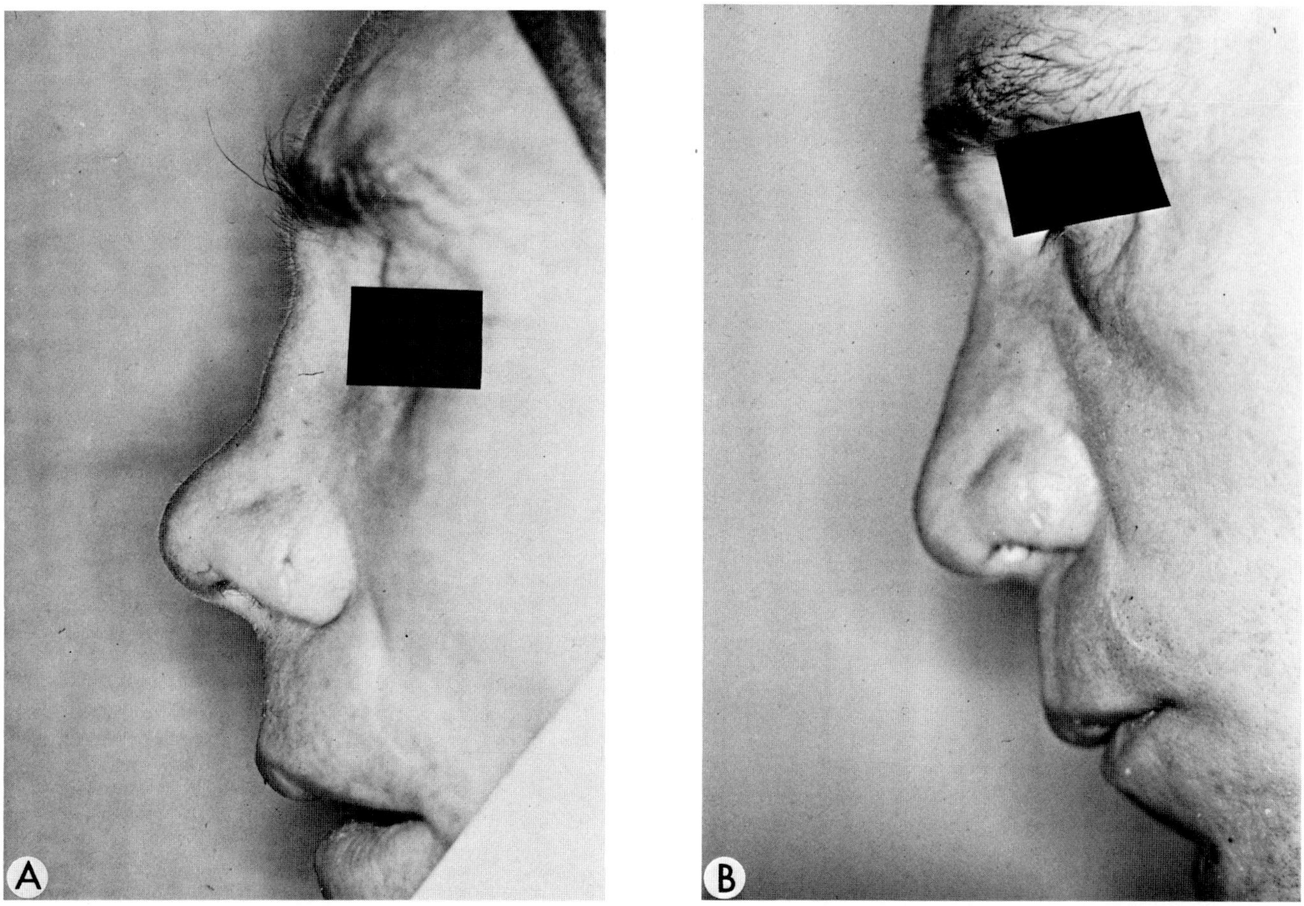

Fig. 3. (A) A very large saddle. (B) This large saddle has been corrected by an appropriate double homologous hump implant.

small implant was placed with the correction noted in Figure 4B.

Comment

While it is recognized that autogenous tissue is preferred the search for other approaches is stimulated by certain inherent well-known difficulties with autogenous bone or cartilage. To enter the iliac crest for cancellous bone or the rib cage for cartilage involves significant additional surgery. Septal cartilage is more readily available but is often impossible to shape properly whereas the preserved nasal hump already has the correct configuration. As was noted in the patient with osteogenesis imperfecta even iliac crest occasionally absorbs and rib cartilage is notorious for curling. In this study preserved homologous nasal hump implants have shown firm adherence to surrounding tissue and aesthetic results thus far have been excellent.

References

1. Bernstein D: Homologous nasal hump implant, Arch Otolaryngol 98:385–386, 1973
2. Smith, HW, Arch Otolaryngol 98:435, 1973

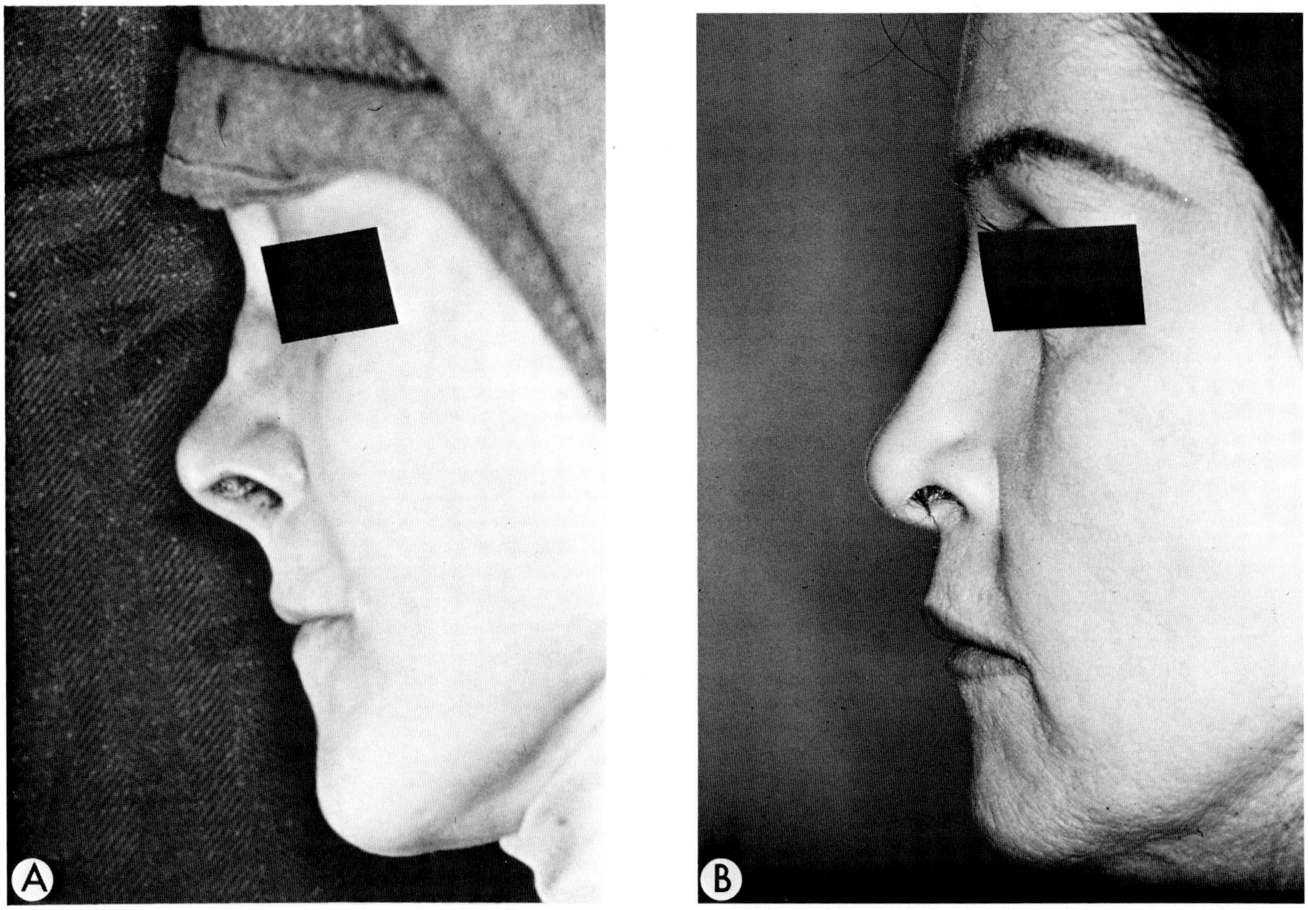

Fig. 4. (A) A small defect which has occurred operatively. (B) A small implant has been placed at this same operation to immediately correct the saddle.

Traumatic Cerebrospinal Fluid Rhinorrhea

Eugene Rontal, Southfield, Mich. and
William L. Meyerhoff, San Antonio Texas

Introduction

Traumatic defects of the cranial vault resulting in cerebrospinal fluid rhinorrhea are serious sequelae of facial and skull trauma. Retrograde contamination by nasal bacteria can lead to meningitis, brain abscess and subsequent death. Therefore, exact anatomic localization of the leakage site and subsequent appropriate treatment are critical to safe management of these patients.

Basically, four areas of leakage can be identified: frontal sinus, cribriform plate, and ethmoid sinus, sphenoid sinus, and mastoid otorhinorrhea. These cases of traumatic cerebrospinal fluid rhinorrhea have been divided into acute and delayed types.[1] The acute onset variety has an immediate onset while the delayed form generally occurs four to six weeks after the initial injury. Depending on the nature of the inciting trauma and the resulting clinical signs and symptoms, each will present with a specific clinical picture. Further, each type of rhinorrhea can usually be delineated by the appropriate x-ray and laboratory studies.

Although many reports have appeared in the literature regarding the problem of cerebrospinal fluid rhinorrhea,[1–4] the recognition of exact anatomic site and subsequent appropriate treatment still remains a therapeutic enigma.[5] It is the purpose of this paper to present a logical approach to the clinical evaluation of traumatic cerebrospinal fluid rhinorrhea, so that the maxillofacial surgeon may better be able to diagnose and treat this condition.

Frontal Sinus

Anatomically, the posterior wall of the frontal sinus lies adjacent to the anterior cranial fossa. A posterior wall fracture with a subsequent tear of the anterior cranial fossa dura will produce cerebrospinal fluid leakage (Fig. 1). If the nasofrontal duct is patent, this fluid enters the nose in the middle meatus. If the duct is disrupted by trauma, the

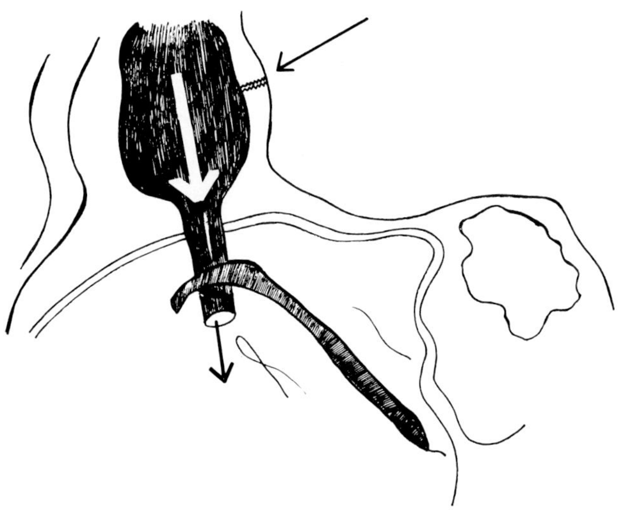

Fig. 1. Path of cerebrospinal fluid through a fracture of the posterior wall of the frontal sinus. Arrows show the direction of flow out the frontal duct beneath the middle turbinate.

fluid will collect in the frontal sinus itself, or follow the lines of fracture to the dependent nasal cavities.

Clinically, most traumatic cerebrospinal fluid leakage in the frontal area is associated with external evidence of trauma. Any laceration of the forehead, eyebrow, or inner canthal area must make the clinician suspect of an underlying frontal sinus fracture. Further, with any proven fracture of the anterior sinus wall, one is obligated to rule out the presence of an associated posterior sinus wall fracture. A clear, watery discharge from the nose associated with this injury makes the diagnosis almost conclusive.

Treatment of acute cerebrospinal fluid rhinorrhea from the frontal sinus area involves reduction of the posterior wall fracture. Prolonged drainage may require an osteoplastic flap exposure and direct repair of the dural tear with elevation and approximation of the posterior wall fragments.[4,5] These cases are commonly done in association with a neurosurgical colleague.

Case Report No 1

A 23-year-old white male was in an automobile accident the evening prior to his admission. The patient was conscious on admission. At that time, head and neck examination revealed a LeFort II fracture, with comminution of the midface and facial lacerations. Profuse cerebrospinal fluid rhinorrhea was noted.

X-rays revealed associated multiple skull fractures, with fractures through the anterior and posterior table of the frontal sinus (Fig. 2). Following preop evaluation, he was taken to the operating room. The fractures were approached through a coronal incision. The fractures of the frontal sinus were identified and repaired from behind. The mucosal contents were carefully drilled away and the frontal sinus was obliterated with fat. The lacerations in the dura were sutured and the coronal flap was replaced. Postoperatively, cerebrospinal fluid abated.

Ethmoid Sinus and Cribriform Plate

The roof of the ethmoid sinus and its cribriform plate lie adjacent to cerebrospinal fluid. The cribriform plate portion is especially susceptible to

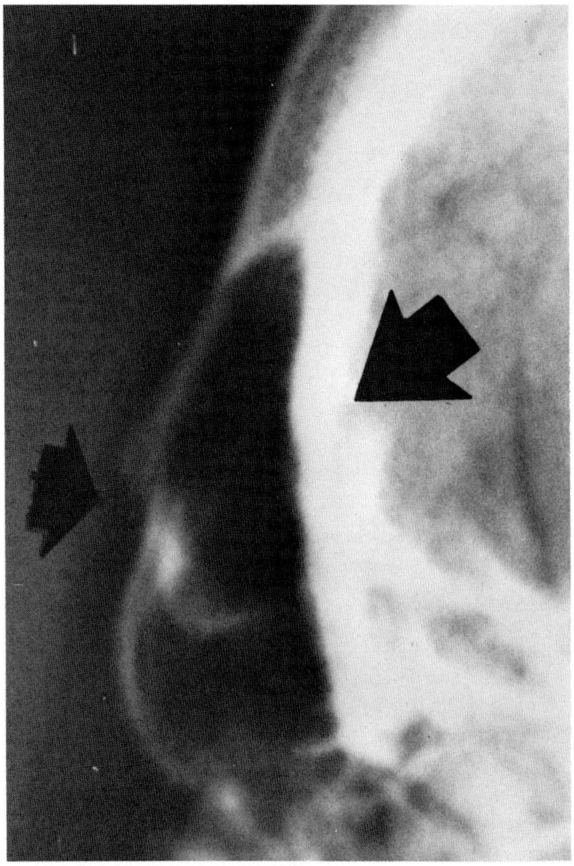

Fig. 2. Arrows indicate fractures in the anterior and posterior walls of the frontal sinus.

fracture due to its fragile structure and the additional weakening by the passage of the olfactory nerves. Trauma to the nasal ethmoid complex is not infrequently accompanied by cerebrospinal fluid leakage.[2] Fluid will drain either from beneath the middle turbinate or from high in the roof of the nose above the superior turbinate (Fig. 3).

Clinically, this site of origin is most commonly associated with complex nasoethmoid fractures or with the LeFort II and III facial disjunctions. Severe comminution of the nasal-ethmoid complex or a mobile mid-third of the face should alert the clinician to this possibility. Occasionally, the cribriform plate can be cracked without displacement of the nasal-ethmoid complex. Again, the clinician should be alerted to this area as a possible source of cerebrospinal fluid leakage, especially with total loss of olfaction. Exact localization may be difficult because of the associated nasal swelling. However, except for reduction of an associated fracture, excessive manipulation of the nose in an acute leakage situation should be avoided, because of the change of subsequent meningitis. Further, fractures of the sphenoid sinus may be associated with this type of fracture.

Treatment of acute cerebrospinal fluid leakage associated with ethmoid roof and cribriform plate is somewhat paradoxical. On the one hand, cessation of acute cerebrospinal fluid rhinorrhea associated with malpositioned external fractures involves reduction of the fracture itself. Frequently, adequate reduction and fixation of the nasal-ethmoid complex and LeFort fractures will be accompanied by stoppage of the drainage. On the other hand, in most cases in which the cribriform plate is fractured without displacement of the nasal-ethmoid complex, conservative management, including bed rest, antibiotics, and avoiding nasal trauma will often be sufficient treatment for the cessation of the cerebrospinal fluid drainage.[3,4]

Sphenoid Sinus

The unusual finding of sphenoid sinus fracture is not uncommonly accompanied by cerebrospinal fluid with drainage. The posterior wall of the sinus lies adjacent to the hypophysis and to the anterior and middle cranial fossa (Fig. 4). Once the fracture has occurred, cerebrospinal fluid will leak from either the sphenoid sinus ostium or from the fracture site into the superior meatus.

Clinically these fractures are usually associated with severe facial trauma. As in the ethmoid area, complex nasal-ethmoid and LeFort II and III fractures are most likely associated with this type of cerebrospinal fluid rhinorrhea. Evidence of an air-fluid level in the sphenoid sinus on x-ray should make the clinician suspect the sphenoid sinus as the site of origin. With severe facial trauma, it is sometimes difficult to distinguish cribriform plate rhinorrhea from the sphenoid sinus. In these cases, tomography of the cribriform plate as well as the various labeling techniques for localization of cerebrospinal fluid rhinorrhea are useful.

Treatment of sphenoid sinus rhinorrhea can be difficult. Conservative management with bed rest and antibiotics is preferred in acute situations.

With prolonged drainage, closure of the leakage site can generally be accomplished via the transethmoid or trans-septal trans-sphenoidal approach.[3,4] Muscle, fascia, and cartilage obliteration of the sphenoid sinus is generally successful in correcting this problem.

Case Report No 2

Ethmoid-cribriform plate and sphenoid sinus fracture. A 19-year-old male was admitted to the hospital following an automobile accident. He had .tensive comminution of the frontal bone and

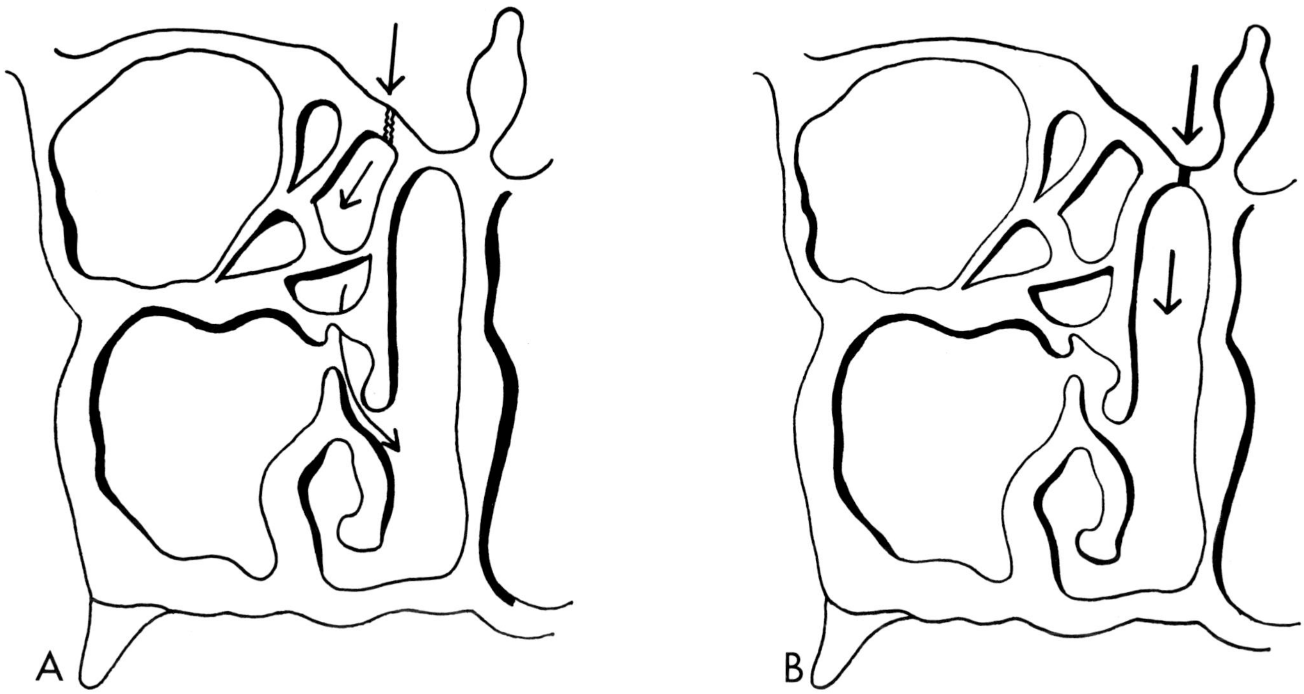

Fig. 3. (A) Path of cerebrospinal fluid drainage from a fracture in the roof of the ethmoid sinus. Leakage will be detected from beneath the middle turbinate in most of these cases. (B) Path of drainage from a fracture of the cribriform plate area. In this case cerebrospinal fluid will be detected high in the cribriform region of the nose.

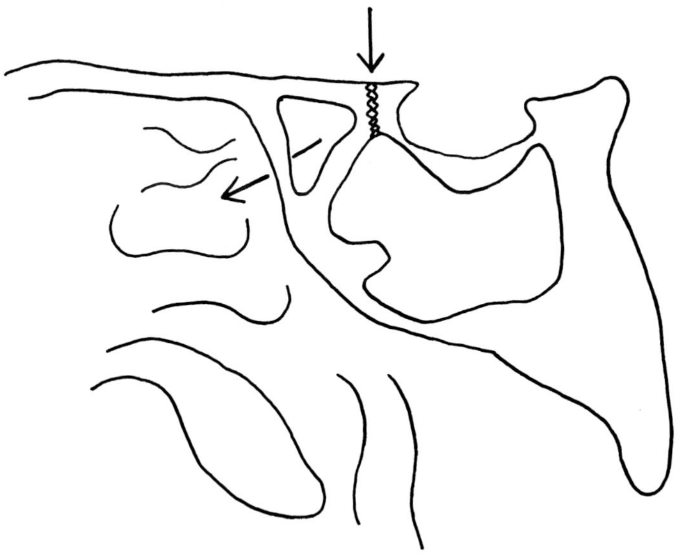

Fig. 4. Path of cerebrospinal fluid drainage from a fracture of the posterior wall of the sphenoid sinus. Leakage will be detected as it exits from the opening of the sphenoid sinus at the speno-ethmoidal recess.

cribriform plate of the ethmoid with associated occipital laceration. Following admission work-up the patient was taken to the operating room and a frontal lobe dural tear was repaired. Postoperatively, he developed amblyopia of the left eye and decreased vision on the right.

Four months later the patient was noted to have persistent cerebrospinal fluid discharge from the right nares. There was no meningitis or nausea and vomiting. X-rays revealed a fracture of the right cribriform plate and sphenoid sinus. One month later a right frontal craniotomy was performed and the suspected fistulous tracts in the ethmoid-sphenoid sinus area were identified. Leakage from these areas was controlled by a muscle-fascia repair. Postoperatively, the cerebrospinal fluid rhinorrhea abated.

Mastoid Otorhinorrhea

The same type of trauma sufficient to cause facial fractures is frequently sufficient to fracture the temporal bone. Both longitudinal and transverse fractures of the temporal bone can cause cerebrospinal fluid rhinorrhea. If the tympanic membrane is left intact following the fracture, then the resultant cerebrospinal fluid leakage drains via the eustachian tube. This eustachian tube drainage will then exit via the nose and present as cerebrospinal fluid rhinorrhea.

With an intact tympanic membrane, the temporal bone as the site of cerebrospinal fluid rhinorrhea may be difficult to diagnose. Associated facial nerve paralysis or hearing loss would certainly make one suspicious of the diagnosis. However, in the absence of these symptoms and signs, the only other finding may be an air-fluid level behind the tympanic membrane or evidence of a hymotympanum. Radiographic evaluation including polytomography of the temporal bone is also extremely useful in elucidating this as the etiologic site.

Treatment in the acute fracture necessitates bed rest and antibiotics. Any attempts to manipulate the ear should be done under aseptic conditions. Generally, the cerebrospinal fluid drainage will stop spontaneously. In those unusual cases of persistent drainage or when another ear procedure has become necessary (i.e., facial nerve decompression), a temporalis muscle fascia obliteration of the middle ear and/or mastoid is indicated. This should only be done after long attempts at conservative management.[3,6,7]

Case Report No 3

Mastoid Otorhinorrhea. A 17-year-old white male suffered multiple contusions and abrasions as well as loss of consciousness in a motorcyle accident. When seen in the emergency room he was comatose with a right hemotympanum and left-beating nystagmus. Aside from his soft tissue findings, no other injuries were identified at this time. The morning after admission, fluid was identified running from his nose onto the pillow with a positive spot test and a glucose of approximately 40 mg %. The presumptive diagnosis at this time was cerebrospinal fluid otorhinorrhea.

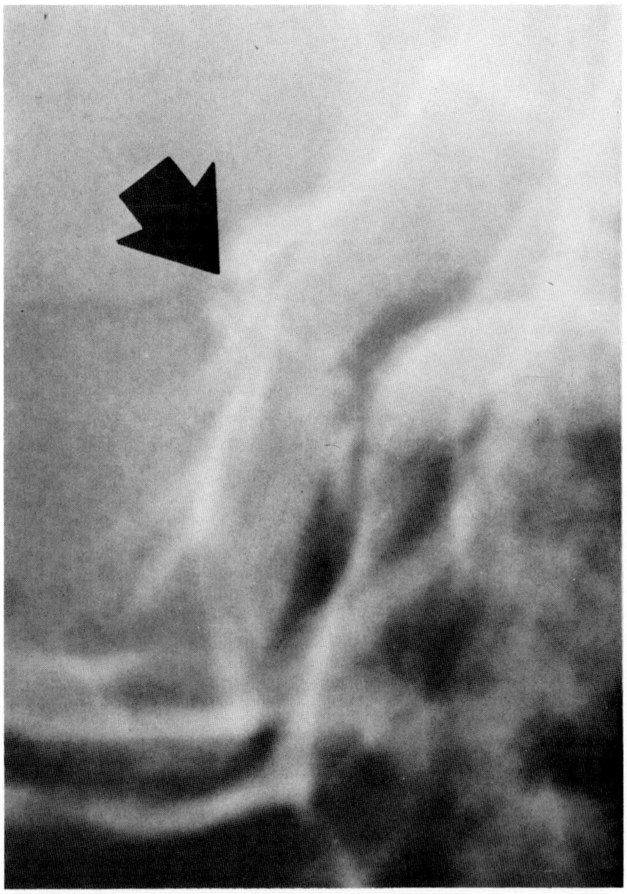

Fig. 5. Stenver's view of the right temporal bone showing a transverse fracture which resulted in a total right facial paralysis.

Admitting x-rays revealed a comminuted but essentially transverse fracture of the right temporal bone (Fig. 5). Approximately 72 hr following admission, the patient regained consciousness and was noted to have a right facial nerve paralysis. Tuning forks suggested a nonfunctioning ear on the right side. Hilger nerve stimulation gave a greater than 3.5 mA difference between the right and left 7th nerves. The cerebrospinal fluid rhinorrhea still persisted. X-rays, including tomograms of the cribriform plate area, revealed no evidence of fracture.

Ninety-six hours following admission the patient was taken to the operating room, at which time a translabyrinthine facial nerve decompression was performed from the brainstem to the stylomastoid foramen. The 7th nerve was found to be totally severed at the geniculate ganglion and a greater auricular nerve graft was placed. The temporal bone itself was extremely comminuted and the labyrinth was lying loose. The cerebrospinal fluid was oozing profusely from the fracture site. The internal auditory canal and mastoid were packed with temporalis muscle and cyano acrylat glue. Postoperatively, the cerebrospinal fluid otorhinorrhea abated. Follow-up has not been long enough to assess facial nerve recovery.

Discussion

The localization of the anatomic site following the diagnosis of cerebrospinal fluid rhinorrhea should be analyzed systemically in terms of frontal sinus, ethmoid and cribriform plate area, sphenoid sinus, and mastoid otorhinorrhea. This four-step process will give a more logical and less random approach to diagnosis. Physical signs and symptoms of cerebrospinal fluid rhinorrhea associated with facial trauma may make detailed x-ray and laboratory studies superfluous. However, prolonged cerebrospinal fluid drainage despite initial treatment, i.e., reduction of the fracture, bed rest, and antibiotics, will necessitate the careful, analytic approach with radiologic and spinal fluid evaluation.

While the presence of glucose makes one highly suspicious for the suspected fluid coming from the subarachnoid space, it is not an absolute test since lacrimal secretion can also contain glucose. Adjunct studies are also necessary to definitively establish the diagnosis. Several clinically useful bedside tests are available. The so-called spot test or ring sign in evaluation of spinal fluid rhinorrhea is one such test. In this evaluation, blood will remain in the center of a cloth saturated with the suspected secretion while the cerebrospinal fluid will form a ring around it. Further, this fluid when allowed to stand on a handkerchief or cloth will not cause the cloth to stiffen. Chemically, when cerebrospinal fluid is allowed to stand, there is no evidence of sediment, it has a specific gravity of 1.004–1.008 and the protein content of the fluid is much greater than that of the nasal secretions.

Once the fluid has been established as being cerebrospinal in origin, certain x-ray studies must be performed. Facial bone and sinus x-rays are mandatory with any facial injury. When cerebrospinal fluid rhinorrhea is suspected, routine mastoid series should also be done, especially the Stenver's and Law's views. Frequently, a fracture of the sinus wall or an air-fluid level will be demonstrable in the frontal or sphenoid sinus. Detailed information of the posterior wall of the frontal sinus, the cribriform plate, and the posterior wall of the sphenoid sinus are usually unobtainable without tomography (Fig. 6). Likewise, although the fracture may be noted on mastoid films, polytomography of the temporal bone is more precise in diagnosing pathology in this area (Fig. 7).

Cerebrospinal fluid rhinorrhea may persist in spite of adequate initial management. In these cases of persistant or intermittant cerebrospinal fluid drainage following head trauma, the exact site of leakage may be difficult to locate. X-rays frequently do not point out a small leakage area, particularly in the cribriform plate region. Subsequent surgical treatment depends heavily on precise localization of the drainage. This problem of anatomic identification has been solved in part by the various examination techniques within the nose itself. The easiest method is to shrink the lining of the nose with cocaine spray and spray it with sulfathiazole powder. Into this dry cavity small cotton pledgets are accurately placed in the suspect areas which include the anterior cribriform area,

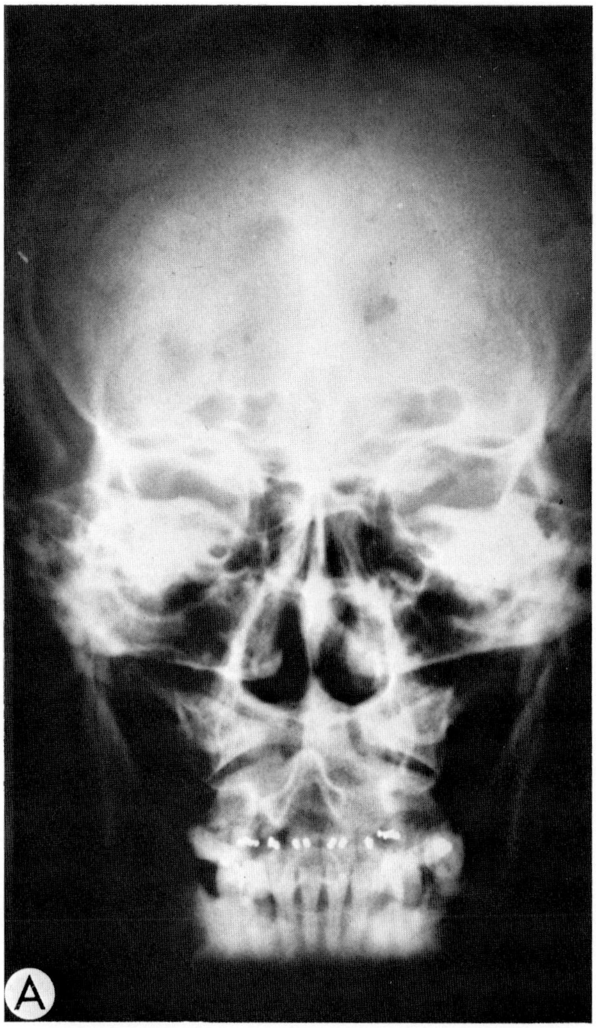

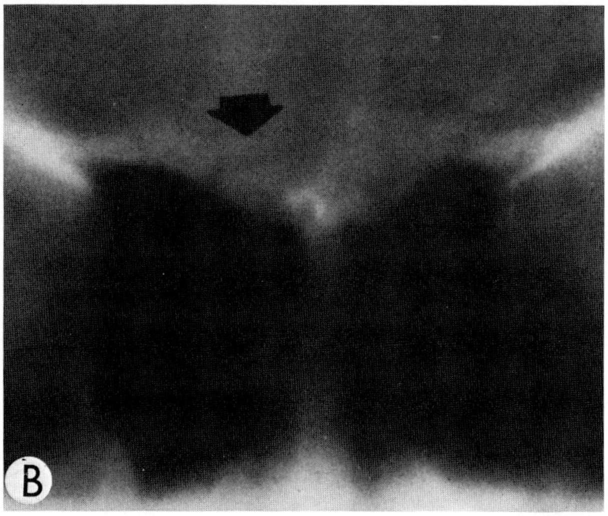

Fig. 6. (A) Routine skull X-ray failing to show fracture. (B) Tomography of the cribriform plate in the same patient showing a fracture posterior to the crista galli.

mid cribriform area, posterior cribriform area, spheno-ethmoidal recess, anterior part of the middle meatus at the frontal infundibulum, and the eustachian tube. The cotton pledgets that become saturated in the specific area would indicate the likely site of drainage.

However, saturation with the fluid itself is not always useful, due to its confusion with lacrimal or nasal secretions. To circumvent this basic problem, modifications of the technique described above have evolved utilizing injected dyes to stain the cerebrospinal fluid. In this method, the cotton pledgets are placed in the nose as previously outlined. A diluted solution of a dye such as indigo carmine or flouroscein is then injected via a lumbar puncture. With the patient in the prone position, the cotton is left in place for approximately 45 minutes and then examined. Specific cotton pledgets that pick up the dye indicate the localization of the cerebrospinal fluid drainage. This cerebrospinal fluid staining technique has been enlarged to include radioactive isotopes which can be evaluated under a scanner and the use of certain monogram dyes which can be studied radiographically.

These tests will generally indicate the precise site of drainage; however, occasionally failures in diagnosis occur. In these most difficult cases, the exact diagnosis may be obtainable only by exploratory surgery.

Prolonged cerebrospinal fluid rhinorrhea, whether delayed or acute requires surgical intervention. Generally speaking, if the drainage persists for over six weeks of conservative therapy, then alternative measures should be contemplated. In the frontal

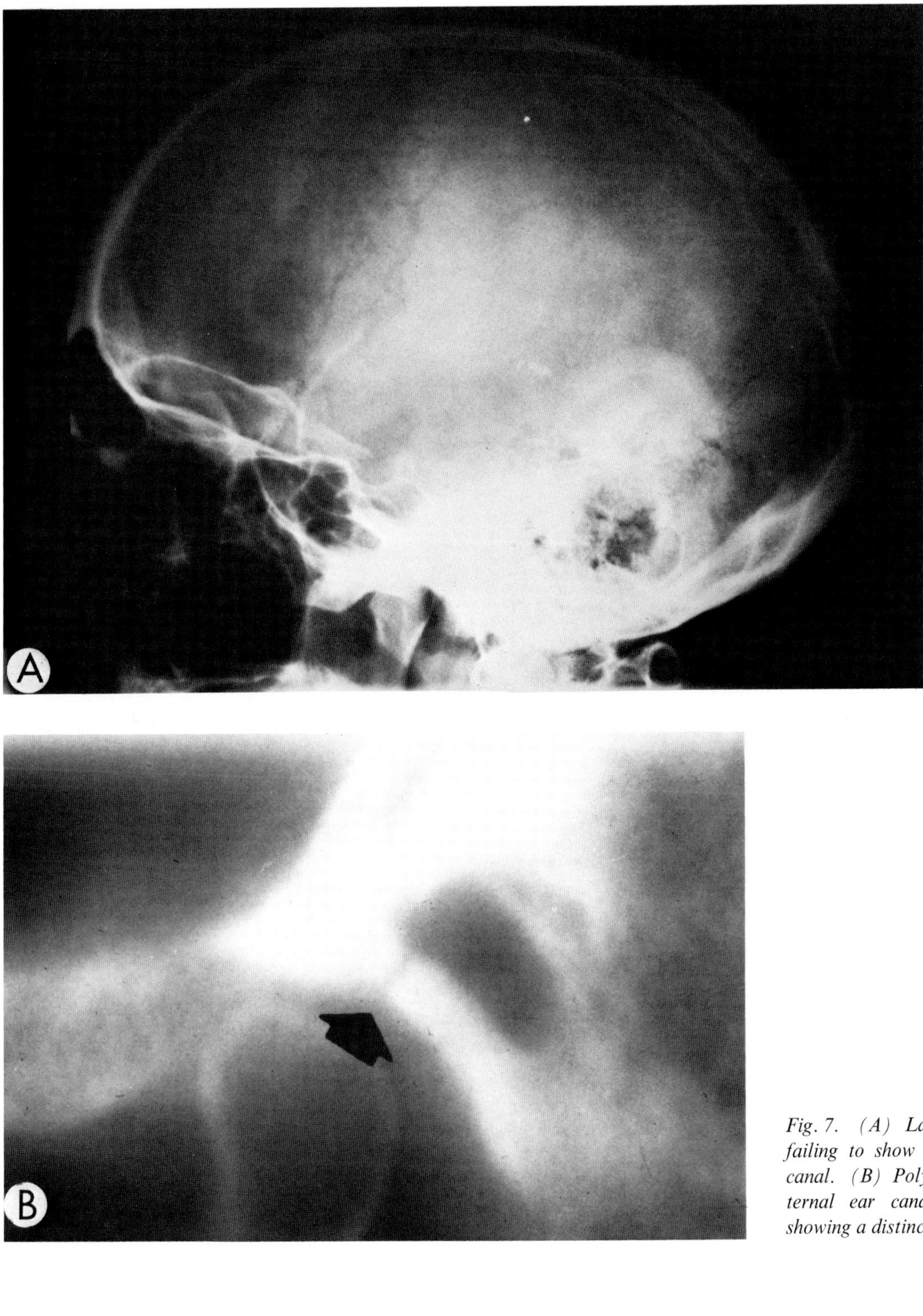

Fig. 7. (A) Lateral view of the skull failing to show fracture of the external canal. (B) Polythomography of the external ear canal of the same patient showing a distinct fracture.

sinus, this involves anterior craniotomy with repair of dural tears. In the ethmoid and cribriform plate area this can be accomplished either through an anterior craniotomy approach or via the ethmoid flap repair advocated by Montgomery. Sphenoid sinus leakage may be approached by craniotomy or through the transseptal-transsphenoidal route. Mastoid otorhinorrhea is corrected by muscle fascia repairs of the middle fossa or posterior fossa dural tears.

Summary

This four-step approach to the diagnosis of cerebrospinal fluid rhinorrhea is presented in an attempt to give the clinician a more precise means of localizing and treating cerebrospinal fluid rhinorrhea which is secondary to trauma.

References

1. Ommaya A: Cerebrospinal fluid rhinorrhea, Neurology 14:106–113, 1964
2. McCoy G: Cerebrospinal rhinorrhea, Laryngoscope 73: 1125–1157, 1963
3. Montgomery WW: Surgery for cerebrospinal fluid rhinorrhea and Otorrhea, Arch Oto 84:538–55, 1966
4. Montgomery WW: Surgery of the upper respiratory system, Vol 1, p 137–168, Lea & Fe, Philadelphia, 1971
5. Jacobson I, Moran AG: Localization of cerebrospinal fluid rhinorrhea Arch Oto 93:79, 1971
6. Blatt IM: Surgical repair for CSF otorrhea due to middle ear and mastoid disease, Laryngoscope 73:446, 1963
7. Anderson T, Hoge R: Cerebrospinal otorrhea Arch Oto 91:19, 1970
8. Crowe HJ, Keogh O, Northfield OWC: The localization of cerebrospinal fluid fistulae Lancet 2:325–327, 1956

Fractures of the Naso-Ethmoid Region—An Anatomical and Mechanical Study

A.D. Cheesman, London, England

The nature of a fracture depends both on the characteristics of the deforming force and on the architectural anatomy of the bone injured. The greater the magnitude of the force, the greater the injury, but equally important is the velocity of application of the force. The energy of a rapidly applied force is dissipated over a small area giving localized comminution of the bone, viz a direct fracture. A more slowly applied force causes the bone to fracture through its weak points over a wider area, viz an indirect fracture. Similarly the area of application of the force affects the injury; a given force acting over a small area causes a localized injury of greater severity. The direction and point of application of the force are particularly important when considering the facial skeleton. Finally the degree of fixation of the skeleton is important, for a blow to the unrestrained head often results in a relatively greater injury to the cervical spine.

The anatomy of the facial skeleton is complex, but for the purposes of the present discussion it is preferable to consider its architectural and functional aspects. Essentially the facial skeleton protects the special sense organs of the head, especially the eye which lies within the bony orbit, the rim of which has considerable strength. Functionally the facial skeleton transmits and distributes the considerable forces of mastication over a wide area of the more rigid cranium. The masticatory forces are transmitted vertically by three main buttresses in the maxillary complex, an anterior canine pillar, a lateral zygomatic pillar, and a posterior pterygoid pillar (Fig. 1). Although these buttresses can withstand considerable vertically applied forces, they are potentially weak to forces applied in other directions. The pterygoid pillar is deeply placed within the head, splinted by muscles, and in the context of this study surgically inaccessible and irrelevant to the discussion. The lateral zygomatic pillar is important as it is the most frequently injured in facial trauma, but its anatomy is relatively simple and several studies have been undertaken in this region.[1] The central canine pillar with its upward extension into the naso-ethmoidal region is of considerable importance clinically because of its complex anatomy and adjacent important structures. The important features of the soft tissue anatomy have been studied in detail by Robinson and Stranc,[2] but little attention has been focussed on the underlying skeletal anatomy and its inherent weaknesses.

Rene Le Fort[3] in his classic study on maxillofacial trauma studied both the characteristics of the deforming forces and the weaknesses of the facial skeleton. Unfortunately his paper was written in French, and despite several very good translations,[4] he has been misquoted in several respects. He demonstrated "lines of weakness" in the facial skeleton rather than "fractures." He pointed out that the facial skeleton did not break cleanly into single fragments, but rather that many fragments resulted, the general direction of cleavage being in one of his three "great lines of weakness." Most important of all, he described his first great line of weakness "the protective barrier of the cranial cavity" (the site of the Le Fort Type III fracture) as passing *through the mid-portion* of the nasal bones (Fig. 2). The upper part of the nasal bones he referred to as being "cranial" with great rigidity, the lower more fragile portion he termed "facial." His "second great line of weakness" (the site of the Le Fort Type II fracture) also traverses the same region of the nose. He further emphasised that there was little risk of damage to the cribriform plate with a fracture passing through his line of weakness; only rarely did the fracture pass through the nasofrontal suture, and in these cases the cribriform plate was invariably fractured.

The purpose of this study is to reemphasize Le Fort's findings, with particular reference to the naso-ethmoid region, by a detailed study of the

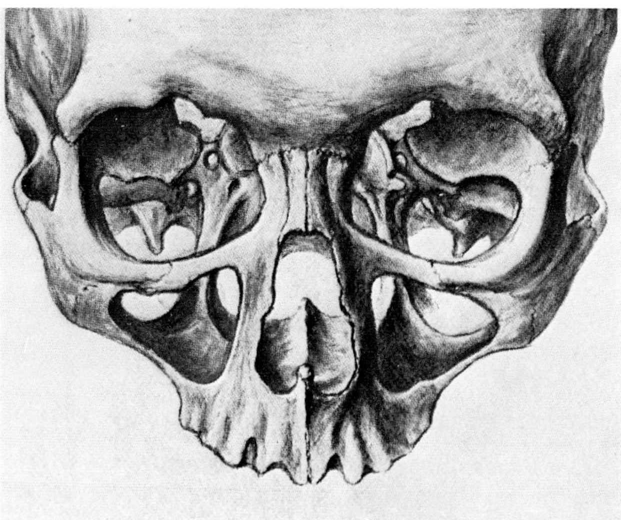

Fig. 1. A schematic drawing of the facial skeleton in which the thin areas of bone have been removed, leaving the main buttresses (after H. M. Shapiro).

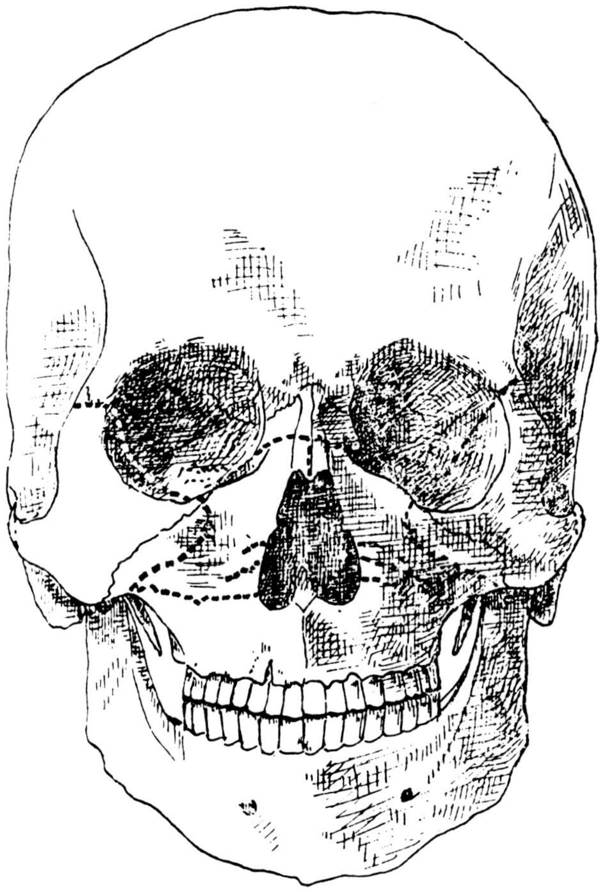

Fig. 2. Reproduction of Le Fort's original illustration showing his lines of weakness (Courtesy Masson & Cie. Paris)

structural anatomy of this region, and demonstration of the weak areas by a mechanical study of the strain patterns resulting from abnormal stresses.

Applied Skeletal Anatomy

The strength of the naso-ethmoid region lies anteriorly in the bones of the nasal pyramid, this constituting the upper part of the canine pillar. Posteriorly the various parts of the ethmoid bone and lacrimal bone contribute little to the region's strength. The structural support of the nasal pyramid has been considered by many workers with reference to rhinoplasty.[5,6] The essential features are demonstrated by consideration of the support of the nasal bones.

The nasal bones articulate medially with each other, and also variously with the frontal, maxillary, and ethmoid bones, and with the septal and upper lateral alar cartilages. A better understanding of the support of the conjoined nasal bones results from considering them as having three distinct regions. The upper third of the nasal bones is very thick, where they have a strong postero-superior articulation with the nasal notch of the frontal bone. The lateral portion of the nasal notch is similarly occupied by the thickened upper end of the frontal process of the maxilla. The adjacent edges of the frontal process and nasal bone also have a strong articulation. This upper third region is very strong (Figs. 3 and 4). The middle third of the nasal bones is much thinner and their lateral articulation is with the slender mid-portion of the frontal process of maxilla. Posteriorly they are supported in turn by the nasal spine of the frontal bone and the perpendicular plate of the ethmoid. The lower third of the nasal bones is fragile, articulating inferiorly with the upper lateral cartilage and posteriorly with the septal cartilage. Laterally their articulation is with the lower part of the frontal process which in this region is again more rigid where it forms the antero-medial aspect of the antrum.

In summary, the upper third region of the nasal pyramid is very strong and closely related to the cranium; this is the region Le Fort referred to as the "cranial portion of the nasal bones." The middle and lower thirds are progressively weaker, but

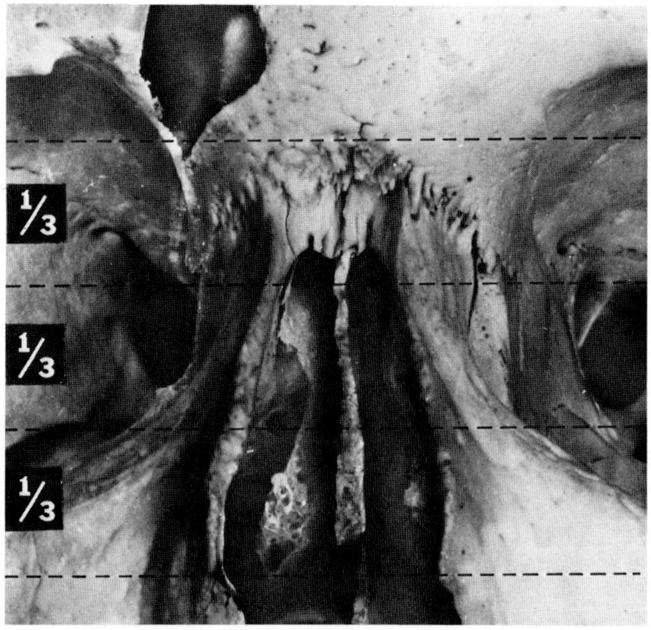

Fig. 3. An anterior view of the nasal region with the nasal bones removed to show their wide articular support from the nasal notch of the frontal bone.

viewed in mechanical terms of structural weakness, the major line of weakness is through the middle third region as this is a relatively weak area adjacent to a strong area. Consequently from an anatomical point of view this must constitute the area through which Le Fort's first and second lines of weakness pass. A simple way of demonstrating this area of weakness is by transilluminating the skull with a light source placed in the region of the nasopharynx. Figure 5 shows such a skull with Le Fort's original lines superimposed. It will be seen that they pass through the weak areas of the facial skeleton. Comparison of this illustration with many similar illustrations in many standard texts will identify some of the misinterpretations of Le Fort's work.

Le Fort in his paper also drew attention to the rarity of a fracture passing through the region of the naso-frontal suture, but clinically we know that such a fracture does occur, particularly as a result of localized trauma. A possible anatomical explanation of this clinical finding can be derived by studying the relative pneumatization of the frontal bone. Figure 4 shows the usual finding in the midline of a skull with moderate frontal pneumatization. Luongo et al[7] have drawn attention to the

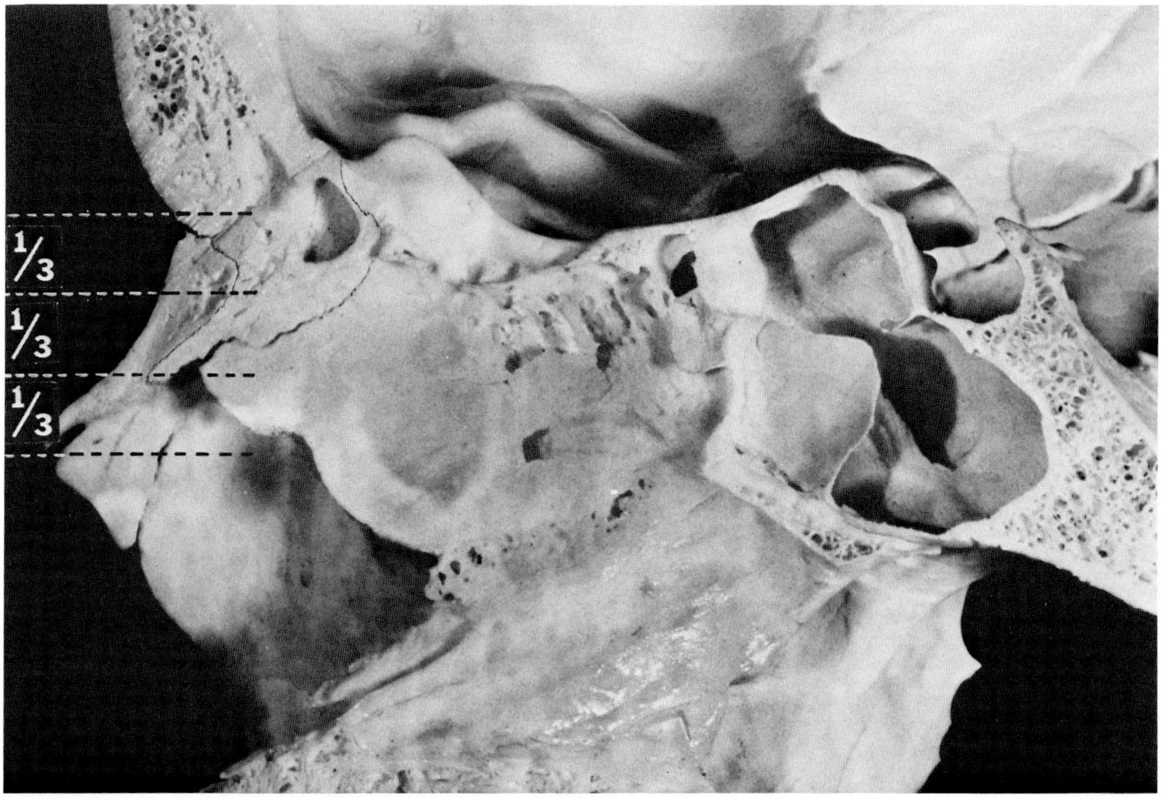

Fig. 4. A sagittal section of the skull with moderate frontal pneumatization. The thick upper third of the nasal bones is seen with the very wide posterior support from the frontal bone. The middle third of the nasal pyramid is supported by the nasal spine of the frontal bone.

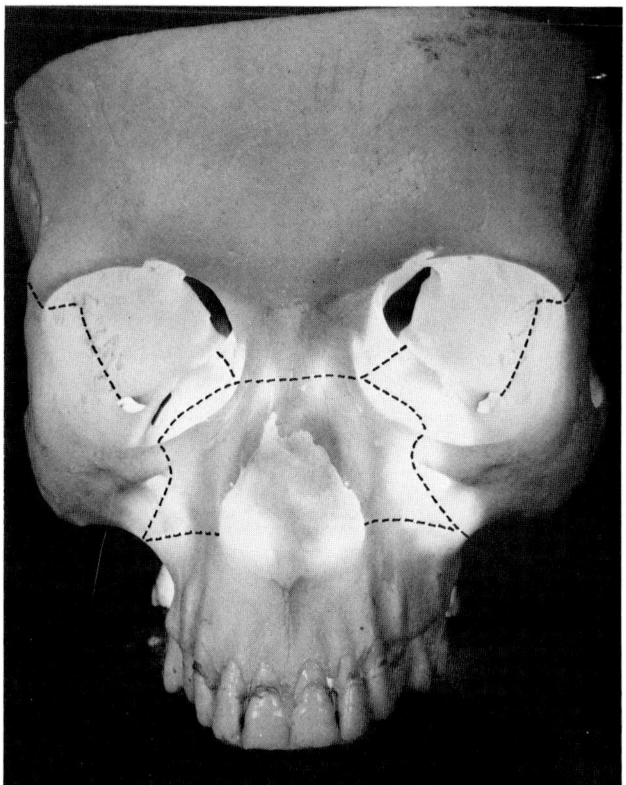

Fig. 5. An anterior view of the skull transilluminated by a light source in the naso-pharynx. The thin areas of bone show greater transillumination. Le Fort's original lines of weakness are superimposed.

extension of frontal pneumatization into the nasal pyramid and discussed its significance in relation to rhinoplasty. Figure 6 shows another bone with a well-pneumatized frontal sinus; in such a skull the support of the upper third of the nasal pyramid is potentially weakened. When such a fracture occurs clinically it is almost invariably accompanied by a fracture of the cribriform plate and c.s.f. rhinorrhoea. Consideration of Figure 7 will explain the anatomical basis of such a finding. It is an anterior view of the ethmoid bone; centrally is the perpendicular plate with its enlarged upper portion, the crista galli. The anterior articulation of the crista galli is with the posterior aspect of the nasal notch of the frontal bone. If a fracture passes through the region of the naso-frontal suture, this strong central part of the ethmoid is driven posteriorly, secondarily causing a fracture of both cribriform plates. The meningeal layer of the dura mater is absent in the region of the cribriform plate, and endosteal layer is readily breached resulting in c.s.f. rhinorrhoea.

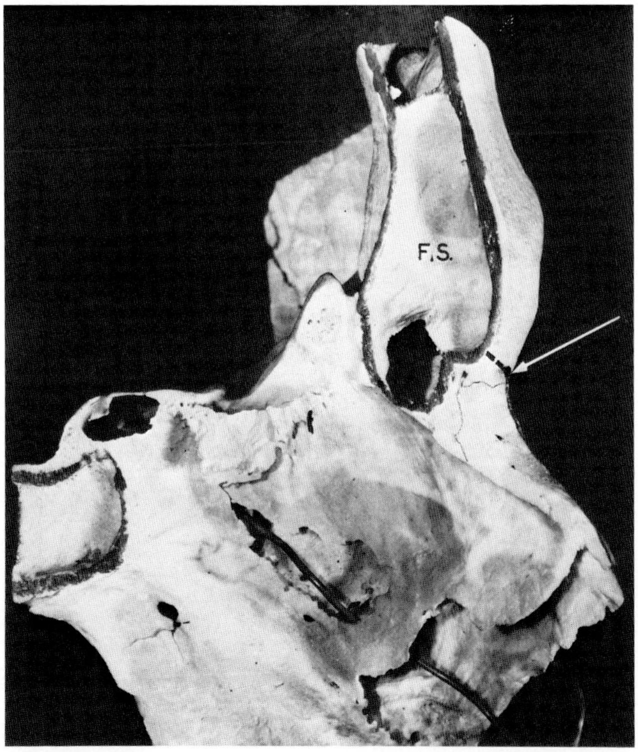

Fig. 6. A sagittal section of the skull showing the weakening of nasal support that results from extensive pneumatization of the frontal sinus. The frontal sinus (F.S.) is outlined and the arrow indicates the considerable reduction in thickness of the frontal bone in the region of the nasal notch (compare with Fig. 4).

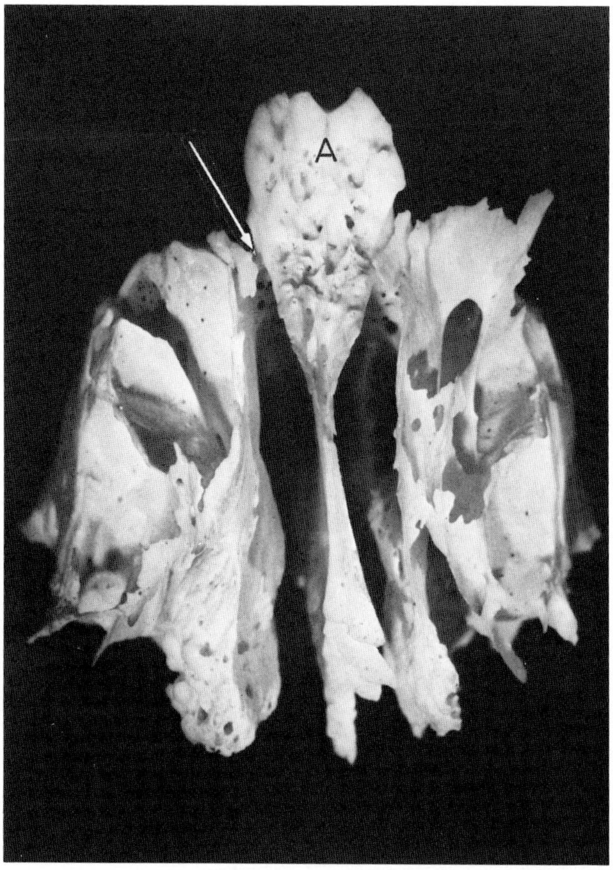

Fig. 7. Anterior view of ethmoid bone. The large articular surface of the criste galli (A) articulates with the posterior aspect of the frontal bone in the region of the nasal notch. The arrow indicates the weak region of the cribriform plate.

Mechanical Analysis of the Stresses and Strains

The areas of weakness in the facial skeleton can be demonstrated by nondestructive techniques of mechanical engineering. The biomechanical analysis of stress and strain in bone has been conducted by many workers, and Evans gives a good review.[8]

Fractures generally result from tensile strains. Tensile strains are best demonstrated by the use of a strain-sensitive coating, and Gurdjian and his co-workers[9] have established the validity of this method in their studies on skull fractures. Clark[6] has used the technique in his analysis of nasal fractures. The general facial skeleton has not been extensively studied due to certain problems, but Hodgson and Nakamura[1] have studied the zygoma in detail and emphasized that the type of fracture produced was dependent on the duration of the force. The present study deals with the analysis of strain patterns in the facial skeleton as a whole. The number of factors involved are extensive and the full results will be published elsewhere. However, certain findings relevant to fractures in the naso-ethmoid region will be demonstrated.

Method

A molten coat of rosin, a strain-sensitive resin, was painted in a thin coat on to a preheated skull. The skull and its coating were then allowed to cool slowly to prevent crazing of the resin. Under standard conditions various forces were applied to the skull.

Findings

On application of the force stresses develop within the bone, and there is some deformation of structure or strain. The brittle resin is very sensitive to tensile strain and cracks develop in it, transverse to the direction of the main strain, appearing first in areas of greatest tensile strain. Fractures occur in the areas of highest tensile strain, the break being in the same direction as the resin cracks. The cracks are detected by careful inspection under oblique illumination, and then their position marked on a photograph of the skull (Figs. 8 and 9).

Antero-Posterior Dynamic Force to Nasal Bridge

The force of a 7 lb weight dropped 6 in. was transmitted in an antero-posterior direction to a mould covering the conjoined nasal bones only. External examination of the skull showed transverse cracks in the resin in the region of the naso-frontal suture. The interpretation of these findings is that a fracture would develop at the naso-frontal suture to a localized dynamic force applied anteriorly on the nasal bridge. Examination of the anterior cranial fossa (Fig. 8) showed resin cracks

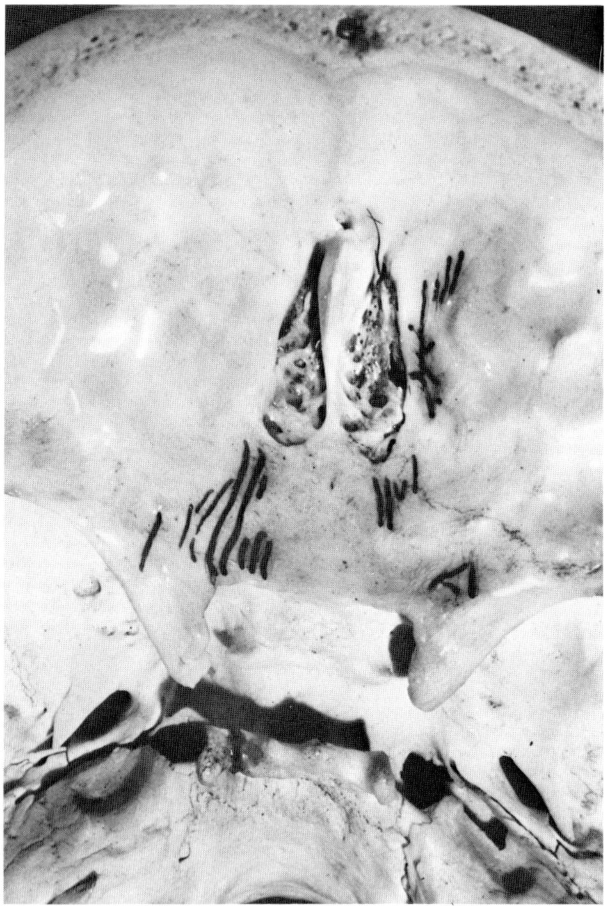

Fig. 8. View of anterior cranial fossa showing orientation of strain cracks following a localised blow to the nasion.

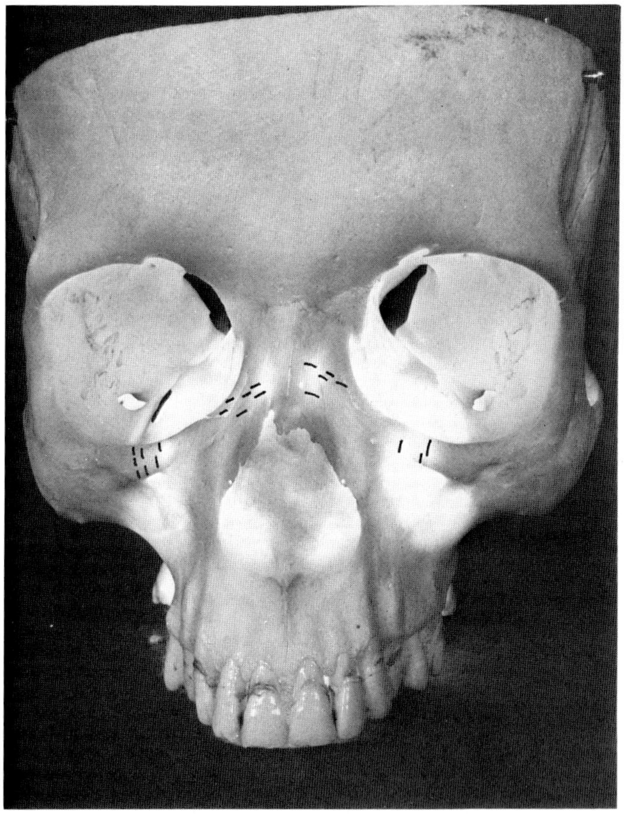

Fig. 9. Anterior view of skull showing orientation of strain cracks following downward blow to the whole middle third of the maxilla.

passing in an antero-posterior direction in the line of the cribriform plate. These cracks are the result of the secondary tensile strain which develops at 90° to the primary compressive strain through the cribriform plate, and demonstrates how a fracture of the cribriform plate occurs in this type of injury.

Oblique Dynamic Force (45° to Upper Alveolus) Applied to the Middle Third of the the Maxilla

Using the same skull, the direction of the force was raised through 45°, and it was applied over a wide area of the middle third of the maxilla. An initial force of 7 lb dropped from 3 in. resulted in oblique cracks in the resin (Fig. 9) over the frontal process of the maxilla and nasal bones on the right side only. Increasing the distance through which the weight was dropped resulted in the further development of cracks disposed along Le Fort's second line of weakness. They were more pronounced on the right side. There were no cracks in the resin in the anterior cranial fossa. The interpretation of this particular experiment is that the indicated type of force would result in a Le Fort II type of fracture with no injury to the cribriform plate region.

Clinical Significance

These studies emphasize that two main types of fracture may result from trauma to the naso-ethmoid region; the respective aetiologies and pathological findings are different, but the principles of treatment are the same for both.

A localized injury to the nasal pyramid, especially of high intensity and short duration tends to cause a localized fracture with disruption of the fronto-nasal suture, fracture of the cribriform plate and c.s.f. rhinorrhoea. This type of injury is relatively uncommon, and generally results from the force of a projectile. Open reduction is invariably necessary, although often facilitated by existing lacerations. This is followed by interosseous fixation and correction of any associated soft-tissue deformity.

More commonly naso-ethmoid injuries follow a road traffic accident or personal violence. In such cases, the force is often cushioned with a consequent lengthening of the impact duration. This results in the facial skeleton fracturing through its inherent weak areas giving the classic Le Fort Type II or III fractures. In such cases, if there is minimal direct damage in the naso-ethmoidal region, closed reduction and fixation is often adequate. However, if there is any doubt regarding the extent of damage in this region, open reduction is again advised.

When performing open reduction it is important to identify and preserve the main bony fragments. This is facilitated by a mental picture of the anatomy previously discussed, and an understanding of the possible fractures that may occur. The important fragments to preserve and return to their normal position are the anteriorly placed bones of the nasal pyramid and medial orbital rim. In practice it will be found that with severe injuries the upper third of the nasal pyramid forms one large fragment, while the frontal processes of the maxillae and adjoining lower portions of the nasal bones form two further fragments, these latter fragments can usually be identified by the anterior lacrimal crest or attached medial canthal ligament.

The bony fragments of the ethmoid, and fragments of the septal cartilage are usually best removed unless they can readily be placed in their correction positions. This debridement serves to preserve nasal and sinus function.

Acknowledgments

I wish to thank Mr. D. Connolly of the Photographic Department for his help in photographing the specimens, and Professor T. Nicol for anatomical advice.

References

1. Hodgson VR, Nakamura GS: Mechanical impedance and impact response of the human cadaver zygoma. J Biomechan 1: 73–78, 1968
2. Robinson TJ, Stranc MF: The anatomy of the medial canthal ligament. Brit J Plast Surg 23: 1–7, 1970
3. Le Fort R: Étude Expérimentale Sur Les Fractures de la Machoire Supérieure. Rev chir de Paris 23: 208–227, 360–389, 1901
4. Le Fort R: Experimental study of fractures of the upper jaw. Translated by Dr. Paul Tessier. The Classic Reprint. Plast Reconstr Surg 50: 497–506, 600–607, 1972
5. Fomon S, Syracuse VR, Bolotow N, Pullen M: Plastic repair of the deflected nasal septum. Arch Otolaryngol 44: 141–156, 1946

6. Clark GM: The principles of the structural support of the nose and their application to nasal and septal surgery. M.S. Thesis, Univ of Sydney, 1968
7. Luongo RA, Luongo RA Jr. Anatomical observations for rhinoplastic surgery. Laryngoscope 68: 1076–1080, 1958
8. Evans, FG: Stress and strain in bones. Charles C. Thomas, Springfield, Ill 1957
9. Gurdjian ES, Lissner HR: Deformations of the skull in head injury studied by the "Stresscoat" technique, quantitative determinations. Surg Gyn Obstet 83: 219–233, 1946

Reconstructive Surgery of the Nose for Neoplasms

James Grant, Memphis, Tennessee

The history of reconstructive nasal surgery dates back to Egyptian and Indian writings which are over 4000 years old. In those days regional pedicle flaps and composite grafts were utilized for reconstructive surgery by an Indian caste of artisans who were assigned the task because of their artistic sense of form and expression. Ultimately, these methods were revitalized by various Italian surgeons during the 15th and 16th centuries; and the work of Tagliacozzi, particularly, corresponds accurately to some of today's methods. Interest in nasal reconstructive surgery lay dormant during the 17th and 18th centuries; however, early in the 19th century, two Berlin surgeons, VonGraefe and Dieffenbach, renewed and perfected the Indian and Italian techniques. Their works preceded efforts by Roe and Weir in the U.S., the former being credited with performing the first rhinoplasty without external skin incisions in New York in 1897. A year later, Joseph, of Berlin, performed the same operation, and in 1931 published his classic composition which is a basic work for modern nasal plastic surgery.

Cancer of the nose is not a rare neoplasm. It accounts for 27 percent of all skin cancers, and occurs primarily in males over 60 years of age. Basal cell carcinoma predominates over squamous cell carcinoma 2 to 1. It can arise from any of the nasal structures or occur as an extension from a contiguous structure. Fortunately, basal cell carcinoma and low grade squamous cell carcinoma of the skin make up the great majority of nasal tumors; and curative efforts are usually effective when consistent with good tumor surgery principles. Effective eradication of the tumor must, however, be combined with the modern-day reconstructive techniques in order to restore facial harmony and function of the organ.

As in other sites of head and neck cancer, the extent, location, and histopathology of the tumor dictate the modalities of treatment and the timing of the rehabilitative efforts in each case. Modern methods of radiation therapy and chemotherapy have been proven effective, alone, and in combination with surgery, in the treatment of superficial nasal skin cancers. However, the modern techniques of plastic and reconstructive surgery are generally preferable to insure disease eradication, avoidance of disfigurement, and preservation of nasal function. Several of the excellent papers and courses in this symposium illustrate the impetus that reconstructive nasal surgery has received from renewed interest in cosmetic rhinoplastic surgery and tissue transfer techniques. Cutaneous lesions, particularly, have provided the surgeon with the opportunity to use regional flaps and composite grafts to successfully restore contour and color to the nose.

The reconstructive efforts used today in nasal surgery have been increasingly successful as anesthetic, pharmacologic, and surgical methods have improved. Research in wound healing, the timing of flap and graft movements, and the understanding of tissue hemodynamics have contributed to this success rate. The nose lends itself to these methods, but requires meticulous care in planning and carrying out these details to insure adequate excision and esthetic results. Immediate reconstruction of the nose varies according to the location of the lesion. The skin over the dorsum and sides of the upper half of the nose is thin and mobile, particularly in the cancer-age-group patient. The skin of the lower half of the nose is thick and adherent to the underlying cartilaginous framework; but both areas are amenable to flap or graft techniques. Proponents of flaps cite the advantages of self contained blood supply, superior cosmetic properties, and enhanced protection from infection and for composite graft reconstruction. Local flaps are most frequently utilized for repair of various sized superficial nasal cancers, and are basically three types: nasolabial advancement flaps, rotational flaps, and transpositional flaps. These three techniques provide the basic elements of sufficient quantities of chromatically matched tissue from donor areas which can be easily hidden in skin folds or preexistent wrinkles. Time limitations prohibit technical description of these methods; the details are provided in the week's courses by Drs. Denecke and Gunter.

Regional flaps are utilized in reconstructive procedures which involve tissue losses too large to be repaired by local flaps or grafts. The skin of the forehead is utilized due to its excellent color match with the nose, and may be the distal portion of a flap made up principally from the forehead or scalp. The base of the flap incorporates at least one of the major facial or scalp vessels, and may be single or bipedicle, thus permitting unusual length-to-width ratios. The disadvantages of these flaps stem from the secondary scarring of the forehead (which can be minimized), and the subsequent procedures necessary for scar revision or flap pedicle return to the donor site. Again, technical details of the procedures are covered in the week's instructional courses.

Composite grafts used to reconstruct the nose are relatively new procedures. Although described in Germany in 1887 by Koenig, the main emphasis was generated by Gillies in England and Brown in the U.S. in the mid-1940s. The auricle is the common donor site and provides a chondrocutaneous graft which supplies the lining and cartilaginous support needed for restoration of the alar or tip areas. Donor sites may also include the opposite side of the nose. Treatment of the donor site as well as the technical procedures of graft removal and suture and dressing techniques are beautifully described in the classic works by Denecke and Meyers and by Claus Walter.

Cases involving extensive loss of nasal tissue are relatively rare; but, as would be expected, are more complex in both reconstructive and tumor surgery requirements. The question of perichondrial or periosteal invasion is paramount as this usually indicates a more aggressive tumor with diffuse rapid extension, often without clinically recognizable evidence of extension. Reconstructive efforts should be postponed for cases that involve the loss of internal nasal lining and nasal structural support to allow histologic verification of resected margins and an adequate period of observation. Indeed, we concur with others that a well constructed nasal prosthesis may be preferable to a prolonged series of reconstructive efforts.

Our interest in nasal prosthetics began as we researched a paper on Carcinoma of the Nasal Septum. While reviewing the sparse literature on this subject and evaluating our own data, it became apparent that regardless of the treatment modality used, the survival rates were poor and often precluded planned reconstructive surgery. The loss of large areas of nasal surface and structure indicated to us that a cosmetic repair which provided early defect coverage but allowed close postoperative observation would be preferable because of the aggressive nature of these tumors. Nasal prosthetics appear to answer that need.

The history of nasal prosthetics closely parallels the history of nasal surgery, also beginning in early Egyptian times. The 16th century found prosthetic concepts revitalized by the French surgeon, Ambroise Paré, a contemporary of Togliacozzi, the famed Italian rhinoplastic surgeon. Paré designed prostheses of silver and pointed out the two major problems reconstructive surgery confronts today: color match and surface-structural replacement. In the late 19th century, interest was increased through the efforts of Martin and Tetamore; and, during the first 50 years of the 20th century, was further enhanced by the adaptation of gelatin-glycerin compounds, and later methyl methacylate and plastics.

The past 25 years have provided an age of technical advances almost comparable to those of surgery, and the preparation and use of nasal prosthetics has correspondingly improved. The technical aspects of nasal prosthetic construction are well described in several texts, and good results have been obtained with various materials.

In summation, immediate or delayed reconstructive surgery for nasal lesions that are amenable to the excellent flap and graft techniques available today must be constantly revised and improved. In patients with lesions that involve extensive loss of nasal tissue, who are unable and/or unwilling to undergo staged reconstructive procedures for personal or surgical reasons, modern day prosthetics should be employed. The use of a prosthesis as a temporary measure in those patients who prefer staged reconstruction to the long term use of a prothesis should also be considered. The combination of these methods will ultimately provide these unfortunate patients with the most rapid and satisfactory return to their places in society.

Surgery of the Nasal Valve

Eugene B. Kern, Rochester, Minn.

Severe nasal airway obstruction with symptoms may result either from apparent anatomic abnormalities or from less obvious nasal deformities. One such subtle yet significant deformity may occur in the nasal valve. The main purposes of this paper are to present (1) a pathologic and a clinical classification of abnormalities in the region of the nasal valve and (2) the principles of precise surgical exposure of the abnormality and the goals of surgical correction.

If a valve is defined as a movable structure that regulates or permits the flow of a gas or fluid, the human nose has a number of valves. The erectile tissues of the turbinates (turbinal valve) and of the nasal septum (septal valve) can regulate the flow of air in the nose; and, therefore, these two tissues are nasal valves. However, the nasal valve is usually referred to as the slitlike opening between the caudal end of the upper lateral cartilage and the nasal septum, which was first described by Mink in 1903.[1] The nasal valve is only a portion of the nasal valve area and should not be confused with the entire circumference of the nasal valve area. The nasal valve area is the narrowest part of the nasal passage and has many synonyms: os internum, ostium internum, limen vestibuli, "valve area," "valve region," and area 2. The nasal valve also has several synonyms, including the liminal valve, "flow-limiting segment," and "liminal chink."

Anatomy of the Nasal Valve Area and the Nasal Valve

The external portion of the nose can be divided into three parts: an upper bony portion, a middle third, which is the roof cartilage or upper lateral cartilage connected as one cartilage to the nasal septum, and a lower third, which is composed of the paired lower lateral or great alar cartilages (or also called the alar or lobular cartilages) (Fig. 1). This skeletal structure is covered by skin, muscles, neurovascular tissues, connective tissues, and mucocutaneous tissues intranasally. The upper lateral cartilage is attached firmly at its proximal end by fibrous tissue beneath the nasal bones. It is also supported caudally and laterally by fibrous tissue,

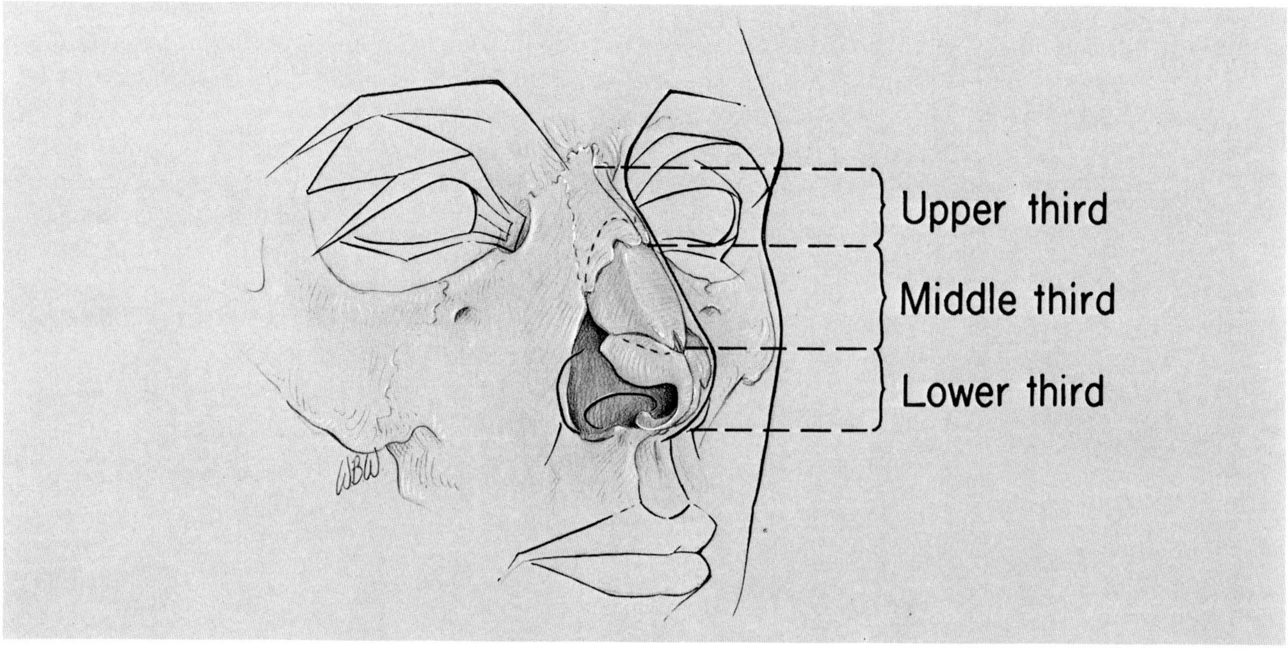

Fig. 1. Skeletal structure of the external portion of the nose is divided into three parts: an upper bony portion; a middle third, which is upper lateral cartilage (roof cartilage); and a lower third, which is composed of paired lower lateral cartilages. Note in the middle third that the upper lateral cartilage is attached beneath nasal bones proximally and beneath lower lateral cartilages distally and extends laterally out to the bony margin of the pyriform aperture formed in part by frontal process of maxilla.

and it extends beneath the lower lateral cartilages and out laterally to the maxilla. Caudally and medially the upper lateral cartilage is separated by a narrow cleft from the nasal septum. The entire nasal valve area extends from the region of the caudal end of the upper lateral cartilage laterally in its relationship to the nasal septum medially, out laterally to the bony point of the pyriform aperture and the soft fibrofatty tissue in this region, and is bounded below by the floor of the nose. The pyriform aperture is that opening in the skull which remains after all of the nasal cartilaginous structures have been removed. Bridger[2] believed that the entire nasal valve area averaged 55 mm^2, whereas Masing,[3] in 1967, calculated the area as 64 mm^2. The narrowest portion of the nasal airway is this opening of the nasal valve area and the specific triangular slitlike portion between the caudal end of the upper lateral cartilage in its relationship to the nasal septum is the nasal valve. The nasal valve angle is measured in degrees and represents the angle between the upper lateral cartilage and the nasal septum and normally ranges between 10° to 15° (Fig. 2).

Alar Muscles of the Nose

Developmentally, the nose pushes through the facial muscle sheet and has two sets of muscles to regulate the external nasal orifice. As in any other part of the body, there are the constrictor muscles and the dilator muscles (Fig. 3). The dilator muscles increase the rigidity of the nasal valve and prevent collapse, whereas the constrictor muscles, when they function, facilitate collapse, or closing the valve. The nasal constrictors are not as important phylogenetically in man as they are in some other forms of life.

Physiology of the Nasal Valve

Bridger,[2] in his classic article on the physiology of the nasal valve, compared the nasal valve to a

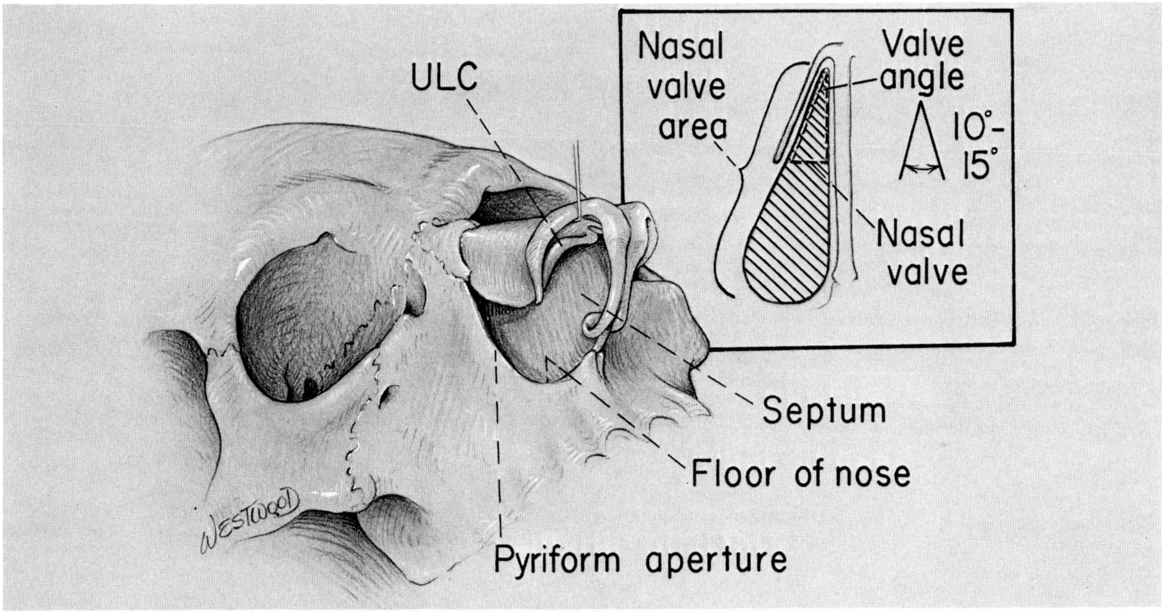

Fig. 2. Nasal valve area is bounded by nasal septum, caudal ends of upper lateral cartilage (ULC), and soft fibrofatty tissue overlying the pyriform aperture and floor of nose. This area is shaped like a teardrop, the slit-like apex of which which is the nasal valve. Inset, nasal valve is slitlike triangular opening at apex of nasal valve area (cross-hatched) and is bounded by caudal end of upper lateral cartilage and nasal septum. Nasal valve angle represents the angle between upper lateral cartilage and nasal septum, and is normally 10° to 15°.

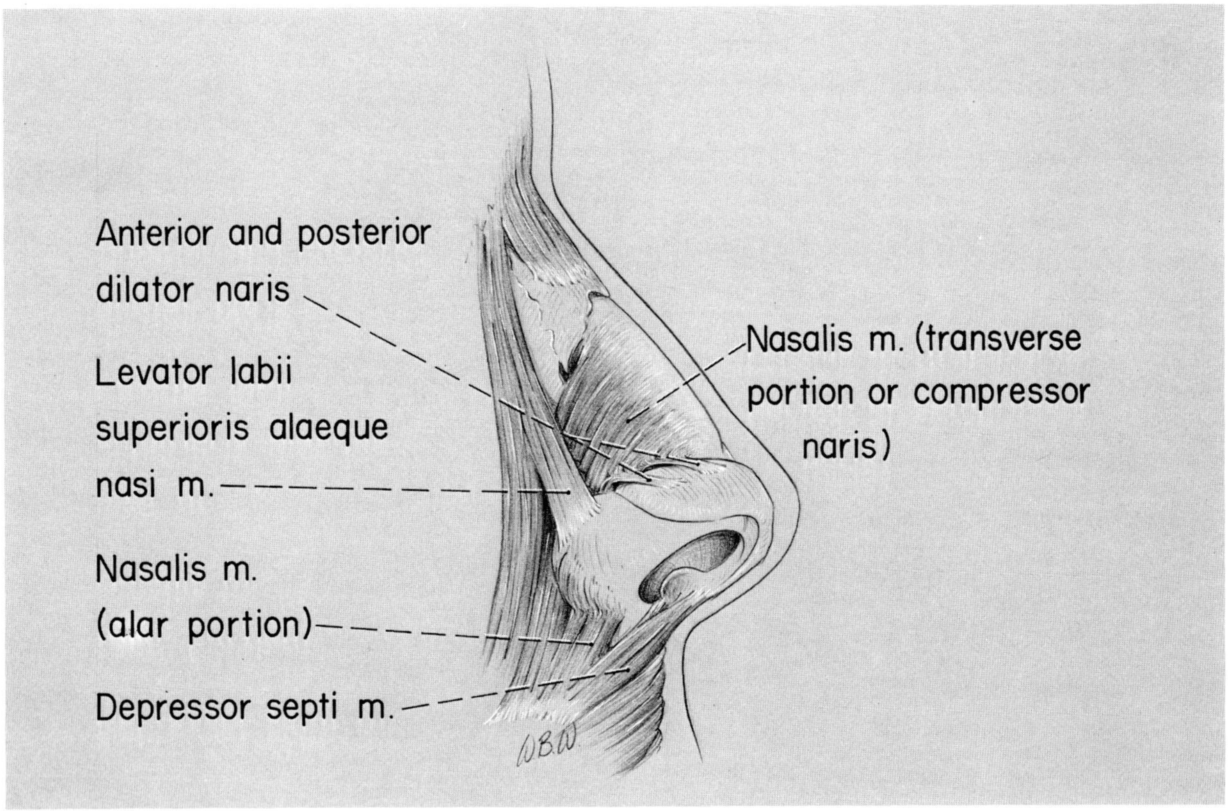

Fig. 3. Alar muscles of nose. Dilator and constrictor muscles of nose. Constrictor muscles (nasalis muscle, transverse portion, also termed "compressor naris muscle") facilitate collapse or closing of nose, whereas all the rest are dilator muscles, which increase rigidity of nasal valve and prevent collapse. The flexible external portion of the nose tends also to resist collapse because of the way the cartilages are sprung open.

Starling resistor. He considered the nose as having a collapsible or flow-limiting segment (nasal valve). His model, therefore, involved a rigid tube—internal nose, with a short collapsible segment—the flexible external nose. The transmural pressure is the difference between the pressure outside the tube (atmospheric) and the intraluminal (intranasal) pressure. The flexible external nose tends to resist collapse primarily because of the way the cartilages are sprung open. Thus, a critical transmural pressure can be reached at which the collapsible segment closes. This occurs when the inside or intraluminal (intranasal) pressure becomes negative from the effect of inspiration (Fig. 4). Bridger[2] has pointed out that a maximal inspiratory effort can increase the flow-pressure curve to a point at which nasal airflow will no longer be increased by a further increase in negative pressure. This finding was compatible with the concept of the nose having a flow-limiting segment or nasal valve.

The complete function of the nasal valve is not known, although Williams[4] has speculated that it

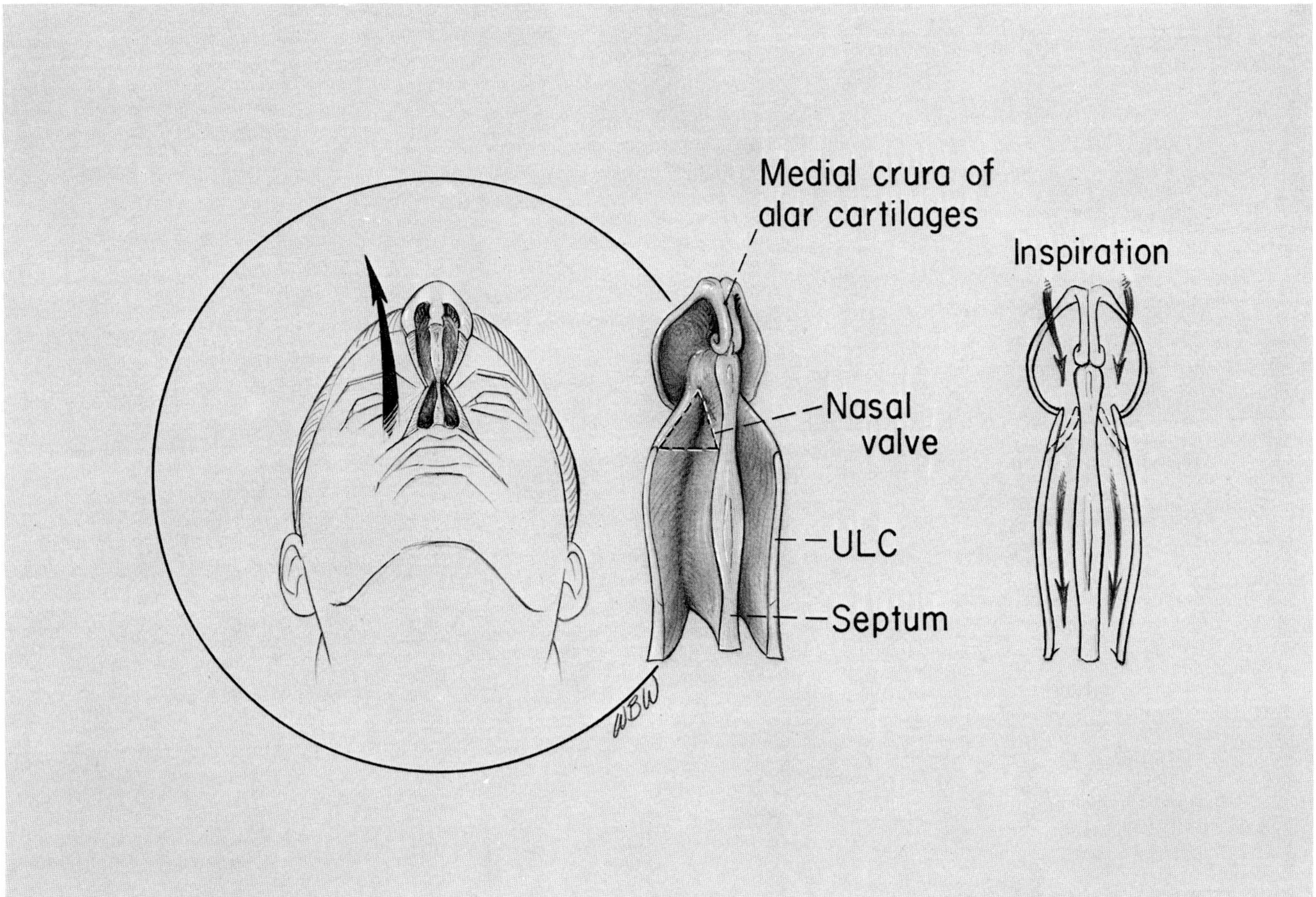

Fig. 4. Physiology of nasal valve. (A) If the nose were dissected free from face, including the lower lateral (alar) cartilages, upper lateral cartilage, and the nasal septum, along with the nasal bones, and this were rotated so that it could be viewed from the undersurface, Figure 4B would be visualized. (B) Undersurface of bony and cartilaginous nasal pyramid with attached lower lateral (alar) cartilages view from floor of nose toward roof into respiratory gutter. Note nasal valve, the specific triangular slitlike portion between caudal end of upper lateral cartilage (ULC), in its relationship to nasal septum. (C) Schematic representation of Figure 4B demonstrating nasal valve as a flow-limiting or collapsible segment that will close when the critical transmural pressure is reached, owing to the effect of increased intranasal negative pressure during maximal inspiratory effort.

functions as an inflow device, controlling the rate and depth of respiration. Hinderer[5] has suggested that the nasal valve controls the inspiratory air currents, changing them from a column to a sheet of air, thereby giving shape, velocity, direction, and resistance to the air currents.

In the Black person (platyrrhine nose), the narrowest part of the nasal passage (the flow-limiting segment) is the area between the nasal septum and the anterior part of the inferior turbinate. Thus, in the Black person, the inferior turbinate probably constitutes the most important inflow regulator, that is, the turbinal valve, whereas in the Caucasian (leptorrhine nose), the nasal valve is probably the most important inflow regulator, accounting for most of the inspiratory resistance to airflow.[5–8]

Pathophysiology of the Nasal Valve

Bridger[2] offers two important concepts in the pathophysiology of the nasal valve. First, the pathologic anatomy produces dysfunction of the nasal valve by causing too early a collapse of this valve during inspiration rather than by changing the total nasal resistance. Second, increased nasal resistance is not a necessary consequence of dysfunction of the nasal valve. Thus, early collapse of an already narrowed nasal valve area seems to be important.

In reviewing his patients who had symptoms of upper airway obstruction but who had not undergone rhinoplasty, Bridger[2] noted that the most common deformity was found in the caudal end of the septum (area 1, Fig. 5), according to Cottle's classification described by Hinderer).[9] He noted that there was deviation and dislocation of the caudal end of the septum and that the deformity was slight at times and seemed to be clinically unimportant. However, on other occasions, the septal abnormality was so significant that it produced deformities of the external nares and nasal tip. He also noted that sagging and depression or twisting and buckling of the upper lateral cartilage also disturbed the relationship of this cartilage with the nasal septum, thereby narrowing the nasal valve.

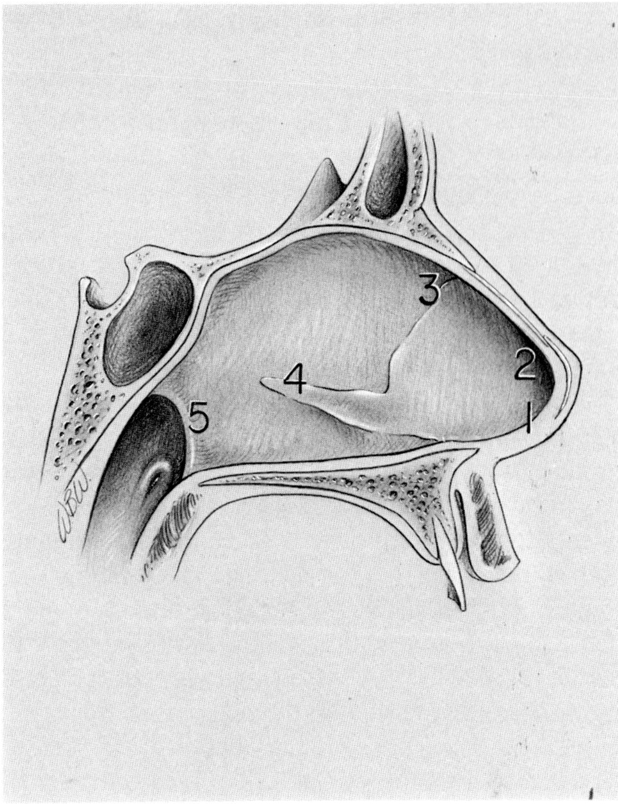

Fig. 5. Areas of nose. Area 1 (vestibular area) is region of caudal end of nasal septum in its relationship to anterior naris. Area 2 (nasal valve area) is bounded by nasal septum, caudal end of upper lateral cartilage, and soft fibrofatty tissue overlying pyriform aperature and floor of nose. This area is shaped like a teardrop, the slitlike apex of which is the nasal valve. Area 3 (attic area) of nasal septum under bony vault of nasal bones. Area 4 (anterior turbinate area) of nasal septum in region of turbinates. Area 5 (posterior turbinate area) of nasal septum in region of choanae.

He stated that these deformities were aggravated by changes in the columella because of retraction or local scars, spurs, and deviations in the maxillary crest and anterior nasal spine—all of which produced asymmetry of the nostrils. He concluded that the pathophysiology of these disturbances essentially was due to the small changes in the size of the nasal valve, which had a marked influence on its collapsibility. Therefore, any abnormality in this nasal valve area could cause early collapse of the nasal valve and thereby cause symptoms.

Clinical Examination of the Nasal Valve

The nasal valve requires careful examination in every patient who has nasal respiratory symtoms in order to rule out a pathologic process in this region (Fig. 6). Frequently, in order to obtain an adequate view of the nasal valve in the male patient, the vibrissae may need to be trimmed. The nasal valve is best examined without a nasal speculum, which may distort the relationship of the caudal end of the upper lateral cartilage to the septum. The tip of the nose can be elevated with a finger, a nasal speculum, or a four-prong retractor, and the nasal valve can be examined with the aid of an adequate source of light. Normally, the caudal end of the upper lateral cartilage should form an angle of 10° to 15° with the nasal septum. A smaller angle is consistent with a symptomatic narrowing of the nasal valve. A larger angle is termed "ballooning" and is normal in the platyrrhine nose, yet it may be associated with nasal symptoms in the leptorrhine nose because of loss of inspiratory control and alterations in nasal resistance.[5]

Thus, the eye, directly or with the aid of a nasal speculum (carefully applied), the four-prong retrac-

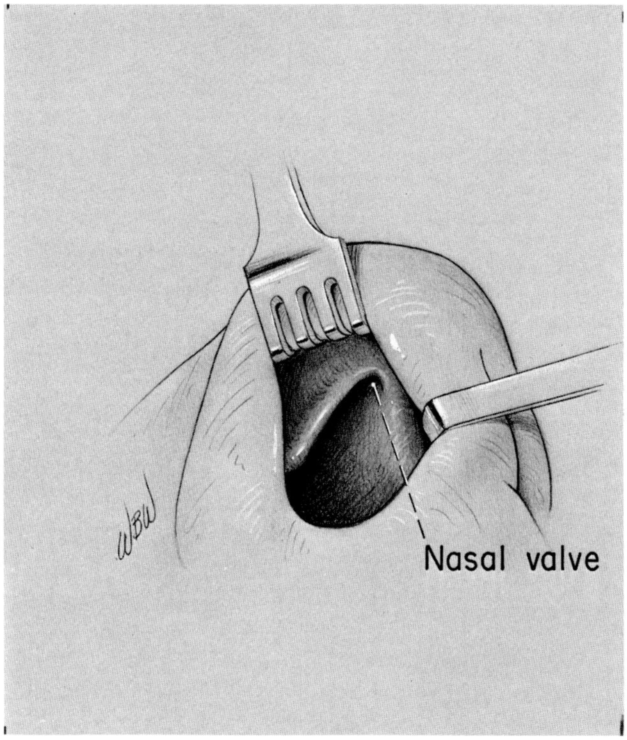

Fig. 6. Clinical view of nasal valve. Note use of four-prong retractor and narrow Nievert retractor to expose nasal valve. When a nasal speculum is used, care must be taken not to obscure nasal valve. Sometimes vibrissae may need to be trimmed in order to visualize nasal valve. Nasal valve is perhaps best examined without any instrument in the nose.

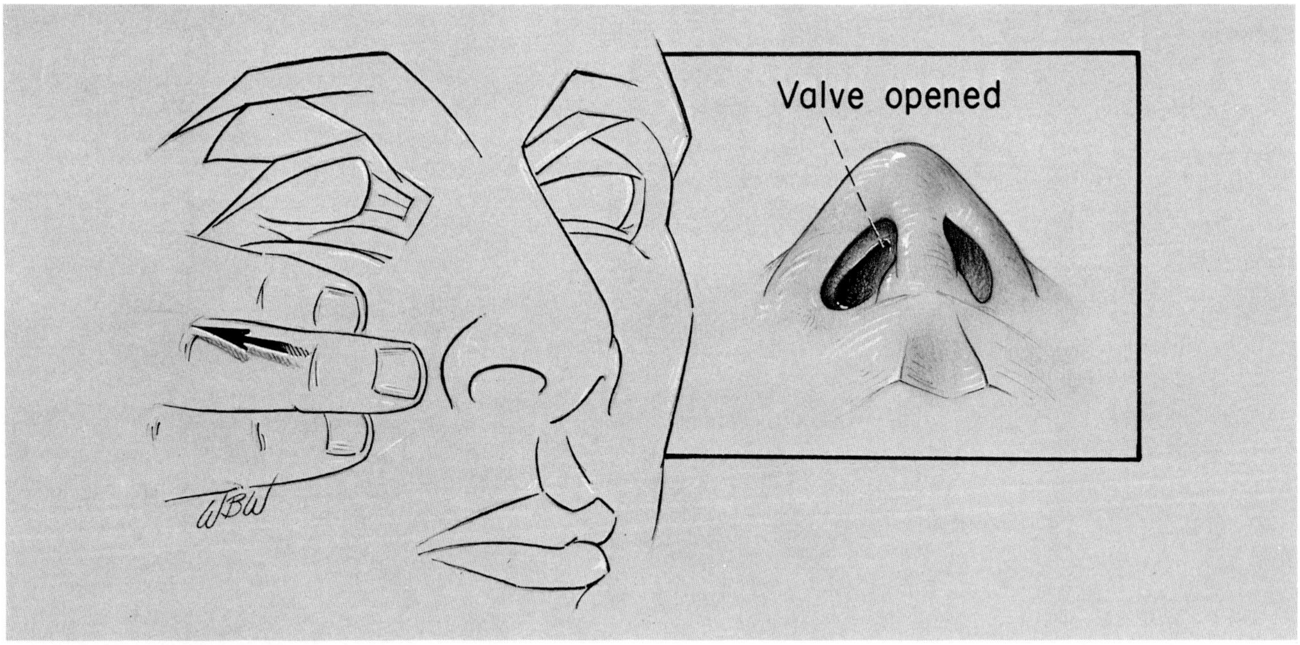

Fig. 7. Cottle test. Cheek is pulled away from midline, carrying upper lateral cartilage away from septum; thus, slitlike angle of nasal valve is opened, and the patient is asked if this improves airflow through the test side. Inset, Cottle sign is positive if this maneuver relieves nasal airway obstruction; if the opposite nasal valve is normal, this may serve as a control for the Cottle test.

tor, or a rhinoscope, may be used to examine this important airflow region, while rhinomanometric examination of the nasal valve also may be carried out by the maximal inspiratory method.[2]

A simple and useful clinical test for confirming the presence of an abnormality in the nasal valve is the Cottle test.[10] While the patient breathes quietly, the cheek is drawn laterally away from the midline opening the nasal valve and the patient is asked if this manuever improves airflow through the test side (Fig. 7). If this relieves the nasal obstruction, the Cottle sign is considered positive and indicates that the abnormality of the nasal valve is a significant factor in the symptomatic nasal obstruction. When this manuever does not markedly improve airflow, the sign is negative. The opposite side if normal may serve as a control. If the nasal valve is occluded by scarring, the patient may have a nasal valve problem with a false-negative Cottle sign. This indicates that the abnormality in the nasal valve (such as scarring of the upper lateral cartilage to the septum) and the resultant airflow disturbance cannot be lessened by performing the Cottle test. A summary of interpretations of the positive and negative Cottle signs is provided in Table 1.

Table 1. Interpretation of Positive and Negative Cottle Sign

Cottle sign	Comment
Positive	Presence of nasal valve abnormality
Negative	Normal nasal valve, with nasal abnormality in another site in nose, or entirely normal nose
False-positive	Can be seen with alar collapse
False-negative	Can be seen with adhesions or stricture of nasal valve

Abnormalities of the Nasal Valve

Nasal valve abnormalities can be classified both clinically and pathologically. The "all inclusive" list is found under pathologic classification (Table 2). The basis of the clinical classification is that nasal valve abnormalities are primarily caused by narrowing of the nasal valve angle from abnormalities of (1) soft-covering mucocutaneous tissues, (2) skeletal supporting tissues, or (3) both (Table 3). The first involves the mucocutaneous coverings and includes such problems as edema, hypertrophy, and scarring, whereas the second involves the nasal septum and the upper lateral cartilage. Probably

Table 2. Pathologic Classification of Nasal Valve Obstruction

- I. Intramural
  - A. Anatomic
    - 1. Mucosal
      - a. Inflammatory
      - b. Hypertrophy
    - 2. Submucosal
      - a. Scar
        - (1) Synechia (adhesions)
        - (2) Stricture
      - b. Hematoma
      - c. Abscess
    - 3. Cartilage
      - a. Septal
        - (1) Absent
        - (2) Thickened
        - (3) Deflected
        - (4) Twisted
      - b. Upper Lateral
        - (1) Absent
          - (a) Complete
          - (b) Incomplete
        - (2) Thickened
        - (3) Deflected
        - (4) Twisted
        - (5) Fixed collapse (secondary to nasal pyramid trauma)
        - (6) Physiologic collapse
  - B. Pathophysiologic
    - 1. Turbulence
- II. Extramural
  - A. External pressure
  - B. Intranasal space-occupying lesions
    - 1. Foreign body
    - 2. Growths

Table 3. Clinical Classification of Nasal Valve Obstruction

- A. Soft-covering mucocutaneous tissues
- B. Skeletal supporting tissues
  - 1. Septum
  - 2. Upper lateral cartilage

the most common causes of nasal valve abnormalities are due to skeletal disturbances produced by trauma and subsequent posttraumatic changes. The septum is probably responsible for most of the abnormalities of the nasal valve, followed in frequency by the upper lateral cartilage and posttraumatic scarring (Figs. 8 and 9).

The clinical problem is to differentiate the normal from the abnormal and to properly locate the existing abnormality, when present. Since the cornerstones of diagnosis are the history and physical examination, a history of previous trauma or surgical intervention with symptoms of rhinologic disturbance is important. Other data from the general history (not related to the nose) also must be considered in the routine otorhinolaryngologic examination. The physical examination must include direct inspection and palpation of external nasal structures, including the nasal spine and septum. Palpation with fingers and a cotton carrier intranasally also may help determine whether the cartilaginous septum is absent, thickened, deflected, or scarred. The upper lateral cartilage also must be examined and evaluated. Once a skeletal abnormality of the nasal valve has been found, surgical intervention probably should be carried out, especially when the patient complains of nasal airway obstruction.

Surgical Approaches to Abnormalities of the Nasal Valve

The principles of surgical correction, enunciated by Hinderer,[5] consist of "undoing or reversing the process of the formation of the deformity. Extensive undermining with freeing the deformed structures, excision of scar tissue and shortening of the isolated caudal end of the upper lateral cartilage is necessary. The preservation of the muscles and the mucosa with excision of excess cartilage with reconstruction of the os internum results in preservation of the valve-like action."

The primary goals of nasal valve surgery essentially are to (1) reconstitute normal anatomy of the nasal valve and (2) improve the airflow without increasing either rigidity or collapsibility of the nasal valve. Injury to muscle, production of scar, narrowing, and collapsibility can be avoided if minimal upper lateral or septal cartilage is resected. If mucocutaneous tissues must be cut in order to approach the abnormality, they must be carefully and gently reapproximated and repaired. It is important to realize that the lower lateral (alar) cartilages constitute an accessory part of the nasal valve because of their intimate association with the upper lateral cartilage; care should be exercised when resecting cephalic margins of lower lateral

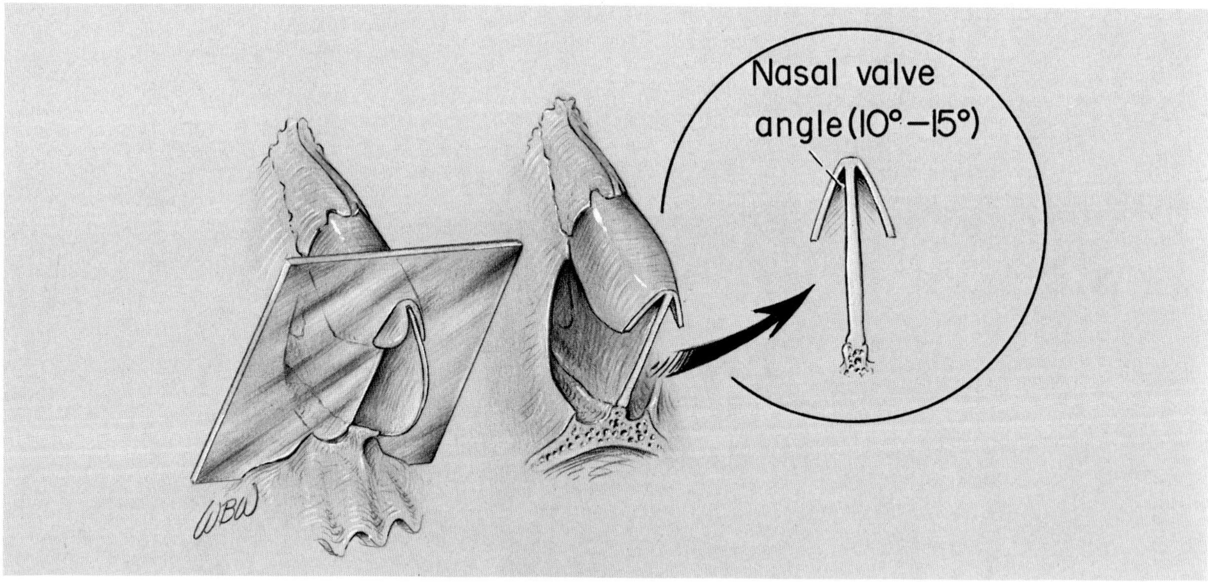

Fig. 8. Schematic representation of nasal valve. Note plane at which caudal end of septum and caudal end of upper lateral cartilage are sectioned so that nasal valve can be adequately visualized. Inset shows nasal valve and angle.

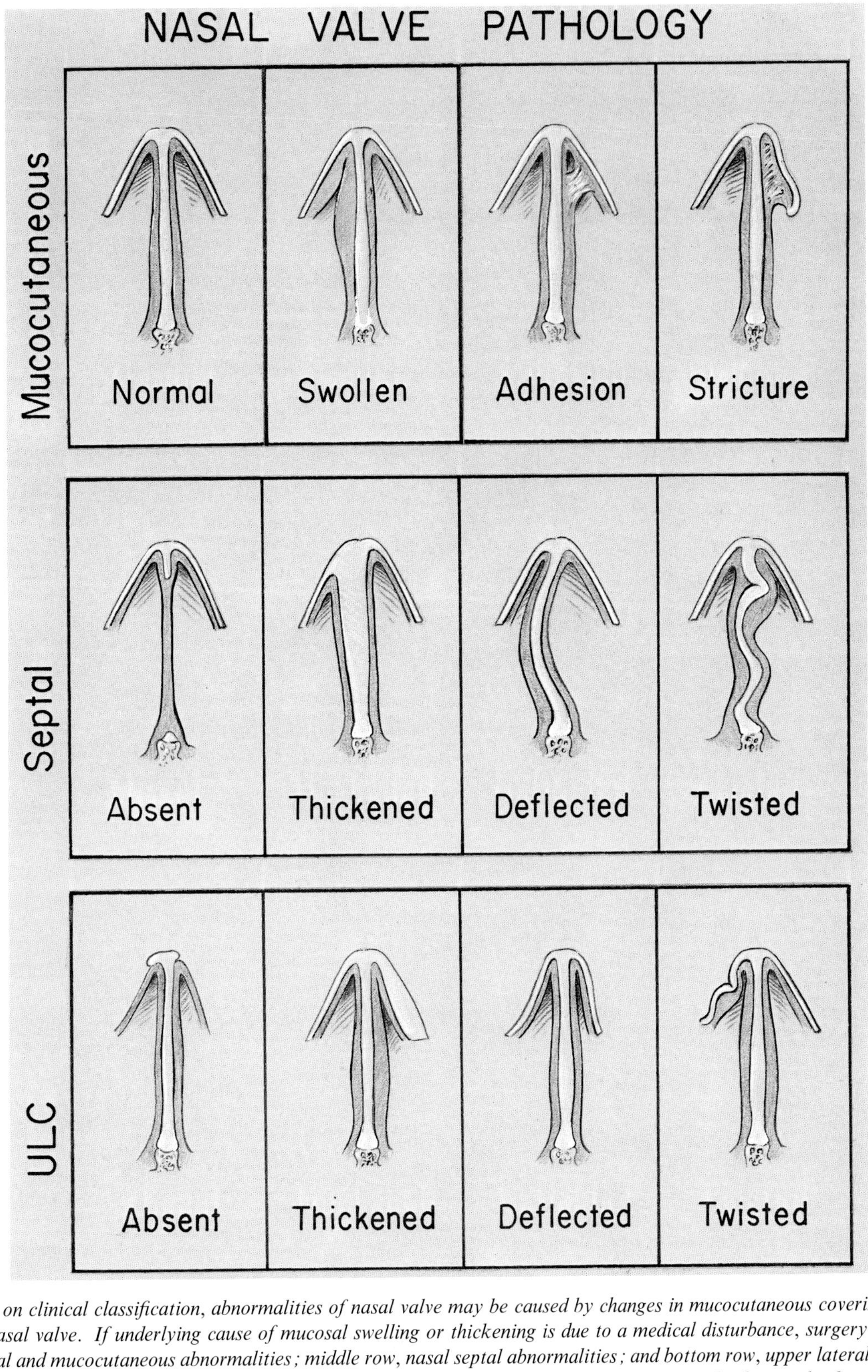

Fig. 9. *Based on clinical classification, abnormalities of nasal valve may be caused by changes in mucocutaneous coverings over skeletal structures of nasal valve. If underlying cause of mucosal swelling or thickening is due to a medical disturbance, surgery is not indicated. Top row, normal and mucocutaneous abnormalities; middle row, nasal septal abnormalities; and bottom row, upper lateral cartilage abnormalities. Such abnormalities can cause fixed or intermittent nasal valve obstruction. Scarring in nasal valve results from surgical or nonsurgical trauma that may produce minimal adhesions or severe stricture of structures of the nasal valve. Some nasal septum abnormalities include absent septal cartilage, thickening of nasal septum, deflection, and twisting. Some upper lateral cartilage abnormalities include absent upper lateral cartilage (unilateral or bilateral, complete or incomplete), thickening, deflected with fixed collapse, fixed collapse (which could have been secondary to trauma and infracture of nasal bone, carrying upper lateral cartilage inward toward the septum), and narrowing the valve angle. Mobile physiologic collapse can occur during deep inspiration (not shown). Twisted upper lateral cartilage cartilage may in itself be the cause of a narrowed valve angle.*

(alar cartilage during tip-modeling procedures in order to avert increased collapsibility of the nasal valve. However, problems of functional nasal valve surgery will exclude the problems of lower lateral (alar) cartilage surgery.

Small deformities in this region can produce significant symptoms. Nasal valve surgery should be exacting, and during the operation, magnification is helpful for precision. Two-power optical loops are extremely useful for the meticulous handling required of the tissues in this region.

A systematic approach to surgery requires that the surgeon be aware of the possible sites and types of abnormalities that may be present (mucocutaneous, septal, upper lateral cartilage, or combinations) and he should have the technical ability to explore the various regions (septum and upper lateral cartilage) and to treat any mucocutaneous disturbance that may be present. This systematic approach involves three types of surgery: (1) septal, (2) upper lateral cartilage, and (3) mucocutaneous (scar).

Septal Surgery

Septal abnormalities that contribute to nasal valve problems may be due to an absent, thickened, deflected, twisted, or a scarred septum or some combination of these. Surgery is carried out in as bloodless field as possible and is facilitated by local and topical (cocaine flakes) anesthesia with a relaxed well-premedicated patient. The anterior tunnels or flaps must be elevated on one side or on both sides so that the caudal end of the septum can be exposed and the abnormalities exposed and corrected. For example, thinning of a thickened

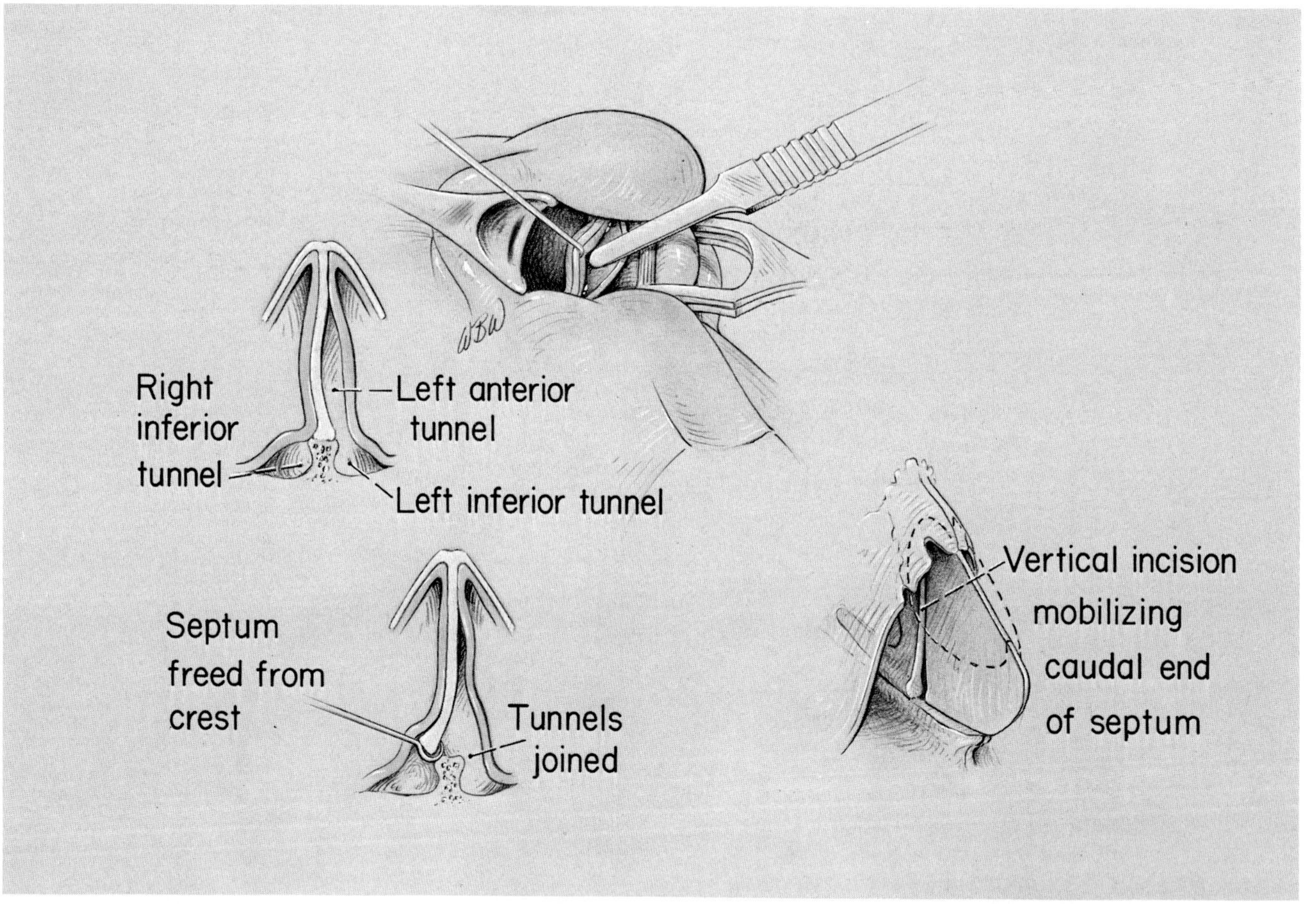

Fig. 10. (A) Right hemitransfixion incision and approach to nasal septum by creation of anterior and inferior tunnels, with joining of left anterior and left inferior tunnels (B and C) to free septum from crest of maxilla and premaxilla. (D) Mobilization of septum is effected by freeing the caudal end of septum from perpendicular plate of ethmoid by a vertical incision.

septal cartilage in this region may be all that is required, and the valve surgery therefore may be quickly terminated. If the septum is more than just thickened or if it presents other problems, the caudal end of the septum may need to be freed and mobilized from the maxillary spine and premaxillary wings, as has been described by Cottle and co-workers.[11] Mobilization can be achieved by making a vertical incision into the quadrangular cartilage anterior to the perpendicular plate of the ethmoid, freeing the caudal end of the septum from its crest, and resecting the dislocated or deflected portions of the septum (Fig. 10). If, by uncovering the septum and freeing it from its posterior and inferior attachments, the deflection is reduced and swings to the midline, relieving the nasal valve obstruction, the surgery can be terminated; however, if a twisted piece of cartilage remains obstructing the nasal valve, then this twisted section can be selectively removed, perhaps by an almond-shaped excision of septal cartilage. If a large piece of cartilage needs to be removed, the septum should be reconstructed by crushing and replacing and fixing the cartilage between the septal flaps. Theoretically, this will avert the problem of flaccidity and early collapse of the nasal valve because of a septal abnormality. The dictum—attempt to reconstitute normal anatomy and avoid increased rigidity and collapsibility—is assiduously followed. At times the only way to correct a severe abnormality requires that the caudal end of the septum be completely removed and replaced. Johnson has illustrated the details of this procedure in a previous communication.[12] In the surgery of the nasal valve region, septal surgery should be considered first, because septal abnormalities probably represent the most frequent cause of nasal valve obstruction. If surgery on the septum does not solve the nasal valve obstruction, the upper lateral cartilage should be explored next.

Upper Lateral Cartilage Surgery

Hemostasis and precision exposure are the keys to surgery of the upper lateral cartilage. Because of the need for accurate surgery in this region, the details of technique will be described. Gray[13] deserves credit for first announcing this detailed technique. The intracartilaginous incision affords the most direct approach to the upper lateral cartilage, and is made, preferably with a no. 15 blade, along the caudal end of the upper lateral cartilage from lateral to medial with the aid of a four-prong retractor and the middle finger of the left hand (if the operator is right-handed). The skin is first incised. The incision is then carried down to a depth of several millimeters into the intercartilaginous aponeurosis between the upper and lower lateral (alar) cartilages (Fig. 11A). If a hemitransfixion or full-transfixion incision had been made for the septal surgery, care is taken not to join the intercartilaginous incision with these incisions; however, should these incisions be inadvertently or deliberately joined (for tip rotation), then accurate suture approximation is required to avoid excessive scarring of the nasal valve. A weighted, single Joseph skin hook, 16 cm,* is placed into the upper lateral cartilage and retracted downward by the operator's left hand while the assistant holds either a four-prong retractor or another upper-lateral-cartilage exposing retractor in his right hand and uses Q-tips or suction in his left hand to remove blood from the field. A no. 66 Beaver knife blade is used on a Beaver chuck handle (3HL) of stainless steel and 6-in. length to reach the perichondrium of the upper lateral cartilage; this not only exposes the upper lateral cartilage but also keeps the overlying canopy of neuromuscular and vascular structures from being injured (Fig. 11B and C). By this technique, the upper lateral cartilage up to and over the nasal bones can be widely undermined in a relatively avascular plane. The upper lateral cartilage may be explored and exposed bilaterally, with minimal injury to any of these overlying structures. The undersurface of the upper lateral cartilage may be exposed, preserving the mucosa, by careful use of the no. 66 Beaver knife blade or a sharp scissors† (Fig. 11D). The caudal border of the upper lateral cartilage or the mucosa itself can be grasped with either a fine mouse-tooth forceps‡ or a 7-in. curved Gerald dressing forceps.**

* Sparta Instrument Co., 305 Fairfield Ave., Fairfield, NJ, 07006

† E. Stumer Co. KG 8702 Lengfeld, Wurzburg, W. Germany. Sharp scissors, Chefarztscheren, 15 cm, angled.

‡ E. Stumer Co. KG 8702 Lengfeld, Wurzburg, W. Germany. Mouse-tooth forceps, Mauseteeth Tweezers, 15 cm, fine.

** Gambole and Merrill, 281 E Street, Boston, MA, 02127. A Gerald tissue forceps, 7-in. curved with teeth 1 by 2, is also available.

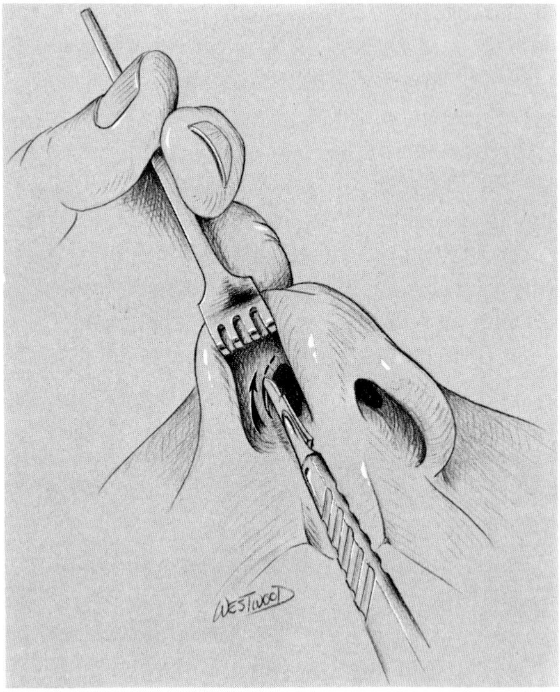

Fig. 11. *(A) Intercartilaginous incision with no. 15 blade carried down just beneath skin.*

Grasping either the skin or cartilage with a forceps facilitates dissection. Thus, the upper lateral cartilage is freed from the mucocutaneous coverings and as much of the upper lateral cartilage as desired may be separated from the septum submucosally by sharp dissection, without injuring the mucosa. The cartilage may be evaluated after it has been precisely exposed, and abnormalities are trimmed in an attempt to reconstitute a "normal" nasal valve with a normal nasal valve angle. Surgery on the upper lateral cartilage is best carried out early in the operation, when the field is dry and the surgeon is not fatigued, probably after the septal surgery and before surgery on the tip and pyramid. The intercartilaginous incision is the most frequently used incision to approach the dorsum of the nose yet, as pointed out by Anderson,[14] the cartilage-splitting incision (cutting through the lower lateral or alar cartilage) can be used as the approach to modify both the dorsum of the nose and the lower lateral (alar) cartilages, without violating the skin or mucosa of the nasal valve.

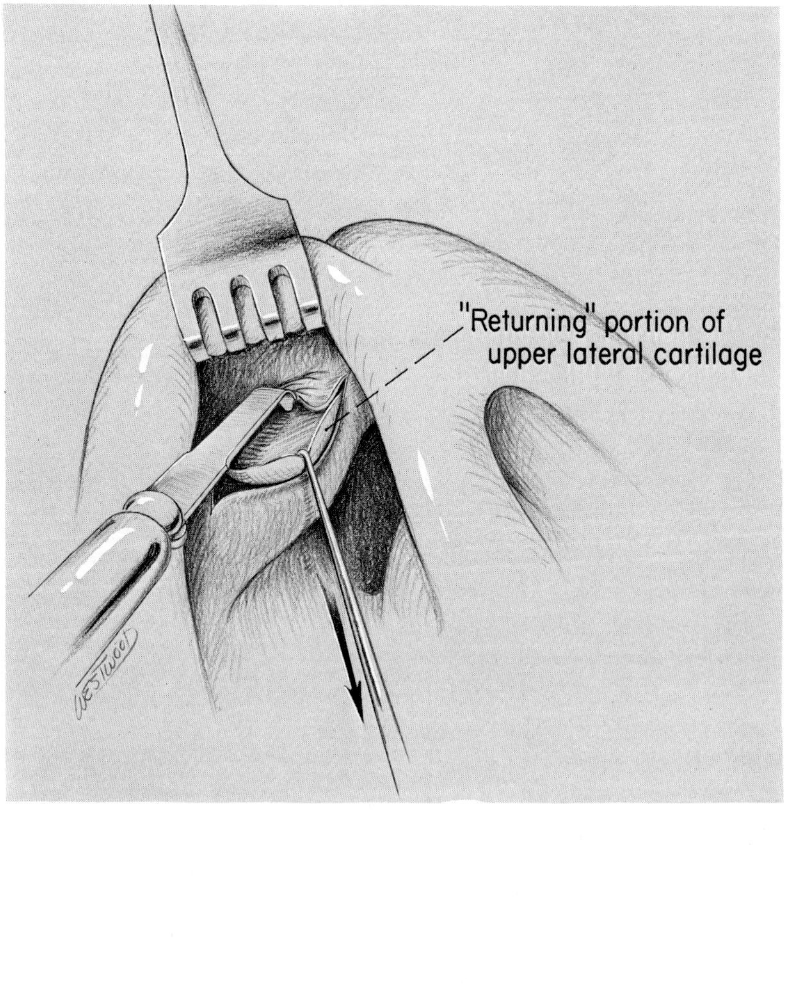

Fig. 11. *(B) Weighted hook is applied to cartilage for counter-traction, and dissection with a no. 66 Beaver knife blade is down to perichondrium.*

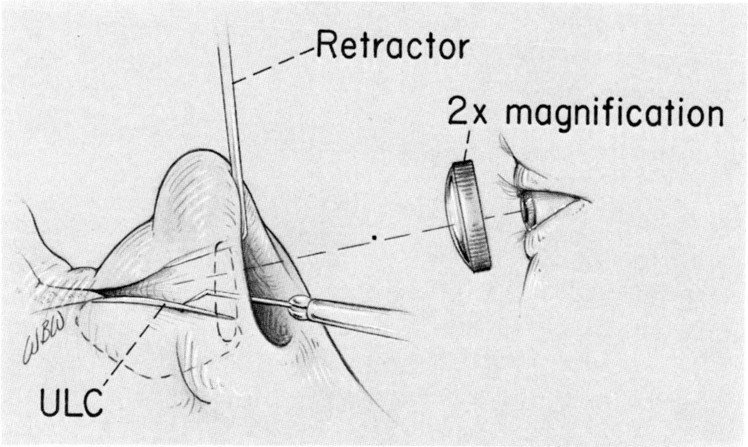

Fig. 11. (C) Lateral view of the surgical field that can be obtained, and angle of no. 66 Beaver knife blade that allows adequate visualization, along with upper lateral cartilage (ULC) retractor used to retract the alar margin of the nostril so roof cartilage can be adequately and widely exposed when necessary.

Thickening or twisting in this region can be adequately managed by resection. Gray [13] believes that some returning (also termed "curling," or "scrolling") of the upper lateral cartilage may be a normal finding. Yet other workers, including Cottle (cited by Hinderer[9]) believe that returning is usually a pathologic finding. "Physiologic" returning of the upper lateral cartilage affords some stiffness to resist collapse, whereas "pathologic" and "excessive" returning may interfere with the flexible valve action of the upper lateral cartilage. In attempting to achieve a normal nasal valve angle and avoiding either increased rigidity or increased collapsibility, the surgeon can use his resourcefulness in reconstituting a normal nasal valve. Resection of the upper lateral cartilage should be conservative so as to avoid mobile inspiratory collapse (Fig. 11E, F). The amount of caudal end of upper lateral cartilage that should be removed is determined, as Hinderer has pointed out, so as to maintain the relationship of the upper lateral cartilage to the caudal end of the septum. Thus, if the septum is being shortened 2 to 4 mm, then resecting 2 to 4 mm from the caudal end of the upper lateral cartilage should be considered. The amount of medial portion of upper lateral cartilage that should be removed is determined by resecting the amount needed to reconstruct a normal nasal valve angle of 10° to 15°. Usually, the removal of a medial triangular section of upper lateral cartilage (base of triangle is caudal and apex is cephalic) can open the nasal valve angle when the upper lateral cartilage is thickened, deflected, or twisted.

After surgery on the upper lateral cartilage, there are times when widening of the nasal valve angle cannot be satisfactorily accomplished by resection of a triangular portion of the upper lateral cartilage because of a congenitally narrowed nose or because of a previous rhinoplasty in which the upper lateral cartilage was carried close to the septum after "hump" removal and infracture. In these cases in which the upper lateral cartilage is collapsed against the septum, the upper lateral cartilage may have to be completely separated from the septum, and medial, lateral, and transverse

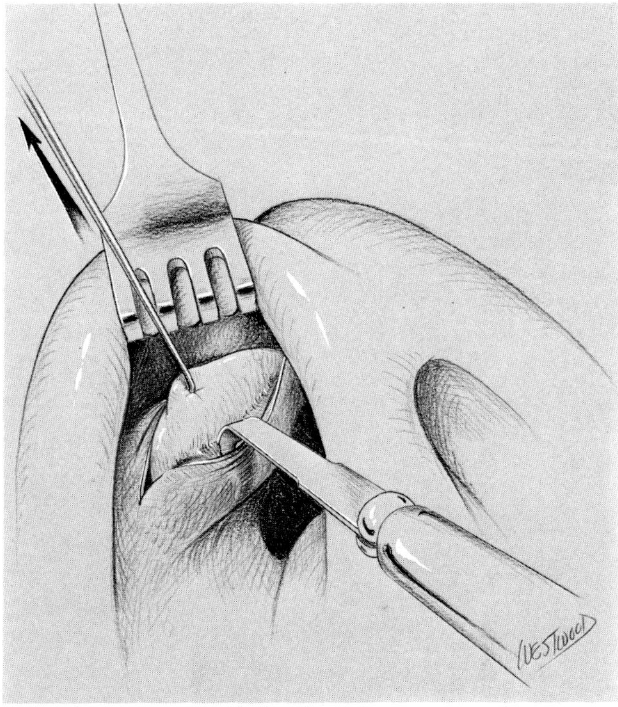

Fig. 11. (D) Undersurface of upper lateral cartilage may be exposed, preserving the skin.

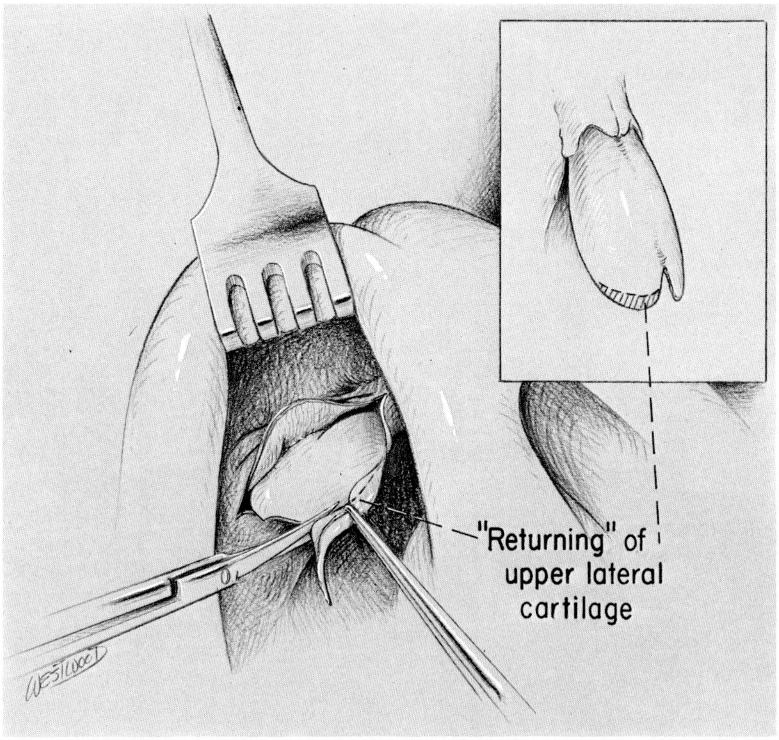

Fig. 11. (E) Resection of caudal end of upper lateral cartilage may be carried out directly, and mucocutaneous tissue can be preserved.

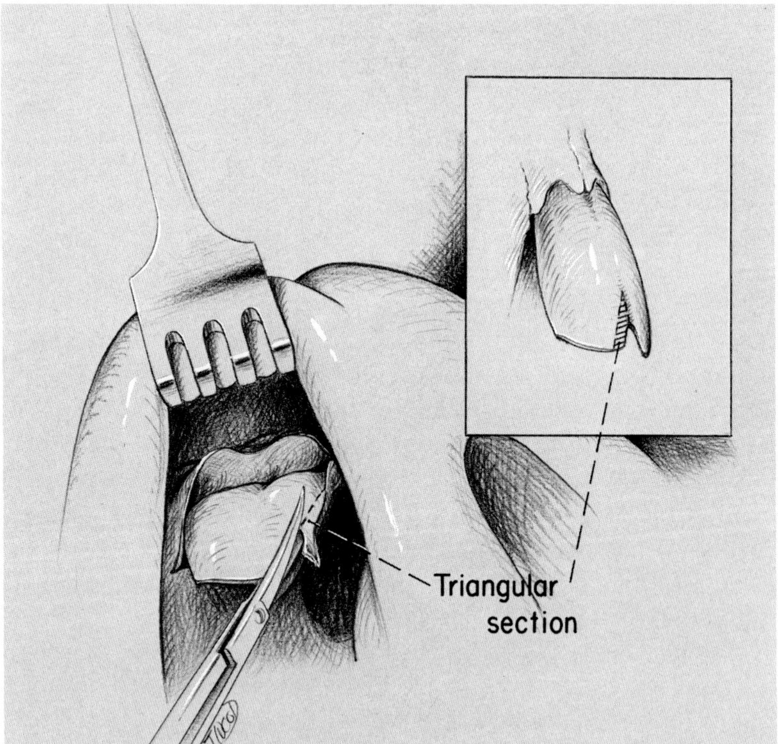

Fig. 11. (F) Medial triangle of upper lateral cartilage can be removed submucosally from its attachment to the septum.

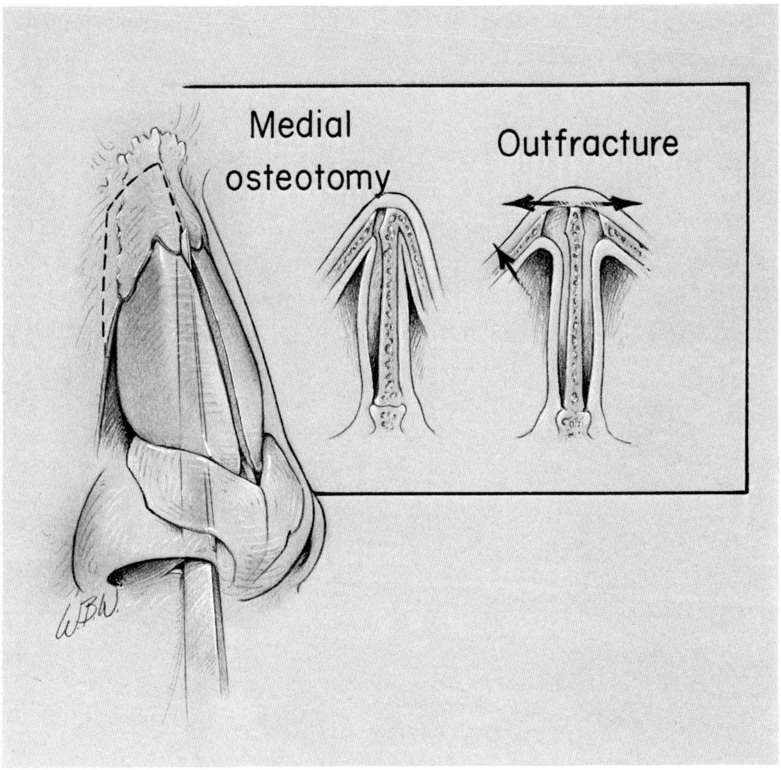

Fig. 11. (G) Upper lateral cartilage can be completely separated from nasal septum submucosally, and lateral, transverse, and medial osteotomies with out-fracture on one or both sides as indicated can be performed to carry the upper lateral cartilage away from septum to open the nasal valve angle.

osteotomies may be required with outfracture, carrying the upper lateral cartilage away from the septum to open the nasal valve angle (Fig. 11G). Undermining the tissue laterally over the frontal process of the maxilla sometimes may produce postoperative scar that can pull the upper lateral cartilage laterally opening the nasal valve angle.

In other words, after septal exploration and upper lateral cartilage exploration, with exposure and resection, if the nasal valve angle is still narrowed, a medial osteotomy with outfracture of the nasal pyramid may be required on one or both sides so that the upper lateral cartilage may be carried laterally. If a "hump" had been previously removed, roof repair will be required, preferably with autogenous cartilage or bone after outfracture.

Special situations or problems may arise that test the surgeon's ingenuity; for example, during nasal septal reconstruction with modification of the external nasal pyramid or during rhinoplasty, modification of the upper lateral cartilage may be required before or after the osteotomies and infracture in order to prevent permanent narrowing of the nasal valve and the nasal valve angle. Thus, a medial triangle of upper lateral cartilage can be removed "prophylactically" in order to maintain a normal nasal valve and prevent a fixed collapse of the nasal valve angle. In the situation of mobile collapse of the nasal valve due either to a nonresilient upper lateral cartilage or previous trauma (surgical or nonsurgical) with partial or complete absence of the upper lateral cartilage either a conchal or septal autograft or even rotation of the lower lateral (alar) cartilage over the remnant of the upper lateral cartilage may be attempted to prevent or lessen the increased collapsibility of the nasal valve.

When the upper lateral cartilage is narrowed for cosmetic reasons, it is important to preserve mucosa and maintain a normal nasal valve, as Bridger[2] has pointed out, "In seven of the people in the symptom group, the symptoms commenced or were aggravated after a rhinoplastic procedure, showing that consideration of the function of the nasal valve is important in nasal surgery."

During treatment of the severely twisted or smashed nose, if "ballooning" or flaring of the upper lateral cartilage is present, the upper lateral cartilage may be separated from the septum submucosally and a section of upper lateral cartilage removed to reconstruct and, in this case, narrow the nasal valve angle to approximate normal.

The intercartilaginous incision should be closed, and the sutures should be placed in the nose after all the steps of the entire operation have been completed. The skin is sutured with 4-0 chromic catgut (Ethicon 744), the sutures being advanced from the mucosa of the upper lateral cartilage and into the skin of the cephalic margin of the lower lateral cartilages.

Scar Surgery

Scar tissue may be present in the region of the nasal valve. There are several techniques that can be used to correct this abnormality. The scar (adhesions) may be lysed if it is thin, and Silastic stents may be introduced into the nasal chamber and sewn in place to prevent recurrence of adhesions. A lining graft such as a buccal mucosa graft may be used if the scar is thick or a stricture is present, and this requires removal of a large amount of tissue. Excision of the scar tissue with placement of mucosa graft can be beneficial in reconstituting a normal" valve. The graft may be sewn with chromic suture or preferably 4-0 plain catgut (Ethicon 1824G) on a straight needle. A Castroviejo (OP7399 V. Mueller), diamond-jaw needle holder can be used. A piece of Silastic sheeting (a medical-grade, silicone rubber subdermal implant material 500-5 nonreinforced from Dow-Corning) may be folded into position and sewn in place with 3-0 black silk, and plastic stents may be positioned to hold the Silastic sheeting against the graft material (Fig. 12). Usually, these are left in place for

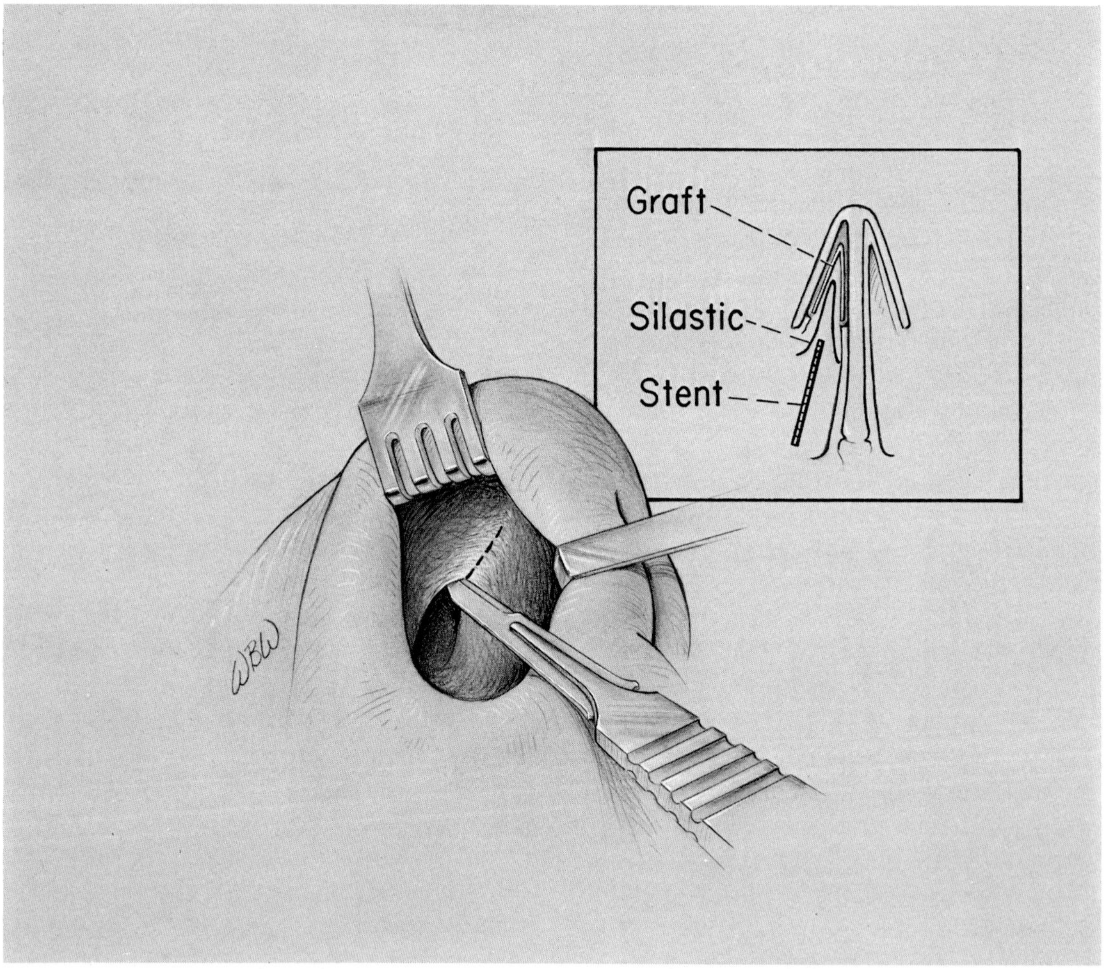

Fig. 12. Scar tissue can be removed and Silastic sheeting folded and sewn, along with plastic stent, to hold a graft in position reconstructing a new nasal valve and preventing further scarring.

3 to 6 weeks. In general, since tissue injury produces scar, the tissues should be handled gently and re-approximated accurately, preserving mucosa, muscles, vessels, nerves, cartilage, and bone whenever possible in order to minimize scar tissue formation.

Results of Surgery

A classification of nasal valve abnormalities, evolved over seven years, facilitates a rational and systematic surgical approach to the nasal septum, upper lateral cartilage, and their mucocutaneous coverings. These surgical techniques and principles can be performed safely and allow adequate and precise exposure, especially in more difficult and complicated cases. The statistical results of these surgical procedures are incomplete at present. To date clinical experience suggests that application of these ideas benefits patients by either preventing or treating abnormalities of the nasal valve. A careful analysis of rhinomanometric data from 1500 patients seen at the Mayo Clinic is currently underway. Nonetheless, continued critical clinical reevaluation, coupled with substantial physiologic data (rhinomanometry), should allow adoption, rejection, or more likely modification of the principles offered by this work.

References

1. Mink PJ: Le nez comme voie respiratorie, Presse Otolaryngol. (Belg), 1903, pp 481–496
2. Bridger GP: Physiology of the nasal valve. Arch Otolaryng 92:543–553, 1970
3. Masing H: Experimentelle Untersuchungen uber die Stromung im Nasenmodell. Arch Klin Exp Ohren Nasen Kehlkopfheilkd 189:59–70, 1967
4. Williams HL: A reconsideration of the relation of the mechanics of nasal air-flow to the function of the nose in respiration. Rhinology 10:145–161, 1972
5. Hinderer KH: Surgery of the valve. Int Rhinol 8:60–67, 1970
6. Dishoeck HAE van: Inspiratory nasal resistance, Acta Otolaryngol 30:431–439, 1942
7. Dishoeck HAE van: The part of the valve and the turbinates in total nasal resistance. Int Rhinol 3:19–26, 1965
8. De Wit G, Kapteyn TS, Bochove W van: Some remarks on the physiology, the anatomy and the radiology of the vestibulum and the isthmus nasi. Int Rhinol 3:37–42, 1965
9. Hinderer KH: Fundamentals of anatomy and surgery of the nose. Birmingham, Alabama, Aesculapius Publishing Company, 1971
10. Heinberg CE, Kern EB: The Cottle sign: an aid in the physical diagnosis of nasal airflow disturbance. Int Rhinol 11:89–94, 1973
11. Cottle MH, Loring RM, Fischer GG, Gaynon IE: The "maxilla-premaxilla" approach to extensive nasal septum surgery. Arch Otolaryngol 68:301–313, 1958
12. Johnson NE: Secondary surgery of the septum. Otolaryngol Clin N Am 7:75–86, 1974
13. Gray VD: Physiologic returning of the upper lateral cartilage. Int Rhinol 8:56–59, 1970
14. Anderson JR: A new approach to rhinoplasty. Trans Am Acad Ophthalmol Otolaryngol 70:183–192, 1966

Microscopic Intranasal Dacrocystorhinostomy (MIDCR)

Ronald Strahan, Los Angeles, Calif.

Introduction

Although the external approach to perform dacrocystorhinostomy for the surgical treatment of obstruction of the tear collecting system at the level of the inferior lacrimal sac or the nasolacrimal duct is successful in more than 90 percent of cases, it has certain disadvantages. These disadvantages encouraged this author to make refinements so that dacrocystorhinostomy can be successfully performed through an intranasal approach. These refinements include the use of a fiberoptic light source for localization of the osteotomy and the use of the operating microscope for absolute control of the surgical field. Since the modern head and neck surgeon has experience with both modalities it is suggested that in certain cases of lacrimal system obstruction the microscopic intranasal route for dacrocystorhinostomy be considered.

Technique

Step 1

Either general or local anesthesia is satisfactory. This author perfers the use of local anesthesia. After the interior of the nose has been cocainized for 10 min with 4 percent cocaine, the columella, nasal septum and lateral wall of the nose are injected with 1 percent Xylocaine with epinephrine 1/100,000 parts. Externally the area adjacent to the anterior lacrimal crest is injected with the same solution. A topical ophthalmic anesthetic solution is dropped into the eye.

A self-retaining medium sized nasal speculum is inserted into the nose and used to expose the lateral wall of the nose to visualize the anterior half of the middle turbinate and that area anterior to the middle turbinate. The straight-look-through operating microscope set at 6× magnification is used to complete the procedure.

Step 2

A nasal mucosal flap based posteriorly is then planned. The following maneuver is executed for localization of the flap.

The anterior lacrimal crest is palpated. A fiber optic light cord is then held against the lacrimal fossa with the light on. The operator is looking into the nose with exposure via the self-retaining nasal speculum. With this maneuver it is quite easy to determine the site of the osteotomy to be performed. Using this as a guide a horizontal nasal mucosal flap based posteriorly is incised with the No.12 Bard Parker knife. A Freer elevator is used to turn the flap posteriorly and it can usually be tucked back under the middle turbinate so that it stays out of the operative field. This exposes the bone where the osteotomy will be performed. The flap usually measures 15 mm in width and 25–30 mm in length.

Step 3

An air powered burr with an angled hand piece is then used to remove the bone from the lateral wall of the nose. Removal of the bone with suction irrigation as frequently used in otologic surgery is employed. The surgeon can reinsure his placing the osteotomy in the correct position by frequently checking the position with the fiber optic light source placed externally. The osteotomy at least 15 mm in width is created and as most surgeons point out the "larger the osteotomy the better."

Step 4

A small lacrimal probe is then inserted in the inferior canaliculus into the lacrimal sac. With light pressure on this lacrimal probe the medial wall of the lacrimal sac is delivered into the osteotomy site. Again, under 6× magnification these maneuvers are very well controlled and executed. A standard otologic sickle knife and single-prong small skin hook is used to fashion a lacrimal flap based anteriorly. The pathology of the lacrimal sac can be inspected via the intranasal exposure with the operating microscope. At this stage it is apparent that the lacrimal sac flap is approximately 1/3 the size of the nasal mucosal flap. Therefore, the nasal mucosal flap is trimmed accordingly. The posteriorly based nasal mucusal flap is then turned into the lacrimal sac and the anteriorly based lacrimal sac flap is turned into the nose and these flaps are packed in position with vasaline gauze saturated with an antibiotic solution.

In the initial 4 cases reported here a small piece of silastic tubing was placed through the superior canaliculus, lacrimal sac, and out the nose and left for 14 days. However, in the other cases this was not employed and did not seem to be essential.

Enough packing is placed in the operative side of the nose so that the area of the dacrocystorhinostomy remains firmly packed for retention of flap position. This packing is removed on the 5th postoperative day.

Postoperative care is minimal. In the initial 3 cases irrigation was performed frequently via the inferior or superior canaliculus, however, this too was abandoned and did not affect long term results.

Table 1. Etiology of Obstruction

No. of cases	Traumatic (Naso-maxillary fractures)	Inflammatory (Recurrent dacrocystitis)	Undetermined
14	6	6	2

Table 2. Microscopic Intranasal Dacrocystorhinostomy

	Postoperative Observation			
No. of cases	More than 24 mos.	18–24 mos.	Less than 18 mos.	Failures
14	7	3	4	1

Material

Fourteen cases of obstruction of the lacrimal system at the inferior aspect of the lacrimal sac and/or the naso-lacrimal duct have been treated with the intranasal approach for microscopic dacrocystorhinostomy. All cases had dacrocystography for localization of site of obstruction. Dacrocystography was performed bilaterally on all patients. The eye was anesthetized with a topical ophthalmic solution. The inferior canaliculus was dilated and a lacrimal canula inserted and the system irrigated with sterile saline. The superior canaliculus was then obstructed with a probe and the radiopaque material (Pantopaque) was injected. Both anterior-posterior and lateral views were obtained.

Table 1 summarizes the etiology of lacrimal system obstruction in this series. In the early stages of performing dacrocystorhinostomy with this technique only trauma cases were considered for surgery. However, after the procedure was perfected obstruction from recurrent dacrocystitis was also satisfactorily relieved with the microscopic intranasal dacrocystorhinostomy. There were 2 cases in which the past history for either traumatic or inflammatory disease was negative.

Of the 14 cases operated with this technique satisfactory results, i.e., relief of obstruction was obtained in 13. One case was considered a failure because the case was lost for postoperative follow-up. Incidently, this case was operated with an angled operating microscope head which is unsatisfactory for this procedure.

The length of postoperative follow-up is depicted in Table 2.

Discussion

Dacrocystorhinostomy performed by the external approach is successful in more than 90 percent of cases. There are, however, certain cases in which incisions on the face should be avoided if at all possible. This author developed the technique presented here of microscopic intranasal dacrocystorhinostomy as a result of a specific challenge presented by his first case. This was a 32-year-old Negro female who had a past history of keloid formation as evidenced by keloids on the lobules of the ear. Following a nasal maxillary fracture she demonstrated on dacrocystography obstruction of the distal 1/3 of the naso-lacrimal duct. After studying the approach described here on several cadaver specimens, this lady was operated with the operating microscope via the intranasal approach. After the success in this initial case, other patients with epiphora from obstruction from the nasao-lacrimal duct were offered both the external and intranasal approach for this type of surgery. Understandably most patients have chosen the intranasal approach.

It goes without saying that if a surgeon is to use this approach he must be competent in intranasal surgical operations. Nasal septal procedures are occassionally necessary to provide adequate exposure. Additionally, in certain patients it is necessary to resect part of the anterior half of the middle turbinate. In all cases of dacrocystorhinostomy the surgeon must be prepared to deal with the anterior ethmoid sinuses.

The microscopic intranasal dacrocystorhinostomy is satisfactory for the surgical treatment of obstruction of the lacrimal system in the inferior aspect of the lacrimal sac or nasal lacrimal duct. The operating microscope and fiber optic light cord add absolute control of surgical field. Fourteen cases of naso-lacrimal duct obstruction have been successfully treated with this technique. If the surgeon is competent in microscopic surgery, he might consider offering the intranasal approach as an alternative to the external approach for certain cases.

Face and Neck

Silicone Implants in Head and Neck Reconstructive Surgery

Robert W. Cantrell and Bruce K. Defiebre, San Diego, Calif.

Introduction

Surgeons have long sought an ideal material for implantation to correct deformities of the head and neck. It is unknown when a foreign material was first used to correct a defect in man. Longacre[1] shows a prehistoric Peruvian skull with a frontal defect repaired with a hammered gold plate. Evidence of healing under the plate indicates some degree of success. Other metals such as silver, platinum, stainless-steel, and chrome–cobalt alloys have been used to repair defects in the head and neck as well as organic materials such as ivory and animal bone.

Human bone or cartilage, either autogenous or homologous, was not used until relatively recently for the same reason some surgeons dislike using it today: a second operation is required in order to obtain the graft. Macewen,[2] in 1878, removed the humeral shaft of a three-year-old boy who had osteomyelitis, and restored the defect with wedges of tibia removed from donor patients. He reported this case in 1881, and it is probably the first recorded case of homologous bone grafting. Macewen does not dwell on the subject of where the donor patients were found, but presumably it was as difficult then to find people willing to contribute a wedge of their tibia as it is today.

A patient with an unsightly defect of the face is generally willing to suffer loss of tissue from elsewhere in the body in order to minimize a visible defect. Donor sites usually chosen are iliac crest bone or costal cartilage.

Many surgeons, however, who have performed such transplants have frequently noted that patients complain more about pain from the donor site than from the primary operative area. A suitable, synthetic material would solve the problem of the necessity for a second operation.

In 1953, Scales[3] listed necessary qualities of synthetic materials to be used as implants. He states the implant must:

1. Not be physically modified by tissue fluids.
2. Be chemically inert.
3. Not excite an inflammatory or foreign-body cell response in the tissues.
4. Be noncarcinogenic.
5. Not produce a state of allergy or hypersensitivity.
6. Be capable of standing up to mechanical strains imposed upon it, as for example, friction when placed in a joint.
7. Be capable of being fabricated in the form required with reasonable ease at a relatively low cost.
8. Be capable of being sterilized.

Rees[4] added to this list:

9. Unchangeable with time, heat, or pressure.
10. Nonsupportive of bacterial growth.
11. Inexpensive.

Plastics

The word plastic means capable of being molded but when applied to a material it refers to any of numerous organic synthetic or processed materials that are mostly thermoplastic or thermosetting polymers of high molecular weight which can be molded, cast, extruded, drawn, or laminated into objects, films or filaments.

Vinyl chloride was polymerized in 1838, styrene in 1839, and methyl acrylate in 1880.[5] Since then hundreds of different plastics have been synthesized, and with the addition of various chemicals, the structure and reactivity of a given plastic can be altered.

Many plastics have found medical application; however, considerable care must be exercised in selecting the proper material. Pure polyethylene may be implanted in man, but polythene (a DuPont product) which contains diacetyl phosphate causes fibrosis. Bakelite, cellulose, polyethylene, polyvinyl chloride, polytetrafluorethylene, polystyrene, nylon, acrylics, and polyester resins have been investigated.[6] Some of these were unsuitable for several reasons; the most serious of which was carcinogenesis. Others, such as polytetrafluorethylene (DuPont's Teflon) or polyester resins (DuPont's Dacron) have been widely used in medicine. A mixture of Teflon granules dispersed in glycerine is used as a paste for injecting vocal cords to improve the voice,[7] and solid Teflon has been used as a bone substitute.[8,9] Dacron and Teflon textiles have been used since the late Forties to replace large blood vessels.[10]

Silicones

The class of plastics known as silicones has found wide medical application.

J. F. Hyde of the Corning Glass Works developed the first flexible silicone resin to seal the voids in fibrous glass cloth during the 1930s, and later, R. R. McGregor at the Mellon Institute developed a series of water white silicone fluids which had properties unlike those of any other liquids.[11] These liquids, known as DC200 Fluids, ranged in viscosity from 0.65 to 1,000,000 centistokes (the viscosity of water being 1 centistoke) at room temperature. These versatile liquids have found multiple uses in industry. Because they are extremely inert and possess many of the properties of Scales's ideal alloplastic substance, they have received wide application in medicine. The Dow-Corning Corporation, one of several companies which manufactures dimethylpolysiloxane, calls their silicone rubber Silastic. They have established the Dow-Corning Center for Aid to Medical Research to test and find new uses for silicone, and to disseminate information to the medical community.[12]

Chemistry

Silicon is a tetravalent, nonmetallic element that occurs in combined form as the most abundant element next to oxygen in the earth's crust. The chemical symbol is Si, and when it combines with two oxygen molecules it forms silicon dioxide (SiO_2) which is also known as silica or quartz, if pure, and flint, if less pure. Beach sand is comprised mainly of small quartz particles, and when melted, it becomes glass.

Starting with silica, SiO_2, the oxygen is removed to form elemental silicon, Si. This inorganic element is one of the least reactive elements known. Through a series of complex chemical reactions, the basic siloxane grouping, SiO, is reacted with various organic materials (R) and formed into chains of organo-silicone compounds:

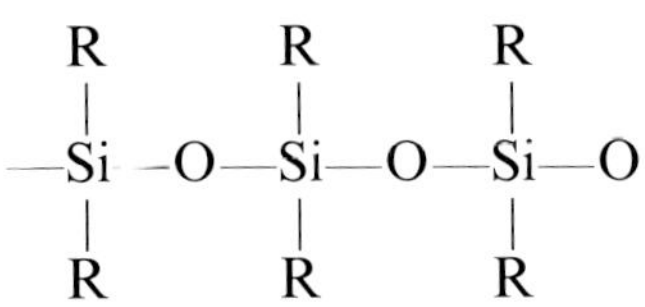

The general formula, R_2SiO, is silicone, so named because of its resemblance to ketone, R_2CO, where silicon is substituted for carbon. Because of the nonreactivity of the silicon, these substances are nearly inert, yet their combination with organic groups gives them elasticity, flexibility and ease of fabrication.

The R group can be almost any organic group, but the methyl group (CH_3) is the most commonly used and the silicones made with this are known as dimethyl polysiloxane,[13] organosilicone, or organopolysiloxane.

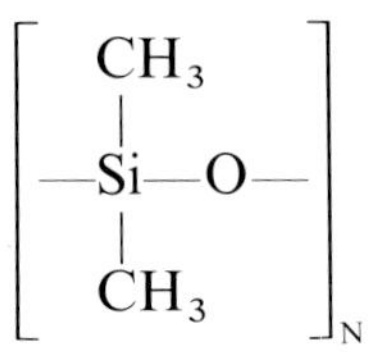

This formula is a clear fluid whose viscosity is determined by the value of N, and the number of cross linkings. If N is 2, the material has a viscosity of 0.65 centistokes, less than water. If N is 130 the viscosity is 350 centistokes, similar to the viscosity of No. 35 motor oil.[13]

It is from the high viscosity (10,000,000 centistokes) formula that medical grade silicone rubber is

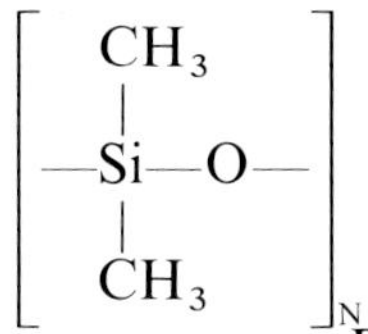

Heat Vulcanizing
High N Value
Silica
Organic Peroxide

Polymer
+
Filler
+
Vulcanizing Agent
Blowing Agent
(if Sponge)
↓
Silicone Rubber
(Cure)

Room Temperature Vulcanizing
Low N Value
+ or −
Stannous Octuate

Fig. 1. Chemistry of Silicone Rubber (From Spiers, A. C., and Blocksma, R.: New Implantable Silicone Rubbers. Plast Reconstr Surg 31:166, 1963. With permission).

made. As a filler to add strength, pure, fine (0.03 micra) silica is added, plus organic peroxides for vulcanizing agents. When this mixture is heated, the long chains are cross-linked, and the material becomes rubbery. Addition of a bubbling agent which will release nitrogen during fabrication results in the formation of sponge. Without the bubbling agent the rubber is solid. The final product is heat cured to drive off volatile products of vulcanization.[14]

If stannous octuate is used as a catalyst, the vulcanization occurs at room temperature (R.T.V.), and the rubbers are capable of being molded or cast as they cure.

Various fillers, antioxidants or hydrocarbon oils, may be added for various desirable industrial properties. These industrial grade silicones should not be used medically as the additives may be reactive and cause inflammation and granulomas. Silicone for medical use must be manufactured in pharmaceutically clean conditions to prevent contamination by extraneous materials. The filler and the catalyst must be pure and nonreactive with human tissue. Materials prepared in this fashion are labeled "medical grade" and these are the only ones which should be used for medical purposes.[13,15] When referring to silicones used medically, the specific type should be listed, e.g., Silastic 382.

Silicones are available as liquids, foams, sponges, resins, and rubbers. The liquids, originally known as Dow-Corning 360 Medical Fluid, are currently called Medical Grade Fluid MDX 44011[4] and are classed as an experimental drug by the Food and Drug Administration.

These compounds are remarkably heat stable, and they can withstand chilling to −80°F or heating to 540°F with little change in their physical characteristics. The fact that they are heat stable allows them to be autoclaved repeatedly if desired. They are unaffected by time; do not crack, crumble or deteriorate. They have been exposed to the sun for 13 years and autoclaved 111 times[15] with no evidence of deterioration.

Tissue will not adhere to silicone. This is useful for drains but can cause problems if an immobile implant is required. In the latter situation, a Teflon or Dacron textile can be glued to the prosthesis with silicone cement, and fibroplastic proliferation into the textile will hold the implant in place. An alternative is to make perforations into the implant which allows the ingrowth of fibroblastic tissue thus immobilizing it.

Carcinogenesis

In 1941, Turner[16] reported three fibrosarcomas in eight rats in which Bakelite was implanted subcutaneously. In 1952, Druckrey and Schmahl[17] reported malignant tumors induced in four of six animals in which cellulose film had been implanted for one year. Oppenheimer et al,[18,19] reported the carcinogenic properties of plastic embedded in rodents. These studies used cellulose, polyethylene, polyvinyl chloride film, Silastic, Teflon film, Dacron film, polystyrene film, and nylon film implanted subcutaneously in Wistar rats. Fourteen of 35 rats developed malignant tumors when Silastic was implanted.[19] Malignancy (usually sarcoma) developed from every type of plastic embedded.

In 1959, Russell and co-workers[20] reported five sarcomas occurring in 299 Wistar rats that survived 300 days after being implanted with polymers in their abdominal wall. One cancer each was associated with polyvinyl chloride film, Silastic 250 and Silastic 2000, and two cancers were associated with Teflon film.

Hueper,[21] in 1964, reported 10 malignancies (carcinomas and sarcomas) in 35 Bethesda black rats after the implantation of pieces of Silastic but no tumor associated with implants of benzoyl peroxide, the catalyst. The previous year, Ben-Hur and Newman[22] injected Silicone fluid into 36 white mice and noted "malignant epithelial tumors" developed in two mice. Grasso and co-workers[23] repeated the experiment using Schofield mice and found no evidence of tumor formation. They then reviewed the tumor tissue described by Ben-Hur and Newman, and considered them to be mammary adenocarcinomas, a common tumor in mice. Ben-Hur repeated the experiment and could find no evidence of tumor.[15]

In 1964, Sternberg and co-workers[24] reported two cases of tumors in apes injected with silicone mixtures and they (Winer et al[25]) further reported three patients who developed benign tumors after receiving large amounts of silicone injected into their breasts. They called these tumors "Siliconomas" but the tumors appeared typical of foreign body granulomas. When exposed to polarized light, the sections showed shiny, silvery crystals which are not present in pure silicone fluid. Apparently medical grade silicone was not used but rather a mixture to which had been added, "1 per cent animal and vegetable fatty acids of unknown types."[4]

Brown and co-workers[26] reported using four synthetics in 600 animals with no cancers occurring and only one fibroma adjacent to a polyvinyl alcohol implant.

In 1954, Dimant[27] reported implanting nine silicone rubber tubes for decompressing hydrocephalus. By 1967 an estimated 150,000 persons had been implanted with silicone rubber hydrocephalus shunt tubes. These tubes are in contact with brain, bone, skin, muscle, and blood, and no tumors associated with their use have been reported.[13]

Tissue Reaction

The initial tissue response to implanted silicone consists of capillary proliferation, infiltration of lymphocytes and occasional neutrophils, followed in 5–7 days by a predominance of fibroblasts.[14] Within eight days after implantation a well-established cellular pseudosheath has developed with evidence of fibroblastic polarity and a deposition of collagen. At one month the fibroblasts have polarized, the cellularity has decreased and the sheath has thinned. After two months the sheath becomes less cellular and the collagen content increases. Fine capillaries grow into the sheath and nerve fibers can be seen in the perisheath tissue. By three–four months, fat has migrated into the perisheath.[28] At three months the capsular thickness varies between 0.2 and 0.8 mm. The average thickness of multiple random samples in Imber's[29] study indicated capsular thickness of 0.2 to 0.4 mm.

If the silicone implant is removed the pocket initially fills with serum and a few erythrocytes. These persist for one–two days. The sheath completely collapses about the fourth day. Complete fusion is apparent by the third week followed by gradual resolution.[28]

Following large doses of injected liquid silicone in rodents, vacuoles can be seen in the retriculoendothelial system (lymph nodes, liver, spleen, kidney, and adrenals). These vacuoles are assumed to be silicone.[4]

There is some evidence that cellular elements of blood will phagocytize silicone fluid. Andrews[30] observed cyloplasmic vacuoles in neutrophils and monocytes in blood collected from a silicone injection site in a patient. These same vacuoles have been observed in peripheral leukocytes and erythrocytes in mice and baboons following silicone fluid administration.[4]

No gross toxicity has been manifested even after administration of massive amounts of silicone fluid in mice, rats, or primates.[31,32]

Medical Uses

Silicones have found application in nearly all fields of medicine. They have been used externally in skin creams to prevent water-borne irritants.[33] Taken internally, they are an active antifoaming ingredient in oral medication for the prevention of flatulance.[34]

Silicones have been used for artificial hearts, heart valves, and heart massagers; to encapsulate drug and electronic devices; for urethras, ureters, penile implants, and testiclular prostheses; artificial finger joints, bone-end plugs to permit weight bearing on the stumps of amputated limbs; as tubes to prevent neuromas of amputated nerves, and to sheath nerve anastomoses. They have been used extensively as urinary catheters, tracheostomy tubes and drainage tubes of all types.[13]

In the head and neck, other than for reconstruction of visible defects, silicones have been used as synthetic dura mater; as lotions to prevent external otitis; as ear plugs (custom-molded or prefabricated) to aid in hearing conservation or to keep water out of the ears which have mastoid cavities or ventilation tubes (some of which are made of silicone).

Silicones as Subcutaneous Prostheses

The area in which silicones are most widely known is in their use as subcutaneous implants.

In 1953, Brown and co-workers[35] discussed the use of silicones in plastic surgery. At that time their use was confined primarily to dermatological preparations. They prophetically stated: "It is thought possible that one of the greatest needs in plastic surgery, that of a permanent subcutaneous prosthesis, may be forthcoming, if these new chemical compounds can be investigated and developed."

During World War II, people in the United States became breast conscious. Whether this was due to publicity given to movie actresses with large breasts or publication of national magazines devoted to baring large breasts as the national standard, breast fixations became widespread. The public aspect of this craze reached its heights in the middle sixties with the "topless dancer" fad which started in San Francisco. There, some performers with 40-in. bustlines, sought augmentations.

The novelty of publicly exposed, large breasts has waned, but many women with small breasts continue to request augmentation mammoplasties.

Free fat grafts and local flaps have been used for breast augmentation but were found wanting due to fat necrosis or scarring. Various synthetic sponges were used which resulted in a pleasing appearance, but with the ingrowth of fibrous tissue and the absorption of tissue fluids, the breasts felt unnaturally firm and frequently rock hard.

In 1963, Cronin and Gerow[36] reported the development, in conjunction with Dow-Corning, of a breast-shaped Silastic bag which was filled with Silastic gel and backed with Dacron mesh to allow firm fixation to the chest wall. Most breast implants today are variations of this idea. From the research necessary to develop a satisfactory breast prosthesis came innovations in the use of silicones in other areas of the body, further demonstrating the remarkable versatility of silicone.

Silicone Nasal Implants

The nose is man's most prominent feature and for centuries the surgeon has attempted to correct nasal deformities. One of the earliest documents in medical literature deals with Susrutu's Indian forehead flap reconstruction of the amputated nose.

Correction of the saddle nose has been attempted by many reconstructive surgeons using such materials as animal bone, ivory, cartilage, and acrylic, to name but a few. Results generally have been unsatisfactory, and it followed that one of the early uses of silicone was as a nasal implant. Here, however, as with other alloplastic materials, the results have been equivocal.

Beekhuis[37] reported in 1964 the use of 24 Silastic 382 nasal implants in 16 patients. Only one was extruded after trauma to the nose. A postoperative infection occurred in another case in the region of the columellar strut, but this was controlled, and the implant had been maintained to that time. The longest follow-up was 15 months.

After submitting the article for publication in September 1963 and prior to publication, Beekhuis added that more implants had been placed with extrusion of "a few more implants." He felt this occurred where too large a piece of Silastic was inserted with inadequate soft tissue approximation or from closure under tension.

In 1966, Farrior[38] discussed synthetics in head and neck surgery and stated that the extrusion rate is high in the nasal septum and columella. He mentioned that silicone was tolerated in two patients where autogenous hip grafts had been absorbed, and a silicone implant for a saddle nose was extruded six months postoperatively following a blow to the nose. The implant was removed and an autogenous hip graft which took readily was inserted into the pocket which had contained the implant.

Milward[39] reported on a six-year survey of 20 patients receiving 76 solid silicone nasal implants in which 36 percent were lost; 85 percent of these within seven months. Antia et al,[40] inserted L-shaped, premolded silicone nasal implants through mid-columellar incisions and reported 18 percent extruded. Flowers,[41] however, utilizing the intraoral approach and a custom implant made in three parts (soft, medium, and firm silicone rubber) was able to obtain good results without extrusion, in 68 patients followed three months to five years.

Our experience has not been as good. Operating independently and using both solid silicone rubber and silicone sponge implants, over a period of several years we have reached the conclusion that silicone implants have limited application in nasal reconstructive surgery. If one does use them, strict patient selectivity and meticulous adherence to the principles governing implants is required.

Ear Implants

Probably the single most difficult structure to reconstruct is the external ear. Tanzer[42] has evolved one of the more successful methods using costal cartilage. Cronin[43] began using a Silastic frame for ear reconstruction in the mid-1960s. In 1968 Cronin, Greenberg and Brauer[44] presented a follow-up study utilizing the Dow-Corning Cronin (Silastic 370) ear frame with D–116 Tricot Dacron mesh sutured over the helical margin in 11 patients and the use of the frame without the mesh in nine patients. Of the 11 where the mesh was used there was one pinpoint exposure. Of the nine patients in which mesh was not used there were three exposures. All four exposures were closed secondarily and remained closed.

Wray and Hoopes[45] reported a series of 16 Silastic ear frame implantations in 1973 in which 81 percent had to be removed. None of these frames had a Dacron cover.

Ohmori et al[46] reported 116 cases with complications that necessitated the removal of the frame in 9.5 percent. They stress five important technical points:

1. Bond the Dacron mesh over the whole rim of the frame.
2. Excavate the conchal area down to the bony area to provide enough spaces for the insertion of the conchal part of the frame without residual tension on the overlying flap.
3. Insert the tail of the frame into the earlobe.
4. Apply continuous suction through a drain tube postoperatively.
5. As part of the dressing, carefully pack the ear crevices with wet cotton to keep the excellent helical and conchal contour.

Our experience with the Silastic ear frame has been minimal and unsatisfactory. Fig. 2 shows a silastic ear frame which became exposed and had to be removed. One of us (B.K.D.) prefers reconstruction utilizing the "expansile framework" of autogenous rib cartilage described by Brent.[47]

Rehabilitation After Maxillectomy

In the performance of a maxillectomy an acceptable cosmetic appearance is possible if the cheek can be held in its normal position. This can be accomplished if a temporary upper plate is made before the operation. Then just prior to the closure, after lining the cavity with skin grafts, the plate is

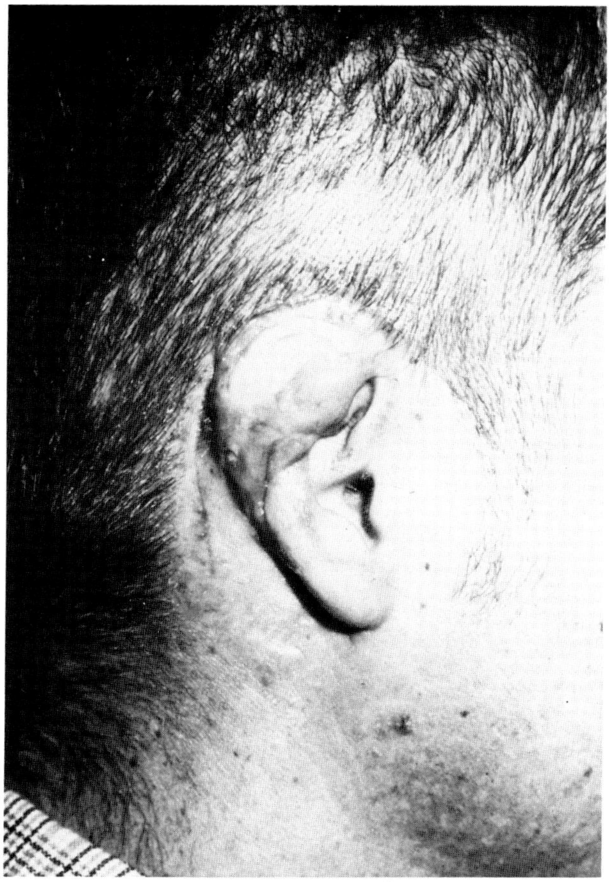

Fig. 2. Exposed silicone ear frame which was later removed.

attached to the remaining teeth, R.T.V. silicone rubber is molded into the cavity. This not only maintains the cheek in its normal position, but it ensures graft survival by maintaining nearly 100 percent even contact between the graft and the graft bed. Additionally, this silicone obturator does not become malodorous the way gauze packing does, and it can be used until the permanent obturator is made some months after surgery. The main disadvantage of this method is the weight of the obturator which sometimes makes retention in the cavity difficult after the swelling of the operation subsides and the obturator has been removed to clean the cavity.

Unfortunately, there is no good way to prevent cheek contraction when the orbital floor is resected. The denture with the obturator cannot be fabricated in such a way as to prevent a deep furrow developing just beneath the eye. Figs. 3A and B show a patient one year following right maxillectomy for adenoid cystic carcinoma of the sinus. It was necessary to resect the floor of the orbit. Note the deep furrow under the eye. A Silastic 382 prosthesis was fabricated. Fig. 4 shows the implant with multiple perforations to allow fibrous tissue ingrowth which will then stabilize it. This was inserted by reopening the Weber-Ferguson maxillectomy incision scar. A pocket was created in the cheek and the implant inserted.

It was necessary to aspirate serum as it collected around the implant for about ten days. After that, the swelling subsided and the outline of the implant was visible. Figs. 5A and B are frontal and lateral photos three months postoperatively.

It is now nearly three years since the Silastic 382 implant was inserted. There has been no evidence of any rejection phenomena. This in spite of 6500 rads of external supravoltage irradiation delivered to a tumor recurrence on the left soft palate one year following the implantation and two years after the initial resection. A portion of the implant was in the irradiated field.

Not all of these cases are successful. In a similar case, a woman desired the depression of the cheek filled in two years following right maxillectomy. A procedure similar to that used in Patient A (Fig. 6) was accomplished. Postoperatively serosanguinous fluid accumulation, discoloration of the overlying skin and extrusion of the inferior portion of the implant occurred. Attempts at trimming the implant and maintaining it were fruitless. The implant was removed three months postoperatively.

Fig. 7A is the immediate post-implant photo. Fig. 7B is the swollen, distorted graft bed with the implant in place three weeks postoperatively. Fig. 8A shows the lower portion of the implant exposed. Fig. 8B is a close-up view showing a small, soft, but sharp edge on the implant. Fig. 9 is the immediate postoperative photo after removing the implant. Violation of several principles governing implants resulted in loss of the implant and an increase in cosmetic deformity.

Reconstruction of the Mandible

Due to motion and major stresses upon the mandible with mastication, silicone rubber is generally not useful for replacement of full or even partial

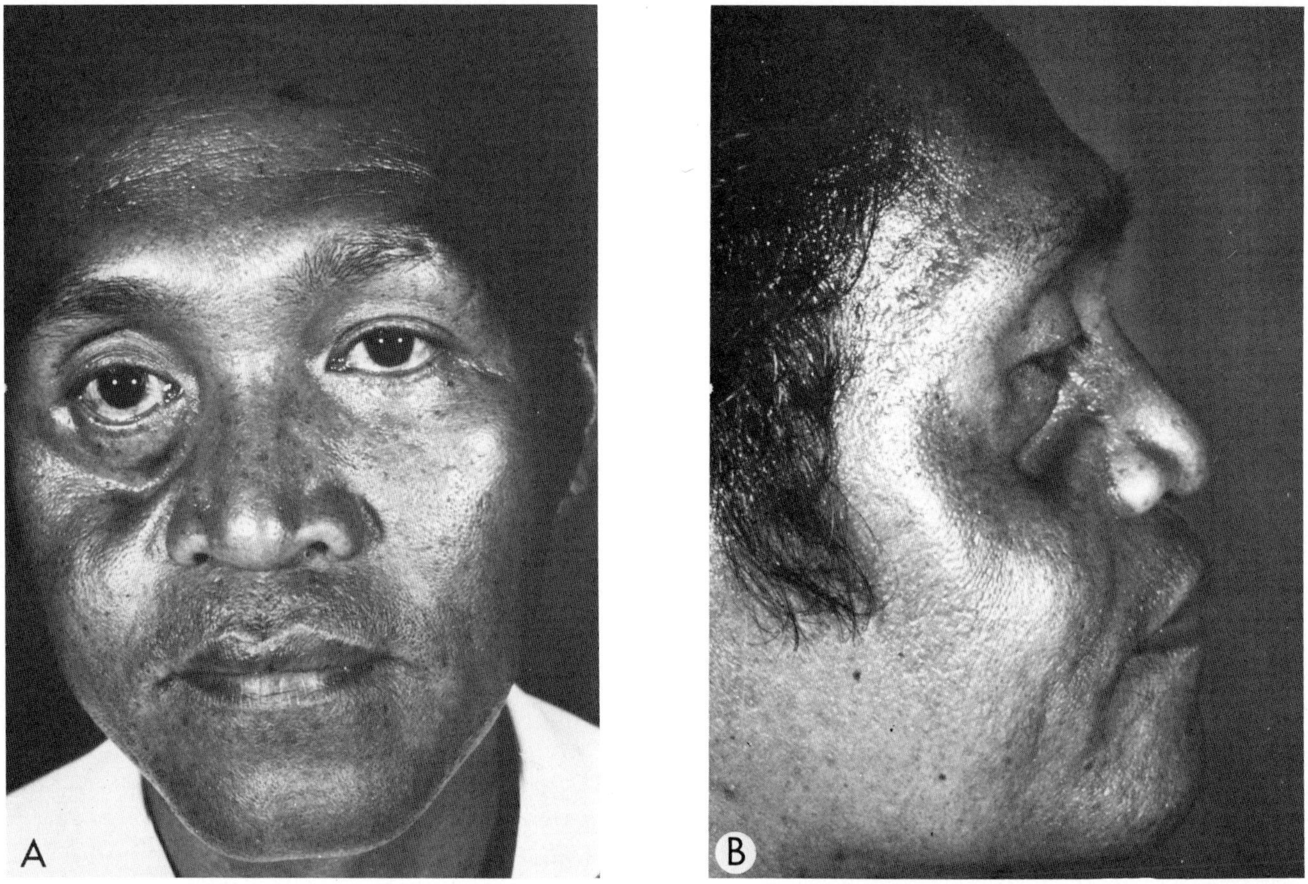

Fig. 3. (A) and (B) are frontal and lateral views of Patient A one year after a right maxillectomy for adenoid cystic carcinoma. It was necessary to resect the orbital floor.

losses. The exception has been the use of a silicone rubber block inserted into the temporo-mandibular joint after resection of the condyle in ankylosis[26] or temporomandibular arthralgia.[48]

The problem in using silicone rubber as a replacement for the body or ramus of the mandible is difficulty in stabilizing the implant since bone will not proliferate into the implant. Swanson et al[49] have achieved remarkable success utilizing a silicone rubber prosthesis, reinforced with wire, containing a tunnel with windows into which autogenous bone is inserted. The windows allow contact of the bone graft with recipient tissue and considerably less bone is needed than when attempting reconstruction solely with carved autogenous bone.

Silicone is readily formed into a custom implant to fill out a depression over the mandible. Fig. 10A shows a depression following multiple fractures of the right mandible with bone and soft tissue loss resulting from a missile fragment. A mask was fashioned and the defect filled with modeling clay to allow formation of an overlay model of dental stone. After removal of the clay, Silastic 382 was poured into the space between the stone models to construct the prosthesis shown in Fig. 10B. Figs. 11A and 11B show the operative approach and the postoperative appearance in this case.

Augmentation of the Chin

Silicone lends itself well to most onlay grafts and several companies presently manufacture various styles of preformed chin implants.[50] These are made in several sizes and can be backed with Dacron felt for adherence to the underlying bone. Fig. 12 is a photograph of a Silastic chin implant developed by Safian.[50]

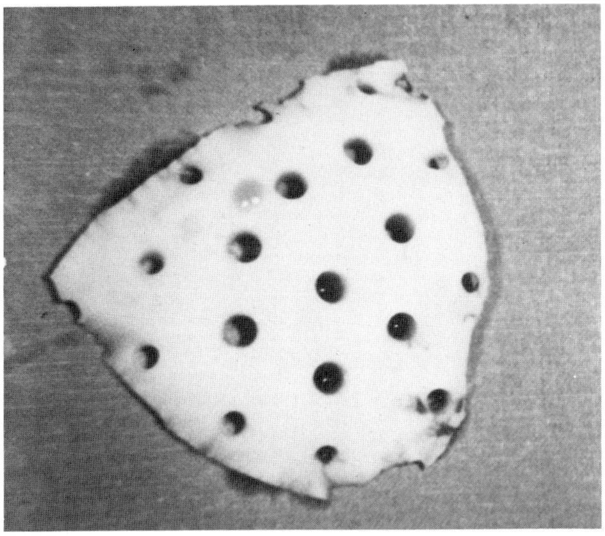

Fig. 4. Silastic 382 cheek implant.

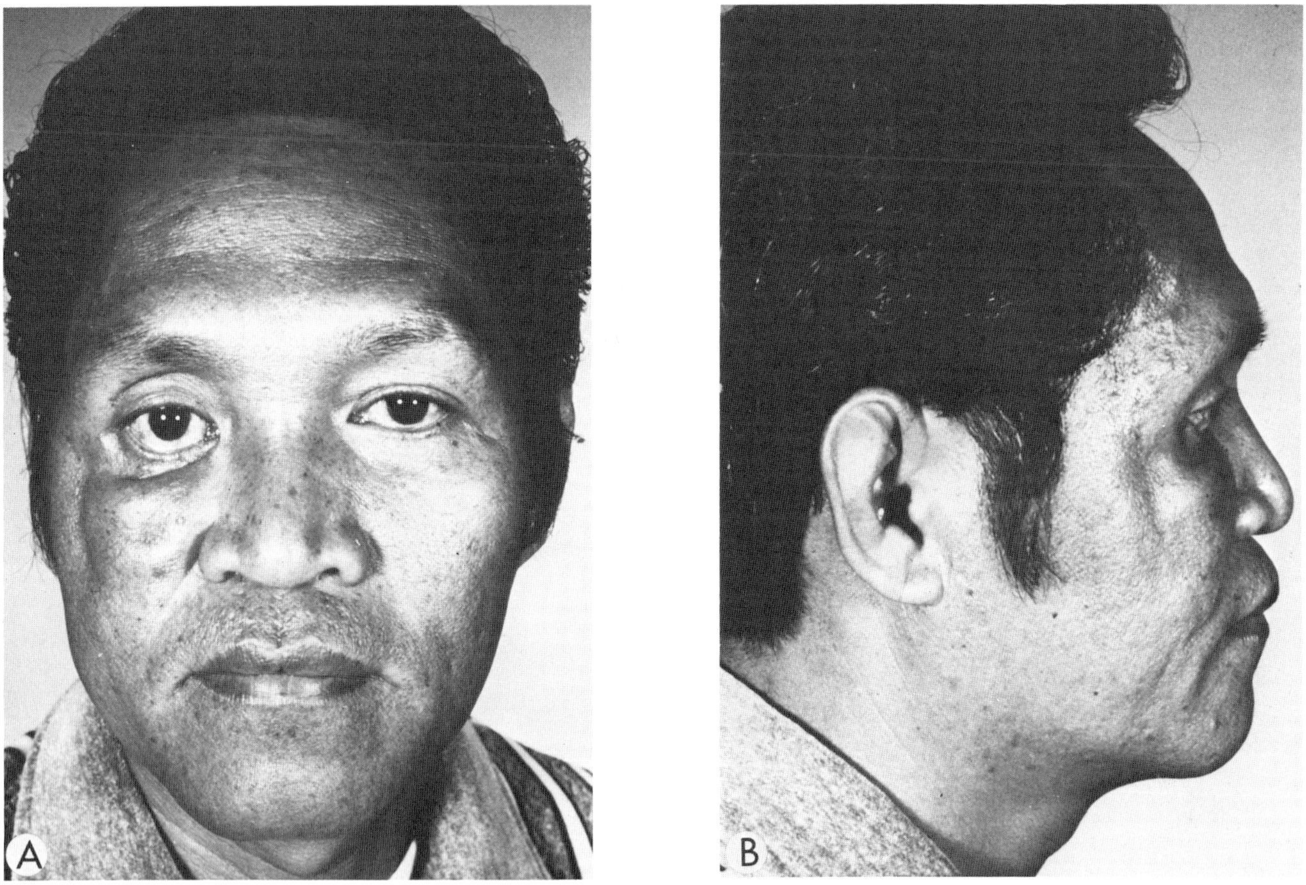

Fig. 5. (A & B) Frontal and lateral photos of Patient A three months after inserting a Silastic 382 check implant.

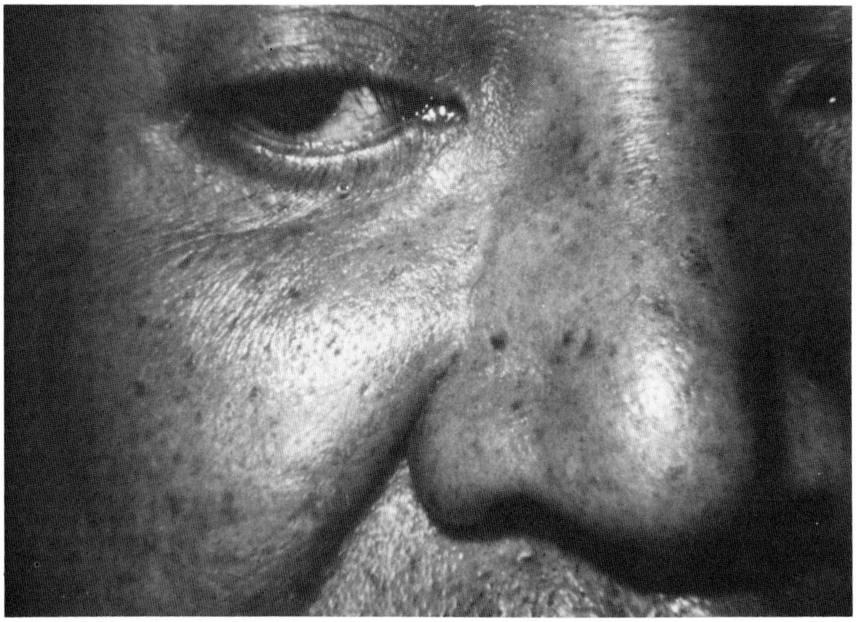

Fig. 6. Frontal view of Patient A thirty months after implant.

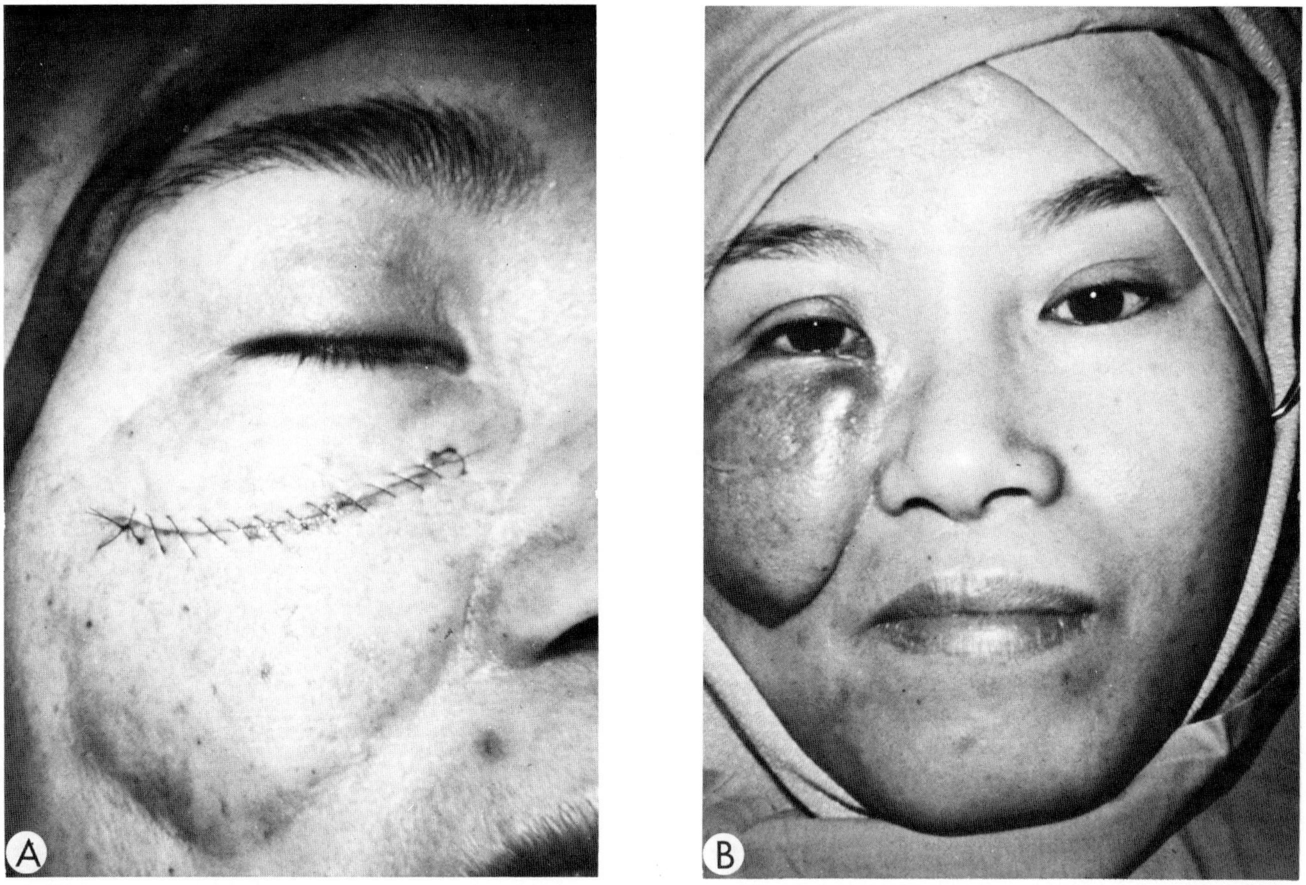

Fig. 7. (A) Patient B immediately postimplantation of a Silastic 382 cheek implant. (B) Patient B two weeks postoperatively showing swelling, and discoloration of the skin over the graft.

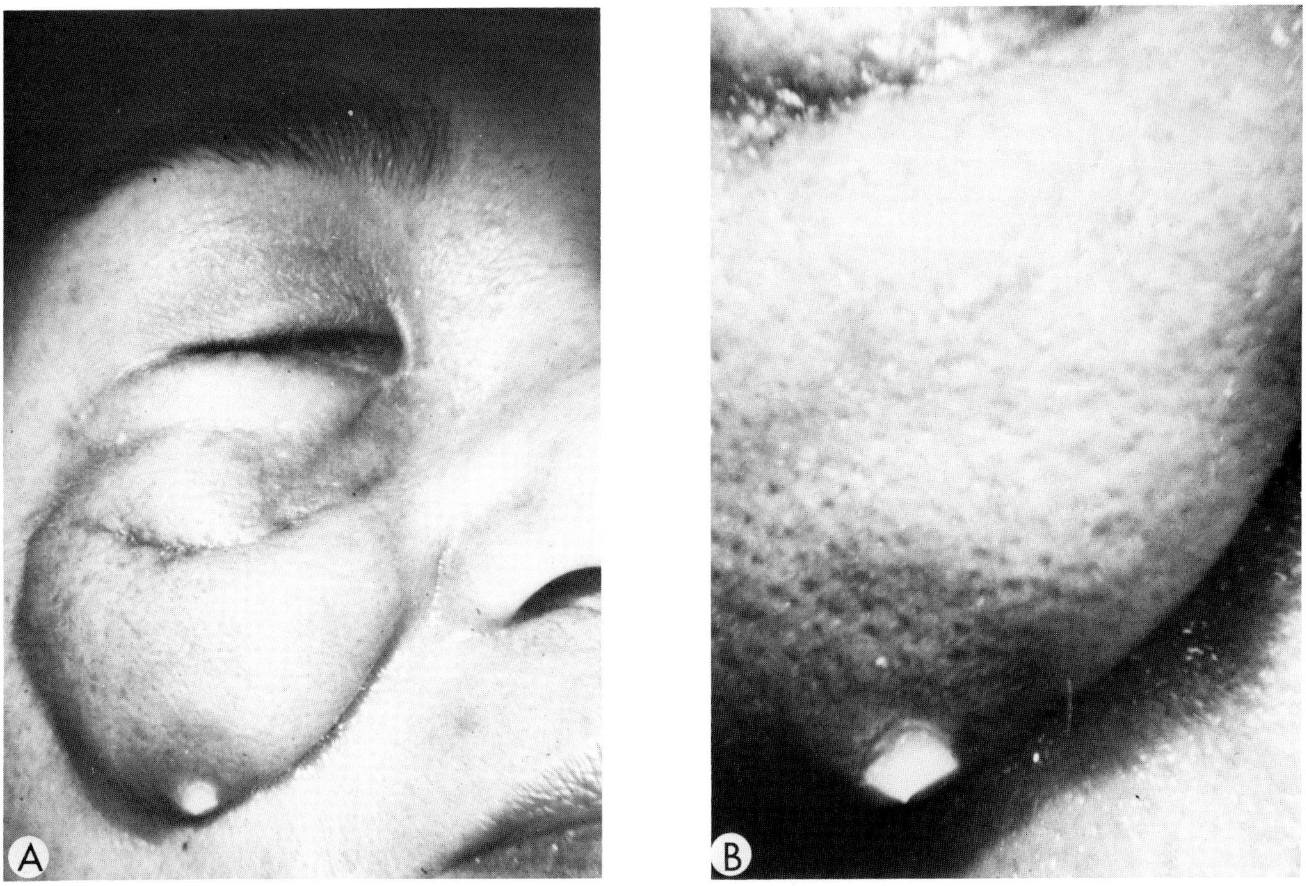

Fig. 8. (A) Frontal view of Patient B with the implant exposed three weeks postoperatively. (B) Close-up of Fig. 8A.

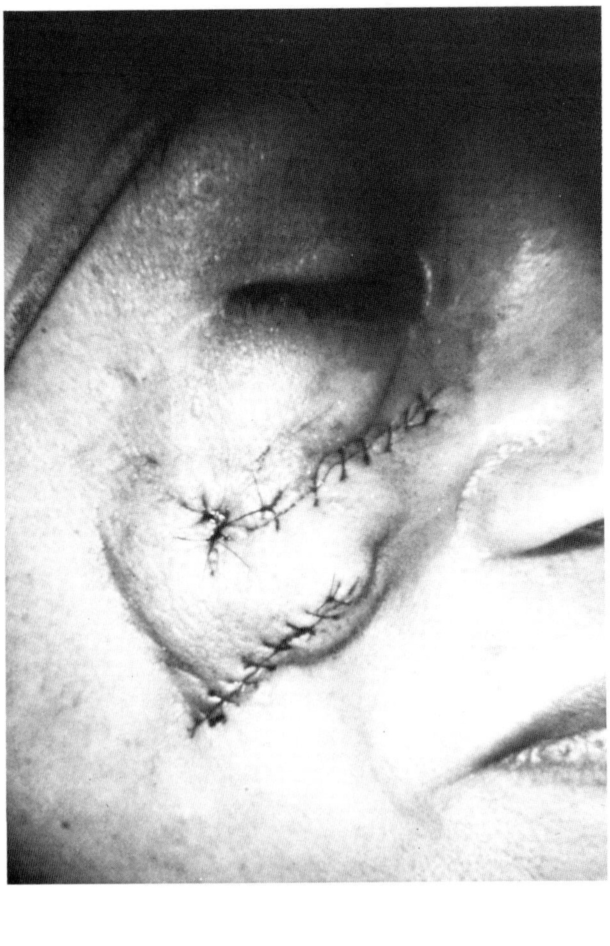

Fig. 9. Immediate postoperative photograph of Patient B after removing cheek implant three months following insertion.

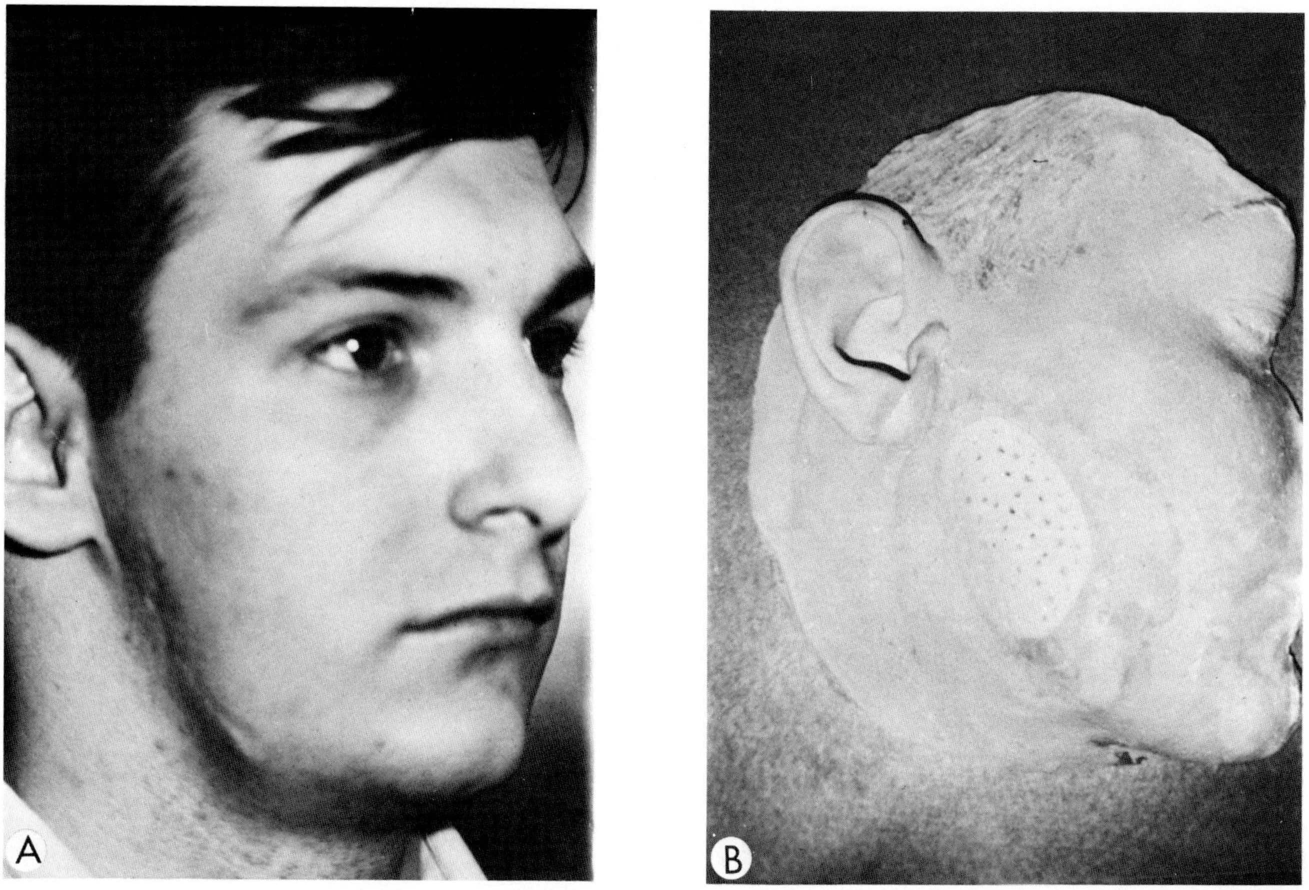

Fig. 10. (A) Depression over right mandible following trauma from a missile wound in Patient C. (B) The dental stone mask filled with Silastic 382.

Converse[51] described an intra-oral approach for bone grafts to the chin in 1950, and Millard[52] has used this approach to make augmentation mentoplasty an adjunct to rhinoplasty in 15 percent of his cases. He utilizes silicone sponge which he carves with scissors at the operating table and inserts through a small stab wound in the labial sulcus. Parkes[53] has also reported successful chin implants with silastic sponge. The problem of bone resorption is minimized by not placing the implant between the periosteum and the mandible.

Silicones as Onlay Implants

A custom implant of Silastic 382 made from a moulage can be used to correct many irregularities and depressions of the face.

Figs. 13A and B show Patient D, a victim of hemifacial atrophy (Romberg's disease). Figs. 14A and B show the results in the treatment of this disease with a moulded Silastic 382 implant. In order for these implants to be successful they must be made with thin margins and they must have multiple perforations to allow for the ingrowth of fibrous tissue. They should be placed on a stable base and fixed in place with nonabsorbable suture or wire to prevent shifting. This limits the use of the solid implant in the treatment of Romberg's disease. It is preferable to use silicone fluid as an adjunct; however, its use is limited by the Food and Drug Administration to only a small number of investigators.[54,55]

Pharyngeal

Blocksma[56] reported success in inserting solid sponge and shredded silicone implants and injecting R.T.V. silicone into the posterior pharyngeal wall

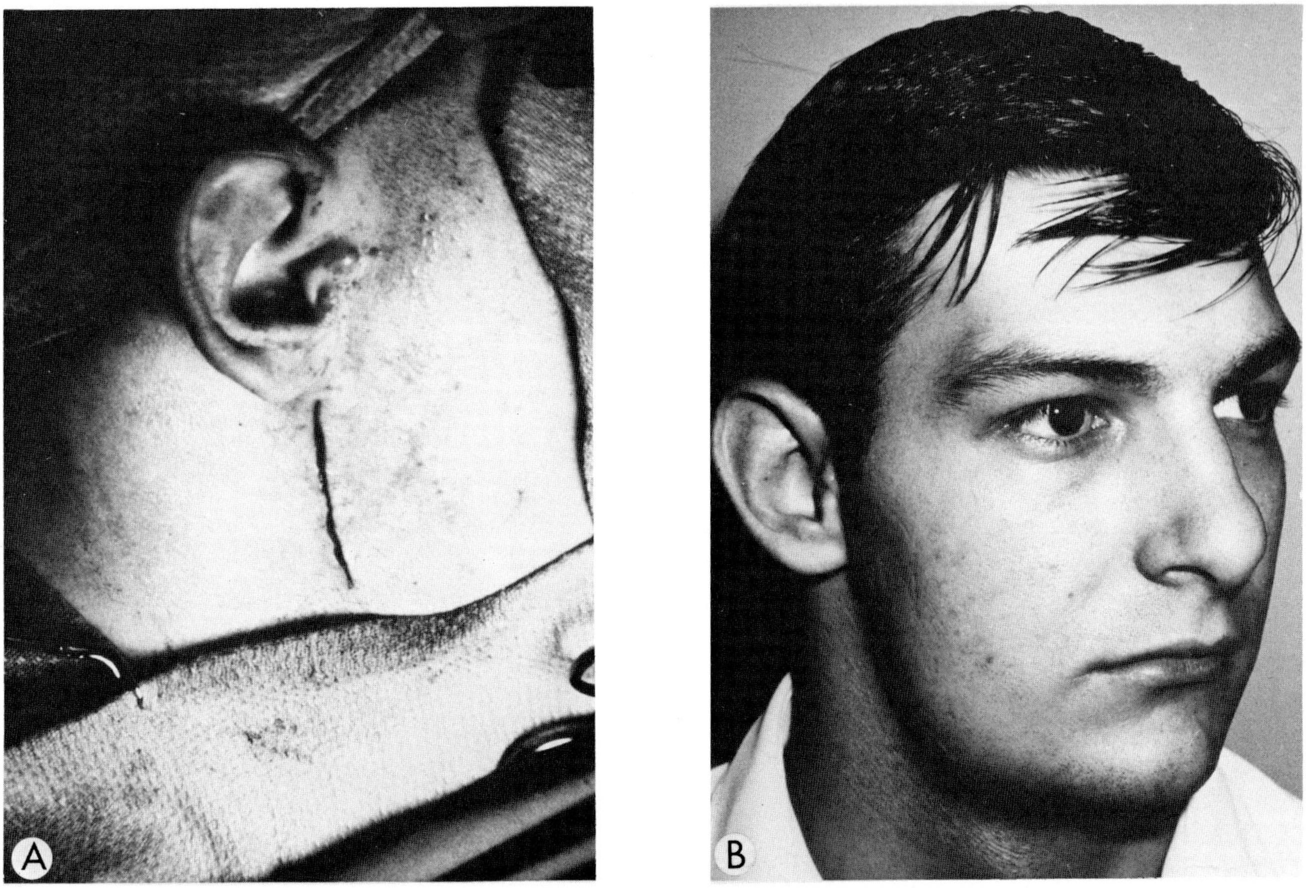

Fig. 11. *(A) The surgical approach for inserting the implant. (B) The postoperative appearance of Patient C.*

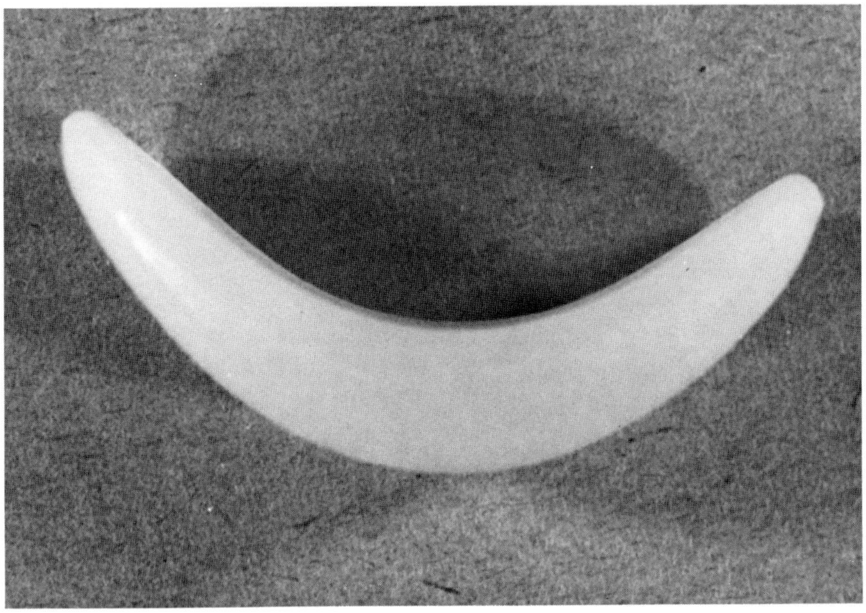

Fig. 12. *A photograph of a Safian-type Silastic chin implant.*

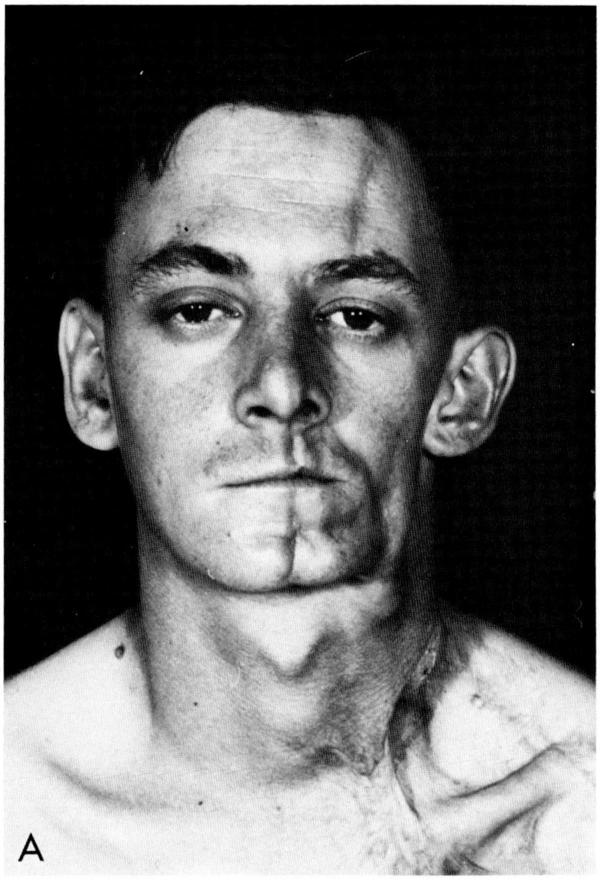

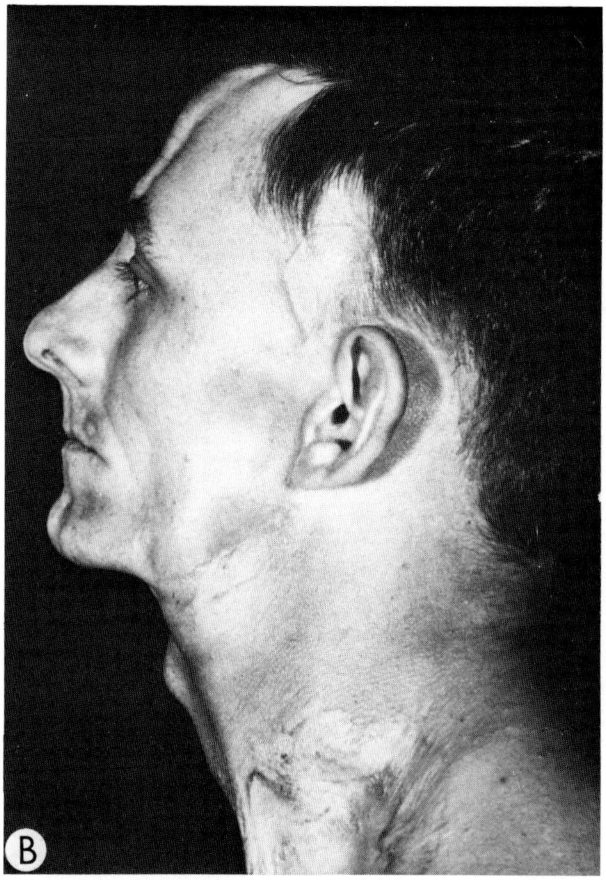

Fig. 13. Frontal and lateral views of Patient D a victim of Romberg's disease.

just above the atlas tubercle to improve speech in velopharyngeal incompetence. The sponge was extruded as well as portions of the shredded silicone but the other implants were tolerated, and speech was improved in 21 of 23 patients.

Discussion

Most silicone used in reconstructive surgery of the head and neck today is either heat or room temperature vulcanized rubber.

The heat vulcanizing rubber has slightly greater tear and tensile strength, but it must be molded prior to surgery or cut to shape prior to implanation.

In order to use the heat-cured silicone, a mask to outline the defect is made of plaster or similar material and the defect filled to normal contours with wax or clay. Another mask is then made, the wax or clay removed and silicone is poured into the defect of the original positive mask and molded with the second, negative mask. Blocks of the material also may be carved to shape at surgery.

The room temperature vulcanizing (R.T.V.) rubber can be mixed with the catalyst, placed in position and molded at surgery, or fabricated in molds as with heat-cured silicone.

Cipcic[57] lists some important principles which can determine the success or failure of implanted silicone prostheses:

1. They should be buried as deeply as possible; preferably under a layer of fat or dermis.
2. Incisions should be placed at a distance from the implanted area.
3. The graft bed must be of adequate size and shape. (We feel it should be ample but not so large as to permit shifting of the implant. A graft bed which is too small will result in a poor cosmetic appearance due to curling of the margins of the implant and pressure necrosis and extrusion may occur.)

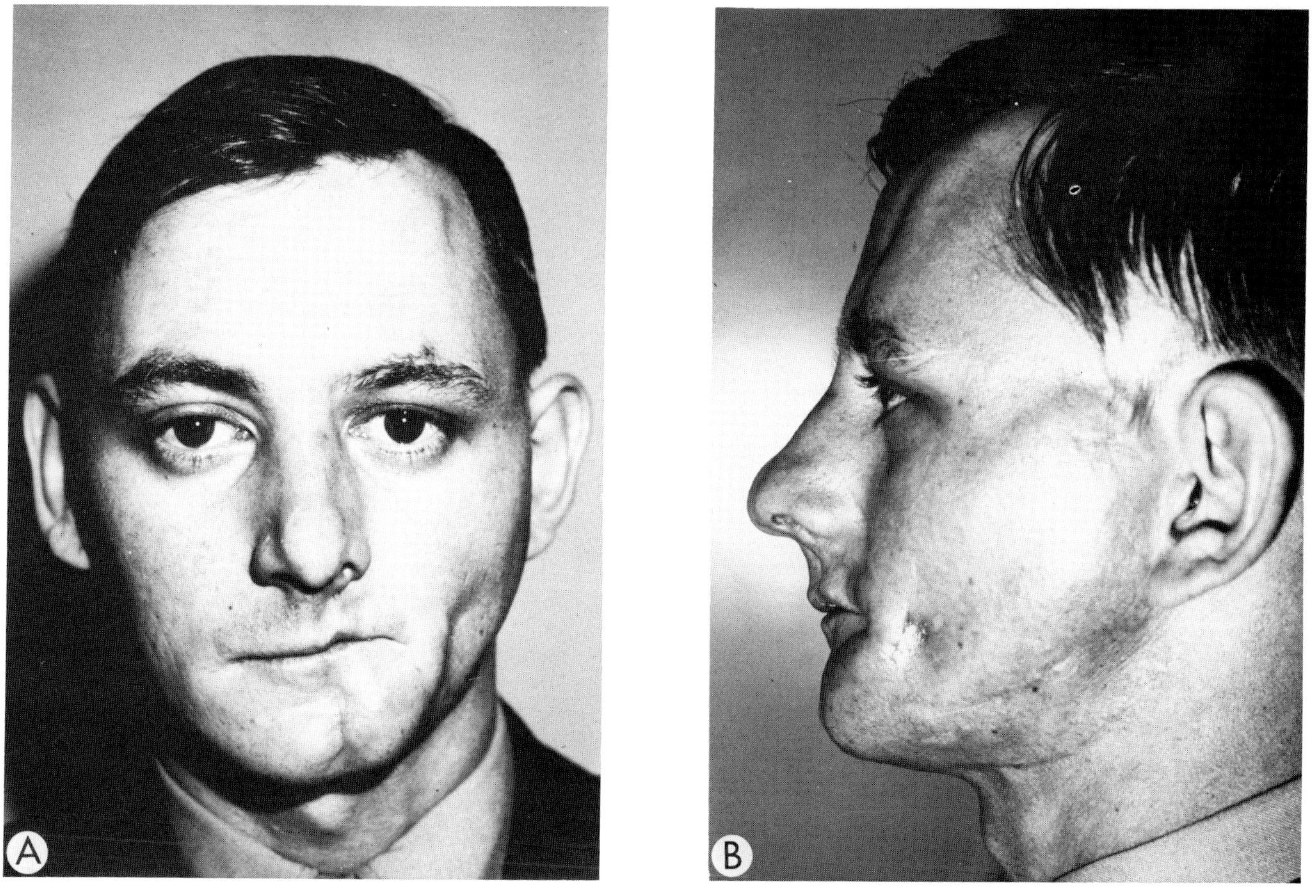

Fig. 14. Postoperative views of Patient D after inserting an onlay implant in his left lateral face.

4. Avoid areas where trauma, motion or tissue tension may cause the implant to extrude.
5. Avoid contamination of the implant with dust, lint or fingerprints prior to insertion. (To this must be added talc or glove powder).
6. All operating room personnel who will be sterilizing the implant must be informed that silicones will not melt when autoclaved (a common misconception). They should *not* be sterilized in a gas autoclave as the implant will absorb the gas which will later diffuse and may be toxic to adjacent tissue.
7. Avoid sharp edges on the implant and fasten securely.
8. Provide multiple perforations of the implant for holding fibrosis.

The rubber silicones have been used widely in medicine, especially for reconstruction of defects about the head or neck characterized by tissue loss. Careful patient selection and adherence to the basic principles of implantation as enumerated here should result in successful rehabilitation of these head and neck defects.

References

1. Longacre JJ: Deformities of the forehead, scalp and cranium, Chapter 19, Volume II, Reconstructive Plastic Surgery. Converse JM, ed, W. B. Saunders Co., Philadelphia, Pa 1964, p 577
2. Macewen W: The growth of bone. J Mackhose, Glasgow, Scotland, 1912
3. Scales JT: Discussion on metals and synthetic materials in relation to soft tissues; tissue reaction to synthetic materials, Proc Royal Soc Med 46:647, 1953
4. Rees TD, Wood-Smith D: Cosmetic facial surgery. Philadelphia, Pa, W. B. Saunders Co. 1973, p 232
5. Plastics, Von Nostrand's Scientific encyclopedia, Ed. 3, Princeton, N.J., D. Van Nostrand Co., Inc., p 1268
6. Bennett T: The use of plastics in otolaryngology, Arch Otolaryn 77:415, 1963
7. Arnold GE: Vocal rehabilitation of paralytic dysphonia: VI Further studies of intracordal injection materials, Arch Otolaryn 73:290, 1961
8. Brown JB, Fryer MP, Ohlwiler DA: Study and use of synthetic materials, such as silicones and teflon, as subcutaneous prostheses. Plast Reconstr Surg 26:264, 1960

9. Small JA, Brown S, Kobernick SD: Teflon and silastic for mandibular replacement: Experimental studies and reports of cases. J Oral Surg 22:377, 1964
10. DeBakey ME, Cooley DA, Crawford ES, Morris GC Jr: Clinical application of a new flexible knitted dacron arterial substitute, Arch Surg 77:713–724, 1958
11. Barondes R deR, Judge WD, Toren CG, Baxter, ML: The silicones in medicine, Mil Surg 106:379, 1950
12. Braley SA: The use of silicones in plastic surgery, a retrospective view. Plast Reconstr Surg 51:280, 1973
13. Braley S: Symposium on synthetics in maxillofacial surgery. I. The silicones for maxillofacial surgery, Laryngoscope 78:549, 1968
14. Speirs AC, Blocksma R: New implantable silicone rubbers. An experimental evaluation of tissue response. Plast Reconstr Surg 31:166, 1962
15. Mullison EG: Current status of silicone in plastic surgery, Arch Otolaryng 83:59, 1966
16. Turner FC: Sarcomas at sites of subcutaneous implanted bakelite disks in rats, J Nat Cancer Inst 2:81, 1941
17. Druckrey H, Schmahl D: Cancerogene wirkung von kunststaff: Folien, Z. Naturforsch 76:353, 1952
18. Oppenheimer BS, Oppenheimer ET, Stout AP, Danishefsky I: Malignant tumors resulting from embedding plastics in rodents. Science 118:305, 1953
19. Oppenheimer BS, Oppenheimer ET, Danishefsky I, Stout AP, Eisich E: Further studies of polymers as carcinogenic agents in animals. Cancer Res 15:333, 1955
20. Russell FE, Simmes MM, Hirst AE, Pudenz RH: Tumors associated with embedded polymers, J Nat Cancer Inst 23:305, 1959
21. Hueper WC: Cancer induction by polyurethene and polysilicone plastics. J Nat Cancer Inst 33:1005, 1964
22. Ben-Hur N, Newman Z: Malignant tumor formation following subcutaneous injection of silicone fluid in white mice. Israel Med J 22:15, 1963
23. Grasso P, Goldberg L, Fairweather F: Injection of silicones in mice. Letter to the Editor, Lancet 2:96, 1964
24. Sternberg TH, Ashley FL, Winer L, Lehman R: Gewebe-recktionen auf injizierte flüssige siliconuver binduggen. Hantartz 15:281, 1964
25. Winer L, Sternberg TH, Lehman R, Ashley FL: Tissue reactions to injected silicone liquids. Arch Derm 90:588, 1964
26. Brown JB, Fryer MP, Kollias P, Ohlwiler DA, Templeton JB: Silicone and teflon prostheses including full jaw substitution: Laboratory and clinical studies of etheron. Ann Surg 157:932, 1963
27. Dimant S: Silicone rubber in surgery. Lancet 267:533, 1954
28. Thompson HG: The fate of the pseudosheath pocket around silicone implants. Plast Reconstr Surg 51:667, 1973
29. Imber G, Schwager RG, Guthrie RH, Gray GF: Fibrous capsule formation after subcutaneous implantation of synthetic materials in experimental animals. Plast Reconstr Surg 54:183, 1974
30. Andrews JM: Cellular behavior to injected silicone fluid: a preliminary report. Plast Reconstr Surg 38:551,1966
31. Rowe VK, Spencer HC, Boss SL: Toxicological studies on certain commercial silicones and hydrolyzable silane intermediates. J Indust Hyg Toxicol 30:332, 1948
32. Ballantyne DL Jr, Rees TD, Seidman I: Silicone fluids: Response to massive subcutaneous injection of dimethylpolysiloxane fluid in animals. Plast Reconst Surg 36:330, 1965
33. Von Kennel J: Dermatology and silicones kosmetische monatschrift, 1:7, 1952
34. Rider JA, Moeller HC: Use of silicone in the treatment of intestinal gas and bloating, JAMA 174:16, 1960
35. Brown JB, Fryer MP, Randall P, Lu M: silicones in plastic surgery. Plast Reconst Surg 12:374, 1953
36. Cronin TD, Gerow FJ: Augmentation mammoplasty. A new "natural feel" prosthesis. Transactions of the Third International Congress of Plastic Surgery. Excerpta Medica Foundation, New York, pp 41–49, 1963
37. Beekhuis GJ: Silicone rubber implants in nasal reconstructive surgery. Laryngoscope 74:1405, 1964
38. Farrior RT: Synthetics in head and neck surgery. Arch Otolaryng 84:104, 1966
39. Milward TM: The fate of silastic and vitrathene nasal implants. Brit J Plast Surg 25:276, 1972
40. Antia NH, Daver BM, Keswani MH, Buch VI: Prefabricated silicone nasal implants. Plast Reconstr Surg 52:264, 1973
41. Flowers RS: Nasal augmentation by the intravial route. Plast Reconstr Surg 54:571, 1974
42. Tanzer RC: Total reconstruction of the auricle. The evolution of a plan of treatment. Plast Reconstr Surg 47:523, 1971
43. Cronin TD: Use of a silastic frame for total and sub-total reconstruction of the external ear. Plast Reconstr Surg 37:399, 1966
44. Cronin TD, Greenberg RL, Brauer RO: Follow-up study of silastic frame for reconstruction of external ear. Plast Reconstr Surg 42:522, 1968
45. Wray RC, Hoopes JE: Silastic frameworks in total reconstruction of the auricle. Brit J Plast Surg 26:296, 1973
46. Ohmori S, Koreaki M, Nakai H: Follow-up study on reconstruction of microtia with a silicone framework. Plast Reconstr Surg 53:555, 1974
47. Brent B: Ear reconstruction with an expansile framework of autogenous rib cartilage. Plast Reconstr Surg 53:619, 1974
48. Hartwell SW, Hall MD: Mandibular condylectomy with silicone rubber replacement. Plast Reconstr Surg 53:440, 1974
49. Swanson LT, Habal MB, Leake DL, Murray JE: Compound silicone-bone implants for mandibular reconstruction. Plast Reconstr Surg 51:402, 1973
50. Safian J: Progress in nasal and chin augmentation. Plast Reconstr Surg 37:446, 1966
51. Converse JM: Restoration of facial contour by bone grafts introduced through the oral cavity. Plast Reconstr Surg 6:295, 1–50
52. Millard DR: Adjuncts in augmentation mentoplasty and corrective rhinoplasty. Plast Reconstr Surg 36:48, 1965
53. Parkes ML: Chin implants with a new plastic compound. Arch Otolaryng 75:429, 1962
54. Ashley FL, Thompson DP, Henderson T: Augmentation of surface contour by subcutaneous injections of silicone fluid. Plast Reconstr Surg 51:8, 1973
55. Rees TD, Ashley FL, Delgado JP: Silicone fluid injections for facial atrophy. Plast Reconstr Surg 52:118, 1973
56. Blocksma R: Correction of velopharyngeal insufficiency by silastic pharyngeal implant. Plast Reconstr Surg 31: 268, 1963
57. Cipcic JA: Silicone implant correction of facial deformities. Laryngoscope 78:565, 1968

Management of Soft Tissue Trauma of the Head and Neck

Jerome C. Goldstein, Albany, N.Y.

An old English proverb states, "Tho the wound be healed, yet the scar remains." Our goal in the repair of soft tissue trauma should be to preserve form and function while minimizing unattractive scarring. The repair of these injuries of the head and neck requires a basic knowledge of anatomy, physiology, and a concern for cosmesis not necessarily required in other parts of the body. The specialist working in this region should be capable of recognizing and repairing anatomic violations involving the patency of the nasal airway, facial nerve branches, salivary gland ducts, nasolacrimal apparatus, eyelid and eye muscles and ligaments, and sinus ostea. The operating microscope is often an important surgical adjunct in these repairs.

Factors to be carefully considered before undertaking the surgical repair of a soft tissue injury include the location and nature of the wound, its size, the amount of tissue loss, the degree and type of contamination, and the general medical situation of the patient. The rich blood supply of the face is actually the surgeon's friend, and a delay of 24 to 48 hr can be permitted if required by other medical problems. Povidone-iodine compresses should be applied to wounds so delayed. Relatively mild injury of the face, if handled inappropriately or without due concern for fundamental cosmesis can yield end results which cause more anguish and suffering than that experienced with the original wound.

The emergency room is rarely the place to repair any but the most minor injuries. The best possible result is accomplished in the best possible environment. This includes proper sterility, light, exposure, assistance, and other accoutrements usually found only in an operating room. This determination obviously is dependent upon local conditions.

The copious blood supply of the face permits a conservatism in debridement unique to this region. Animal bites can be closed primarily, and grossly devitalized tissues need not be widely excised. This is not to infer that one can be careless in wound cleansing. In fact, the choice between local and general anesthesia can be dependent upon whether local anesthesia will permit the vigorous scrubbing and decontamination required. Wounds with ground-in dirt and grease must be scrubbed with a brush to remove all gross particles lest subsequent tattooing result. Hypodermic needles and the point of a #11 blade can be helpful in "picking out" larger particles. Ether is sometimes used to dissolve grease. Occasionally the direction of the laceration can be changed to parallel, rather than cross, wrinkle lines at the time of debridement.

Proper techniques in suturing are fundamental to obtaining the optimal scar. Delicate instruments (Fig. 1), gentle handling of tissues, and fine suture material with small swedged-on needles facilitate these closures. Figure 2 illustrates the basic techniques of layered closure to obliterate dead spaces and shows the subcuticular suture. Knots should be inverted to lessen skin reaction. Perpendicular insertion of needles into the skin is emphasized in Figure 3.

Jagged lacerations can often best be closed with careful preservation of the sharp convexities and concavities. A debridement which would result in a straight line closure is avoided if it crosses rather than parallels wrinkle lines. As justification for this, one should recall that the treatment of an unsightly straight line scar on the face is to break it up into a "W-plasty" or "zigzag-plasty." A jagged laceration often provides the opportunity of accomplishing this at the time of primary repair. The straight line portions of a larger laceration can be

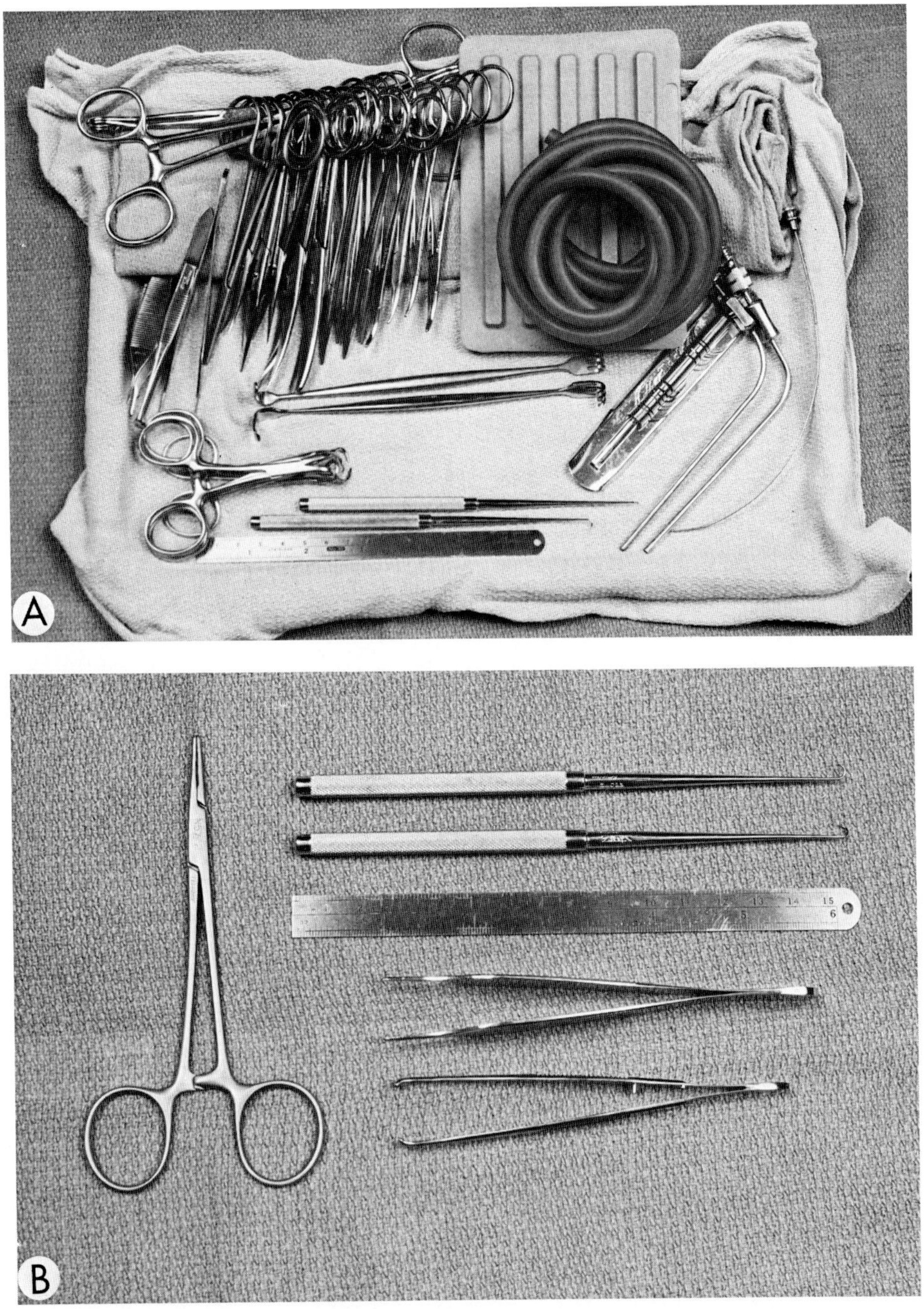

Fig. 1. (A) "Minor Plastic Tray" with instruments sufficient to handle the injuries described in this paper. (B) Close-up of Webster needle-holder, skin hooks, forceps and ruler contained on this tray.

satisfactorily closed with a subcuticular suture. This saves time and gives a superior result. A 4-0 suture is delicate, yet strong enough to avoid breaking on pull-out. 5-0 and 6-0 nylon on tiny "plastic surgery" needles are used for interrupted sutures. Sutures should be placed close together and not more than a millimeter or two from the edge of the wound. Lacerated mucosal surfaces are loosely approximated with chromic sutures except when adjacent to vermillion borders, where they are closed with nylon just as if they were skin.

Micropore tape is helpful in reenforcing a delicate wound closure, especially in children. Removal of interrupted sutures is started on the second or third postoperative day. Micropore tape is reapplied following this removal if the wound is dry. Systemic antibiotics are used in all patients with animal bites, with grossly contaminated wounds,

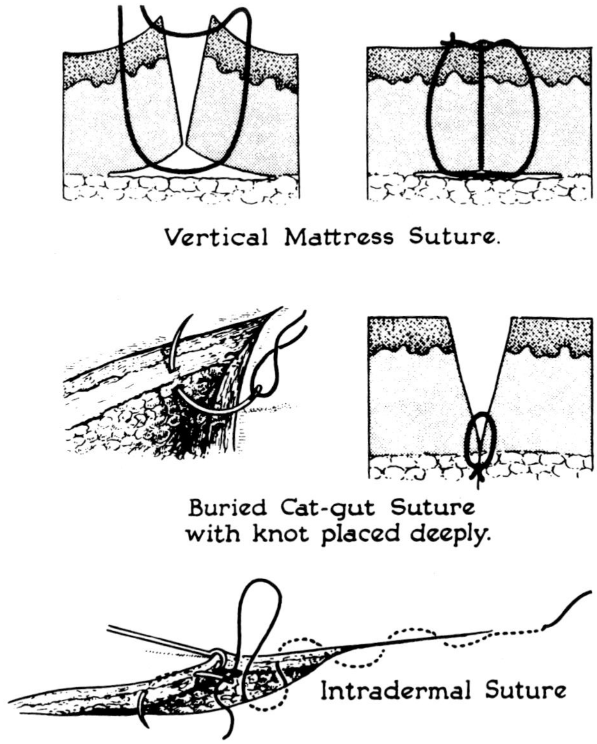

Fig. 2. From: McGregor, I.A., Fundamental Techniques of Plastic Surgery, Churchill Livingstone, 5 ed. p. 22.

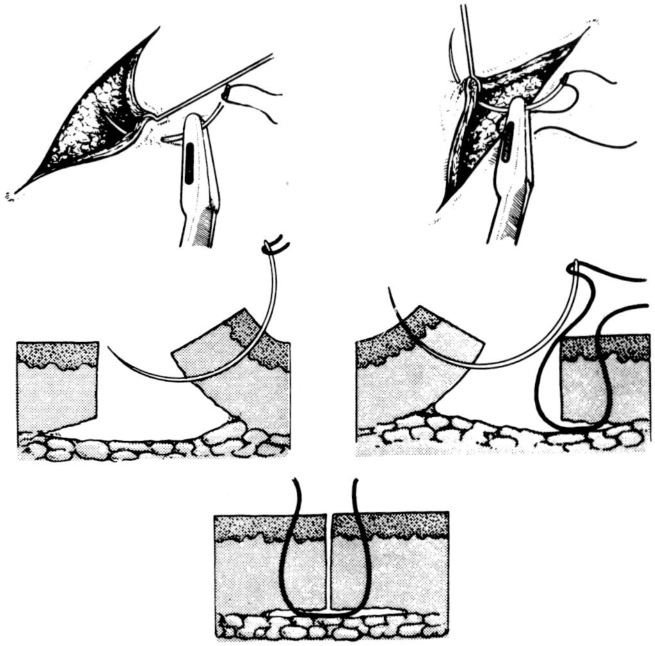

Fig. 3. From: McGregor, I.A., Fundamental Techniques of Plastic Surgery, Churchill Livingstone, p. 21. Note that the suture should be inserted such that the bite taken is wider at the depth than at the surface. This causes eversion of the margins.

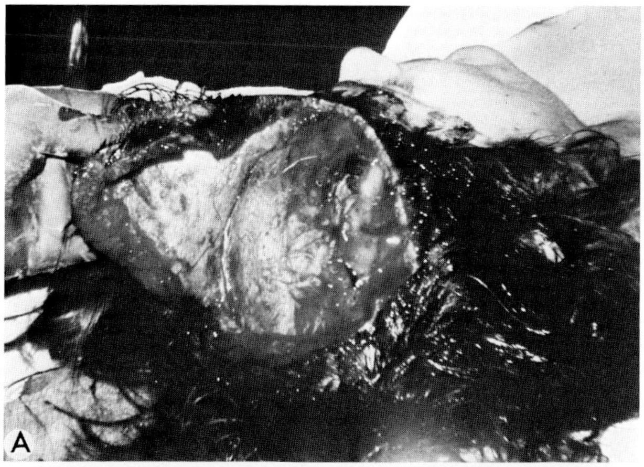

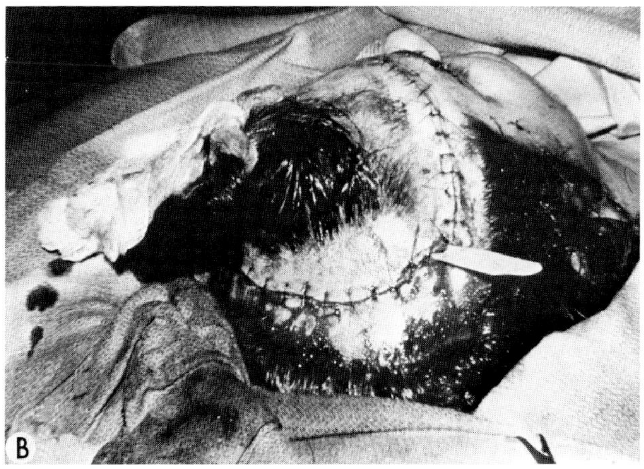

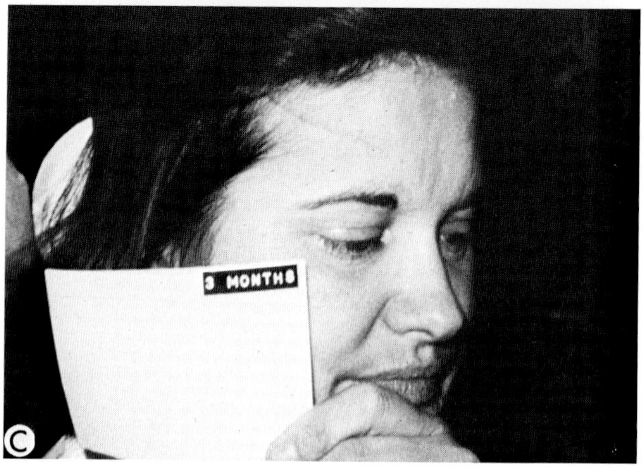

Fig. 4. Scalping wound from automobile accident. See text for details.

and with lacerations communicating with mucosal surfaces. In addition topical antibiotic ointment (Pfizer's Terramycin) is applied postoperatively to grossly contaminated or weeping wounds. The status of tetanus immunization is ascertained and appropriate therapy given.

Almost every head and neck surgeon has a collection of terribly mutilating facial injuries. It is not the purpose of this presentation to add to this catalog of horrors, but rather to illustrate one surgeon's experiences with the more commonly encountered variety of wounds, and to illustrate the foregoing principles and techniques which can consistently produce good results.

The cases presented are pure soft tissue injuries not associated with underlying fractures. However the principles and techniques illustrated here are directly applicable to more extensive injuries whenever they are encountered. When fractures are present, they should be managed through the associated lacerations whenever possible without compromising exposure, rather than adding to the number and variety of soft tissue wounds that must then be closed.

Figure 4 illustrates a scalping wound. This type of injury often extends to the pericranium. The entire scalp need not be shaved but only that area one or two centimeters on each side of the suture line. Deep sutures are rarely necessary here. 3-0 or 4-0 suture material can be used to reapproximate the wound. Deep bites are taken with the large needles affixed to this size suture and should include the underlying muscle. These wounds are prone to accumulate fluid and so should always be drained. When the laceration extends onto the forehead, the previously described soft tissue techniques using smaller sutures are appropriate.

Figure 5 illustrates the technique of subcuticular suture and the tiny bites taken to reapproximate vermillion borders.

Figure 6 illustrates the assortment of facial wounds not infrequently seen in passengers involved in automobile accidents. If endotracheal anesthesia is used, the tube should not be fixed, but rather be free to move about thereby avoiding distortion. The variety of wounds here are handled wherever possible with linear closure using subcuticular sutures. These sutures may either be tied upon themselves, split shot can be used to secure

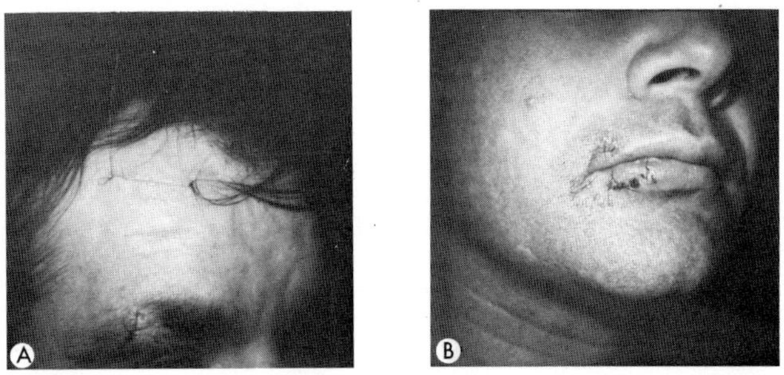

Fig. 5. (A) Subcuticular forehead suture on the third postoperative day. Free ends are secured by knots. (B) Same patient with 6-0 nylon interrupted sutures closing lacerations of both lips.

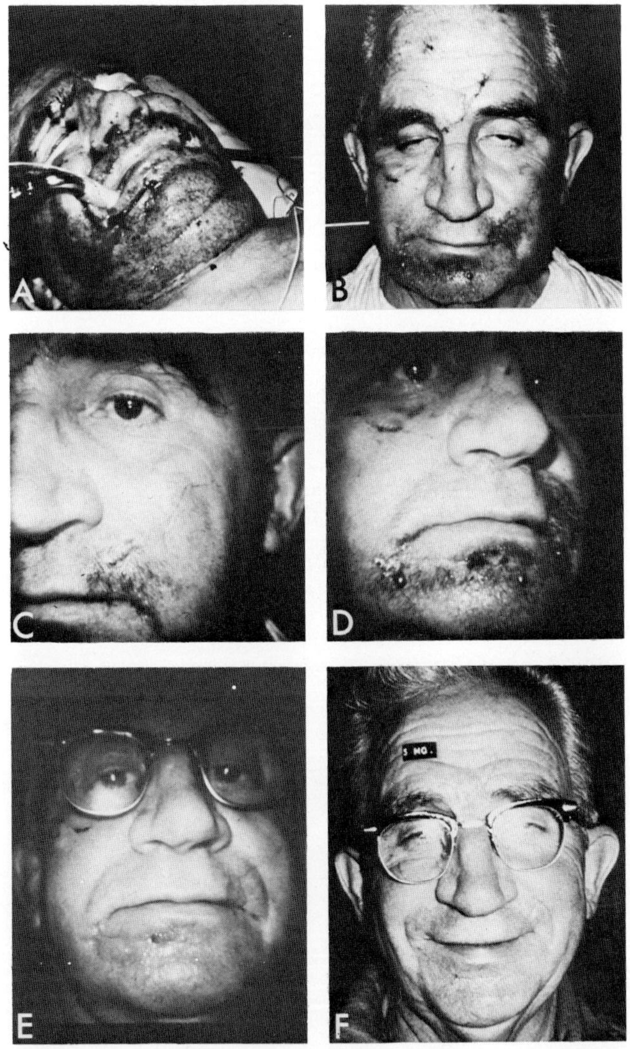

Fig. 6. (A) A patient with a variety of facial wounds resulting from an automobile accident. (C) Subcuticular suture five days postop with the ends left free. (D) Split shot was used to secure the subcuticular suture in the lower lip. (E) After removal of all the sutures on the tenth postoperative day. (F) The result at five months.

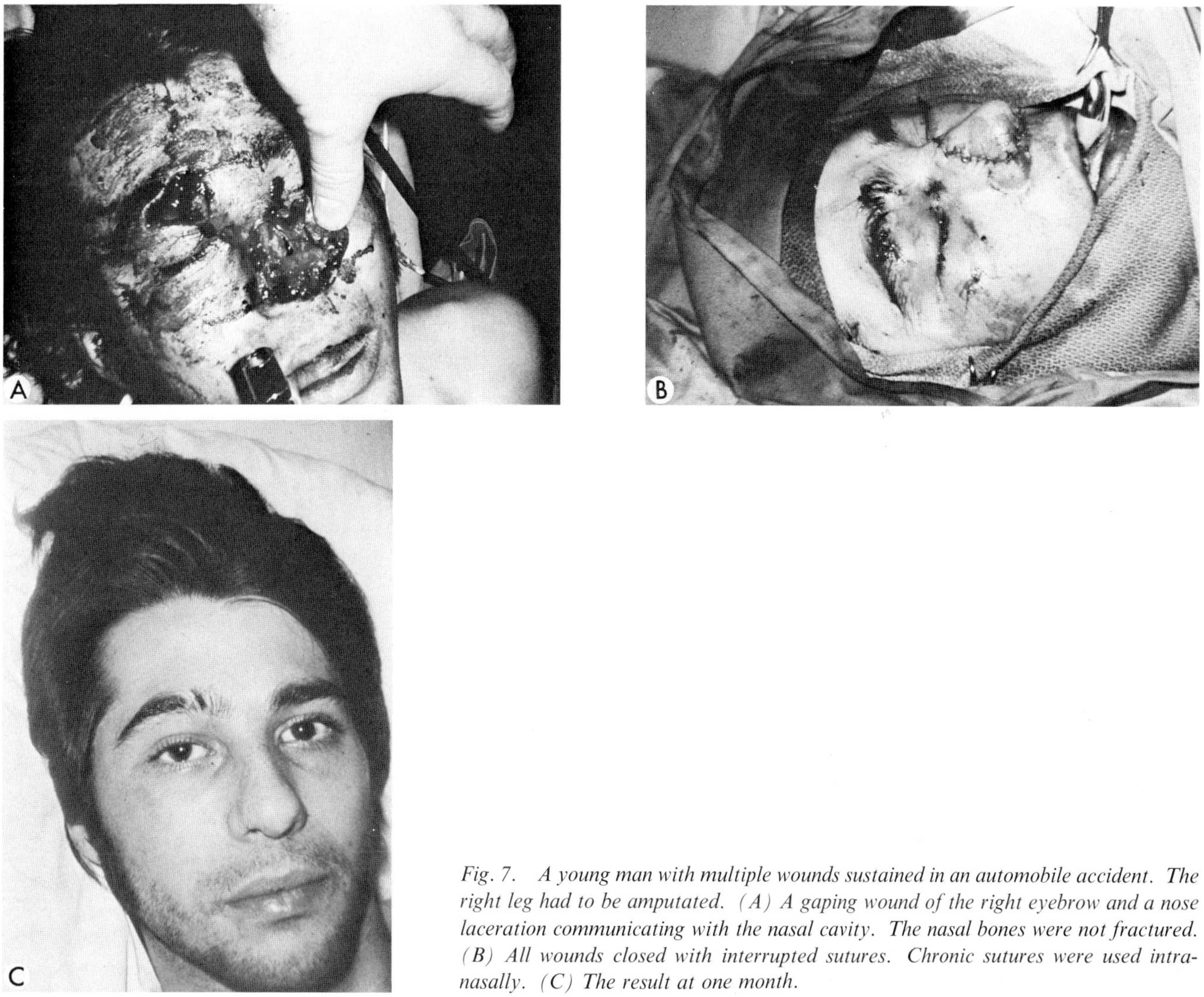

Fig. 7. A young man with multiple wounds sustained in an automobile accident. The right leg had to be amputated. (A) A gaping wound of the right eyebrow and a nose laceration communicating with the nasal cavity. The nasal bones were not fractured. (B) All wounds closed with interrupted sutures. Chronic sutures were used intranasally. (C) The result at one month.

the ends, or the ends may be left free, depending upon wound tension. If the closure is meticulous then later revision is rarely necessary.

Figure 7 shows an unfavorable laceration crossing the nasal dorsum. Careful layered closure and interrupted suture technique yields an acceptable result.

Figure 8 illustrates again the technique of subcuticular closure of an oblique jagged forehead laceration. This closure is reenforced by "double twists" of 5-0 or 6-0 nylon. These simple surgeon's knots are removed on the second postoperative day while the subcuticular sutures are left in for ten days to two weeks depending upon the amount of reaction present.

Figure 9 shows another automobile accident victim with an eyebrow and eyelid laceration. An eyebrow is never shaved because of the possibility of its failure to regrow. These oblique lacerations favor the formation of edema fluid postoperatively and this stays until the lymphatic circulation reestablishes itself. Note in the four month picture that the eyebrow, although not shaved, has now become sparse and will take another two to three months to regrow to normal.

These wounds must go through the natural sequences of wound healing that apply to lacerations or surgical incisions anywhere on the body. The first few weeks the scars become hypertrophic, red, and indurated. Gradually, as the months pass,

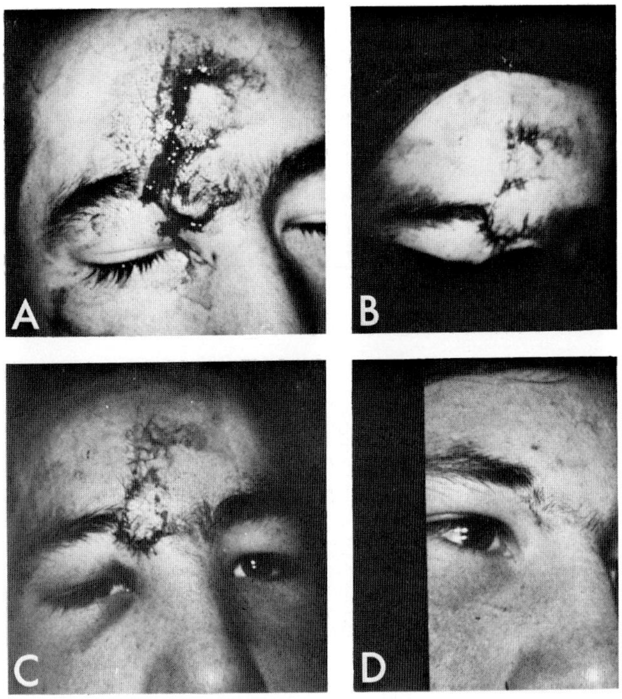

Fig. 8. See text for details. (D) Seven weeks post injury.

the scar becomes softer, more pale, and gradually involutes. It is rarely advisable to revise a scar before a year, and even more rare to revise one before six months. An exception to this rule is shown in Figure 10. This illustrates the problem of the tiny trapdoor laceration. This type of flap stays edematous for a prolonged period. If not significantly improved six months after the injury, I then excise the scar converting it to a linear closure.

Figure 11 demonstrates primary closure of a wound with significant loss of tissue. This too was the result of an automobile accident. Figure 1B illustrates rotation and advancement of local tissue. Antibiotic ointment appears to facilitate healing. The four month follow-up picture demonstrates the excellent result obtained by using local tissue.

Figure 12 demonstrates a dog bite. Vigorous cleaning under local anesthesia preceded the subcuticular closure shown in Figure 12B. This was reenforced with interrupted sutures which were removed in the office three days later (Fig. 12C).

Figure 13 illustrates another dog bite with significant loss of tissue. Although one-quarter to one-third of the lower lip was lost, primary closure was obtained (Fig. 13B). The child returned two days later as shown in Figure 13C. He fell off a swing and broke open the repair. Primary closure was again performed, this time reenforced with micropore tape, and the six month results are shown in Figure 13F and G.

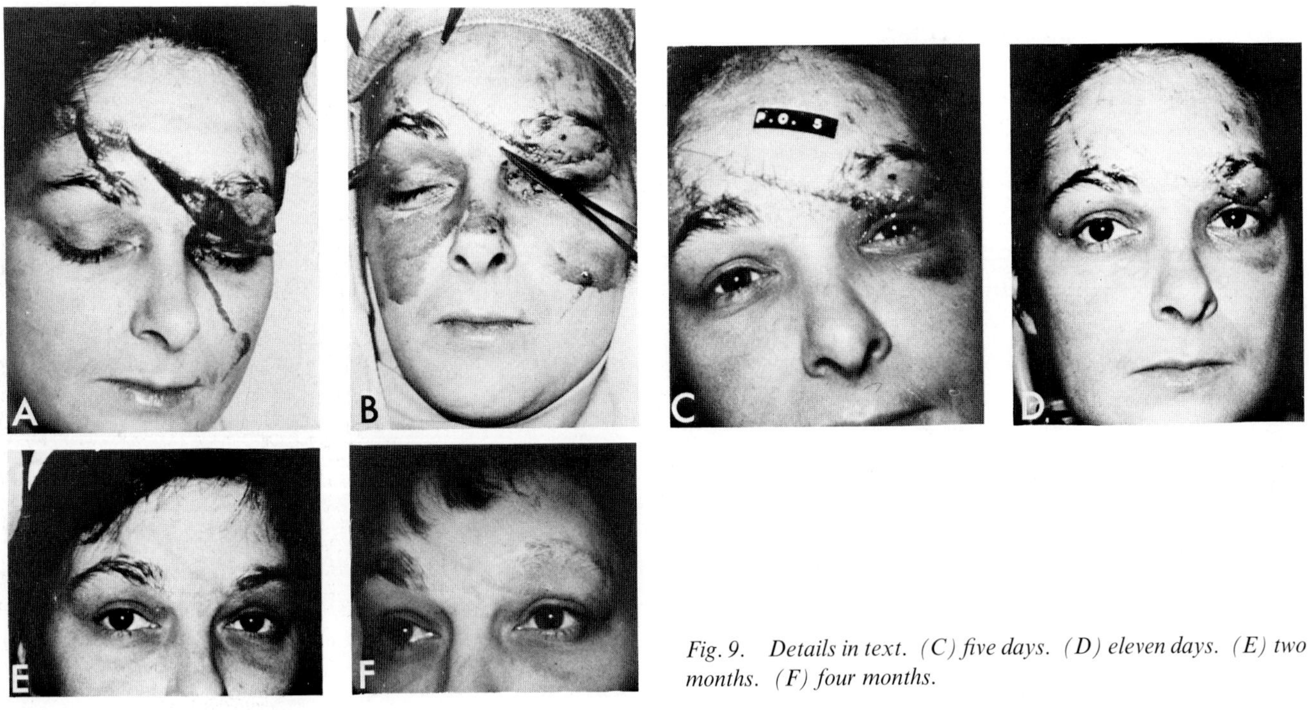

Fig. 9. Details in text. (C) five days. (D) eleven days. (E) two months. (F) four months.

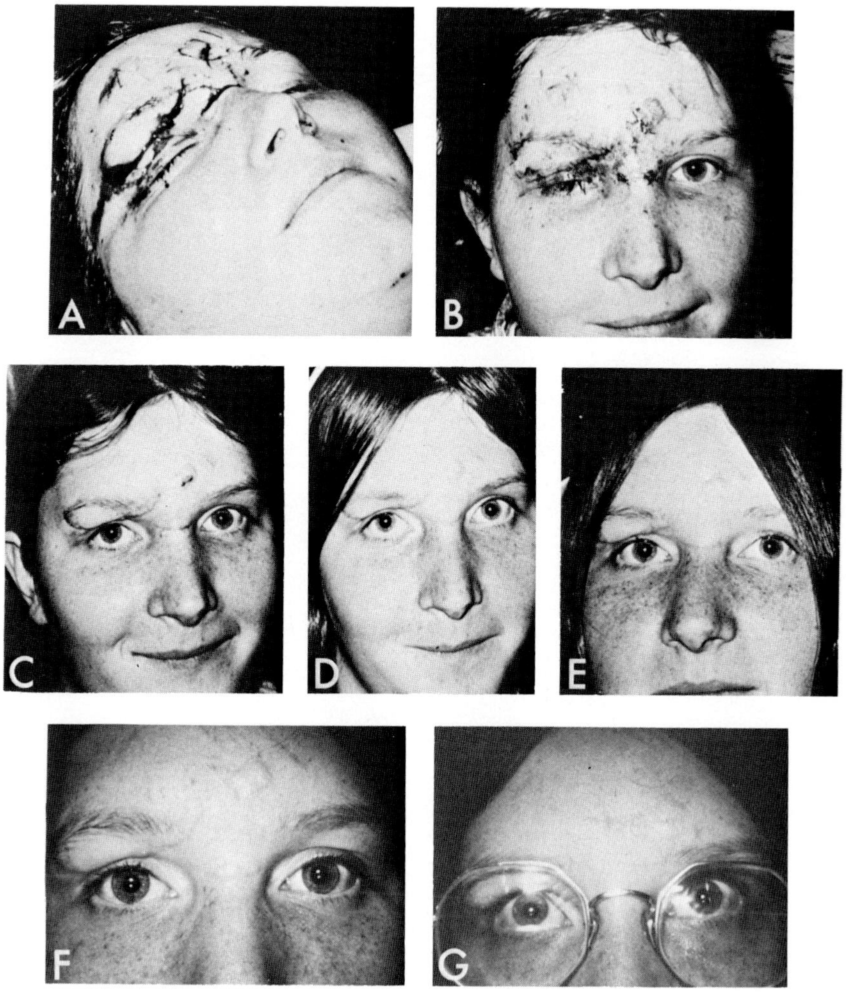

Fig. 10. Injuries sustained in automobile accident. (C) two weeks. (D) seven weeks. (E) three months. (F) six months, patient admitted for revision of "trapdoor". (G) six weeks post-revision.

Figure 14 shows a four-year-old boy whose face was bitten by a horse. His maternal grandfather was "a bleeder." This boy "perhaps bruised easily" but was not thought to be a bleeder. In fact another otolaryngologist had him scheduled for an adenoidectomy two weeks hence. A standard bleeding profile was drawn in the emergency room and every parameter was two or three seconds prolonged. With the reassurance of the hematology consult, the child was taken to the operating room where primary closure was performed. Half-way through the second wound, profuse bleeding followed every needle insertion. Fresh frozen plasma did not prevent a significant hematoma. Postoperative investigation revealed a classic Factor VIII deficiency. The resultant scar-distortion is shown in Figure 14D. Needless to say the adenoidectomy was cancelled.

Shakespeare wrote, "What wound did ever heal but by degrees?"[2] The productive, collagen, and maturation phases characterize the healing of all wounds. The described techniques of careful cleansing, delicate handling, preservation of tissue, and meticulous closure, combined with the rich vascular supply of these tissues, should result in fine, thin, cosmetically acceptable scars.

References

1. McGregor IA: Fundamental techniques of plastic surgery: Edenburgh and London, Churchill Livingstone, 5th edition, 1972
2. Othello II, iii, 377

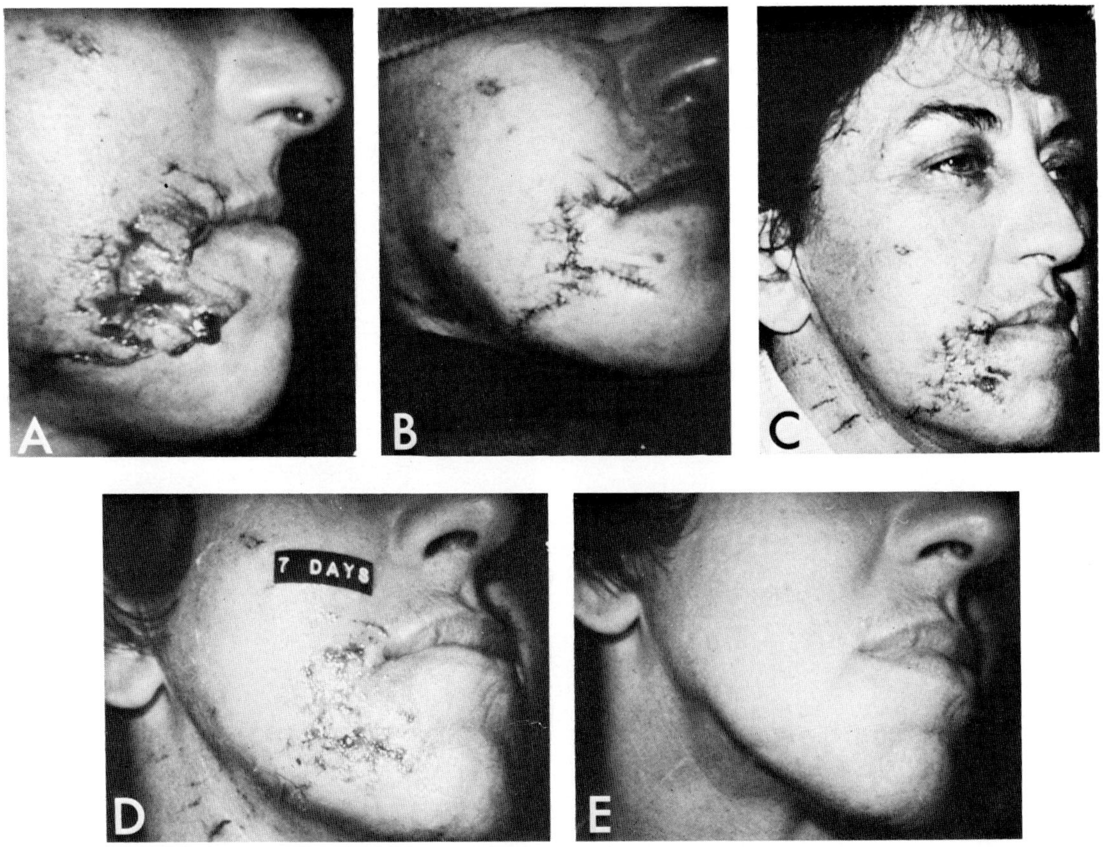

Fig. 11. Details in text. (C) four days. (D) seven days. (E) four months.

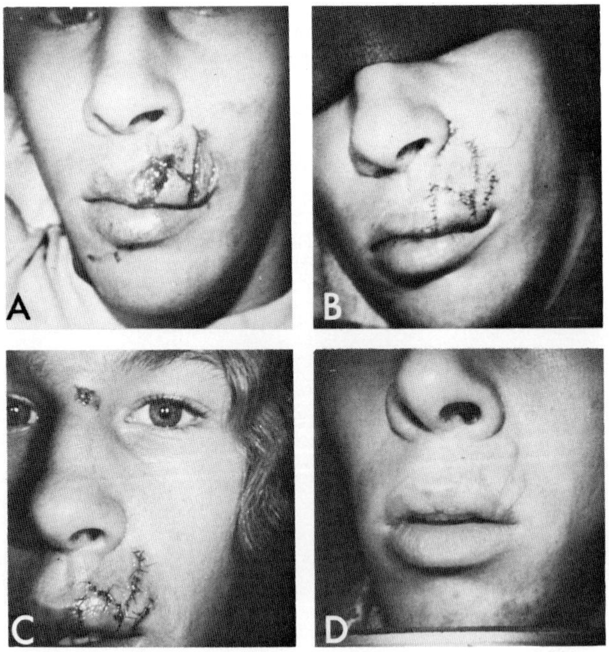

Fig. 12. Dog bite. (C) three days. (D) three weeks.

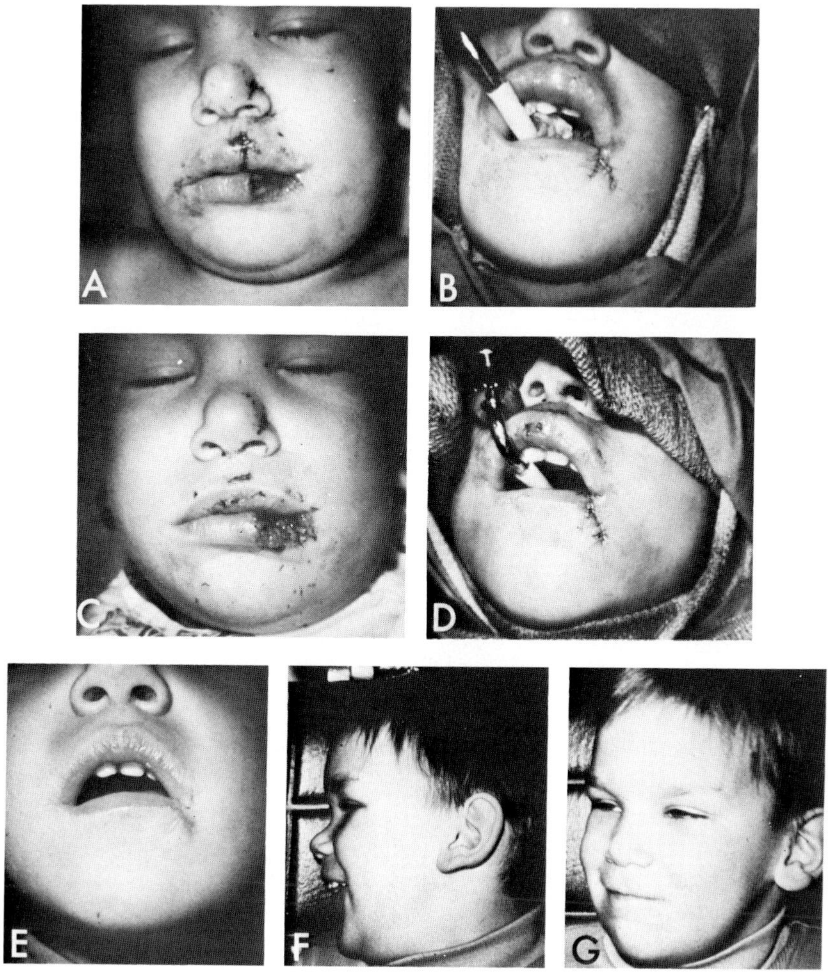

Fig. 13. Dog bite with loss of approximately one-fourth of lower lip. (B) Primary closure. (C) Wound broken open two days later when child fell off swing. (D) Reclosure. (E) One month. (F,G) six months.

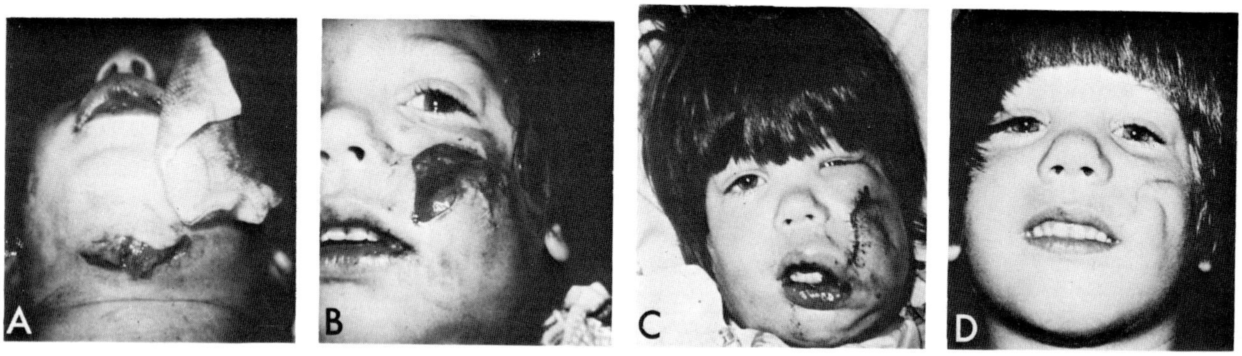

Fig. 14. Horse bite in undiagnosed hemophiliac. (A,B) Wound in emergency room 2 h after injury. (C) Second postoperative day. (D) Three months postop.

Rotational Flap for Neck Dissection and Cervical or Facial Skin Replacement

Ray Smith, Oklahoma City, Oklahoma

Extension of primary or metastatic cancer to facial or cervical skin necessitates excision of the involved area and some surrounding normal skin to provide an optimal chance for cure. Small defects often can be closed by simple advancement of adjacent skin; however, larger defects often require a skin graft or a flap to achieve primary repair. If the extirpative procedure includes a radical neck dissection, as is almost always the case when cervical skin is removed, a flap is employed to provide adequate carotid artery protection. When other considerations outweigh cosmesis, excised facial skin can be replaced with split thickness skin unless bone is exposed, under which circumstances more substantial coverage is desirable. When flaps have been utilized to replace facial or cervical skin, patients have usually faced the expense and inconvenience of multistaged procedures.

In 1970, Nickell et al,[1] described a large rotational flap that was employed in conjunction with a horizontal "T" incision to allow performance of a radical neck dissection and the primary replacement of excised cervical skin. Smith et al[2] later reported the use of a modified Schobinger incision and a large rotational flap to permit replacement of facial skin after excision of a parotid tumor in combination with neck dissection. We have now used large rotational flaps to replace facial skin in five patients and to repair cervical defects in six patients. Colleagues have told me of two additional cases in which the flap was employed to provide facial skin coverage.

Surgical Technique

When using the rotational flap to replace facial skin in combination with neck dissection, the Babcock and Conley[3] modification of the Schobinger[4] incision has been employed. The horizontal "T" incision, described by Nickell et al,[1] is favored when a cervical defect is repaired. In either situation the vertical limb of the incision is extended down over the anterior chest to the level of the axilla, after which the incision is curved medially just above the nipple and is continued to the lateral border of the sternum, (Fig. 1). A thoracic defect necessitating a skin graft may remain after rotation of the flap; however, the likelihood of such a defect is decreased if the incision is kept lateral over the superior chest.

The cervical skin can be elevated superficial or deep to the platysma muscle. Toomey and Lell[5] have reported evidence that the chances for cervical flap survival are improved if the platysma layer is retained, but principles of tumor resection may dictate inclusion of the platysma muscle in the neck dissection specimen. The thoracic portion of the flap is elevated deep the fascia overlying the pectoral muscles. Some type of carotid artery protection has been employed in every case.

Blood Supply

The thoracic portion of the large medially based rotational flap receives an excellent blood supply from perforating branches of the internal mammary artery. As described by Calcaterra et al[6] the most constant of these vessels, which emerge about one centimeter lateral to the lateral border of the sternum, are those in the second and third intercostal spaces. Superiorly, the flap derives nutrition from vessels crossing from the opposite side of the neck; however, recent studies have demonstrated that this horizontal blood supply is less than one

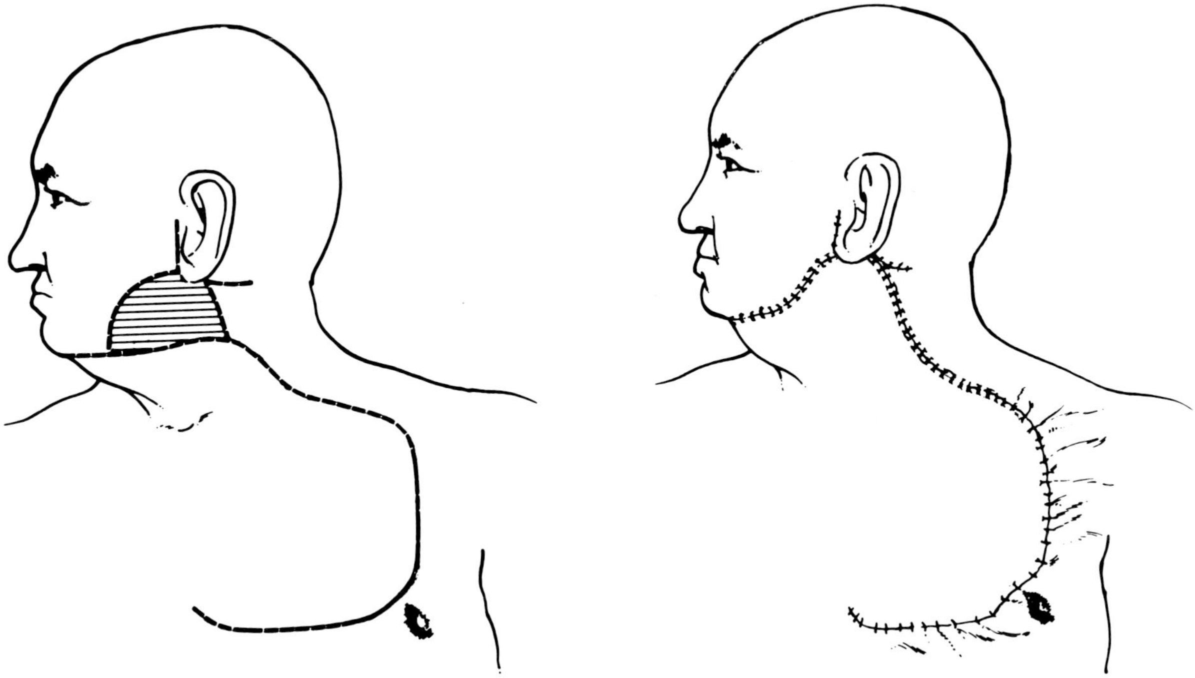

Fig. 1. *(Left) Flap design for neck dissection and rotation into 6 cm facial defect. (Right) Flap rotated superiorly. (Reproduced with permission of Arch Otolaryngol from Arch Otolaryngol 99: 122–124, February, 1974.)*

might expect.[7] Branches from the thoracoacromial artery are severed during elevation of the thoracic portion of the flap.

Clinical Material

The cases reviewed include 11 patients treated by the author and residents from The University of Oklahoma Health Sciences Center and from The University of Florida College of Medicine, Otolaryngology programs. Two additional patients, who were treated by Dr. Phillip Andrews, Fort Myers, Florida, and by Dr. Layton Runkle, Norman, Oklahoma, are also included.

Results

Individual cases are reviewed in Tables 1 and 2. Of the seven flaps that were used to repair facial defects, three healed with no tissue loss. Two patients developed superficial skin necrosis of the distal 2 cm of their flaps, but the defects healed without additional reconstructive procedures. Full thickness loss of the superior 5 cm of the flaps occurred in two cases.

One patient in whom the flap failed was a 74-year-old female with squamous cell carcinoma of the buccogingival sulcus that extended through the external skin. Resection of the tumor created a large full thickness cheek defect that was repaired with a forehead flap to line the oral cavity and the cervical rotational flap that was advanced 7 cm to provide external coverage. Following debridement of the necrotic flap, the remaining defect was covered with a split thickness skin graft, providing satisfactory coverage but poor cosmesis (Fig. 2). Although this patient had a tracheotomy, every effort was made, including suturing the tube to the skin, to prevent pressure on the flap from the tracheotomy tube tapes. Since the wound was not infected, the best explanation for failure of the flap was that too large a flap was elevated in too superficial a plane for the available blood supply in this elderly lady.

The other failure occurred in an 81-year-old male with a previously irradiated squamous cell carcinoma of the parotid gland that extended through the skin. The superior 5 cm of a flap that

Table 1. Rotational flaps for cervical defects.

LARGE ROTATIONAL FLAPS

Cervical Defects:

	PATIENT	AGE	DIAGNOSIS	PRIOR RT.	PLATYSMA WITH FLAP	DISTANCE ADVANCED	RESULT	STATUS LOCAL DISEASE	PATIENT STATUS	COMMENT
1.	A. G.	80	Metastatic squamous cell Ca. (LARYNX)	No	Yes	8 c.m.	No tissue loss	Controlled	NED - * 33 Mo.	
2.	J. N.	54	Metastatic squamous cell Ca. (PHARYNX)	Yes	Yes	5 c.m.	No tissue loss	Tumor in Jugular Foramen at surgery	Dead of Disease 12 Mo. Post-Op	
3.	R. G.	71	Metastatic squamous cell Ca. (TONSIL)	Yes	Yes	5 c.m.	Primary Healing	Unknown	Dead of metastasis 10 Mo. Post-Op	Fell 2 weeks after discharge - superior incision separated.
4.	H. S.	63	Metastatic squamous cell Ca. (LIP)	No	Lower Flap Only	5 c.m.	No tissue loss	Controlled	NED 1 Yr.	
5.	C. S.	52	Metastatic Papillary Ca. (THYROID)	No	Yes	4 c.m.	No tissue loss	Controlled	NED 1 Yr.	
6.	D. H.	54	Metastatic squamous cell Ca. (MAXILLARY SINUS)	No	Yes	4 c.m.	1 c.m. superior loss	Tumor to base of skull at surgery.	NED 1 Yr.	Patient considered alive with disease without visible tumor at present.

* NED - No Evidence of Disease.

Table 2. Rotational flaps for facial defects.

Facial Defects:

	PATIENT	AGE	DIAGNOSIS	PRIOR RT.	PLATYSMA WITH FLAP	DISTANCE ADVANCED	RESULT	STATUS LOCAL DISEASE	PATIENT STATUS	COMMENT
7.	T. W.	61	Recurrant mucoepedermoid Ca. (PAROTID)	Yes	Yes	7 c.m.	No tissue loss	Local Control	Dead of Disease 28 Mo. Post - Op	Died of intra-cranial metastasis
8.	L. H.	55	Metastatic melanoma (PAROTID NODES)	No	No	6 c.m.	No tissue loss	Controlled	Died of brain metastasis 3 Mo. Post - Op	
9.	F. C.	74	Squamous cell Ca. (BUCCO-GINGIVAL SULCUS)	No	No	7 c.m.	Failure necrosis superior 5 c.m.	Local Recurrance	Dead of Disease 12 Mo. Post - Op	
10.	W.M.	60	Recurrant melanoma (PREAURICULAR SKIN)	No	No	10 c.m.	Superficial skin loss superior 2 c.m.	Controlled	NED - 7 Mo.	
11.	J. M.	81	Squamous Cell Ca. (PAROTID) Persistent Post RT.	Yes	Lower Only	7 c.m.	Failure necrosis superior 5 c.m.	Post-Operative death- 23 days	Post-Operative death - 23 days	Cause of death bronchopneumonia, chronic obstructive lung disease, old tuberculosis.
12.	R. C.	71	Mucoepidermoid Ca. (PAROTID)	No	Yes	10 c.m.	Superficial skin necrosis superior 2 c.m.	Controlled	NED - 9 Mo.	Patient treated by Phillip Andrews, M.D.
13.	R. M.	70	Metastatic Melanoma (PAROTID NODES)	No	No	6 c.m.	No tissue loss	Controlled	NED 9 Mo.	Patient treated by Layton Runkle, M.D

* NED - No Evidence of Disease

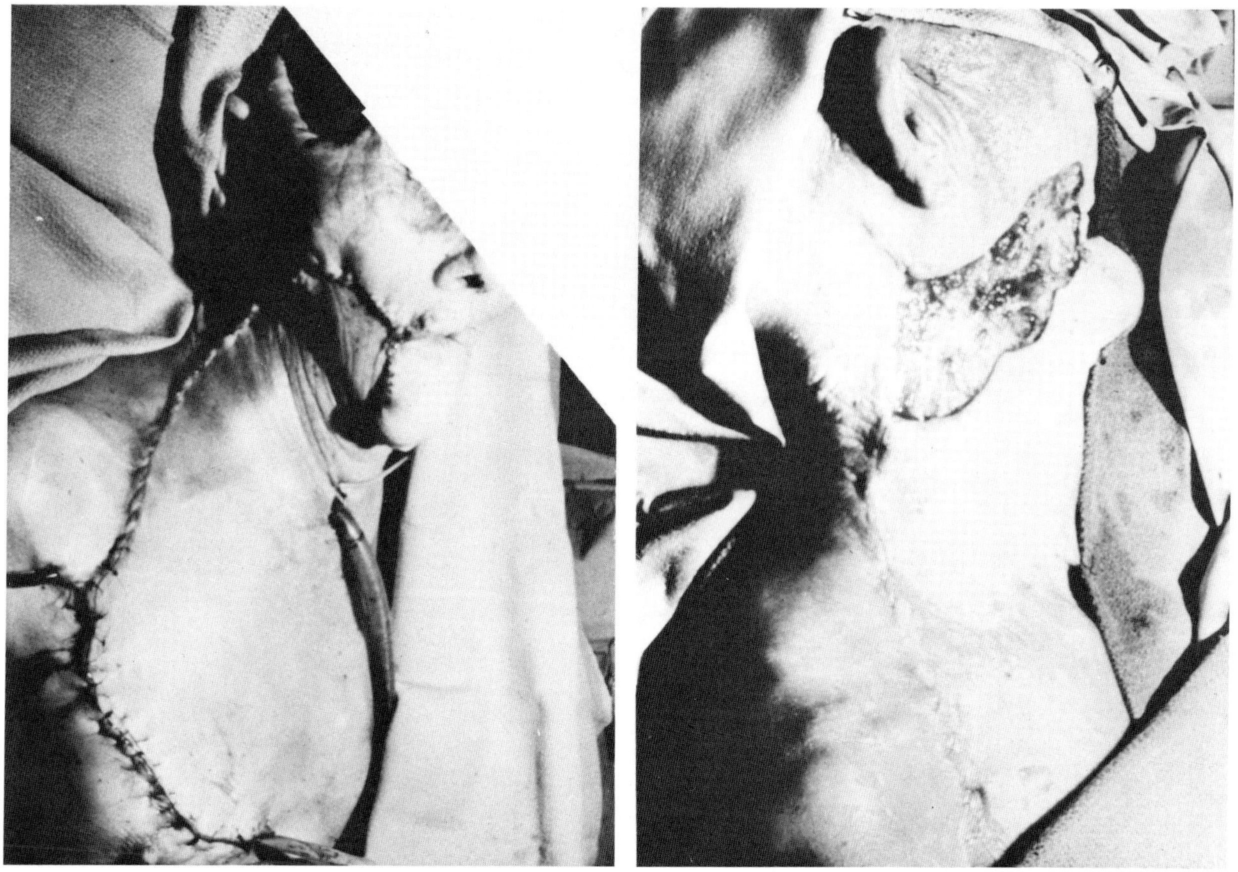

Fig. 2. Flap Failure. Patient number 9, Table 2. (Left) Flap advanced 7 cm superiorly and anteriorly to oral commissure. (Right) Defect after debridment of necrotic superior 5 cm of flap.

was advanced upward into a 7 cm defect necrosed. Again, inadequate flap nutrition rather than infection or some other cause appeared responsible for loss of the flap. This patient died of pulmonary complications on the twenty-third postoperative day.

Both facial flaps that developed superficial skin necrosis were advanced 10 cm superiorly. One flap was elevated superficial and one deep to the platysma muscle (Figs. 3 and 4).

Primary healing occurred in all but one of the patients in whom the flap was used to replace cervical skin (Fig. 5). Necrosis of the superior 1 cm of a flap that was elevated 5 cm to the mastoid tip occurred in a 54-year-old female who developed a cervical metastasis from a maxillary sinus squamous cell carcinoma. This patient had received prior radiation therapy to the superior neck. The defect that remained after debridement of the necrotic tissue slowly healed and necessitated no additional reconstructive procedures. Another patient (71-year-old female) whose flap appeared to be healing well after a radical neck dissection fell one week after discharge from the hospital and had separation of the suture line along the superior border of the flap. Healing of the resultant raw area was extremely slow, and the defect eventually was covered with split thickness skin. This elderly lady had received prior radiation therapy and also presented nutritional problems because of difficulty swallowing after sacrifice of the hypoglossal nerve.

In summary, seven patients' flaps healed primarily with no complications. Three flaps displayed some necrosis but healed without additional procedures. One patient had separation of an apparently healing suture line after trauma, causing a defect that was closed with a small split thickness skin graft. Two flaps were total failures.

The short follow-up period does not permit any conclusions in regard to the curability of this diverse

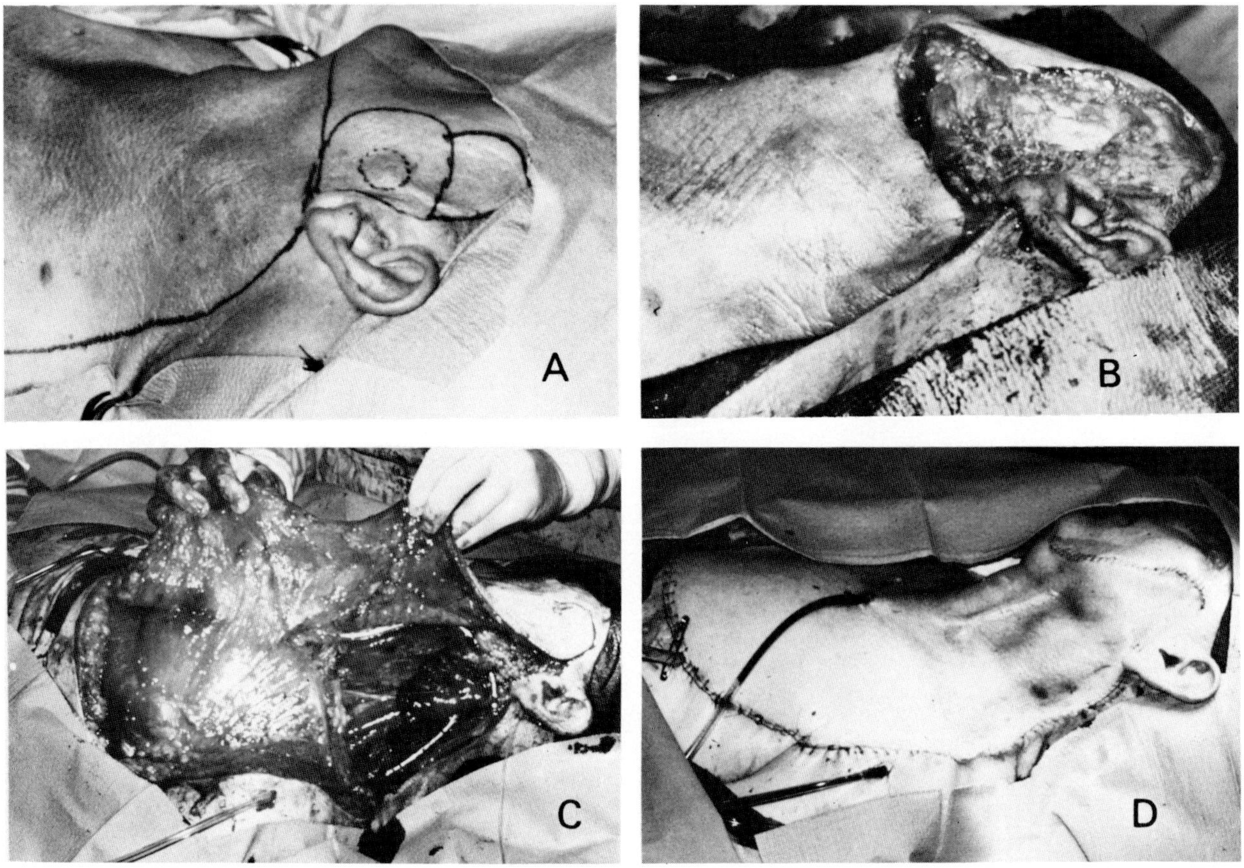

Fig. 3. Patient number 10, Table 2. (A) Planned incisions marked. (B) 10 cm defect after excision of melanoma, underlying parotid gland and prior skin graft. (C) Flap elevated and superior portion sutured into defect. (D) Flap sutured in place.

group of patients; however, a perusal of the tables does indicate an overall poor prognosis for these patients with tumor adjacent to or extending through the skin. Only seven of the thirteen patients are still alive and one of them almost certainly has persistent tumor.

Comments

Although experience with this flap has increased, only impressions rather than conclusions can be drawn from these few cases. The rotational flap as described by Nickell et al[1] for the replacement of cervical skin appears to be a fairly reliable flap that can be advanced up to 9 cm superiorly. Necrosis of the posterior superior (distal) portion of one flap that was advanced to a higher position than most, is not surprising. Babcock and Conley[3] reported some necrosis of the same area in 11 of 50 patients in whom they used an anteriorly based cervical flap for neck dissection. Carotid artery exposure did not occur in our patient nor in those reported by Babcock and Conley; however, we have elected to cover the carotid artery with levator scapulae muscle or dermis in every case.

As might be expected, the rotational flap has proved less reliable for the repair of facial defects than for cervical ones. Levator scapulae muscle overlying the carotid artery was exposed in one patient in whom the flap failed, accentuating the need for carotid protection in these patients. Although some superficial necrosis occurred in two patients, the resulting cosmesis was similar to what would be anticipated with a split thickness skin graft.

When the flap has been rotated into a facial defect, it has appeared that a portion of the posterior neck would not be covered. We have been able

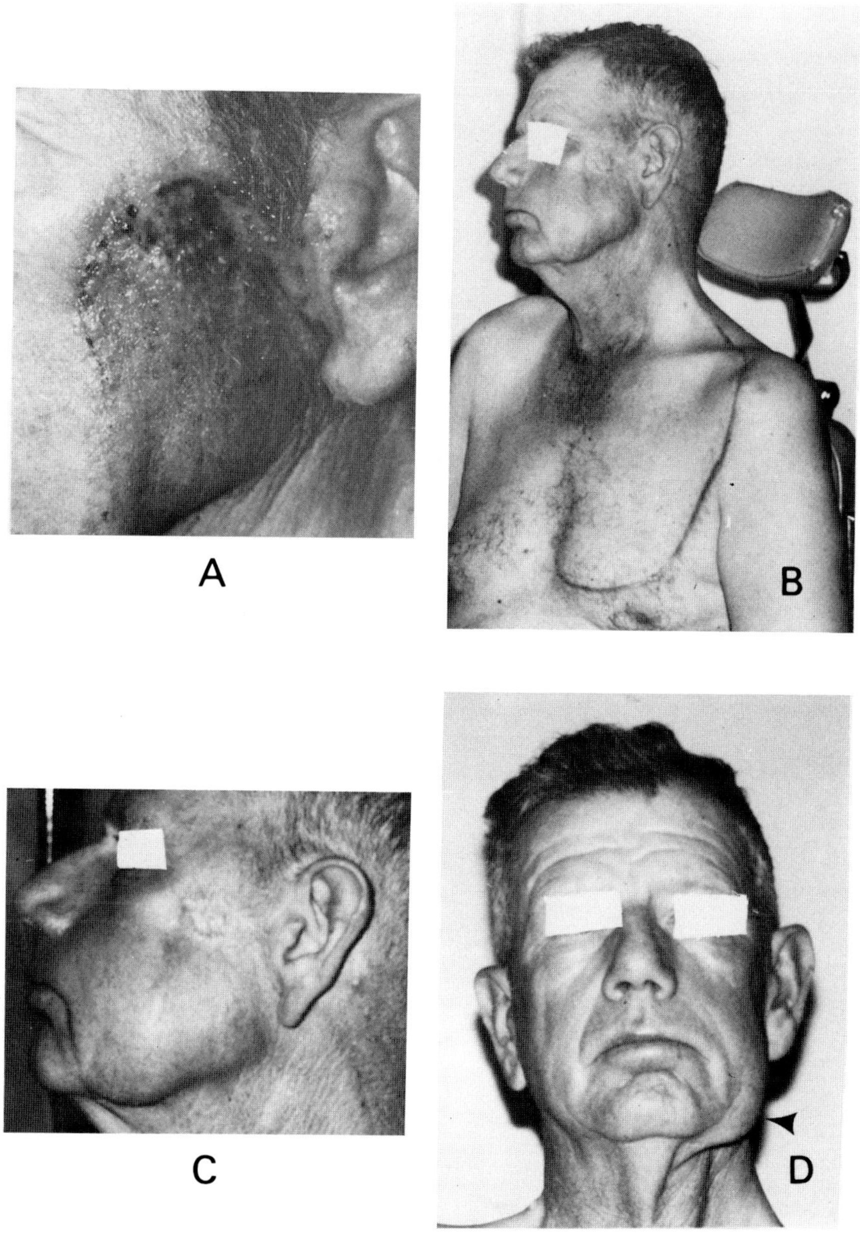

Fig. 4. Same patient as in Figure 3. (A) Early superficial skin necrosis (seventh postoperative day) of superior 2 cm of flap. (B) Healed flap 8 weeks after surgery. (C) Contracture of superior portion of flap. (D) Bunching of tissue over mandible (arrow) just anterior to healed flap.

to close this potential defect by advancing skin posterior to the neck dissection.

The obvious major advantage of the large rotational flap for facial or cervical skin replacement is the availability of a relatively simple one-stage procedure to repair fairly large defects. A disadvantage that deserves consideration is that one has eliminated the possibility of using a medially based deltopectoral (Bakamjian) flap on the same side.

As with other cervical skin flaps, the large rotational flap is not as sturdy as the commonly employed chest flaps. Advancement of the flap more than 7 cm superiorly, prior radiation therapy, physiologic advanced age, and elevation superficial to the platysma muscle all appear to tax the flap's viability. The flap can be used with reasonable assurance to replace cervical skin and provides a useful technique for the repair of some facial defects. When using the flap, particularly when advancing it onto the face, the surgeon must remain aware of the decreased predictability of cervical skin flaps and of the possible need for an alternative plan.

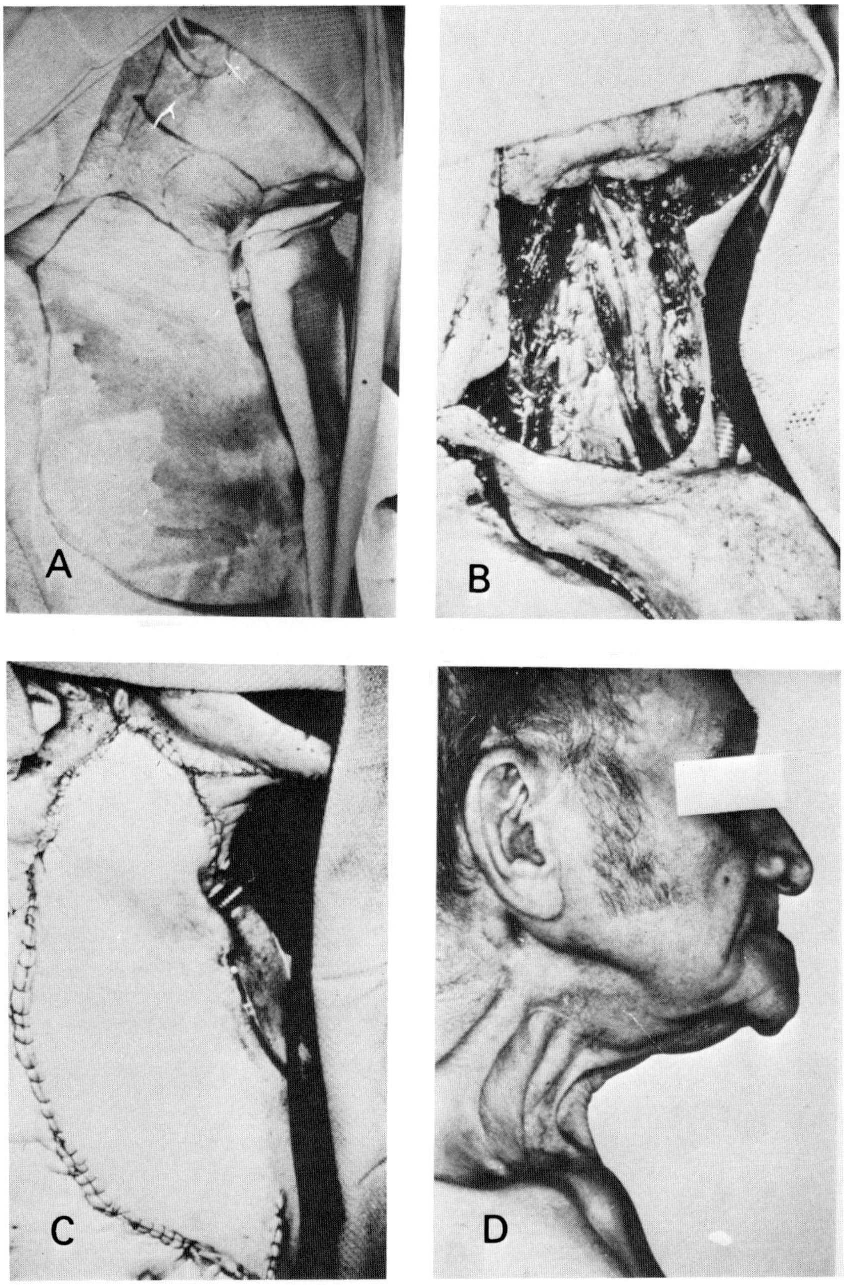

Fig. 5. Patient number 1, Table 1. (A) Planned incisions for flap and removal of involved skin. (B) Defect after neck dissection. (C) Flap sutured in place. (D) Healed flap, six months after neck dissection.

References

1. Nickell WB, Furlow LT Jr, Jurkiewicz MJ, Herrero FA: Multipurpose flaps for primary reconstruction of large head and neck defects. South Med J 63:297–300, 1970
2. Smith R, Black FO, Teachey WS: Large rotational flap for neck dissection and facial skin replacement. Arch Otolaryngol 99:122–124, 1974
3. Babcock WW Jr, Conley J: Neck incision in block dissection. Arch Otolaryngol 84:554–557, 1966
4. Schobinger R: The use of a long anterior skin flap in radical neck resections. Ann Surg 146:221–223, 1957
5. Toomey JM, Lell W: The roll of platysma in the survival of cervical skin flaps, in Conley J, Dickinson JT (eds): Plastic and reconstructive surgery of the face and neck, New York, Grune and Stratton, 1972, pp 129–131
6. Calcaterra TC, Cherney EF, Saffouri M: Cutaneous vascular anatomy of pectoral skin flaps. Ann Otol 82:691–695, 1973
7. Hetter GP: Neck incisions relative to the cutaneous vasculature of the neck. Arch Otolaryngol 95:84–87, 1972

Facial Paralysis: Principles of Intratemporal Surgical Management

Malcolm D. Graham, Los Angeles, Calif.*

Contemporary surgical exposure of the facial nerve has as its aims adequate exposure of the facial nerve at any point in its course, with preservation of hearing and vestibular function, without further injury to the facial nerve and the necessity for producing a mastoid cavity. Today it is surgically possible to expose the facial nerve from the brainstem to its terminal branches in the face. A decade of experience has shown that if the operator is armed with intimate anatomical knowledge of the temporal bone and middle and posterior fossas, and if the principles of facial nerve surgery outlined are meticulously adhered to, these aims may be accomplished.

A system of surgery will be described in detail with discussion of the advantages, disadvantages, and techniques of operation. By utilizing the appropriate procedure of combination of procedures, the otologic surgeon will realize his goals of predictable and safe surgical exposure of the facial nerve.

Principles of Facial Nerve Surgery

Knowledge of Anatomy

It is imperative that the surgeon contemplating partial or total exposure of the facial nerve be familiar with the course of the nerve throughout its intratemporal course. The facial nerve in its vertical, or mastoid, segment is familiar to most surgeons experienced in surgery for chronic ear disease and the horizontal, or intratympanic, portion is to those performing stapedectomy. However, to obtain satisfactory exposure with the preservation of function, extended study and dissection in the temporal bone dissection laboratory are required.

Facility with Microscopic and Drill Techniques

For surgery to be successful within the confines of the temporal bone, magnification as provided by the Zeiss surgical microscope is of extreme importance. Facility with varying magnifications and knowledge of drilling techniques and various drill motor capacities are essential. Experience with their use and knowledge of the capabilities, hazards, and advantages of cutting and diamond drills are imperative.

Experience with Suction Irrigation

In order to successfully operate upon bone adjacent to the facial nerve sheath as well as to preserve vital structures of the labyrinth, continuous suction irrigation is essential not only for cleansing of the operative field of blood, bone chips, and bone dust, but also to keep the operative field cool and thereby preserve the facial nerve and adjacent structures from inevitable heat damage.

Experience in Intracranial Neuro-otologic Surgery

As described later, when employing the middle cranial fossa, translabyrinthine, or retrolabyrinthine surgical approach to the facial nerve, it is obvious that the middle and posterior cranial fossa areas are invaded. Therefore, detailed knowledge of the anatomy for these areas is imperative prior to contemplating surgery on the facial nerve in these areas. Should bleeding occur, the surgeon must be totally familiar with methods of clipping, packing, and electrocoagulation in order to safely conclude the operation. Cerebrospinal fluid escape

* Sponsored by the Otologic Medical Group, Inc., and the Ear Research Institute, Los Angeles, California.

at the termination of the procedure must be controlled and effective methods must be fully understood.

It is essential, therefore, for the surgeon contemplating extensive exposures of the facial nerve to be fully conversant with otologic and neuro-otologic surgery. This can only be gained by repeated dissections in the temporal bone dissection laboratory and continuing experience in surgery of the temporal bone.

Structures at Risk

In addition to an appreciation of the course of the facial nerve within the temporal bone, a full understanding is required of all structures within or adjacent to the temporal bone.

Auditory System

The ossicles so intimately related to the tympanic portion of the facial nerve may easily be dislocated or traumatized in exposing the facial recess or during the actual decompression of the facial nerve. Should the drill contact the intact and mobile ossicular chain, the vibrations may result in a significant and irreversible sensorineural hearing loss. Likewise, following entry into the perilymphatic spaces of the cochlea by instruments or during removal of areas of bone erosion and fistulization, serious loss of cochlear function may result.

Vestibular System

As in the cochlea, invasion of the semicircular canals or vestibule may produce not only disturbances of balance but serious sensorineural hearing loss as a result of instrumentation or during removal of diseased tissue involving or adjacent to the facial nerve.

Jugular Bulb

As has been recently emphasized,[1] the jugular bulb may be at risk in any surgical procedure involving the temporal bone, particularly when one is proceeding medial to the plane of the mastoid segment of the facial nerve. The jugular bulb may ascend high and medial to the facial nerve, and occasionally up to the level of the inferior crus of the posterior semicircular canal or even directly underneath the internal auditory canal. Should this structure be injured during surgery upon the facial nerve, profuse venous bleeding is inevitable. If bleeding is not readily controllable by extraluminal packing, more definitive control will be required, necessitating proximal extradural packing of the sigmoid sinus and distal ligation of the internal jugular vein. Such action will decrease the amount of bleeding and also prevent central propagation of thrombosis or the packing used to occlude the jugular bulb.

Constant awareness and utilization of the diamond drill and suction irrigation when in close proximity to the jugular bulb usually prevent this serious complication.

Sigmoid Sinus

Constant awareness of the possibility of variations in the location of the sigmoid sinus usually insures against inadvertent damage to this structure. It must be appreciated that the sigmoid sinus may be superficial under the mastoid cortex or deep if pneumatic air cells pass lateral to this structure, or it may lie far anteriorly, almost adjacent to the posterior wall of the external auditory canal. With constant suction irrigation and awareness of these variations it will usually be possible to avoid this structure even while skeletonizing it in order to allow deeper entry into the mastoid segment. Should bleeding occur, the management would be identical with that previously described for control of bleeding from the jugular bulb.

Dura

Both the middle and posterior fossa dura may be encountered during surgery upon the facial nerve. Even with the use of constant suction irrigation the cutting drill will tear the dura and probably result in cerebrospinal fluid leak and prolapse or herniation of the cerebellum or temporal lobe. Therefore, care must be exercised in approaching these rather substantial linings of the intracranial fossae. If the diamond drill is used with constant suction irrigation, tearing can usually be avoided.

Leakage of cerebrospinal fluid may be controlled by extradural packing with muscle or

Surgicel. The dural will tolerate electrocoagulation, provided the current is at low intensity.

Surgical Technique

Transcanal Transtympanic Approach

The transcanal transtympanic surgical approach performed via either the endaural or the postauricular route offers limited access to the horizontal portion of the facial nerve above the oval window and stapes. Because of the limitations imposed by the size of the external auditory canal, access is necessarily limited and indications are few for exposure of the nerve by this route.

The patient is placed supine on the operating table with the head turned so that the involved ear is uppermost. With the patient under premedication, 1 percent Xylocaine with epinephrine is injected in the routine stapes fashion and a large tympanomeatal flap is elevated. Some posterior superior bony currettage may be performed to afford greater visualization of the facial nerve, and the incus may be extracted to allow visualization of the nerve in this area. Limited decompression may be performed from the geniculate ganglion to the pyramidal eminence. Other surgical procedures upon the facial nerve are not feasible via this limited approach. Prior to replacement of the tympanomeatal flap, the incus is replaced, preferably transposed onto the head of the stapes, since this usually yields better hearing results than replacement in the anatomical position. The tympanomeatal flap is replaced and ointment or packing is placed in the external auditory canal.

Transmastoid Approach

The postauricular transmastoid approach is utilized for surgical exposure of the facial nerve in its entire horizontal and vertical portion from the geniculate ganglion to the stylomastoid foramen. This approach is favored when hearing and balance function are serviceable, for it allows maintenance of the normal anatomy and physiology of the ear.

With the patient under general anesthesia and after the postauricular incision is made in the usual fashion, a complete simple mastoidectomy is performed, the horizontal and posterior semicircular canals, digastric ridge, middle fossa dural plate, sigmoid sinus, and fossa incudis being identified (Fig. 1). The posterior bony canal wall is thinned down and the facial recess developed; this is a triangular area of bone bordered externally by the chorda tympani nerve, medially by the upper half of the descending portion of the facial nerve, and superiorly by the bone that forms the fossa incudis (Fig. 2). When this recess has been opened sufficiently, it is possible to see the pyramidal eminence,

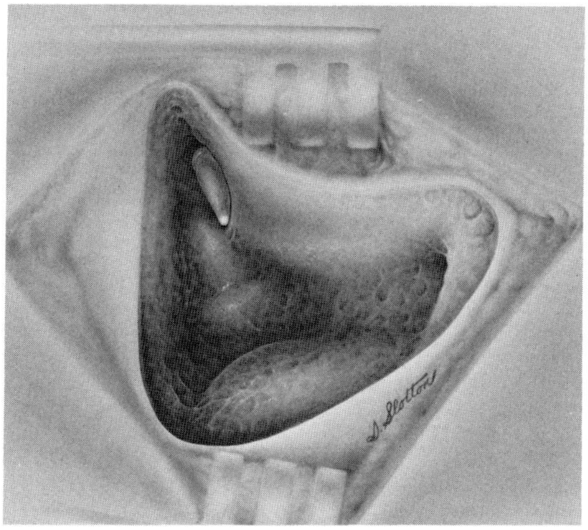

Fig. 1. Transmastoid approach, right ear, surgeon's view. A complete simple mastoidectomy has been performed. The horizontal and posterior semicicular canals, middle fossa dural plate, sigmoid sinus, fossa incudis, and digastric ridge are identified.

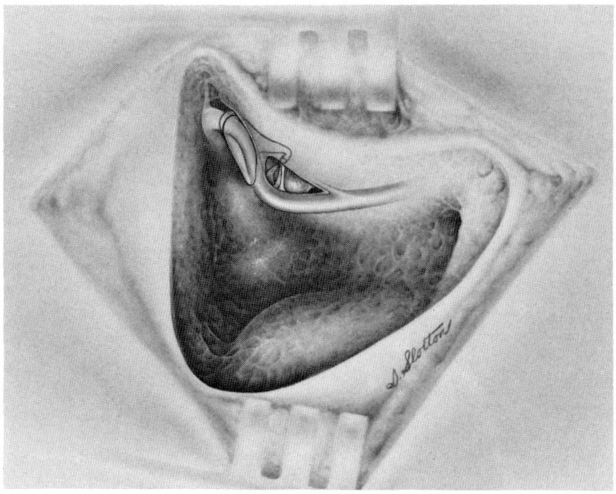

Fig. 2. Transmastoid approach. The posterior bony canal wall is thinned, and the facial recess developed. This is the triangular area of bone bordered externally by the chorda tympani, medially by the upper half of the descending portion of the facial nerve, and superiorly by the bone which forms the fossa incudis.

the oval and round windows, the stapes, and the horizontal process of the facial nerve as far anteriorly as the cochleariform process. Access to the facial nerve between the cochleariform process and the geniculate ganglion is obtained between the body of the incus, the horizontal semicircular canal, and the middle fossa dura superiorly. Care must be taken at this point to identify and preserve the ampullated end of the superior semicircular canal. Once the exposure of the facial nerve has been accomplished, the bone over the entire nerve accessible by this approach is thinned down to eggshell consistency with the diamond drill and constant suction irrigation. In order to gain maximal exposure of the nerve, bone is thinned down anterior and posterior to the nerve in its vertical course so it may be uncapped to its maximal diameter (Fig. 3). This thin bone is then removed with a small

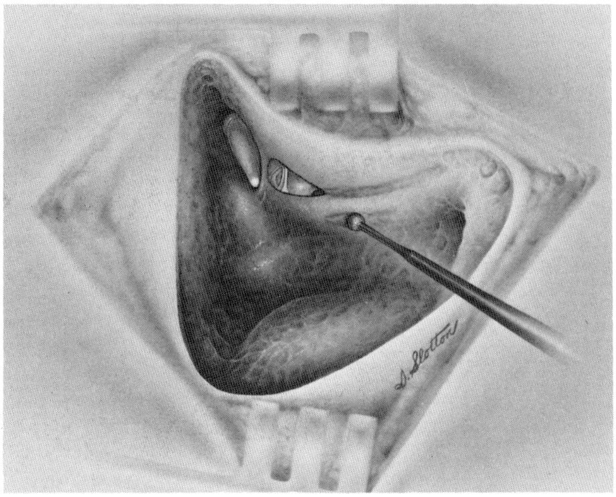

Fig. 3. Transmastoid approach. Once the exposure of the facial nerve has been accomplished, the bone over the entire nerve accessible by this approach is thinned down to eggshell consistency with the diamond drill and constant suction irrigation.

dental excavator or sickle knife in the vertical portion and with a small sickle knife through the facial recess beneath the long process of incus in the horizontal section (Fig. 4).

After complete unroofing of the facial nerve from the geniculate ganglion to the stylomastoid foramen, a Von Grafe cystotome knife is used to open the descending portion of the facial nerve and a Zeigler needle knife to open the sheath of the horizontal and labyrinthine portion of the facial nerve (Fig. 5).

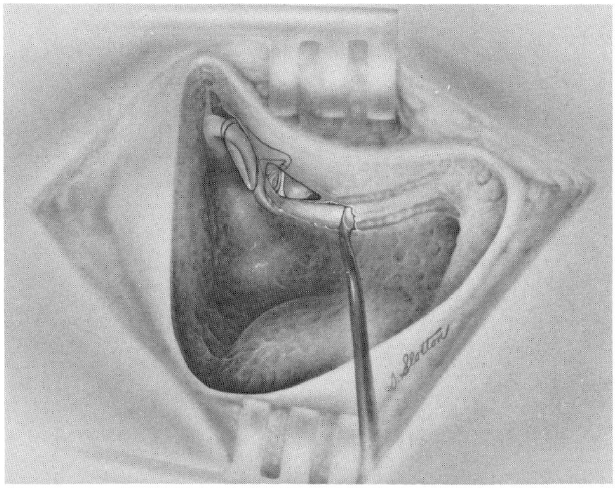

Fig. 4. Transmastoid approach. The thin bone overlying the facial nerve is removed in the horizontal and vertical portion.

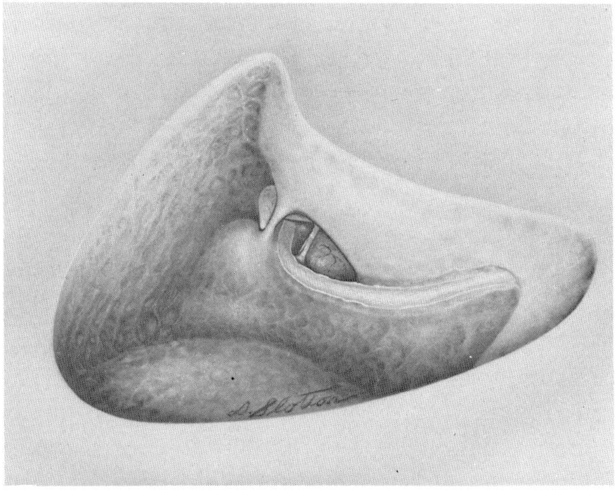

Fig. 5. Transmastoid approach. The facial nerve sheath is incised from the geniculate ganglion proximally to the stylomastoid foramen distally.

Upon completion of the intended procedure upon the facial nerve, the postauricular wound is closed with 3-0 interrupted catgut sutures subcutaneously without drainage.

Middle Cranial Fossa Approach

The middle cranial fossa surgical approach to the facial nerve is indicated for exposure of the facial nerve in its course through the internal auditory canal and labyrinthine portions of the facial nerve. Utilization of this approach is indicated when serviceable hearing and vestibular function is present, and it may be used as the definitive procedure or in combination with the postauricular transmastoid approach for total decompression of the facial nerve.

The patient is placed upon the operating table in a supine position with the head turned slightly away from the side of operation. General anesthesia is employed, a half-head shave is performed, and the area draped. The skin is infiltrated with 1 percent Xylocaine with epinephrine, and an incision is made from approximately 2 cm in front of the tragus of the ear vertically and curving slightly posteriorly to end approximately 4 cm above the superior aspect of the helix. The plane between the skin and the temporalis muscle is developed by blunt dissection; the skin is reflected and held in place with self-retaining retractors. The exposed temporalis muscle is incised in the direction of the fibers, and the attachment of the temporalis muscle and temporalis fascia to the zygomatic arch is incised parallel to the zygomatic arch and at right angles to the direction of the fibers of the temporalis muscle. This maneuver is very important if one is able to obtain access via the subtemporal approach. By limiting the incision to the muscle and fascia at the zygomatic arch, the ascending branch of the facial nerve can be avoided. The temporalis muscle is stripped from the underlying calvarium over an area approximately 4 by 4 cm. A self-retaining retractor is then placed beneath the temporalis muscle, exposing the underlying bone. A rectangular temporal bone flap is removed by use of a dental drill and the microscope (Fig. 6). It is important that the base of the bone flap approximate the level of the floor of the middle cranial fossa. The anterior-posterior dimensions of the bone flap should lie two thirds in front and one third behind the external auditory canal.

Following removal of the temporal bone flap, the dura is exposed and bleeding from the diploic bone of the skull is controlled with bone wax (Fig. 7). Arterial bleeding from branches of the middle meningeal artery coursing over the surface of the dura is controlled by electrocoagulation.

The House-Urban self-retaining dural retractor is inserted between the edges of the craniectomy incision (Fig. 8). The dura is then carefully elevated from the floor of the middle cranial fossa, and the blade of the retractor is placed between the dura and bone floor. In elderly patients the dura may be quite thin and adherent to the bone floor and may be opened, resulting in profuse leakage of

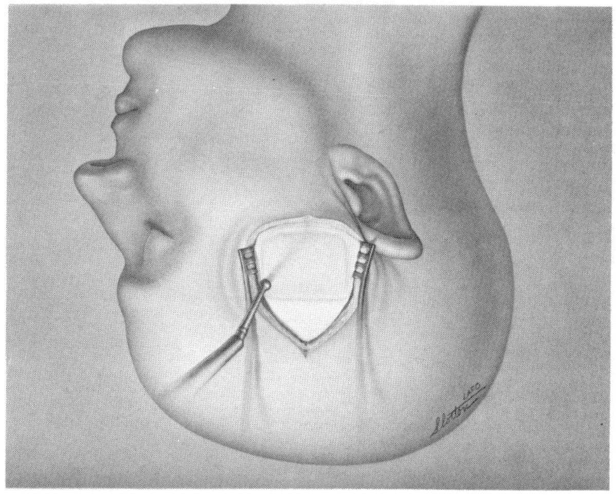

Fig. 6. Middle cranial fossa approach, right ear, surgeon's view. The skin and temporalis muscle are incised vertically and a rectangular temporal bone flap is removed by use of the dental drill and microscope.

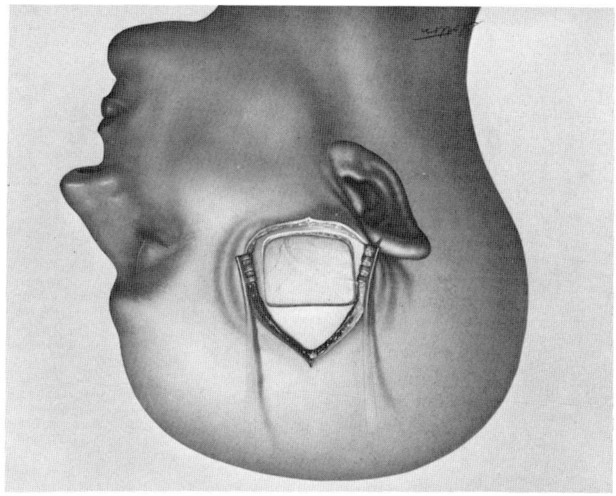

Fig. 7. Middle cranial fossa approach. The anterior posterior dimensions of the bone flap should lie two thirds in front and one third behind the external auditory canal, and the base of the bone flap should approximate the level of the floor of the middle cranial fossa.

cerebrospinal fluid. If this occurs, the opening in the dura is protected by a cottonoid pledget.

The first important landmark that must be identified is the middle meningeal artery (Fig. 9). This artery emerges from the foramen spinosum and is a basic landmark for all middle fossa surgery. Directly medial lies the thin tegmen of the eustachian tube. Lateral to the artery is the roof of the temporomandibular joint. With this focus firmly fixed, dural dissection is carried posteriorly to uncover the arcuate eminence and the ridge of the

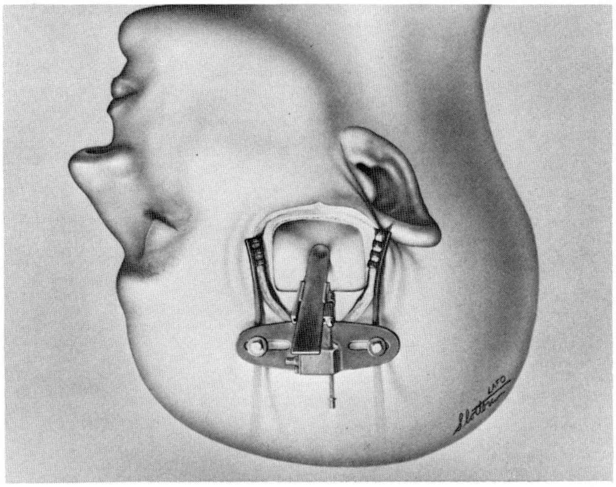

Fig. 8. Middle cranial fossa approach. Upon removal of the temporal bone flap, the dural is elevated and the House-Urban self-retaining dural retractor is inserted between the edges of the craniectomy.

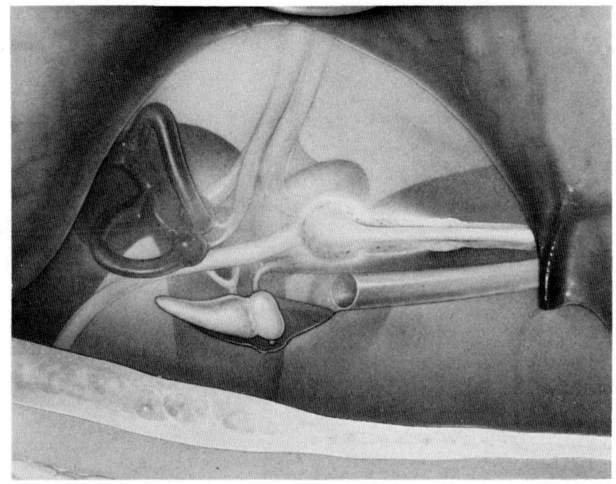

Fig. 9. Middle cranial fossa approach. The first important landmark that must be identified is the middle meningeal artery. Medial to this lies the greater superficial petrosal nerve, which if followed posteriorly leads to the geniculate ganglion.

petrous pyramid. Slightly anterior to the arcuate eminence, and posterior and lateral to the middle meningeal artery, lie the greater and lesser superficial petrosal nerves as they enter the middle cranial fossa. The retractor blade is then withdrawn slightly and advanced posteriorly, where a second landmark, the arcuate eminence, is located. The dura is carefully elevated over the dome of the arcuate eminence, and the blade of the retractor is advanced so that it fits over the ridge of the bone that corresponds to the superior petrosal sinus. The dura is then dissected free between the arcuate eminence and the middle meningeal artery. This step must be performed very carefully, because if the bony covering of the geniculate ganglion is dehiscent, the ganglion may be injured.

By approaching from behind and stripping the dura away anteriorly, it is possible to find a third major landmark, the greater superficial petrosal nerve, without injury to the ganglion. The retractor blade is now placed medial to the geniculate ganglion and as near to the superior petrosal sinus as possible. The greater superficial petrosal nerve serves as a guide to the geniculate ganglion. Once this ganglion has been exposed, the position of the lateral end of the internal auditory canal is fixed (Fig. 10). Here the labyrinthine portion of the facial nerve is exposed as it runs from the geniculate ganglion medially to the lateral extent of the internal auditory canal. In addition to running medially from the geniculate ganglion, the facial nerve runs posteriorly, displaced slightly in this direction by the basal turn of the cochlea. The bone is now removed over the facial nerve. Now the dissection can be carried medially toward the opening of the internal auditory canal into the posterior fossa by removing the usually thick bone covering the internal auditory canal.

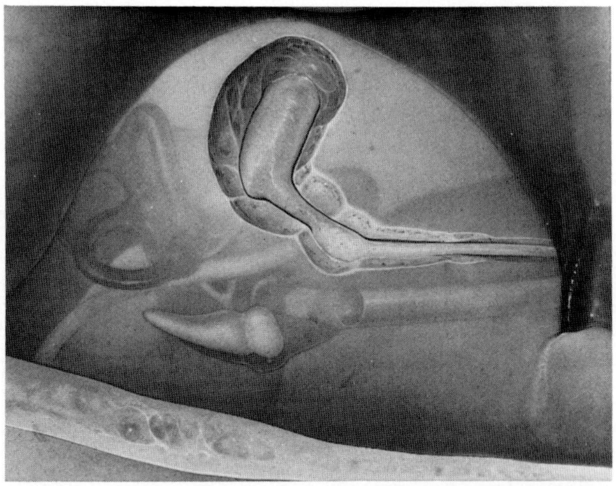

Fig. 10. Middle cranial fossa approach. Once this ganglion has been exposed, the position of the lateral end of the internal auditory canal is fixed. The labyrinthine portion of the facial nerve is then exposed as it runs from the geniculate ganglion medially and posteriorly to the lateral extent of the internal auditory canal.

Once the dura is exposed, the triangular piece of bone in the lateral extent of the canal is identified (Bill's bar), separating the anterior superior facial nerve compartment from the posterior superior vestibular nerve compartment. Once these landmarks have been identified, the dura is incised posteriorly over the superior vestibular nerve in order to make the incision away from the facial nerve and to leave an anteriorly based dural flap over the facial nerve to protect the structure (Fig. 11).

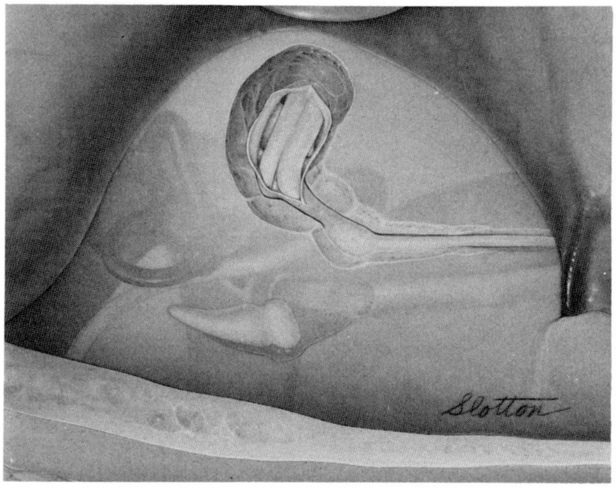

Fig. 11. Middle cranial fossa approach. Once the dura is exposed, the triangular piece of bone in the lateral extent of the canal is identified (Bill's bar) separating the anterior superior facial nerve compartment from the posterior superior vestibular nerve compartment. The dura of the internal auditory canal may now be incised.

Should this approach be combined with the postauricular transmastoid approach, bone lateral to the geniculate ganglion over the epitympanum may be removed, thereby connecting the two approaches and affecting total exposure of the facial nerve (Fig. 12).

Upon completion of the procedure, all bleeding points are controlled and a plug of free temporal muscle is placed over the internal auditory canal to prevent postoperative cerebrospinal fluid leakage. The dural elevator is removed slowly and the temporal lobe allowed to re-expand into its normal position in the middle cranial fossa. The previously created temporal bone flap is reinserted and the temporal muscle and temporalis fascia are brought together in layers. The skin and fascia are brought

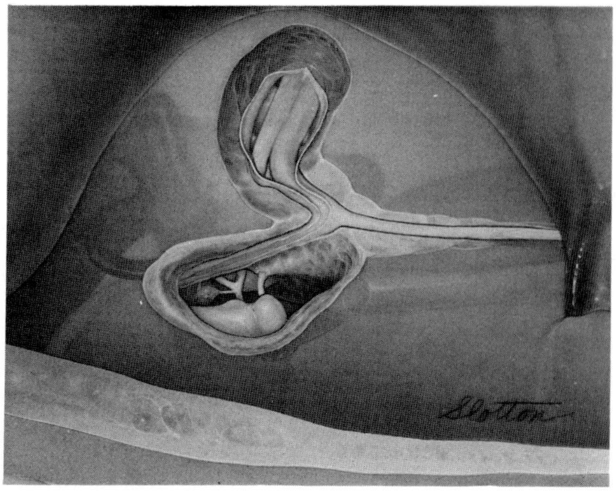

Fig. 12. Combined transmastoid middle cranial fossa approach, middle fossa portion, right ear, surgeon's view. Note here the full exposure of the facial nerve from the internal auditory canal through its labyrinthine portion down to the more distal tympanic segment.

together with either subcutaneous 2-0 chromic catgut sutures or interrupted wire sutures. Drainage is not used; a dry sterile dressing is placed over the wound and the patient is observed in the intensive care unit overnight.

Combined Transmastoid-Middle Cranial Fossa Approach

This combination of surgical approaches is utilized when serviceable hearing and vestibular function are present and when total exposure of the facial nerve is required (Fig. 13).

With the patient under general anesthesia, initially the transmastoid exposure is accomplished and then either by extension of the postauricular incision anteriorly and superiorly or by a separate incision the middle cranial fossa approach is used.

Upon completion of the transmastoid part of the total exposure, it is helpful if a small perforation is made in the epitympanic tegmen just lateral to the geniculate ganglion. This perforation remains extradural, and upon elevation of the middle fossa dura during the second half of the operation this hole is readily identifiable from above, aiding considerably in more rapid clarification of landmarks.

The details of each of the postauricular transmastoid and middle cranial fossa approaches to the facial nerve are as outlined earlier in this discussion.

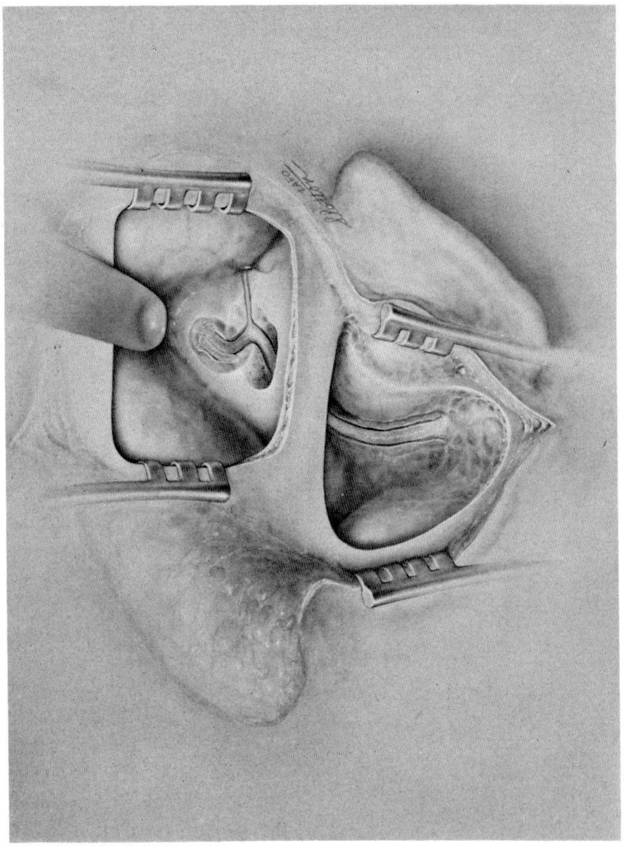

Fig. 13. Combined transmastoid middle cranial fossa approach, transmastoid portion, right ear, surgeon's view. The facial nerve from this view reveals its entire course from the internal auditory canal to the stylomastoid foramen.

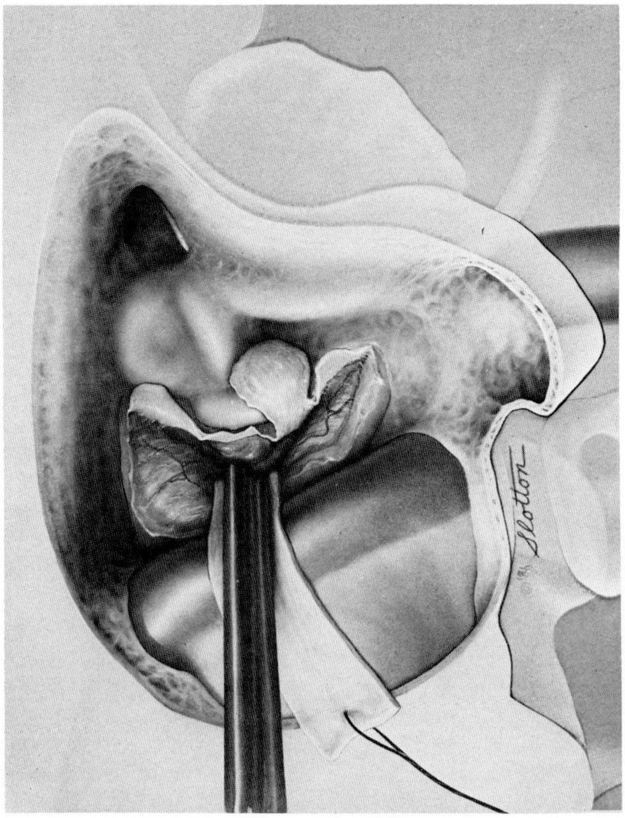

Fig. 14. Retrolabyrinthine approach, right ear, surgeon's view. Note a wide simple mastoidectomy has been performed with removal of bone over the sigmoid and posterior fossa dura. An incision is made in the dura parallel to and anterior to the sigmoid sinus, carefully preserving the endolymphatic sac and reflecting the structure anteriorly.

Retrolabyrinthine Approach

The retrolabyrinthine approach to the posterior fossa course of the facial nerve is useful when access to this area is required in a patient with useful hearing and balance function.

The patient is placed supine on the operating table with the head turned so that the involved side is up. Under general anesthesia an incision is made over the mastoid cortex. The skin and soft tissues are reflected off the mastoid cortex and adjacent lateral suboccipul. With the self-retaining forceps in position and utilizing the operating microscope, the air dirll, and constant suction irrigation, a complete mastoidectomy is performed and the bone over the lateral suboccipul, sigmoid sinus, and posterior and middle fossa dura is removed as far medial as the posterior semicircular canal. The jugular bulb is skeletonized inferiorly and the middle fossa plate superiorly. The posterior bony external auditory canal is preserved and the facial nerve identified inferior to the lateral semicircular canal.

An incision is made in the dura parallel to and anterior to the sigmoid sinus, thereby carefully preserving the endolymphatic sac, which is reflected anteriorly. The dural and endolymphatic sac are held in place with sutures fixed to the surrounding soft tissues (Fig. 14).

The subarachnoid space is then opened and cerebrospinal fluid is released from the lateral cystern. The cerebellum falls posteriorly, and usually minimal retraction is necessary to expose the exiting nerve roots in the cerebellopontine angle. The trigeminal nerve lies anterior and superior to the seventh and eighth cranial nerves. The ninth and tenth cranial nerves are seen inferior to the seventh and eighth nerves (Fig. 15).

The brainstem and adjacent blood vessels are readily visualized. All bleeding must be controlled prior to closure of the dura with continuous silk suture. A free graft of temporalis muscle is used to plug the defect in the mastoid and to prevent cerebrospinal fluid leakage. The skin and soft tissues are brought together in one layer with 2-0 interrupted subcutaneous chromic catgut sutures or interrupted wire sutures without drainage.

The patient is returned to the intensive care unit for observation overnight. The typical postoperative course is four to five days.

Translabyrinthine Approach

The postauricular translabyrinthine approach for exposure of the facial nerve affords total exposure of the facial nerve from the posterior fossa proximally to the stylomastoid foramen distally. This approach affords through one incision maximal exposure of the facial nerve. However, because the vestibular labyrinth is exenterated, the procedure is reserved for patients without serviceable hearing or balance function.

The patient is placed supine on the operating table with the involved side uppermost. The postauricular area is shaved and draped. Under general anesthesia an incision is made approximately 1 to 2 cm behind the postauricular crease, extending from 1 cm above the superior aspect of the helix to 2 cm behind the tip of the mastoid. It is important not to incise too close to the postauricular crease, for it is more difficult to remove bone posteriorly through a more anteriorly placed incision.

The skin is held in place with self-retaining retractors, and the plane between the temporarlis fascia and the subcutaneous tissue is developed by blunt dissection. The soft tissues are stripped off the mastoid forward to the external auditory canal and posteriorly to the lateral suboccipút. By use of a large cutting burr, air drill, and constant suction irrigation, a wide mastoidectomy is performed. The opening is extended forward above the external auditory canal into the epitympanum. The antrum is exposed and the middle ear identified. The facial nerve is skeletonized in its course through the mastoid to the stylomastoid foramen (Fig. 16). The

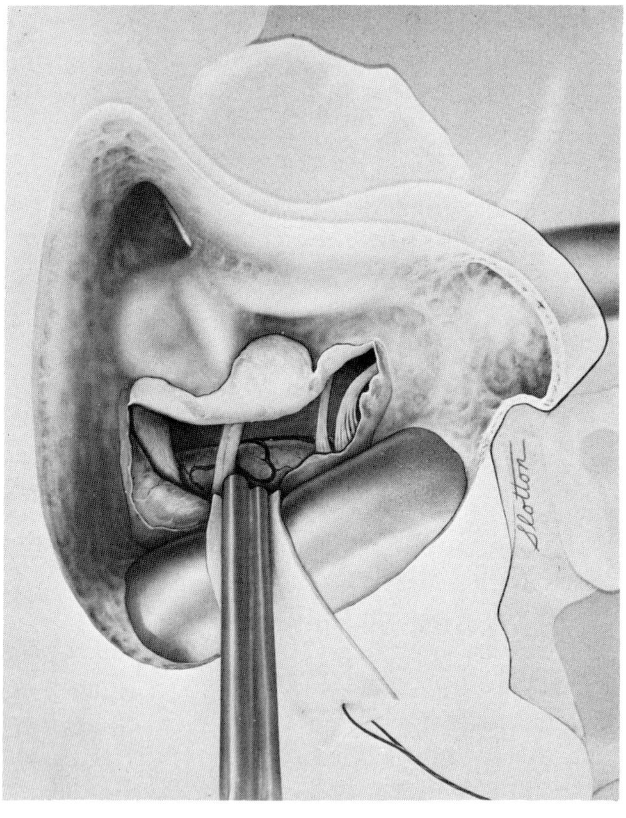

Fig. 15. Retrolabyrinthine approach. The subarachnoid space has been opened, the cerebrospinal fluid is released, and the cerebellum falls posteriorly exposing the fifth, seventh, eighth, ninth, and tenth cranial nerves as they emerge from the brainstem.

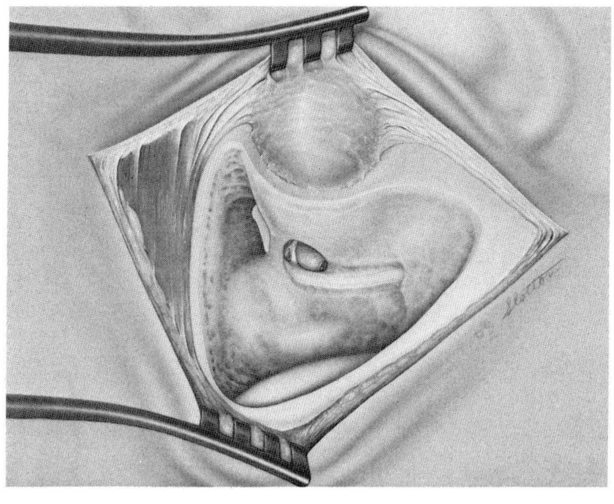

Fig. 16. Translabyrinthine approach, right ear, surgeon's view. A wide simple mastoidectomy is performed; the facial nerve is skeletonized in its course through the mastoid to the stylomastoid foramen.

genu of the facial nerve is identified, and a thin layer of bone is left over the facial nerve at this point to protect the structure. Posteriorly, the superior petrosal and sigmoid sinuses are exposed, again leaving a thin shell of bone over these structures for protection.

A labyrinthectomy is then carried out. The fibers of the superior vestibular are identified as they enter the vestibule. The bony removal is then carried out along the superior vestibular nerve to the internal auditory canal. The entrance of the facial nerve into the internal auditory is exposed by careful removal of bone above the superior vestibular nerve with a diamond burr. A definite bar of bone (Bill's bar) lies between the superior vestibular nerve and the facial nerve. The facial nerve is then completely exposed from the posterior fossa to stylomastoid foramen with the diamond drill under constant suction irrigation. The incus and head of the malleus are removed in order to expose the facial nerve in the tympanic portion. However, the tympanic membrane is left intact. All bone is then removed with the diamond burr and constant suction irrigation from the internal auditory canal to the stylomastoid foramen (Fig. 17). Access to the posterior fossa, if required, may be obtained by removing the layer of bone previously left over the sigmoid sinus and posterior fossa dura.

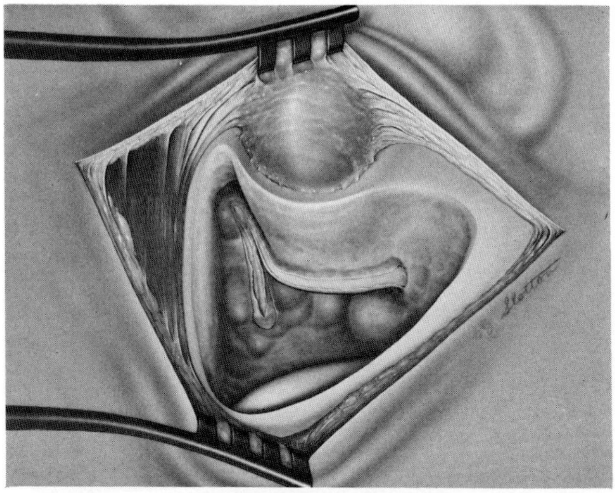

Fig. 17. Translabyrinthine approach. A labyrinthectomy has been carried out and the internal auditory canal skeletonized. The entrance of the facial nerve into the internal auditory canal is exposed by identification of the superior vestibular nerve canal. All bone is removed and the facial nerve is thus exposed from the internal auditory canal to the stylomastoid foramen.

Upon completion of the procedure, all bleeding must be carefully controlled. Abdominal fat or a temporalis muscle plug is used to fill the mastoid and epitympanum in order to prevent leakage of cerebrospinal fluid. The wound is then closed with 2-0 subcutaneous interrupted chromic catgut sutures without drainage. A mastoid dressing is applied and the patient is returned for observation overnight in the intensive care unit.

Summary

Lesions producing facial nerve palsy may occur within the temporal bone anywhere between the internal auditory canal and the stylomastoid foramen. Surgical exposure of this nerve may be necessary for decompression, grafting, rerouting, or removal of such lesions as acoustic tumor, meningioma, facial nerve neuroma, and cholesteatoma.

Contemporary surgical exposure of the facial nerve has as its aim adequate exposure of the facial nerve at any point in its course, with preservation of hearing and vestibular function, without further injury to the facial nerve and the necessity for producing a mastoid cavity.

When hearing and balance function are present, the transcanal-transtympanic approach to the horizontal segment of the facial nerve offers limited access to the facial nerve in its tympanic course. Wider exposure is obtained by postauricular transmastoid exposure of the tympanic and mastoid portions of the facial nerve. The middle fossa approach to the facial nerve offers access to the internal auditory canal and labyrinthine portions of the nerve, whereas the retrolabyrinthine approach offers access to the facial nerve in the posterior fossa. Total facial nerve exposure with preservation of hearing and balance function is obtained by the combined transmastoid and middle cranial fossa approach. In individuals who have lost all function of hearing and balance, the postauricular translabyrinthine approach offers total exposure of the facial nerve within the temporal bone and posterior fossa.

The aim of this discussion was to present in succinct fashion a systematized approach to surgical exposure of the facial nerve within the temporal bone and posterior fossa.

Acknowledgments

Sincere gratitude is expressed to Mrs. Arleen Valentin for help in manuscript preparation, and to Mr. Dan Slotton for his very excellent artwork.

Reference

1. Graham MD: The jugular bulb. Its anatomic and clinical considerations in contemporary otology, Arch Otolaryng 101:560–64, 1975.

Animal Bites to the Head and Neck

Robert H. Mathog, Leonard H. Wurman, and Deborah Pollak, Minneapolis, Minn.

Animal bites are common causes of human injury. Reported cases in the United States per year reach 600,000, but estimates to include nonreported injuries may approach two million.[1] This is not surprising in that Americans have about twenty-five million dogs and twenty-five million cats, and that the numbers continue to grow at a rapid rate.[2]

It is well known that a large number of these animal bites are to the head and neck. Injury to this region poses problems of management similar to other sites of the body, but also some that are unique to the facial areas. Often there is a question of rabies, and many of the decisions regarding these bites must deal with the isolation of the animal, anti-rabies therapy and tetanus toxoid. On the other hand bites of the head and neck must be especially evaluated and treated for the prevention of deformity. There is frequently a dilemma of choosing methods in wound debridement and closure. Such decisions may involve a choice of direct suturing techniques, grafts, or flaps.

It is the purpose of this paper to evaluate head and neck bites in an urban community—Minneapolis—and to compare this experience with that of other localities. Bite injuries will be analyzed for the incidence, cause, site, and effectiveness of medical and surgical treatment. The rationale of administering or withholding therapy for rabies will also be evaluated.

Incidence

During the period from January 1, 1971 to January 1, 1974, 5078 cases of animal bites were reported to the Division of Public Health in Minneapolis. The population at this time was about 436,000 indicating that there were 630 bites per 100,000 people.

In this group of reported cases, 397 (or 7.8 percent of all cases) had an injury to the head and neck area. This accounted for 417 bites since in some patients there were multiple areas of injury. One-third of all head and neck bites occurred in the area of the cheeks, while almost one-quarter of the bites were noted on the lips (Table 1). Other areas less involved were the scalp, ears, eyelid, nose, and neck.

Cause of Bites

Most animal bites were inflicted by a family dog or at least a dog known in the neighborhood. As shown in Table 2, dogs accounted for 86 percent of the bites. The cat inflicted a smaller number of bites, while a few were ascribed to the bat, squirrel, mouse, monkey, gerbil, fox, rat, and "pet" bear.

Usually bites to the head and neck were provoked. They occurred frequently while an individual was playing with or removing food from an

Table 1. Head and Neck Bites Distribution of Sites

Sites	Number	Percent
Scalp	28	6.7
Forehead	12	2.8
Ear	31	7.4
Nose	32	7.6
Eyelid	53	12.7
Lip	81	20.6
Cheek	154	36.9
Chin	12	2.8
Neck	14	3.4
	417	100.0

Table 2. Cause of Bite 397 Cases

	Number	Percent
Dog	342	86.0
Cat	40	10.0
Bat	7	1.7
Squirrel	2	0.5
Others	6	1.8
Mouse, Monkey, Gerbil		
Fox, Rat, "Pet" Bear		

Table 3. Age Distribution

Years	Number	Percent
0–1	8	2.0
1–5	179	45.1
6–10	106	26.7
11–15	31	7.8
15 and over	37	9.4
Unknown	36	9.0
	397	100.0

animal. Occasionally they resulted from injuring the animal or disturbing a litter. Provocation as a cause of the bite was also reflected by the predominance of bites in young children. About three-quarters of the bites occurred in children between the ages of one and ten years and about half in those individuals between the ages of one and five years (Table 3).

Evaluation of Treatment

In order to obtain an analysis of medical and surgical management in head and neck bites, 75 selected patients were evaluated at the University of Minnesota affiliated hospitals. Two additional cases from the University of Iowa* were included to illustrate other types of injuries.

Medical Treatment

In most of these 77 detailed cases, the animals that inflicted the bites were not felt to be rabid. Consequently, antirabies treatment was usually withheld while the animals were being observed. In this group where the animal could be observed, none of the animals ever did develop rabies.

There were however several cases where rabies could have been transmitted. These were in bites by unprovoked dogs (3 cases) or in wild animals that could not be observed following the injury (4 cases). In both types of cases, four of the patients were started on antirabies therapy, while three of the patients were observed. Vaccine and serum were administered to one patient injured by a squirrel and to another bitten by an unprovoked strange dog. Vaccine alone was administered to one patient with a bat bite and to another with a dog bite. In this group of seven patients, none developed rabies. Complications were rare in that only a minor local reaction developed in one patient who received antirabies vaccine.

Documentation of the administration of tetanus toxoid or a history of immunization for tetanus was noted in more than one-half of the cases (44/77). No patient in the series developed tetanus.

In general antibiotics were infrequently used for the prevention of infection. If an antibiotic was given to a patient, penicillin was the drug of choice. In spite of the sporadic use of antibiotics, infection was observed in only two cases as a complication of initial therapy.

Surgical Treatment

In the 77 cases, 56 were lacerations, 12 were abrasions or puncture wounds, and 9 were avulsions. All wounds were treated with standard

* Separate cases demonstrating avulsion of the nose and lip are courtesy of G. E. McFarland, M.D., Iowa City, Iowa.

techniques. Initially the wounds were irrigated with saline or antiseptic solutions. Benzalkonium chloride (zephiran) was used on ten patients. Wounds in other patients were cleaned with irrigations of saline, phisohex, hydrogen peroxide or betadine. Only one patient had mechanical debridement of the wound and only one patient had antirabies serum instilled directly into the wound.

Abrasions, scratches, contusions and puncture wounds were generally treated by open techniques. These less severe wounds were managed by irrigation with saline and cleansing with antiseptic materials. Such areas were frequently covered with antibiotic ointments and subsequently healed without significant scar formation.

The other deeper wounds, comprised of lacerations or avulsions, were treated with closed methods. These techniques usually included suture approximation of tissues to relieve tension on the wound edges. Infection was not observed in any of the cases treated in this fashion, and scarring was minimal.

With regard to avulsed injuries, specific repair depended upon the site and extent of the injury. Where there was minimal loss of tissue, advancement techniques were useful for closure. In more extensive wounds skin grafts and local flaps were necessary.

An example of management in a laceration-avulsion of the cheek was demonstrated by the injury in Figure 1. In this case a 6-year-old boy was bitten by his grandparents' dog. The laceration involved the left lower cheek. Facial function was intact and exploration of the wound within two hours of the bite revealed a noninjured salivary duct system. Following irrigation with saline and aqueous zephiran, the wound was closed with absorbable subcutaneous and nonabsorbable subcuticular and cuticular sutures. In spite of the placement of three drains, the patient developed a superficial wound infection and later, widened scars. These areas were eventually revised with excision and zigzag techniques.

Another example of this type of wound was demonstrated by a laceration-avulsion of the midface area in a 4½-year old boy bitten by his own dog (Fig. 2). Lacerations extended from the bridge of the nose to the medical canthal ligaments bilaterally. The nasal bones examined through these flaps were noted to be fractured in several areas. It was suspected that the upper canalicular system was injured on the right side. Surgical correction involved exploration of the canalicular system and direct open reduction of the naso-ethmoid fracture. The avulsion was repaired by advancement of adjoining soft tissues. Since only the superior canaliculus was injured, the functional and cosmetic results were excellent.

A similar bite was also observed in another child who had provoked a "family" dog (Fig. 3). In this patient the laceration extended through the nasal soft tissues separating the upper lateral cartilages on the left from the nasal bones. After adequate cleansing of the wound, subcutaneous

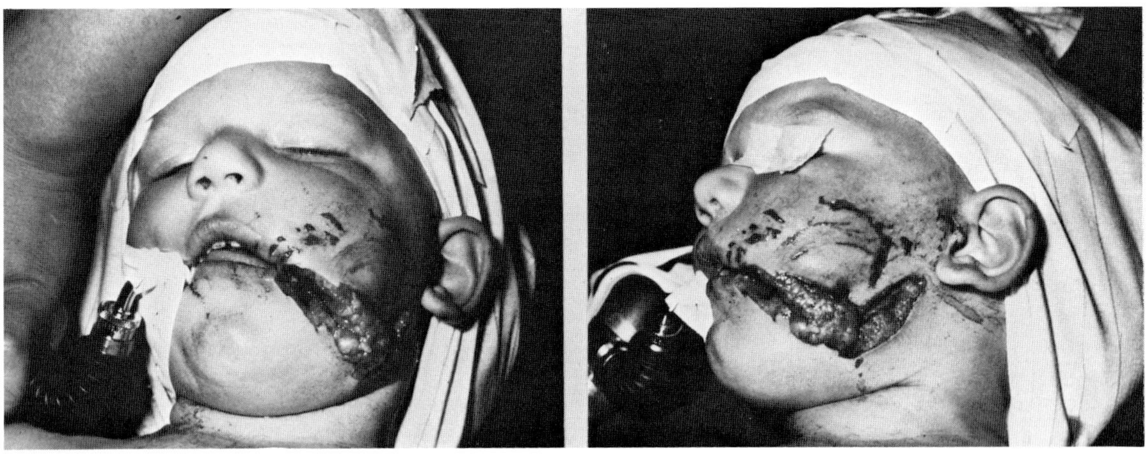

Fig. 1. A dog bite characterized by a laceration-avulsion of the cheek in a 6-year-old boy. The parotid duct and facial nerve were not injured.

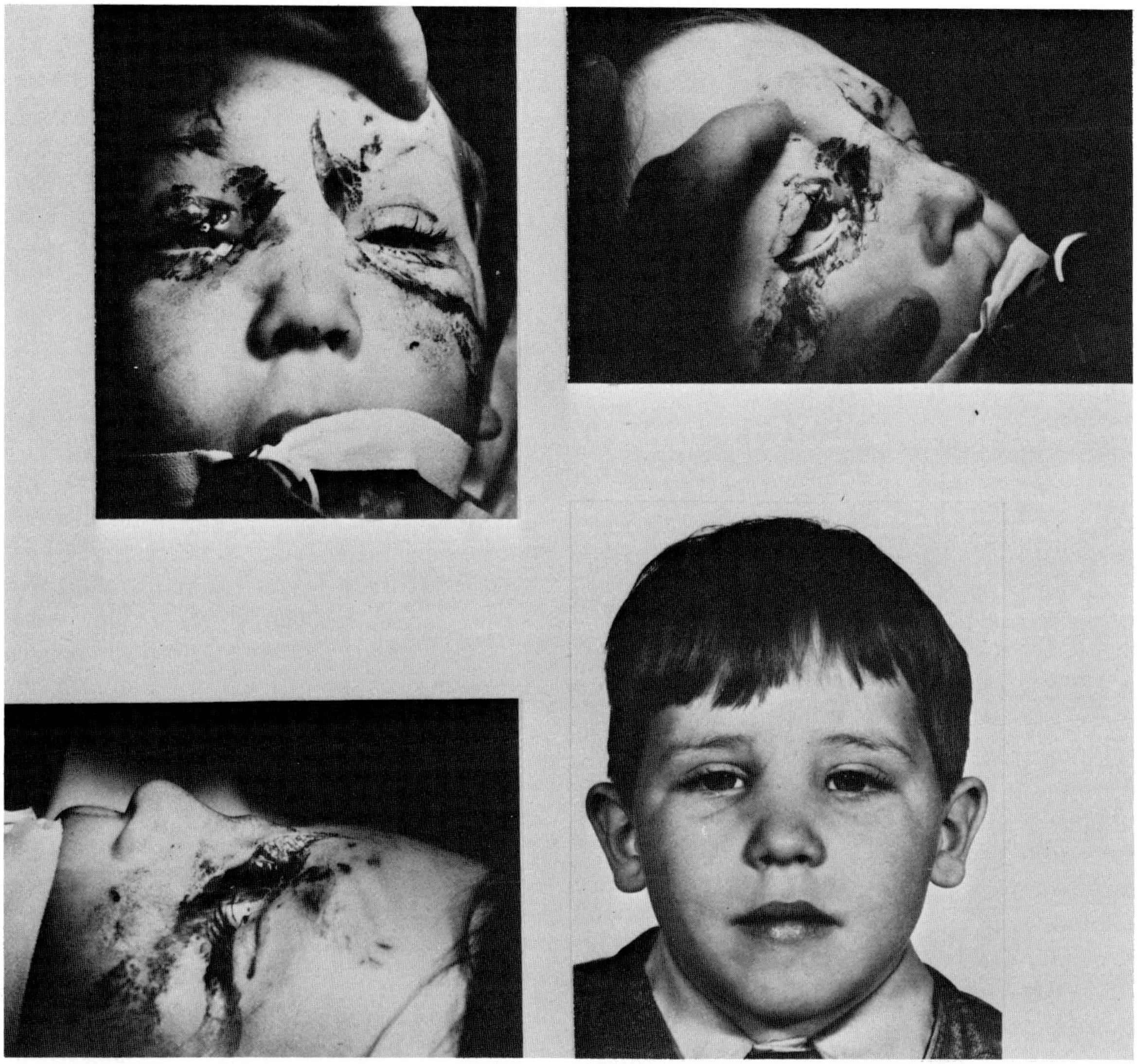

Fig. 2. Laceration-avulsions of the midface in a $4\frac{1}{2}$-year old boy as a result of a dog bite. Medial canthal ligaments, nasal bones, and the right superior canaliculus were displaced at the time of injury.

and skin tissues were approximated to provide a satisfactory cosmetic and functional result.

In some cases, where there was loss of tissue, advancement was not possible. In one bite involving the cutaneous and subcutaneous tissues of the auricle, skin advancement was extremely difficult (Fig. 4). For this defect involving the helical rim, a full-thickness graft was chosen as a method of treatment.

In two other cases with large avulsions, local flaps were used to correct the deformities. One 5-year-old boy, who sustained avulsion of the lip, had an immediate flap reconstruction. As shown in Figure 5, the Abbe-Estlander type of flap was utilized for repair of the defect. In another case of a severe injury to the nose, initial treatment was primary closure. This occurred in a young boy, who 15 years later, underwent surgical reconstruction of the alar and columellar defect with staged naso-labial flaps (Fig. 6).

Discussion

Upon evaluation of these animal bites, in a community such as Minneapolis, it was apparent

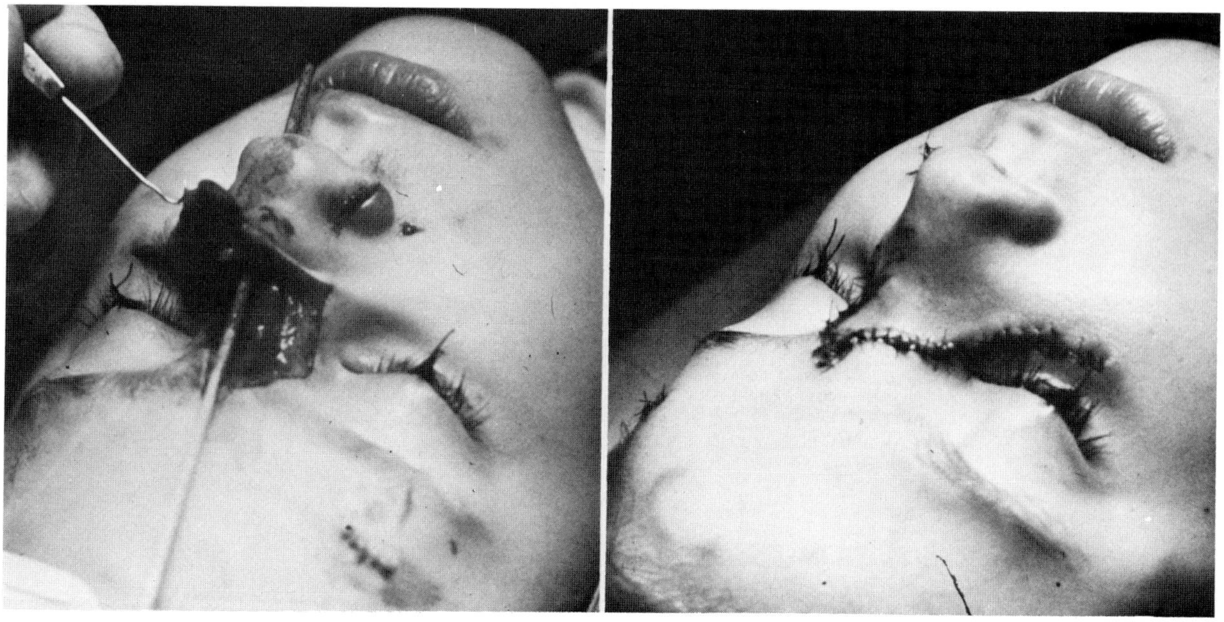

Fig. 3. A dog bite characterized by a laceration-avulsion of the nose in a 5-year-old girl. The upper alar cartilage on the left was separated from the nasal bones.

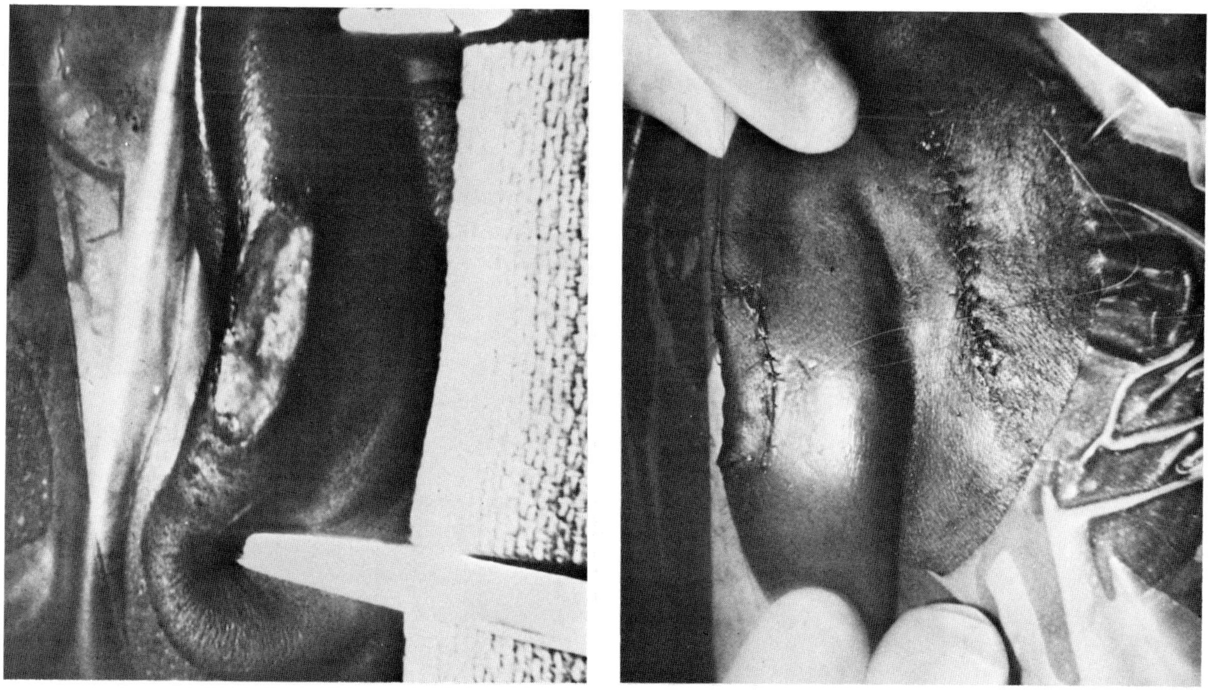

Fig. 4. Avulsion of the helical rim as a result of a dog bite. The wound was repaired with an immediate postauricular full-thickness skin graft.

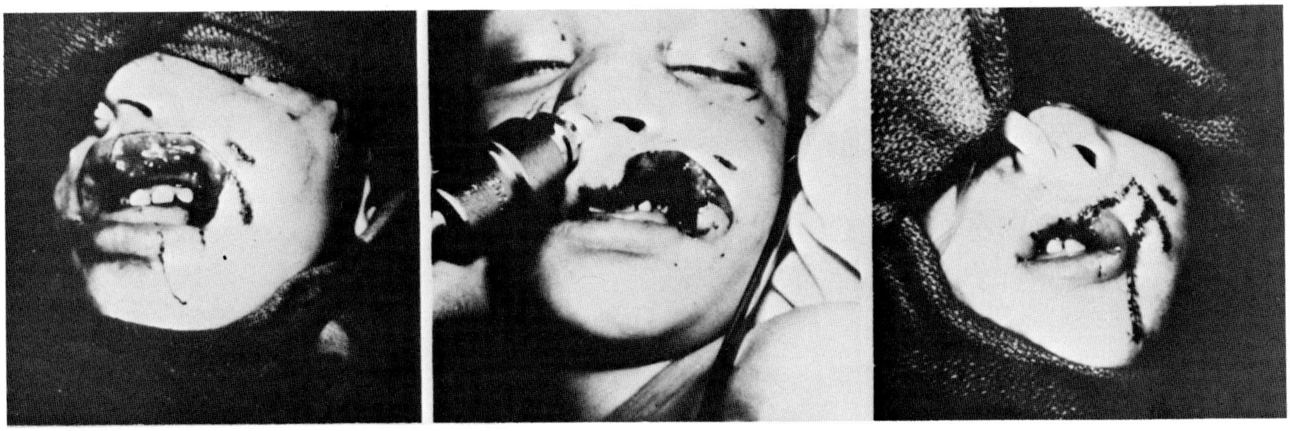

Fig. 5. A dog bite of the lip in a 5-year-old boy necessitating an Abbe-Estlander flap for immediate reconstruction. (Courtesy of G. E. McFarland, M.D.)

that there were a larger than expected number of injuries. In fact, this was about twice that reported in other urban areas. It was possible that this rate reflected a larger number of pets, but because of strict guidelines established by the Health Department, the increased incidence probably was due to a more accurate reporting of injuries.

The relative incidence of head and neck bites as a percentage of total bites was much less than the 25–30 percent reported by Ford[3] and Sokol.[4] This was difficult to explain, but possibly the lowered incidence was a function again of improved reporting and recording, especially of minor injuries to other parts of the body.

The high occurrence of dog and cat bites in children confirmed the reports of Scarcella and others.[1,2,4,5] This predilection for children could have been explained by their small stature.[5] Another possible explanation, as shown by the present study, was the tendency of the child to accidently provoke the animal.

Most bite lesions were located on or very near the lip area. Barclay[6] reported this as a particular type of dog bite injury. In his cases, the animal struck at the individual while that person was kissing the animal. On the other hand, the cheek and lips are obvious protruding parts of the head and neck and therefore, would be more prone to injury.

As expected all cases were evaluated as to whether to institute antirabies therapy. Several considerations were the available types of therapy and the complications of the therapy.

Two recommended methods or combinations were available—serum for immediate passive immunity, and vaccine for active immunity.[7,8] It is well known that the administration of horse serum has been associated with serum sickness, but recently the availability of human rabies immunoglobulin has reduced this complication.[9] Likewise, neural tissue vaccine has also been associated with a high incidence of reaction, but the newer duck embryo vaccine has caused only a few dermatologic, neurologic and allergic problems.[10,11]

According to the guidelines of the World Health Organization,[7,8] there should be more concern for the head and neck bite which has been accompanied by a shorter period of incubation. In such cases they have suggested that the patient be started on a course of anti-serum; then if on observation, the animal develops rabies, the vaccine should be given. Recommended dosages are 40 IU of equine antirabies serum intramuscularly, or one-half intramuscularly and the other half into the wound. If necessary the vaccine should be administered as 21 daily doses subcutaneously (followed by two booster doses). If one were to reduce the incidence of serum reactions, it should be possible to substitute equivalent human rabies immunoglobulin at 15–40 IU/kg.[9]

All of these recommendations are useful, but for urban and local conditions, they require modifications. Most of the bites in the Minneapolis area were from dogs or cats. Since most infectious rabies bites reported in the United States were from

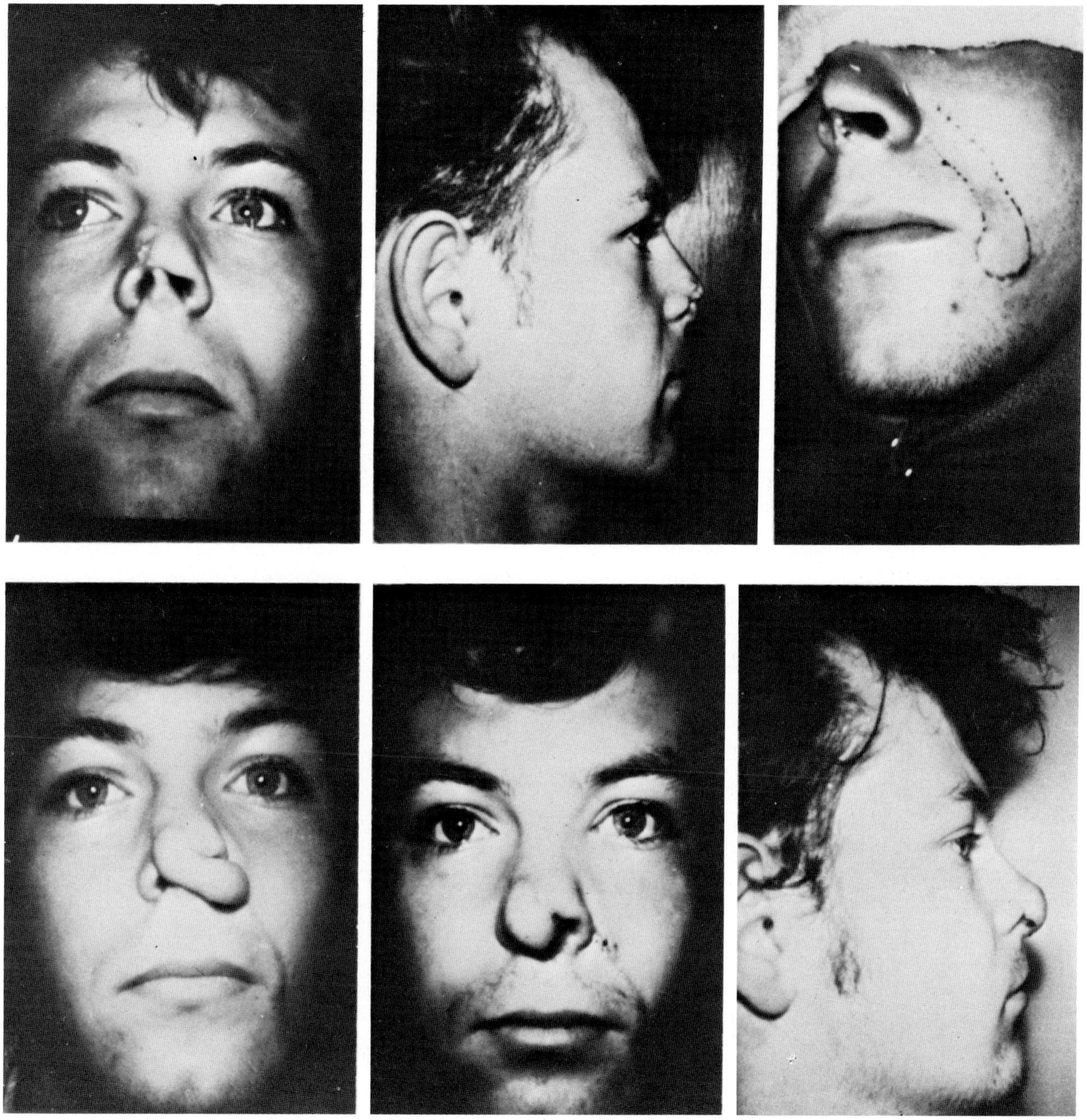

Fig. 6. Staged naso-labial flap reconstruction of alar-columellar defects occurring 15 years earlier as a result of a dog bite. (From McFarland GE: Reconstructive flaps in otolaryngology. Laryngoscope 84:1267–1275, 1974.)

a skunk or raccoon,[8] household pets were considered as unlikely vectors. Other animals that could carry rabies, but were not implicated in this series, were the fox, cattle, horse, sheep, bobcat, coyote, and especially the vampire bat from South America.

Another consideration was, that since strict animal codes require vaccination for rabies, it was unlikely that the dog or cat could carry the virus. Thus, only in the case of an unprovoked dog bite or one in which a wild animal escaped after the attack, was it felt that there was a significant risk of rabies. This was one of the reasons for the infrequent use of vaccine and antiserum in the present series.

In a few cases suspected of possibly developing rabies, the animal involved in the bite was killed and evaluated for Negri bodies in the nerve tissues. Negative findings were confirmed by innoculation of suspected brain tissue supernatant into the cerebrum of mice for transmission of disease. Since it is well known that 1–20 percent of the rabid animals may not have these histologic findings, this test has been largely supplanted by a fluorescent antibody assay.

With regard to the prophylactic use of antibiotics and tetanus toxoid, their rationale could not be substantiated by the present study. Only a few patients received antibiotics; others did not, and there was infrequent infection in both groups. Pasturella species infection, reported with bites of domestic animals,[12] also was not observed.

No patient developed tetanus. It appeared unlikely that the organism causing tetanus would be a normal inhabitant in the animal's mouth, or that contaminated clothing would be involved in an injury to the head and neck area.

Debridement of the wound was carried out in all cases. Benzalkonium chloride, as recommended by others was used in ten cases as a form of rabies prophylaxis.[3,13] Since this treatment carries minimal risk, it probably should have been used in every case. Necrotic tissues at the wound edges did not seem common and mechanical debridement was rare. Most wounds, even the avulsion type had clean edges. Only one wound was injected or swabbed with antiserum as suggested by Kaplan et al.[9]

Surgical management of the injury was accomplished by simple direct closure, advancement of adjacent tissues, split-thickness grafts and local flaps. Completely avulsed or amputated pieces of tissue would have been replaced, but this situation was not observed in this series.[14,15] The specific type of repair for avulsion depended upon the site and extent of injury.

Avulsions of the auricle were treated with full-thickness grafts, but these could also have been reconstructed using other techniques. One method could have been a wedge excision with direct closure but this would have reduced the size of the ear. Other methods for large avulsions could have employed postauricular transposition flaps, chondrocutaneous flaps,[16] or the temporary burying of the helical rim underneath the postauricular skin.[17] Composite grafts from the opposite ear could have been used,[18] but this procedure probably should be performed only as an alternate technique after primary healing. Advancement of tissues over the cartilages have been described but this would have required extensive postauricular undermining to relieve tension of the wound edges.

Lip lesions were common types of wounds. Frequently they were simple lacerations and were closed directly. Musgrave and Garrett[19] reported excellent results with healing by secondary intention. Barclay[6] recommended wedge excision of the wound, and actually this would have been applicable in several of the cases where there was maceration of tissue. In one case there was a large avulsion of the lip which required initially an Abbe-Estlander flap. This provided a satisfactory functional and cosmetic result. Postoperative scarring was not a problem in any of the cases, and revision was unnecessary in any of the patients treated in these various ways.

Laceration-avulsions of the nose, when possible, were closed primarily. If there was a severe avulsion of this area, this was corrected initially by advancement of local tissues. Although not necessary in any of these cases, the advancement techniques could have been augmented by shortening the nose. In one case where primary closure resulted in deformity of the ala and columella, the defect was corrected later by nasolabial flap reconstruction. Scarcella[2] also reported a case with similar reconstruction techniques. Immediate composite grafts recommended by Wynn[20] were felt to be with risk and were not used on any patients. Split-thickness or full-thickness grafts, although often used temporarily, were not considered cosmetically acceptable as definitive treatment in younger people.

Injuries to the eyelids required special techniques of reconstruction. Although Silverman and Obear reported avulsions of upper and lower lids and methods of reconstruction,[21] in this series no patients required repair of avulsed tarsal plates or medial canthal ligaments. One patient did require evaluation and repair of the lacrimal system and closure of a full-thickness defect in the lid. Obtaining anatomical continuity by placing tissues into their normal position was sufficient from a functional and cosmetic standpoint.

Avulsions and lacerations of the broad areas, i.e., cheek, forehead, chin, and neck areas were repaired by direct closure or by advancement. Loss of tissues in these areas was not great and did not pose any serious problems of reconstruction. Evaluation of the parotid duct and facial nerve was performed in one patient where the injury extended through the glandular tissues of the cheek. Interestingly, this patient was one of the few who developed cellulitis in the area of the wound.

Conclusion

According to this analysis of animal bites, there appear appropriate measures for evaluating and treating head and neck bites in an urban community. In general the animals can be isolated and observed for changes in health while the patient is being treated for the bite. Rabies prophylaxis probably can be instituted when the bites are unprovoked and created by wild carnivores, i.e., skunk, fox, coyote, raccoon, and bat. Vaccination of the biting animal and the presence of rabies in the geographic region are important considerations. If the bite is unprovoked and the animal cannot be observed or identified, then treatment should be instituted within 48 hr. Such antirabies treatment can probably be accomplished with rabies equine or human immune serum and duck embryo vaccine.

Although infection is usually not a problem, all wounds should be irrigated thoroughly to remove foreign materials. Zephiran is suggested in the irrigation process to provide some prophylaxis of rabies. Prophylactic antibiotics may be used in cases with wounds that are open for long periods of time, or where there is severe tissue damage. Most wounds can be closed primarily but treatment of avulsed tissues will depend upon the location and severity of the wound. This may include techniques of skin grafts, advancement and local flaps.

Acknowledgments

The authors would like to express their appreciation to F. G. Gunlaugson, M.D., Division of Public Health, Minneapolis for assisting in the collection of the animal bite data.

References

1. Klein D: Friendly dog syndrome. NY State J Med 66:2306–2309, 1966
2. Scarcella JV: Management of bites. Early definitive repair of bite wounds. Ohio State Med J 65:25–31, 1969
3. Ford WJA: The treatment of dog bites and the rabies problem. Am J Surg 93:676–681, 1957
4. Sokol AB, Houser RG: Dog bites: Prevention and treatment. Comments from a surgeon's viewpoint. Clin Pediatr 10:336–338, 1971
5. Mayers SP, Beachley RG: A survey of dog bites in Arlington. Va Med Mon 82:317–319, 1955
6. Barclay TL: Dog bites of the face. Br J Plast Surg 9:34–37, 1956
7. Expert Committee on Rabies, Second Report. WHO Tech Rep Ser 321, 1966
8. Public Health Service Advisory Committee on Immunization Practices. US Dept HEW 21:25, 1972
9. Hattwick MAW, Rubin RH, Music S, Sikes RK, Smith JS, Gregg MB: Postexposure rabies prophylaxis with human rabies immuneglobulin. JAMA 227:407–410, 1974
10. Mathison DA: Active rabies immunization in an individual hypersensitive to duck embryo vaccine. J Allergy and Clin Immunol 50:246–251, 1972
11. Rubin RH, Hattwick MAW, Jones S, Gregg MB, Schwartz VD: Adverse reactions to duck embryo rabies vaccine. Ann Intern Med 78:643–649, 1973
12. Torphy DE, Roy CG: Pasturella multocida in dog and cat bite infections. Pediatrics 43:295–297, 1969
13. Kaplan MM, Cohen D, Koprowski H, Dean D, Ferrigan L: Studies on local treatment of wounds for the prevention of rabies. WHO 26:765–775, 1962
14. Grabb WC, Dingman RO: The fate of amputated tissues of the head and neck following replacement. Plast Reconstr Surg 49:28–32, 1972
15. Potsic WP, Naunton RF: Reimplantation of an amputated pinna. Arch Otolaryngol 100:73–75, 1974
16. Millard DR: The chondrocutaneous flap in partial and auricular repair. Plast Reconstr Surg 37:523, 1966
17. Curtin JW, Greeley DW: Human bites of the face. Early treatment and late reconstructive repair. Plast and Reconstr Surg 28:397–404, 1961
18. Brandt FA: Human bites of the ear. Plast Reconstr Surg 43:130–134, 1969
19. Musgrave RH, Garrett WS Jr: Dog bite avulsions of the lip. A conservative concept. Plast Reconstr Surg 49:294–296, 1972
20. Wynn SK: Immediate composite graft to loss of nasal ala from dog bite. Plast Reconstr Surg 50:188–191, 1972
21. Silverman JP, Obear MF: Delayed primary repair of totally avulsed upper and lower eyelids. Am J Ophthalmol 70:230–233, 1970

The Double-Breasted Vest Technique of Scar Repair

Ronald Strahan, Los Angeles, Calif.

Introduction

Tension is one of the most important factors which adversely influence the character and width of a scar. Surgeons experienced in scar revision surgery recognize certain areas of the body as being notorious for poor scars. In most of these areas, tension is a constant factor as a result of body movement, i.e., flexion, extension, rotation, and muscle expansion. In these areas, a simple linear closure of a wound will be subject to this unrelenting tension and the result is the spreading of the scar to an undesirable width.

Conversely, hairline scars are the usual result if tension is absent from the wound closure during the healing period. It follows that if the tension of the edge-to-edge skin approximation of the wound can be eliminated by placing the tension at an offset position in the subcutaneous closure, a hairline scar might be possible in body areas subject to constant tension. The double-breasted vest technique of scar repair was designed with this in mind, and has been helpful in preventing the spread of scars in unfavorable locations.

Several authors have published descriptions of variations of the double-breasted vest technique for scar repair. However, Millard[1] is given the credit for adding the refinements to this surgical procedure that made it so useful. This author has added his indications to those suggested by Millard. Also, in Millard's description of this technique for scar repair, he only referred to those scars that were favorable for linear closure. This author has combined the double-breasted vest technique with the maneuvers of W-plasty and geometric design closure for excellent results in special circumstances of scar repair.

Operative Technique

Step No. 1. If the long axis of the scar for revision lies in agreement to the lines of relaxed skin tension, a fusiform excision of the scar is marked. For purposes of discussion, one side of the scar shall be marked right and the other side left (Fig. 1). The dermal-scar flap to be developed will remain attached to the right side of the scar excision. The subcutaneous closure, which alleviates the tension of the epithelial closure, will occur on the left side. The epithelium is dissected from the scar, leaving the dermal-scar component intact. Although the incision on the left side is made with the knife perpendicular to the skin edge, it is helpful later in the closure if the incision on the right side is made on a bias, as illustrated in Figure 2.

Step No. 2. At the left side of the scar, an incision is made through the dermis into the underlying subcutaneous fatty tissue. The undermining on the left side of the incision has a bias direction and is carried away from the skin edge, slightly more than the width of the scar (Fig. 3).

Step No. 3. The dermal-scar flap which remains attached to the right side of the scar, is undermined perpendicular to the skin surface to a point directly underneath the right side of the scar incision. Here the undermining is carried on a bias into the subcutaneous tissue, illustrated in Figure 4 by the broken line. On the right side of the scar excision, at a point where the denuded dermal flap joins the normal skin, an incision is extended on the bias to a depth that matches the skin thickness of the opposite edge. This is illustrated in the lower portion of Figure 4.

Step No. 4. The flap of the scar sheet is then advanced across the wound into the area undermined underneath the left side. The scar sheet flap

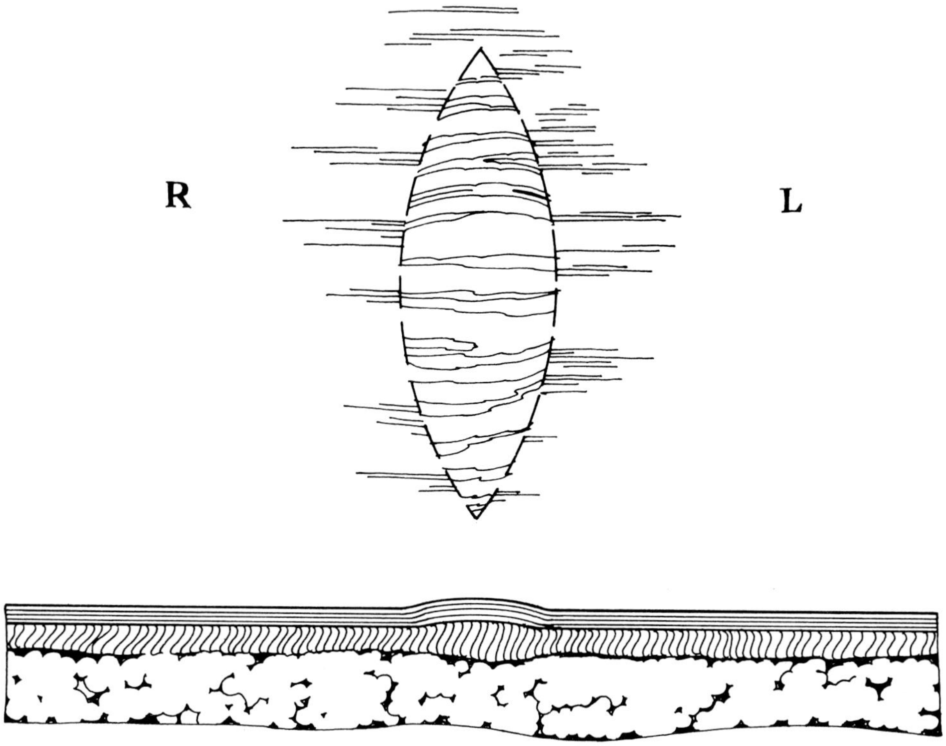

Fig. 1. Hypertrophic, widened scar situated in agreement with lines of relaxed skin tension.

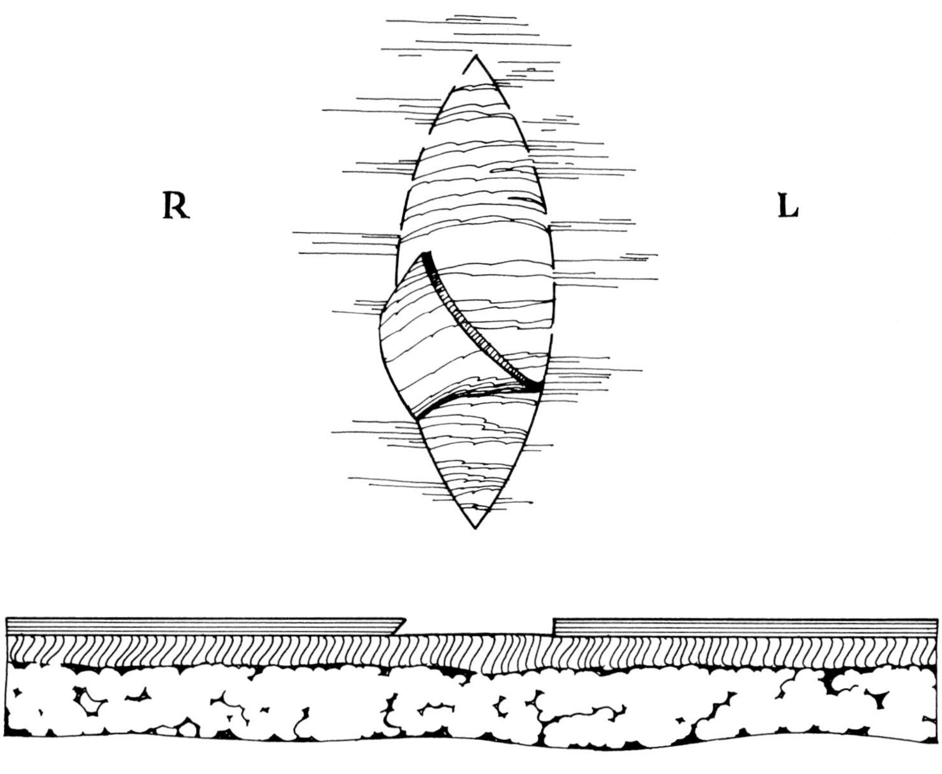

Fig. 2. Fusiform excision of scar.

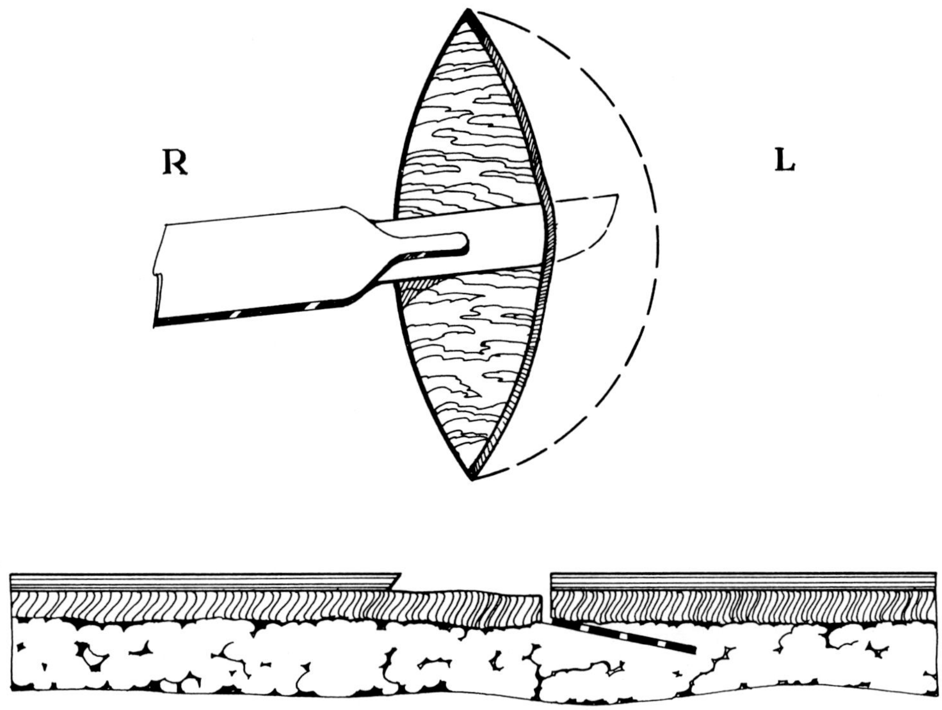

Fig. 3. Bias direction of undermining on the left side. Extent of undermining is greater than original scar width.

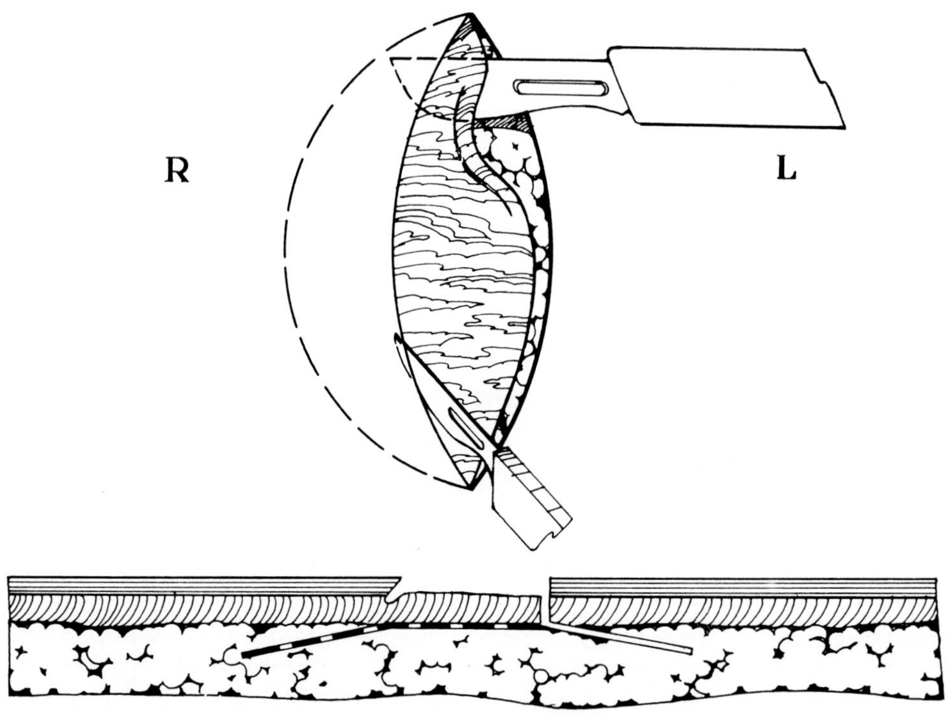

Fig. 4. Development of the dermal-scar flap. Bias direction of undermining on the right side of scar. Redefining the skin-scar junction on right. Thinning of the left side of excision site.

is sutured to the subcutaneous tissues and underneath surface of the dermis at a point that will allow the opposing skin edges to literally oppose each other without any evidence of tension. This author prefers the use of Dexon for this maneuver, however, other authors have used a nonabsorbable colorless suture. The skin edges are inspected and if the left edge is thicker than the right it is thinned with fine curved scissors. This is illustrated in the bottom part of Figure 5. The skin edges are approximated with a subcuticular nonabsorbable suture which is removed in 8 to 10 days. Cross-taping with paper tape is recommended for 3 weeks.

The name "double-breasted vest approach" was coined because of the similarities of this technique with the underbuttoning and the outside buttoning of the double-breasted vest. The scar flap which is sutured to the underneath of the opposite side is analogous to the underbuttoning. This is the most important maneuver of the procedure, as it places all the tension on the closure at the subcutaneous level and away from the skin closure. The skin closure is the outside buttoning. The healing between the scar sheet flap and the overlying dermis, i.e., the "dermal imbrication" ensures against tension being exerted on the actual visible skin scar.

Indications

Millard suggested that the double-breasted vest principle be considered for scar repair under certain conditions. This technique should be considered: (1) if the long axis of the scar is in agreement with the lines of relaxed skin tension, and (2) if the scar occurs on certain areas which make notoriously poor scars as a result of constant tension from flexion, extension, rotation, and muscle expansion. He identified these areas as the anterior chest and the arm or leg.

This author has obtained satisfactory results using the double-breasted vest technique in the primary revision of scars of the back of the neck. Additionally, this technique is most satisfactory for the repair of face and anterior neck scars if the long

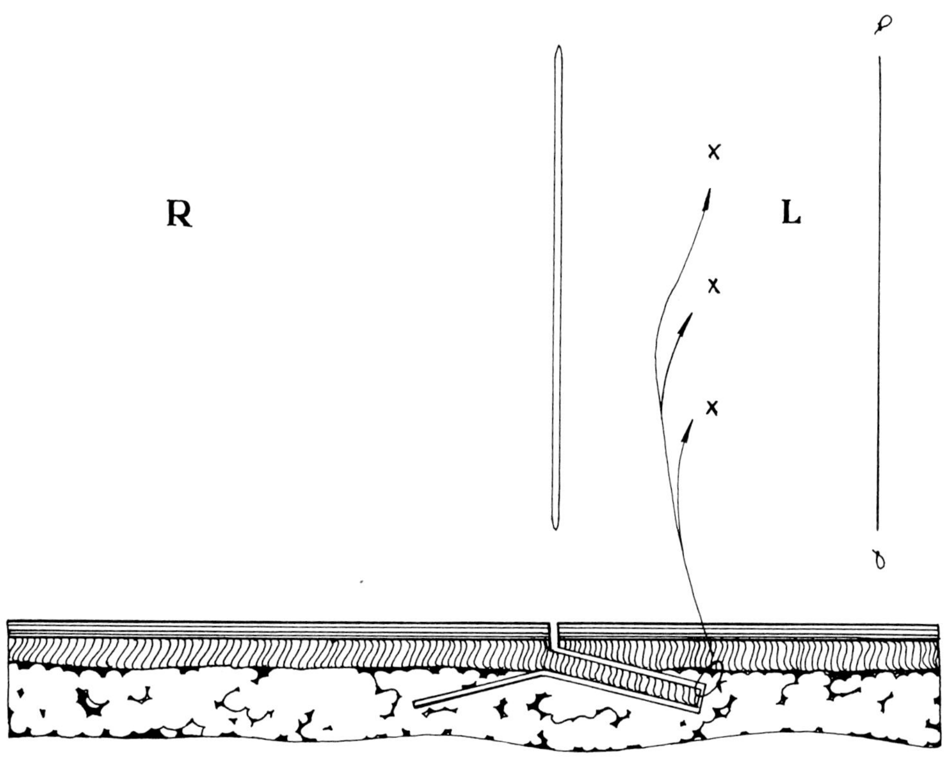

Fig. 5. The scar flap is sutured to the dermis, making the skin closure tension free. Note the thinning of the left side to match the right side.

axis is in agreement with the lines of relaxed tension after regular revision procedures have failed, i.e., as a secondary scar revision technique.

One of the most exciting and interesting aspects of mastering the double-breasted vest technique of scar repair, is that it can be combined with the W-plasty and the geometric design closure maneuvers. This author has utilized these techniques for repair of scars both on the face and extremities, when tension is a problem. The only requirement for combining these procedures is that the scar sheet flap must remain attached to one side of either the W-plasty or geometric design closure (Fig. 6). If the surgeon finds the use of the scar sheet flap awkward, individual tethers of the scar sheet can be constructed and individually sutured to the underside of the dermis of the opposite side of scar repair. Notice that if individual tethers are used in conjunction with the W-plasty they can be constructed from either side of the scar excision (Fig. 7).

References

1. Millard DR: Scar repair by the double-breasted vest principle. Plast Reconstr Surg 45:616–619, 1970

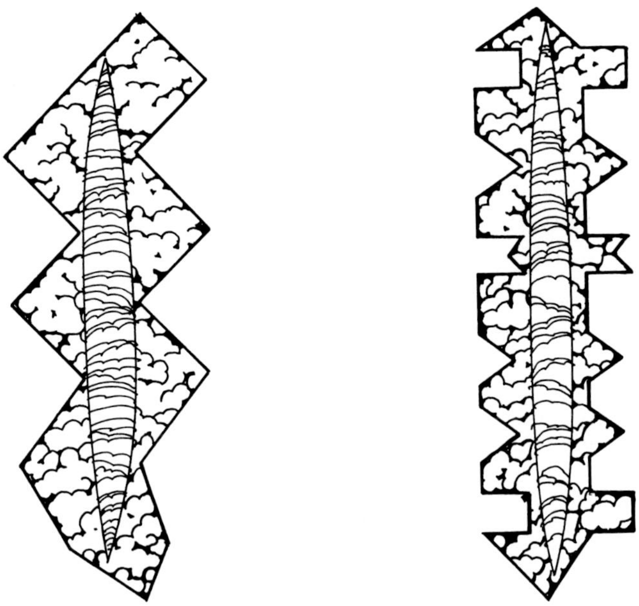

Fig. 6. Double-breasted vest approach combined with W-plasty and geometric design closure. Scar sheet left attached to one side of scar excision site.

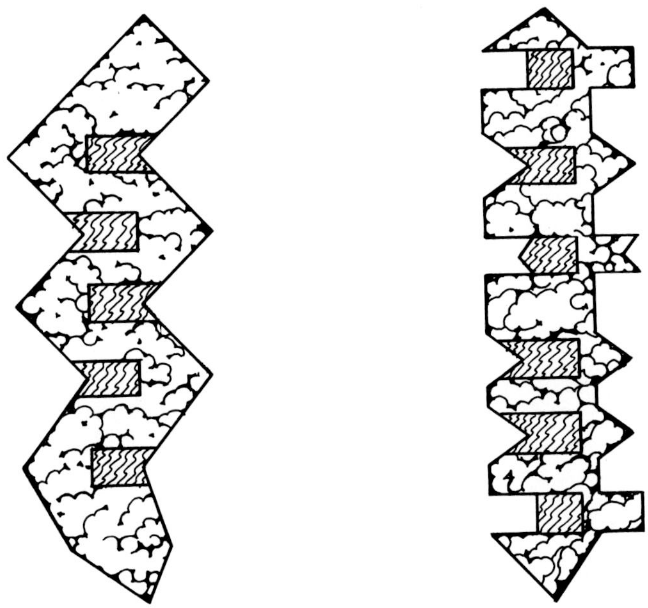

Fig. 7. Individual tethers of scar flaps used with W-plasty and geometric design. Tethers can originate on either side of wound for ease of handling.

Microscopic-Controlled Excision of Cutaneous Tumors

Samuel J. Stegman and Theodore A. Tromovitch, San Francisco, Calif.

When one of the standard therapeutic modalities—surgical excision or radiation therapy or curettage and desiccation—fails to eradicate a cutaneous tumor, treatment of that recurrence with any of these same modalities carries a surprisingly low cure rate. A study out of New York Medical Center by

Menn and Robins, in which complete follow-up data for a large number of cutaneous tumors was tabulated, standard treatment of the recurrent tumors had a cure rate of only around 50 percent.[1] By in large, these recurrences develop because the extent of cutaneous tumors, particularly the basal cell carcinoma, is difficult to judge clinically. The basal cell carcinoma and some squamous cell carcinomas have the proclivity to spread along perichondrium and periosteum, to follow neurovascular bundles, and to spread throughout scar tissue without displaying definate surface changes. As well, there are histologic types of basal cell carcinoma which often do not have distinct clinical borders.

Routine sectioning of skin specimens for pathologic examination is illustrated in Figure 1. The vertical surface of one side of each of these sections is cut by the microtome and thus visualized under the microscope. This approach is adequate to detect the margins of a solid tumor. However, this technique can fail to detect all of the tumor when it is a morphea or sclerosing type (Fig. 2), a multicentric superficial budding type, (Fig. 3), or has finger-like strands (Fig. 4).

To treat these difficult and recurring tumors, a method has been designed, based on Mohs' zinc chloride chemosurgery to examine the entire base and all lateral surfaces of every surgical specimen.[2] This method is called microscopic-controlled excision. Briefly described, under local anesthesia the clinically obvious tumor is curetted or excised in bulk. Around this defect sections are planned and excised so as to obtain specimens which will fit onto a cryostat objective holder and which can be pressed out flat as shown in Figure 5, so that the microtome blade cuts the entire under surface. Thus, microscopic examination of all of the specimens is equivalent to examination of the entire cut surface of the base and the sides of the suspected tumor. The specimens are color coded on two adjacent edges

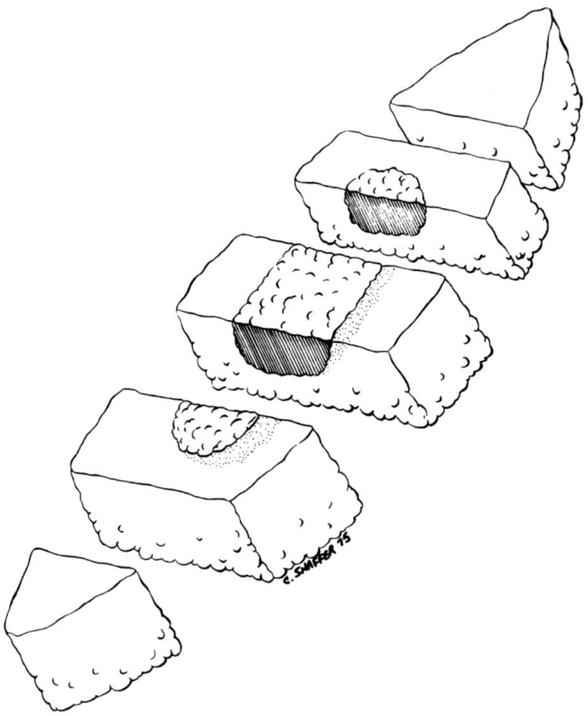

Fig. 1. Standard histopathology sectioning of a nodular, cystic, or adenoid basal cell epithelioma. If the margins are tumor free, usually the entire tumor has been excised.

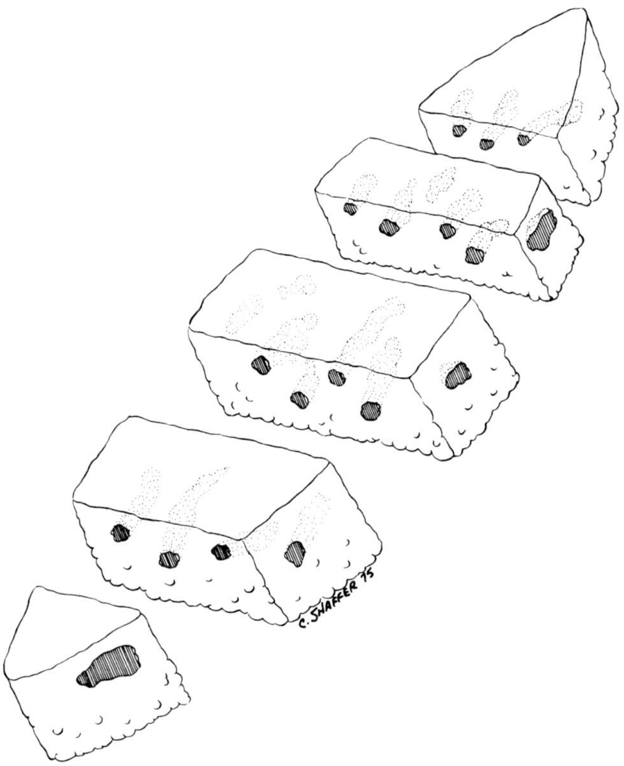

Fig. 2. Standard histopathology sectioning of a morphea or sclerosing basal cell epithelioma. If the margins are tumor free, many times tumor still extends beyond the surgical excision.

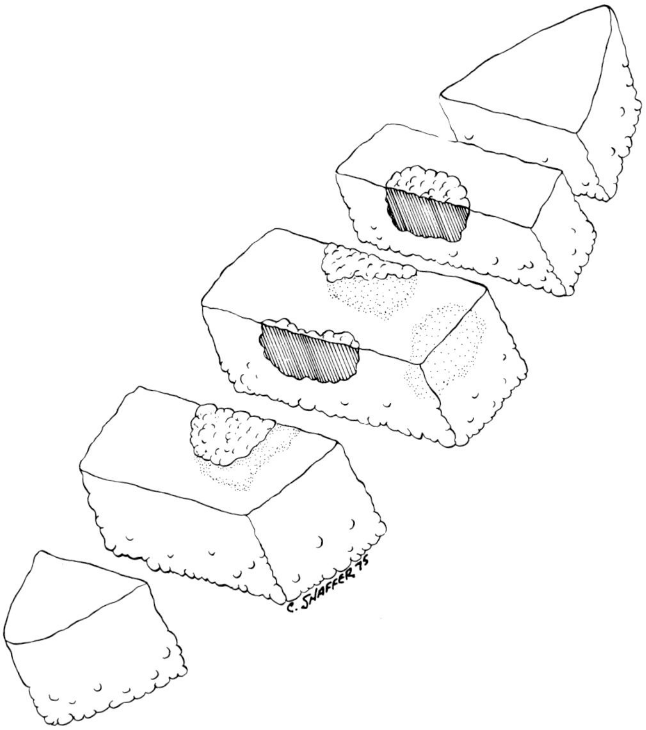

Fig. 3. Standard histopathology sectioning of a multicentric or superficial budding basal cell epithelioma. If the margins are tumor free, tumor may still be present at the lateral borders.

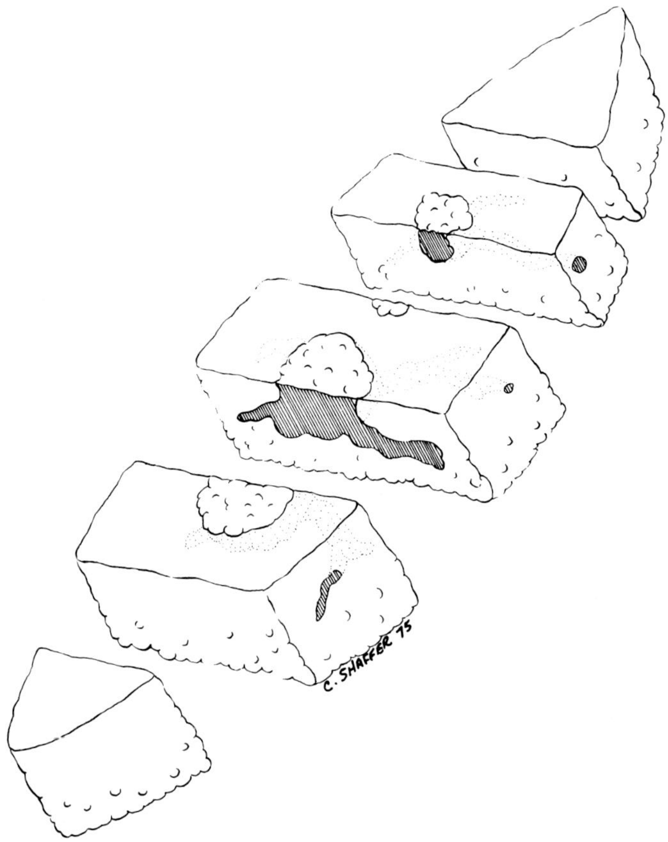

Fig. 4. Standard histopathology sectioning of a basal cell epithelioma which has long fibroepitheliomatous strands. Tumor free margins does not insure that the entire tumor has been excised.

with red and blue dyes which withstand the freezing and cutting and remain visible under the microscope (Fig. 6). This color coding in conjunction with a schematic drawing of each section and its anatomical position on the patient provides the surgeon with exact knowledge of the location of any remaining tumor (Fig. 7). Repeat sections are taken at once, usually after only 30 min to 1 hr, and are marked, mapped, flattended, frozen, sectioned, and microscopically examined in a like manner until all tumor is traced out and excised. As many as four repeat cuttings can be taken in any given working session. If necessary, the surgery can continue on into the following day.

An assistant using a suction apparatus keeps the operative field clear while the tissue is being cut, then hemostasis is achieved by pinpoint electrodesccation and large bleeders are ligated with sutures.

Microscopic-controlled excision is perfectly acceptable for tumors on the trunk and extremities but is especially valuable for tumors which dive deep into areas such as the nasal labial fold or the medial canthus. Microscopic-controlled excision is indicated for tumors in the post auricular area, on the pinna, and on the forehead which are often incompletely treated because they spread beyond what is considered clinically to be an adequate margin for the placement of a radiation field or a surgical border. This method is designed for the sometimes necessary 3rd, 4th, 5th, or however many repeat cuts are needed to achieve total tumor destruction.

Microscopic-controlled excision has been used by us at the University of California Medical School, San Francisco, for approximately 10 years and preliminary data of over 300 cases with a three to seven year follow up indicate that the cure rate is greater than 97 percent for basal cell carcinomas which had already recurred at least once after one or several of the standard treatment modalities.[3]

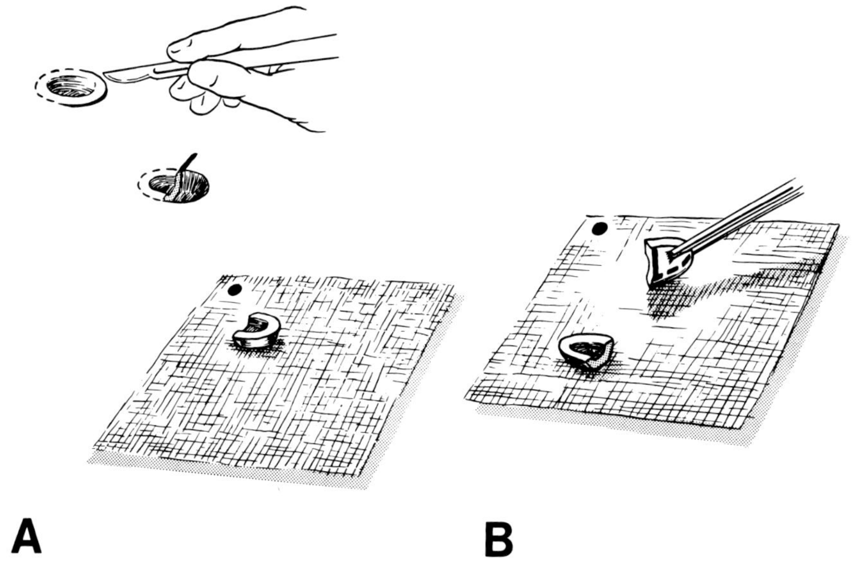

Fig. 5. (A) Excision of the first section for histologic examination of the base and lateral margins. (B) Color coding of the specimen. Red dye is represented by the solid line and blue dye by the dotted line.

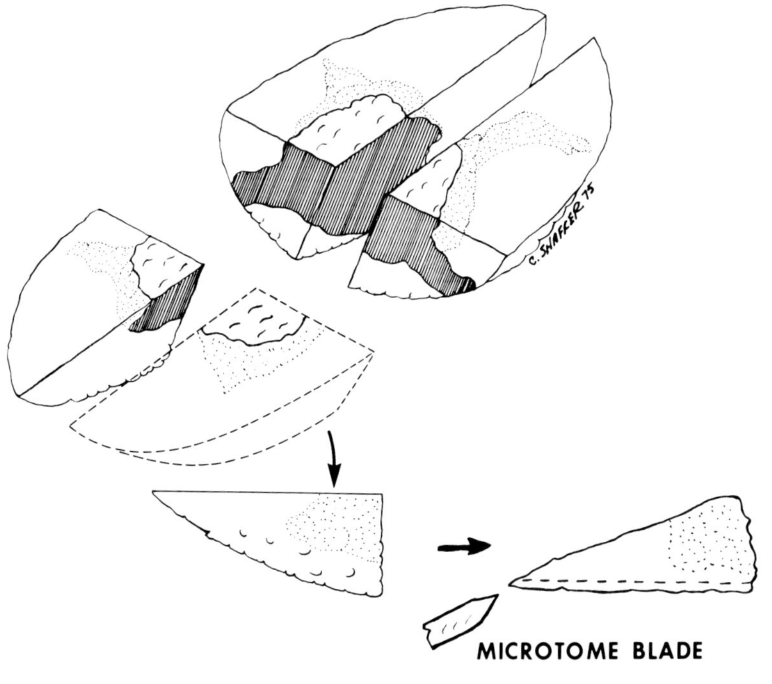

Fig. 6. The microscopic-controlled excision sections for any cutaneous tumor. The entire base and lateral walls are examined microscopically. Insert: one specimen has been pressed down to illustrate how the lateral walls are captured by the cryostat blade.

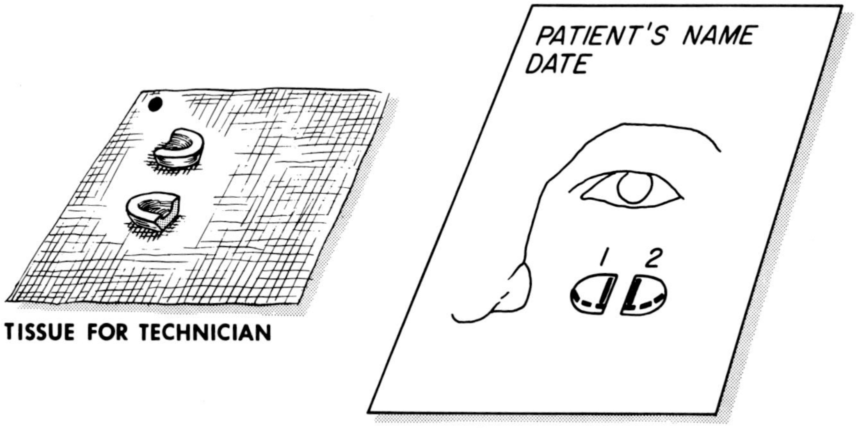

Fig. 7. Coded tissues and the accompanying diagrammatic map.

These cure rates are comparable to Mohs' chemosurgery and are far better for recurrent tumors than has been obtained by surgical re-excision or radiation therapy.[4]

The method has two features of prime importance for the facial plastic and reconstructive surgeon. First, a minimum of normal tissue is sacrificed. This reduces needless loss of important cosmetic structures or facial tissues and prevents unnecessary nasal or ear perforations.

Second, immediately upon completion of tumor removal, the wound can be repaired by the most advantageous manner. For the elderly, closure by simple secondary intention is often the wisest choice. However, primary closure, side to side, or with flaps and grafts can be performed at the same surgical sitting as the tumor excision itself.

Microscopic-controlled excision meets the criteria for present day surgical cancer therapy by providing. (1) A high five year cure rate for those difficult and recurring tumors. (2) The absolute minimal sacrifice of uninvolved and cosmetically important tissues. (3) A method not requiring hospitalization or general anesthesia. (4) Immediate cosmetic repair of the defect.

References

1. Menn H, Robins P, Kopf AW, Bart RS: The recurrent basal cell epithelioma. Arch Dermatol 103:628–631, 1971
2. Mohs FE: Chemosurgery in cancer, gangrene and infections. Charles C. Thomas, Springfield, Illinois, 1956
3. Tromovitch TA, Stegman SJ: Microscopically controlled excision of skin tumors, Arch Dermatol 110:231–232, 1974
4. Mohs FE: Chemosurgery for the microscopically controlled excision of skin cancer. J Surg Oncol 3:257–267, 1971

The Scarf Flap: an Innovation in Cervical Facial Reconstruction

C. Thomas Yarington, Jr., Seattle, Wash.

Flaps have been used in reconstruction of defects in the head and neck since antiquity. Cutaneous rotation flaps from the forehead, the neck, and face, and the chest have been widely used throughout this century with, during the past two decades, the innovation of composite flaps of bone and cartilage. Research into the physiology of flaps, their healing characteristics, circulation, and the limitations of design have led to many innovations and advances in reconstructive efforts following extirpative surgery of the head and neck. One of the flaps which has been a part of the surgeon's armamentarium for some time, has not had wide popularity because of certain limitations in its use. This is the "nape of the neck" flap. This flap frequently based on the posterior occipital arteries and the small perforating arteries of the posterior cervical skin is a useful flap, but frequently considered of limited size and, therefore, infrequently used in the reconstruction of lesions of the anterior neck and jaw. The purpose of this presentation is to draw attention to a flap which has been referred to as the "scarf flap", which is a derivative of the nape of the neck flap. While not an original concept, it seems that an increased awareness of this flap would be beneficial and several innovations made possible by its use are to be presented.

The flap is nourished by the perforating vessels of the scapular circumflex arterial system as well as the posterior occipital vessels. In our experience, the flap is best delayed at least once, and frequently we have utilized this process to implant split-thickness skin grafts which are frequently helpful in reconstructive efforts of the oral cavity or closure of fistulas of the neck.

One of the most versatile and rewarding procedures which this flap allows is reconstruction of the cervical esophagus following ablative surgery for cancer of the laryngopharynx. As seen in Figure 1, a cutaneous tube may be created from lateral neck skin to replace the cervical esophagus

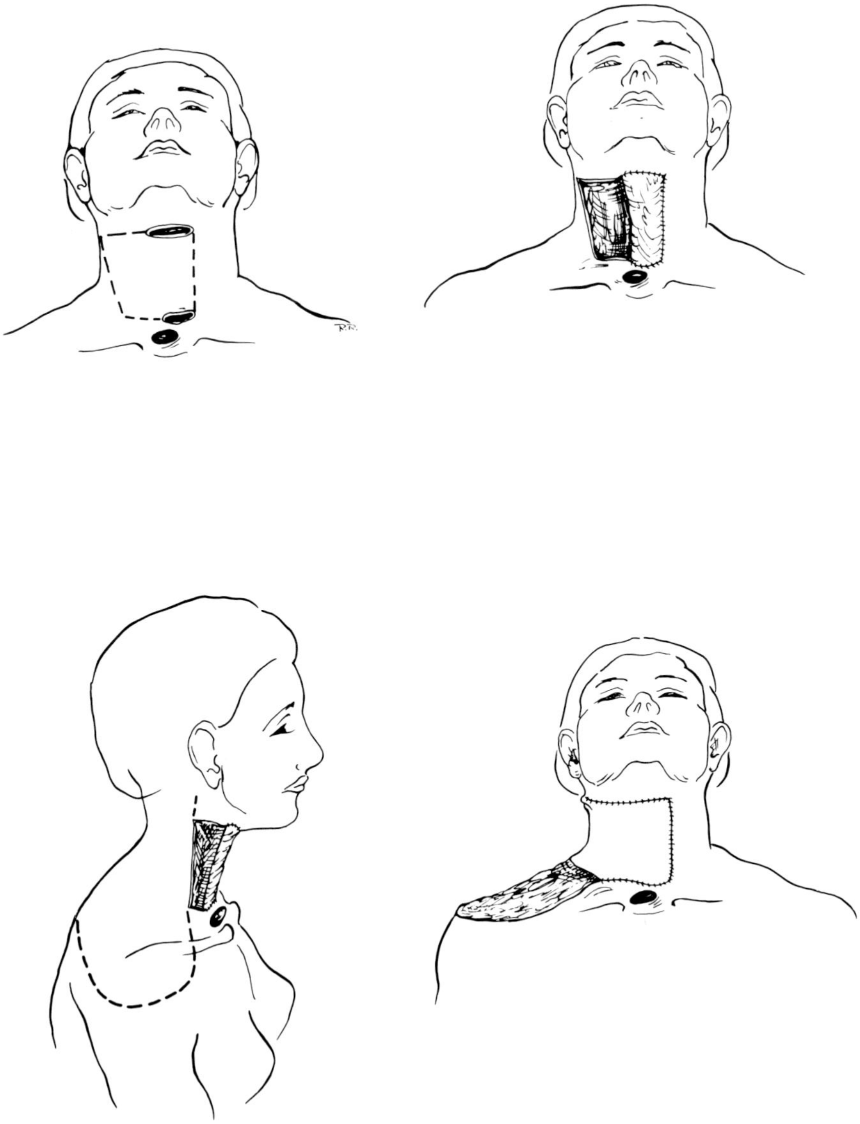

Fig. 1. The four steps for construction of a new cervical esophagus using a lateral neck flap and "scarf flap" as described in the text.

by bridging the gap between a pharyngostoma and esophagostoma. The raw surface created by elevation of this flap and the outer raw surface of the newly created tube may then be covered in one stage by elevation and rotation of a scarf flap as demonstrated. This procedure may frequently be accomplished in one stage, and as seen in Figure 2,

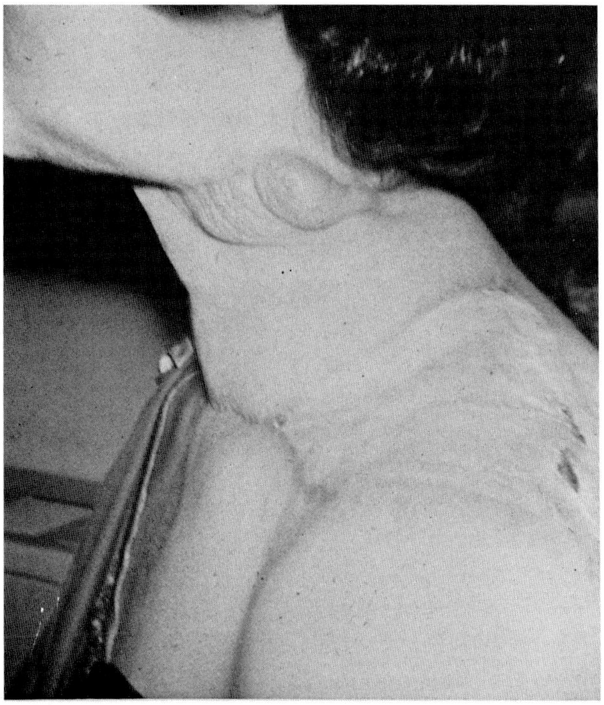

Fig. 2. A patient who has had a reconstruction as depicted in Figure 1, showing the neck flap and healed skin graft on the donor site.

the donor site is repaired with a split thickness skin graft. The end result is cosmetically acceptable, allows a one stage reconstruction of the cervical pharyngoesophagus, and, in our hands, has been the most consistently successful mechanism for reconstruction of this area.

A second area in which we have had rewarding experience with this flap is in reconstruction of the chin and anterior floor of the mouth. An example of this can be seen in Figure 3, illustrating a patient who has been cured of carcinoma of the floor of the mouth with the use of excessive radiation therapy. This resulted in complete loss of the soft tissues of the floor of the mouth, alveolus, labial alveolar sulcus, and all the soft tissue attached to the anterior two-thirds of the mandible bilaterally.

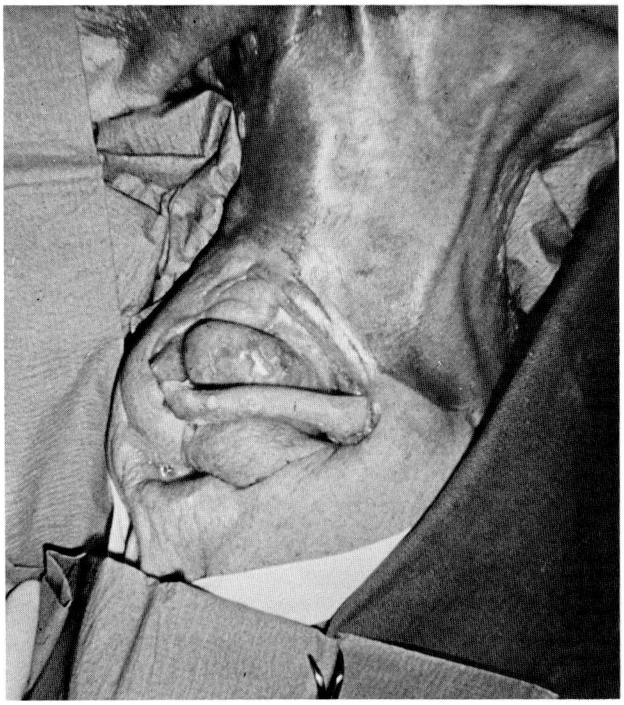

Fig. 3. A patient with loss of the floor of the mouth and mandible requiring reconstruction.

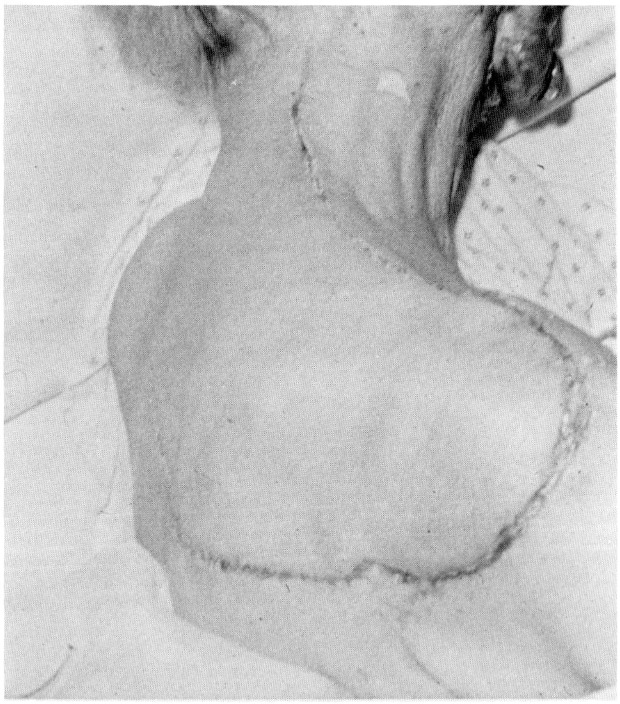

Fig. 4. The large scarf flap utilized to reconstruct the defect shown in Fig. 3.

The radionecrotic mandible required excision and the floor of the mouth was reconstructed using a large scarf flap as demonstrated in Figure 4. This large flap was initially elevated and a split-thickness skin graft placed on the under surface to form the lining for the new anterior floor of the mouth. The placement of the graft is illustrated in Figure 5. At a second stage the flap is rotated into position and the healed skin graft forms the new internal lining of the floor of the mouth and small rotation flaps of buccal mucous membrane are elevated from lateral to medial to bridge the area between the split-thickness graft and the cutaneous surface of the flap and form a vermillion of a newly created lower lip. This stage is illustrated in Figure 6. Following stabilization of the new blood supply to the distal flap, the pedicle is transsected and the proximal portion of the separated distal flap inserted into the submental tissue of the neck closing the oral cavity. The newly created floor of the mouth and chin structures, although without bony support, provided a water-tight oral cavity and allowed adequate speech and complete nutrition compatible with that of an edentulous individual.

Clearly, other uses of this flap will become apparent to the observer as they have to the author.

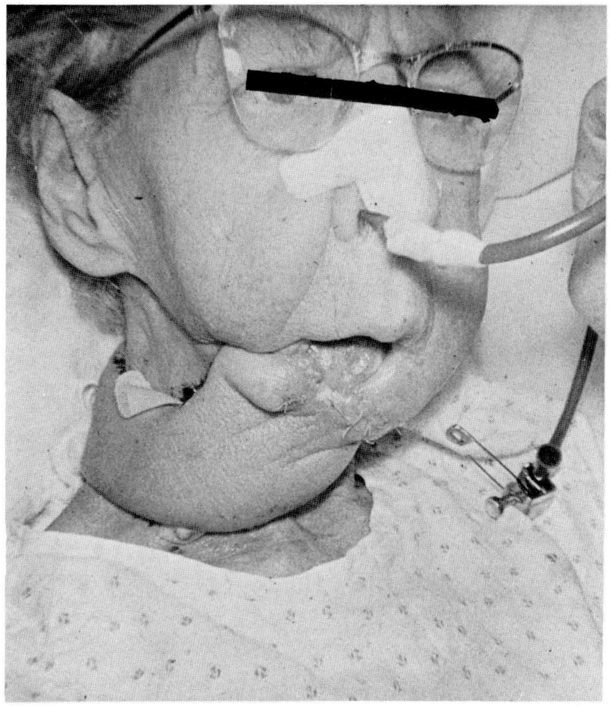

Fig. 6 This demonstrates the initial status after rotation of the flap and reconstruction of the floor of the mouth and chin.

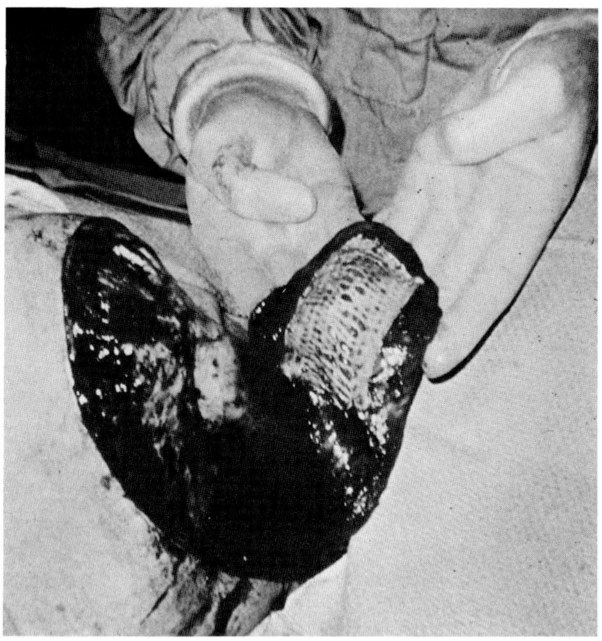

Fig. 5. A large split thickness graft was inlaid on the flap seen in Fig. 4 at the time of its initial delay.

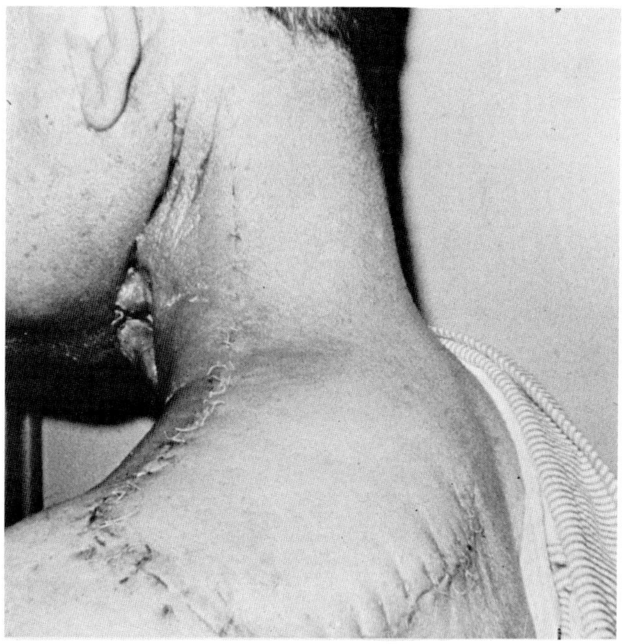

Fig. 7. The end result of reconstruction of the defect seen in Figure 3.

The flap can be used in large dimensions, with the tip extending out over the posterior surface of the upper arm, or as a long, narrow shoulder flap. The flap may be elevated and rotated about the neck much as a scarf is wrapped around the neck and used in the reconstruction of those areas of the neck, lower face, and chin which a scarf might cover. From this we have coined the term "scarf flap." Variations in the length and width of the flap may be easily achieved to suit the the problem that is being rectified while maintaining an adequate ratio of not greater than 3:1 for length to width (Fig. 7).

Summary

A derivation of the nape of the neck flap has been presented and it is suggested that this flap might be utilized for a variety of reconstructive tasks about the head and neck. Examples of its use in closure of the cervical esophagus and in reconstruction of the anterior floor of the mouth and chin have been presented. While it usually requires a delay, it is a versatile and useful flap which is appropriate for any of the areas of the neck and mandible which might be covered by a scarf.

Orbit

Surgery of the Orbit and Lacrimal System (Panel)

Allen M. Putterman:

The following is a synopsis of the presentations at the plenary session on surgery of the orbit and lacrimal system at the Second International Symposium on Plastic and Reconstructive Surgery on the Head and Neck. Dr. Morton Goldberg initiated the presentations with a paper titled "Use of the Retinal Cryoprobe in the Surgical Management of Orbital Tumors." The paper was written by Drs. Allen Putterman and Morton Goldberg and will soon be published in the American Journal of Ophthalmology.

Four cases were described in which the retinal cryoprobe facilitated the removal of orbital and adnexal tumors. The retinal cryoprobe was used in Case 1 to apply traction to an optic nerve glioma without tearing it. It was not necessary to place toothed forceps or clamps into the substance of the nerve. Traction also facilitated taking frozen and conventional histopathologic specimens. There was no significant bleeding from the sites of the tumor removal. In Case 2, the cryoprobe allowed moderate traction to be applied to a cavernous hemangioma without tearing its capsule and aided in intracapsular delivery. Progressive circumferential reapplication of the cryoprobe tip along the course of blunt dissection of the tumor was found to be an advantageous method of removing the tumor. In Case 3, the cryoprobe application allowed much more pressure to be exerted over a medial canthal cystic mass than would forceps or clamps. The progressive circumferential reapplication used in Case 2 was valuable in this case also. When the cyst was severed, the cryoprobe application sealed the opening and allowed removal of the cyst in its entirety, decreasing the risk of reoccurrence. In Case 4, the circumferential reapplication of the cryoprobe allowed moderate traction to be applied to a hemangiopericytoma facilitating separation of about 50 percent of the tumor from the surrounding tissue. However, when marked traction was applied to the tumor to separate tight adhesions to the superior orbital tissues, the capsule ruptured. This demonstrated that use of the cryoprobe is not without potential complications. However, it was evident that grasping the tumor with forceps or other instruments would have caused rupture of the capsule with much less traction than that induced with the cryoprobe.

In all four cases, the cryoprobe application had no apparent effect on the microscopic detail of the histopathologic sections.

In summary, the retinal cryoprobe was a valuable instrument in the surgical management (biopsies and excisions) of orbital and ocular adnexal tumors in four patients. The strong bond between the cryoprobe tip and the tumor allowed moderate traction to be applied to the tumor, facilitating its removal. The ice ball that encompassed the communication of the cryoprobe tip and the tumor helped prevent rupture of the tumor and cyst wall.

Dr. Putterman's presentation stressed the treatment of enophthalmos after blow-out orbital floor fractures and exophthalmos caused by thyroid disease by eyelid, rather than orbital surgery. Before discussing the treatment of enophthalmos after blow-out orbital fractures, he remarked on the nonsurgical management of blow-out fractures. A paper titled "Nonsurgical Management of Blow-out Fractures of the Orbital Floor" (Putterman AM, Stevens T, Urist M, Amer J Ophthalmol 77: 232, 1974) reported on 57 patients with radiographically proved pure blow-out fractures of the orbital floor who were followed without surgery despite the severity of their fractures and symptoms. Although 50 percent of the patients had visually handicapping diplopia at their first examination, none of the patients had visually handicapping diplopia four to six months later. None of the patients developed cosmetically unacceptable enophthalmos, although about 20 percent of the patients did develop measurable enophthalmos of 3 mm or less which was cosmetically acceptable and did not require surgical treatment. Also, infraorbital anesthesia decreased with time. Since most patients with blow-out fractures will be asymptomatic and cosmetically acceptable without surgery, since the surgical treatment of blow-out orbital floor fractures has multiple complications, including blindness, since it is possible to successfully treat visually handicapping diplopia and cosmetically unacceptable enophthalmos in the few patients in whom this exists after four to six months, the authors advocate that all pure blow-out fractures of the orbital floor be followed without surgery for four to six months after trauma. If after this time visually handicapping diplopia persists, it can be treated by extraocular muscle surgery usually on the uninvolved eye.

If cosmetically unacceptable enophthalmos exists after four to six months, it can be treated in one of three ways:

1. A thick Silastic orbital floor can be implanted if downward sinking of the eye is present. The implant is carved from a block of Silastic to match the deformity of the orbital floor. The thickness of the implant directly below the eye is equal to the millimeters of downward sinking of the eye. Posteriorly the implant is usually made several millimeters thicker than the part below the eye and anteriorly it is usually tapered to 2 to 3 mm. When the anterior aspect of the implant is sutured downward to the inferior orbital rim, a teeter-totter effect is created in which the posterior aspect of the implant is elevated, thereby pushing the eye upward and outward. A patient with total loss of the orbital floor secondary to a blow-out fracture with 6 mm of enophthalmos and 5 mm of downward displacement of the eye was presented to demonstrate surgical achievement of cosmetic acceptance with the Silastic implant.

2. If enophthalmos is associated with a narrow palpebral fissure, elevating the upper eyelid with a Müller's muscle-conjunctival resection ptosis procedure widens the palpebral fissure and creates the illusion of enophthalmos resolution without invading the orbit. This procedure takes advantage of the principle that when the eyelids are opened widely, an exophthalmic appearance exists and when the eyelids are partially closed, an enophthalmic appearance exists. The "Müller's muscle-conjunctival resection blepharoptosis procedure" is an operation devised by Dr. Putterman and Dr. Urist and will soon be published in the Archives of Ophthalmology. It consists of applying a clamp designed by Dr. Putterman and produced by Karl Ilg and Company to 8 mm of conjunctiva and Müller's muscle above the superior tarsal border. The tissues held in the clamp are severed from the tarsus after a suture is run distal to the clamp connecting the remaining conjunctiva and Müller's muscle to the tarsus. The patients with enophthalmos associated with a narrow palpebral fissure whose upper eyelids elevate to an acceptable position after the instillation of 10 percent phenylephrine to the upper ocular fornix are candidates for this procedure. Phenylephrine stimulates the sympathetically innervated Müller's muscle and gives the surgeon an approximation of what can be accomplished through strengthening the muscle by resection and advancement. There has been a high correlation between the upper eyelid level after the phenylephrine test compared to that after the Müller's muscle-conjunctival resection procedure, thus making it an accurate test for choosing surgical candidates.

3. If enophthalmos is associated with a deep supratarsal sulcus, excising an ellipse of skin and orbital fat from the contralateral upper eyelid leads to symmetric deep supratarsal sulci and cosmetic acceptance.

Exophthalmos after thyroid disease that is associated with visual loss is treated with steroids initially and, if vision has deteriorated and does not improve, by an orbital decompression. Orbital decompression is rarely necessary for exophthalmos after thyroid disease that is not associated with visual loss. It is recommended for those few patients with severe unilateral exophthalmos or severe bilateral exophthalmos without eyelid retraction. The preferred method is Ogura's procedure of removing the orbital floor and medial wall through a Caldwell-Luc approach and allowing the orbital contents to prolapse into the maxillary and ethmoid sinuses. The frequent complication of diplopia after an orbital decompression makes the procedure disadvantageous for patients who have only a cosmetic problem.

Most patients with thyroid exophthalmos have associated eyelid retraction and can be successfully treated by lowering the upper eyelid through the excision of Müller's muscle and the stripping and recession of the levator aponeurosis. This procedure narrows the palpebral fissure and creates the illusion that the exophthalmos has resolved. (This is the opposite idea to widening the palpebral fissure in patients with enophthalmos after blow-out fractures to create the illusion of exophthalmos.) The procedure was fully described in "Surgical Treatment of Upper Eyelid Retraction" by Dr. Putterman and Dr. Urist (Arch Ophthalmol 88:665, 1972). The procedure consists of providing sensory without motor anesthesia and gradually lowering the upper eyelid by a step-by-step excision of Müller's muscle and stripping and recession of the levator aponeurosis. The patient is sat up frequently during the procedure until the eyelid level and arch are satisfactory, thereby adding to the predictability of the postoperative result.

In summary, this presentation stressed the treatment of enophthalmos after blow-out fracture by a Müller's muscle-conjunctival resection blepharoptosis procedure to create the illusion of enophthalmos resolution, and the treatment of exophthalmos after thyroid disease by the controlled excision of Müller's muscle and stripping and recession of levator aponeurosis to create the illusion of exophthalmos resolution, both performed through eyelid surgery without invading the orbit.

Dr. Lup Q. Pang presented his technique for external dacryocystorhinostomy. He stressed minimizing hemorrhage during the procedure by using local anesthesia achieved with an infraorbital and supratrochlear nerve block, nasal mucosal cocaine, and subcutaneous infiltration. An incision is made 2 to 4 mm from the medial canthus to avoid incising the angular vessels which are 8 mm nasal to the medial canthus. A layer-by-layer dissection at the incision site is performed until periosteum is reached. Retractors are used to aid in hemostasis. The periosteum is reflected with the nasal lacrimal sac wall. The anterior lacrimal sac flap is fashioned to be twice the size of the posterior flap. The anterior and posterior lacrimal flaps are then sutured to the anterior and posterior nasal mucosa flaps.

Dr. Ronald Strahan presented a patient with a lacrimal sac tumor. He stressed that the diagnosis be anticipated in patients with recurrent dacryocystitis and a progressive enlargement of the medial canthal area. Palpation of a firm mass and dacryocystography can aid in substantiating the diagnosis. The case presented had infiltration into the orbital tissue and required an orbital exenteration.

Dr. Strahan also presented a technique for intranasal dacryocystorhinostomy. The advantage of this approach is that it avoids a visible scar which can be quite noticeable in those blacks who tend to keloid formation. The procedure is facilitated by the use of an operating microscope. A fiberoptic light applied externally between the anterior and posterior lacrimal crests points out the intranasal site for the osteotomy. Nasal mucosa and lacrimal sac flaps are allowed to fuse together by placing Vaseline gauze packing between them.

Dr. Byron Smith stated that acute dacryocystitis can lead to closure of the common canaliculus by edematous folds of lacrimal sac mucosa falling against the common canaliculus. The common canaliculus can be opened in these cases and the pain relieved by aspirating the contents of the lacrimal sac.

Lipiodol injection is not recommended in dacryocystography because interstitial extravasation from the lacrimal excretory system can create a granuloma which has to be removed surgically. The surgeon himself should be responsible for dacryocystography injection since the occurrence of false passages is quite high when this responsibility is delegated to assistants.

Dr. Smith stated that he has been successful in surgically treating canalicular obstructions by suturing the canalicular walls to the conjunctiva. He recommends that the pigtail probe not be used in lacrimal surgery as it is a dangerous instrument that can cause false passages and secondary obstructions. Teflon tubes are left in the repaired canaliculi for three to four months postoperatively to act as stents to prevent reoccurrence of the obstruction. Dacryocystectomy is rarely necessary in the treatment of chronic dacryocystitis and dacryocystorhinostomy is usually indicated.

The presentation at the plenary session of the surgery of the orbit and lacrimal system consisted of many interesting ideas which should be useful to all attending the session.

Immediate Rehabilitation of the Orbit Following Radical Exenteration

Ronald C. Hamaker, Indianapolis, Ind. and
John Conley, New York, N.Y.

A maxillectomy causes minimal deformity and is easily rehabilitated with a palatal prosthesis. However, maxillectomy with orbital exenteration has resulted in a gross orbital defect. Many modifications have been made to improve this cosmetic deformity and rehabilitate the patient. Such techniques as excising the eyelid lash margins with direct approximation as well as tarsal plates preserving eyelids totally, have been described.[1,2]

In all of these techniques, the patient resorts to wearing a black eyepatch, frosted unilateral lens, or an ocular prosthesis attached to the glasses.

This paper presents a technique which allows for an immediate ocular prosthesis and rehabilitation at the time of surgery. The technique when successfully accomplished has allowed the patients to eliminate their black eyepatch which has been the customary hallmark of orbital exenteration.

The decision to remove the orbital contents is frequently made prior to surgery by means of radiographic tomography and clinical examination. Orbital exenteration is required in approximately 45 percent of paranasal sinus malignancies. When clinical examination or roentgenography are not sufficient to justify initial orbital exenteration then an exploration of the orbital floor and medial wall is required to make that decision.

The lateral rhinotomy incision is extended superiorly and laterally through the eyebrow to approximately two-thirds of the brow's length (Fig. 1). The subconjunctival space is infiltrated elevating the conjunctiva from the globe (Figs. 2, 3). An incision is then made around the limbus (Fig. 4). The subconjunctival plane is dissected to the level of the tarsal plate. This elevation is done in a

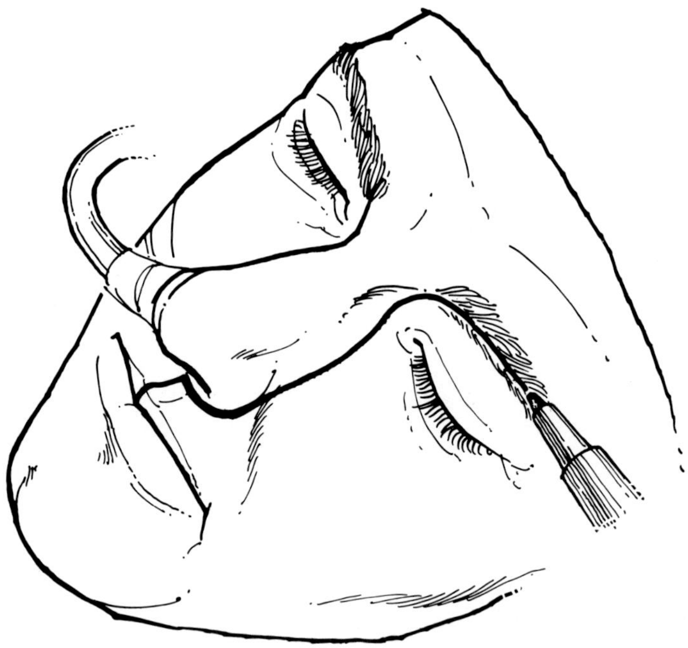

Fig. 1. The incision is carried through the eyebrow to the lateral one-third.

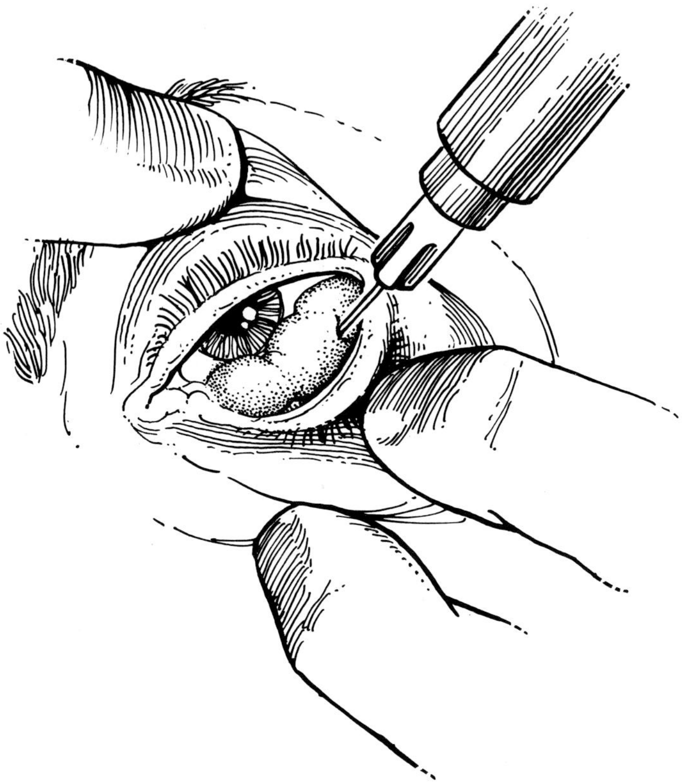

Fig. 2. Infiltrate in subconjunctival plane elevating the conjunctiva from the globe.

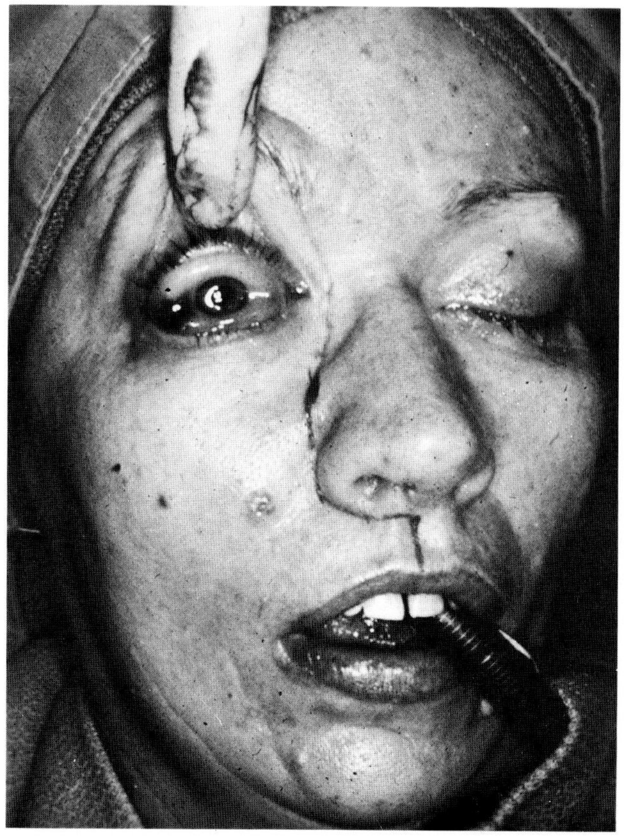

Fig. 3. Conjunctiva elevated in preparation for dissection.

radial fashion from the iris. The medial canthus is then dissected, incising and elevating the medial canthal ligament with the orbicularis muscle, tarsal plates, conjunctiva of the globe, and overlying eyelid skin. The plane of dissection is between the orbicularis muscle and orbital septum. This elevation is joined with that previously done over the face of the maxilla. Thus a large facial flap is raised, based laterally with its limitation of reflection being the lateral extension of the brow incision superiorly and the posterior extension of the buccogingival incision inferiorly as the flap's pivot points. The lateral canthus continuity with the lateral orbital rim is preserved (Fig. 5). The neuromuscular system of the lids is intact.

The standard maxillectomy with exenteration of the orbit is performed. At completion the conjunctival defect (area of iris and pupil) is closed. A split thickness skin graft is used to line the cavity and the undersurface of the reflected orbital-facial flap (Fig. 6). The flap is then returned for closure, wire suturing the medial canthal ligament to the remaining nasal bone or to the opposite medial canthus as in a canthoplasty operation (Fig. 7). This stabilizes the orbicularis muscle and palpebral fissure into a normal position. At the completion of closure and packing of the maxillo-orbital defect, an orbital disc prosthesis with color match may be inserted (Fig. 8).

The most obvious contraindication to this technique is tumor extension through the orbital septum into the eyelid. This would require excision of the eyelid en toto for an adequate margin. Usually when the orbit is involved without skin involvement, the tumor extension is deep to the confining limits of the orbital septum. Preservation of the medial canthus may be contraindicated in large ethmoid malignancies or extension into the area by a maxillary carcinoma. In this case the technique does not need to be totally abandoned.

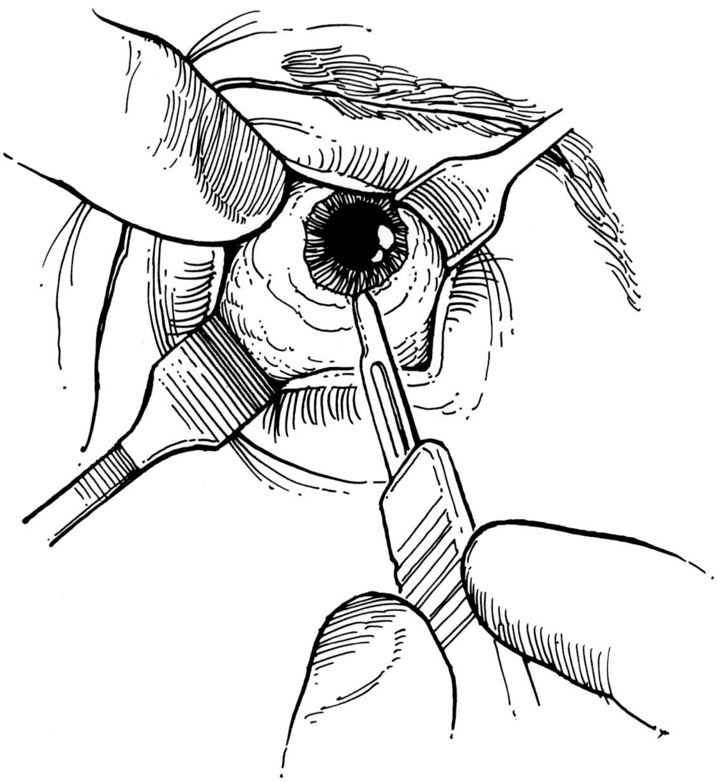

Fig. 4. Incision is made about the limbus for dissection of the conjunctiva.

Elevation of the flap in the medial aspect can be undertaken anterior to the ligament and on approaching the lacrimal punctum the dissection can be carried through the orbicularis to the orbital septal plane. An excellent result has never been accomplished when the medial canthus was resected. However, the accomplishment is still superior to a large orbital defect.

One of the most disappointing complications of this technique has been the development of fistulae along the conjunctival closure line or in the medial canthal area (Fig. 9). This occurs primarily in heavily irradiated tissues either preoperative or postoperative. This problem can be reduced by inserting a portion of the temporalis muscle and fascia through the lateral orbital wall posterior to the orbital rim to reinforce the closure line and medial canthus.

Edema of the upper lid requires up to six months for improvement. This occurs with lateral extension of the dissection and irradiation (Fig. 10). Ptosis is created by the procedure and may require multiple adjustments in the ocular prosthesis to improve the cosmetic appearance.

The preservation of the conjunctiva permits immediate reconstruction of the eye socket. The technique presented allows for orbicularis oculi function as the innervation is preserved. There is good visualization for ablative surgery. The rehabilitation is far superior to that of previous described techniques in reconstruction of this area. It has been carried out on fourteen patients with 90 percent success in nonirradiated cases and 40 percent success in irradiated cases.

References

1. Harrison DFN: The natural history of some cancers affecting the head and neck. J Laryngol Otol 86:1189–1202, 1972
2. Kimmich HM: Radical palliative surgery about the orbit. Arch Otolaryngol 94:338–346, 1971

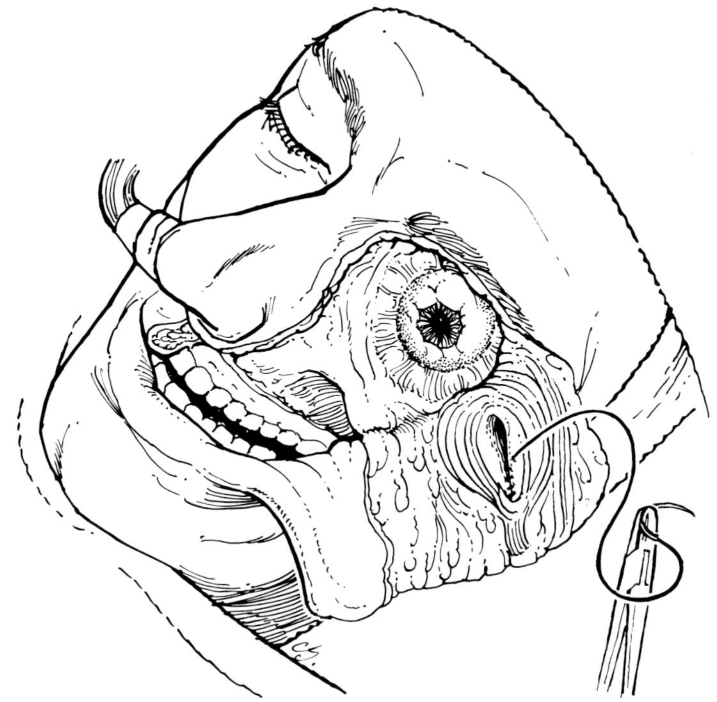

Fig. 5. Reflection of the flap with the orbicularis muscle and medial canthal ligament preserving the orbital septum for resection. The conjunctival limbus incision is closed. The lateral canthal ligament is preserved.

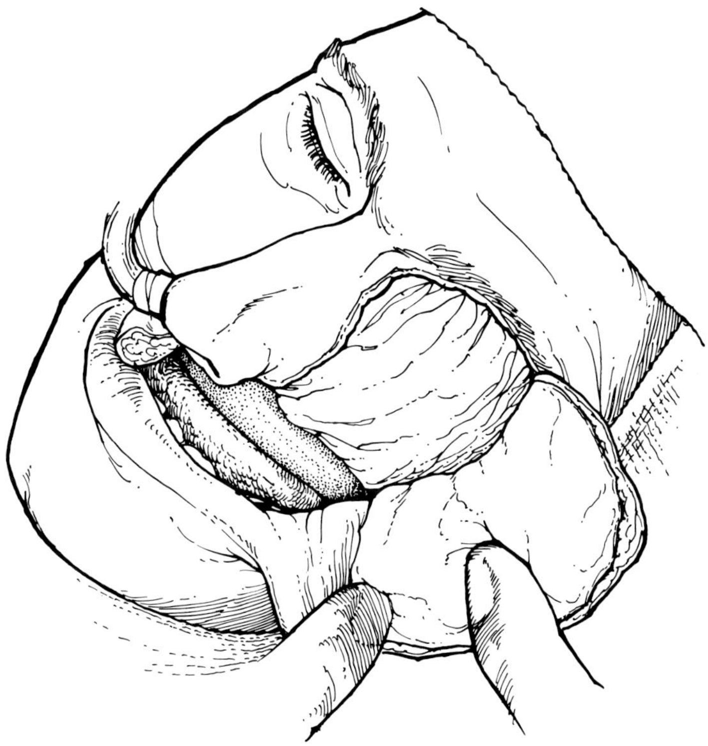

Fig. 6. A split thickness skin graft is applied to under surface of flap covering raw surface and conjunctival closure line.

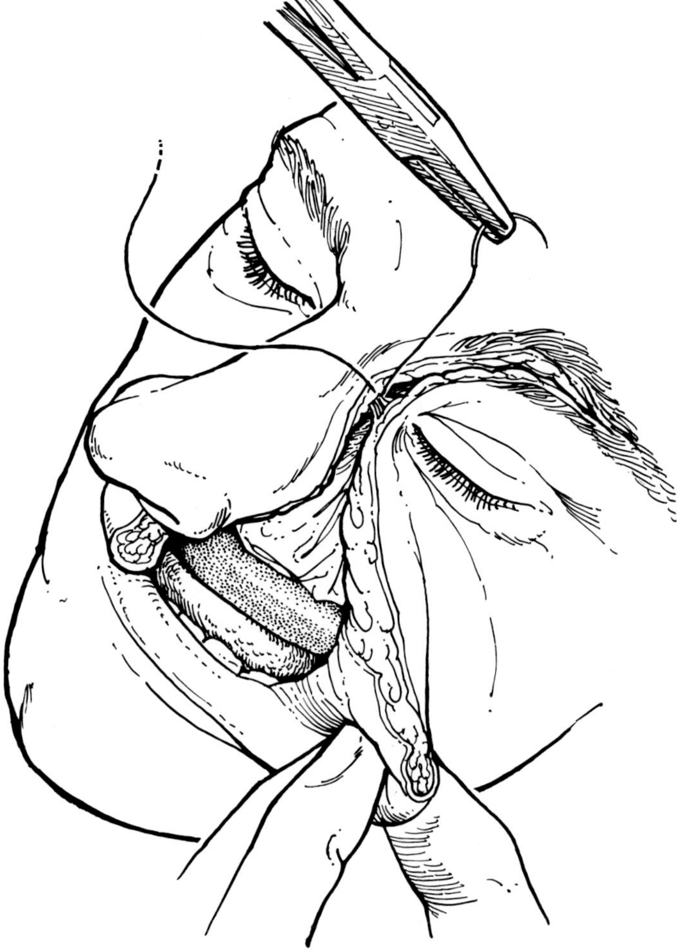

Fig. 7. Medial canthal ligament is repositioned with wire suture to the original area or by through and through wire to the opposite medial canthus.

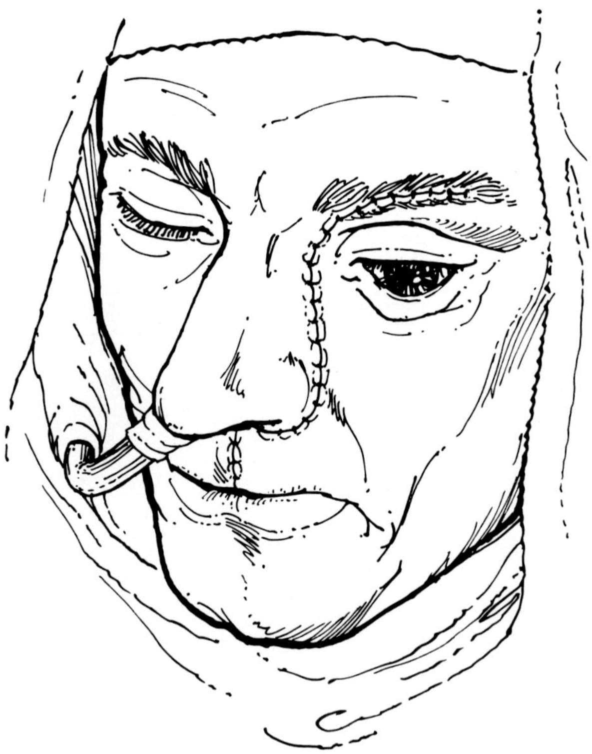

Fig. 8. Incision closed and ocular prosthesis inserted.

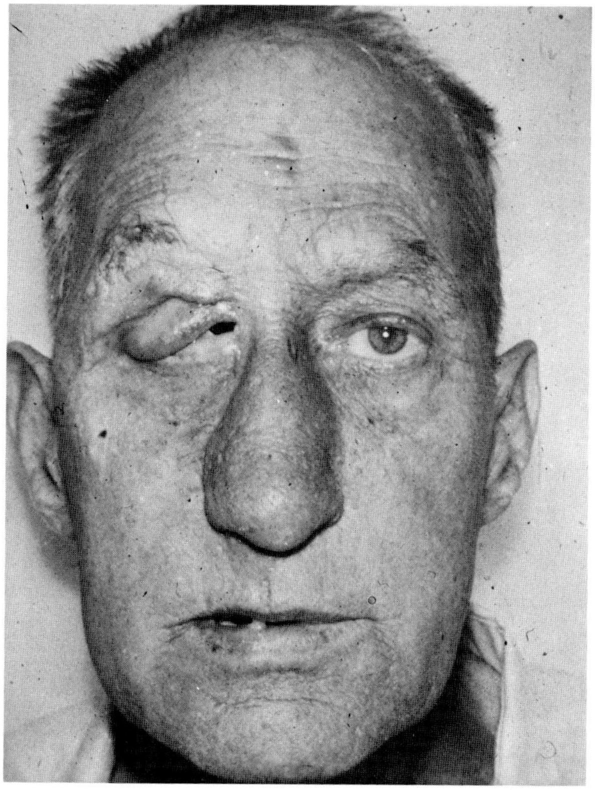

Fig. 9. Case of undifferentiated carcinoma treated with preoperative radiation, and postoperative chemotherapy and radium implant for residual disease. Had fistula requiring black eye patch for cosmesis.

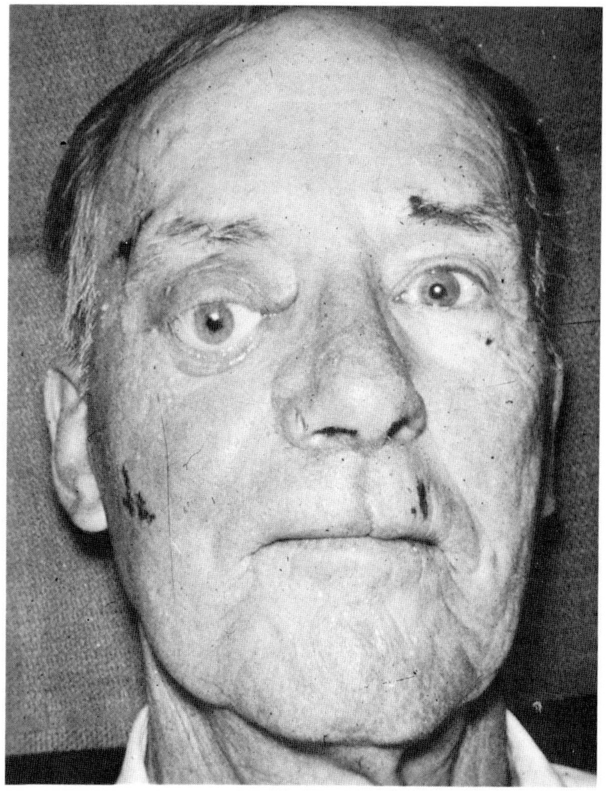

Fig. 10. Patient six weeks postoperative maxillectomy and orbital exenteration for squamous cell carcinoma. Shown is the edema in the upper lid associated with postoperative irradiation. This improved and the prosthesis adjusted for better cosmesis.

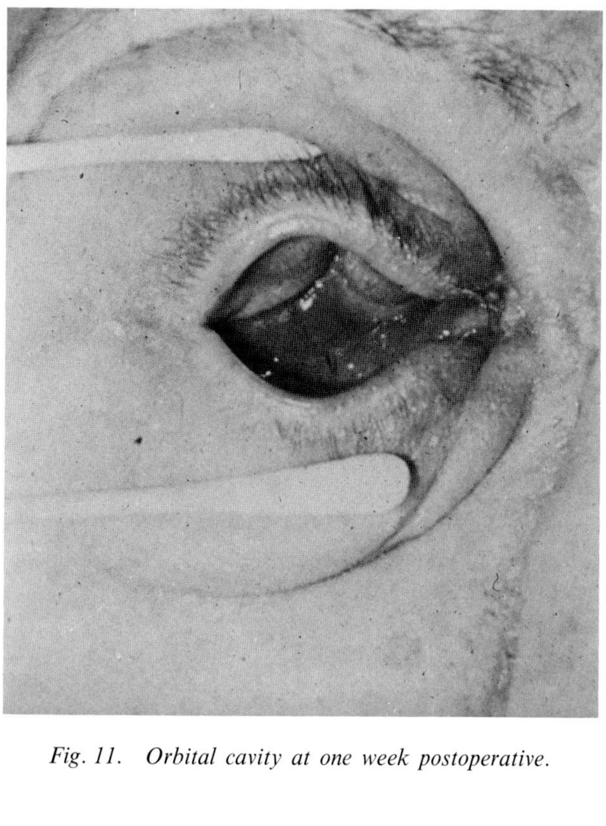

Fig. 11. Orbital cavity at one week postoperative.

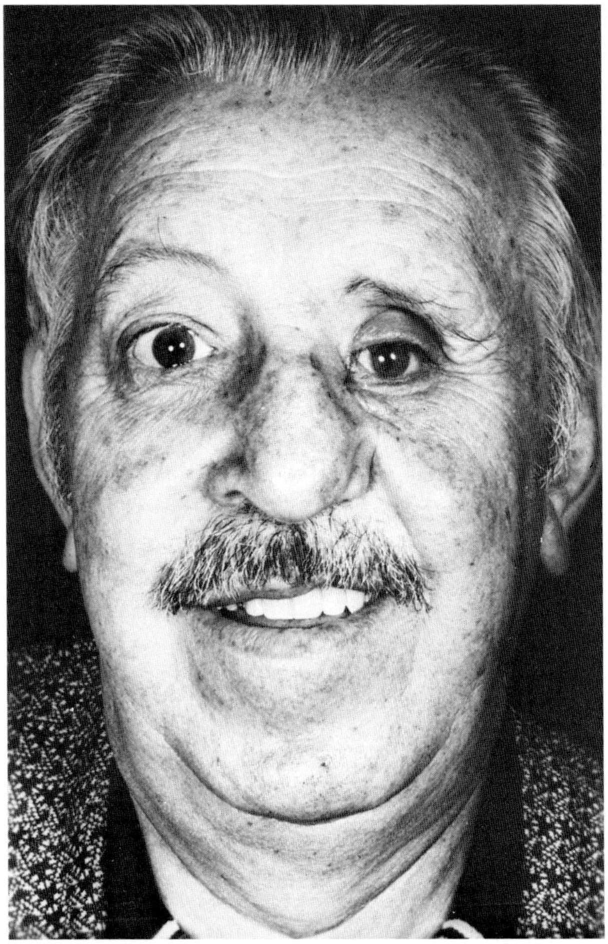

Fig. 12. *Patient one month postoperative for melanoma of lacrimal sac requiring maxillectomy, ethmoid and orbital exenteration.*

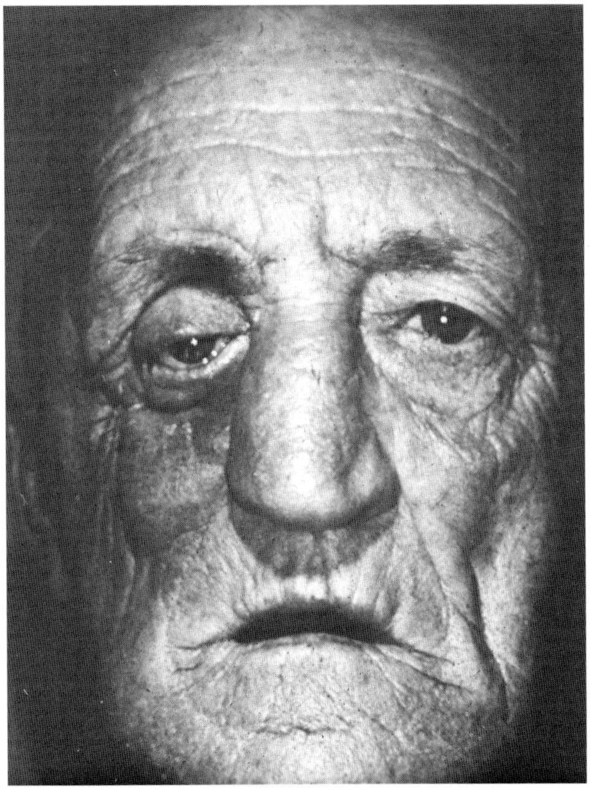

Fig. 13. *Case of squamous cell carcinoma of the maxillary sinus extending into the orbit. Our technique has been used by others with good results (Courtesy of Dr. D. E. Schuller and Dr. W. H. Saunders).*

Treatment of the Traumatized Orbital Floor

William L. Meyerhoff, San Antonio, Tex., Kent Wilson, Minneapolis, Minn., and Thomas Christiansen, Philadelphia, Penn.

Introduction

Fractures of the facial skeleton which involve the orbital floor are not uncommon in the experience of reconstructive surgeons who care for facially injured patients. Because of the orbital floor's proximity to the globe, the paranasal sinuses, and the soft tissues of the face, several disciplines may become involved in the management of orbital floor fractures. Reports of orbital floor fractures, their diagnoses and treatment, are numerous and date back to the original description by MacKenzie in 1844.[1] The volume of work in this area gives evidence to the confusion surrounding the proper approach to the patient with the traumatized orbital floor, especially in regard to fundamental differences in the frequencies with which surgical therapy is undertaken.

In 1962, Patterson and Dupre, in discussing facially injured patients, stated, "it is relatively easy for an orbital floor fracture to be overlooked and in many of these cases, after the initial crisis is over, the ocular complications of diplopia and enophthalmos may persist as the major cause of disability." They concluded by saying, "treatment is directed toward freeing the orbital contents from the fracture site and the restoration of the orbital floor and this must be carried out within the first seven to ten days before irreversible changes occur".[2] Reeh and Tsujimura supported this concept in their 1966 article saying, "this fracture must be recognized and treated at once, or assuredly within a period of seven days." And, they added, "late treatment of blowout fractures is discouraging".[3] McCoy et al, in an analysis of 91 patients with midfacial injury involving the orbital floor concluded that orbital floor exploration was indicated whenever orbital floor involvement was suspected.[4]

The opposite end of the therapeutic spectrum is represented by Putterman et al, who emphatically advocated, "no patient with pure blowout fracture be operated on immediately but be kept under observation for 4 to 6 months or longer to observe the rate of improvement".[5] Most authors have taken a more intermediate position and suggest that surgical treatment of fractures involving the orbital floor be reserved for those cases exhibiting incarceration or impingment of extraocular tissue, displacement of orbital contents, and comminution or malposition of the fracture segments. Surgical intervention should be accomplished within two weeks of injury to minimize enophthalmos and persistent diplopia.[6–11]

In an attempt to clarify some of these differences, a retrospective study of facial fractures involving the orbital floor was undertaken. It is felt that the study population represents a satisfactorily broad spectrum of orbital floor fractures to yield valid conclusions regarding therapeutic approach.

Materials and Methods

During the five year period from January, 1969 to December, 1973, over 300 patients with orbital floor fractures presented for treatment at the two county hospitals affiliated with the University of Minnesota Medical School. Management of these injuries was directed by the attending staff and residents of the department of Otolaryngology except in 13 cases of pure blowout fracture which were managed by the Ophthalmology Service.

Several of the patients were excluded from the study population because of follow-up failure or death from associated injury. This left a total of 272 patients with 295 orbital floor fractures for study. The age range of these patients was 30 months to 84 years with a mean age of 34.5 years. Males outnumbered females by more than 3 to 1 with fractures occurring in 206 males and 66 females (Table 1). By far, the most common precipitating event was motor vehicle accident accounting for 44 percent of the injuries while fractures resulting from a direct blow from a fist accounted for 28 percent. The remaining 28 percent of injuries were secondary to a variety of other causes (Table 2).

The total of 295 orbital floor fractures (272 patients) was subdivided on the basis of anatomical involvement: (1) pure blowout accounted for 35 fractures, (2) tripod zygoma fractures with linear

Table 1. Incidence of Facial Fractures Involving the Orbital Floor

Number of Patients	272
Number of Fractures	295
Age Distribution	3 mos.–84 years
Average Age	34.5 years
Number of Males	206
Number of Females	66
Ratio Males: Females	3.1

Table 2. Etiology of Facial Fractures Involving the Orbital Floor

Motor Vehicle Accidents	44%
Altercation	28%
Other	28%

fracture of the orbital floor accounted for 137 fractures, (3) tripod zygoma fractures with comminution and displacement of the orbital floor accounted for 87 fractures, (4) LeFort II and III midfacial fractures with orbital floor involvement accounted for 32 fractures, and (5) medial maxillary fractures accounted for 4 fractures (Table 3, Figs. 1–5). From a therapeutic standpoint the fractures were divided into two groups, those that were treated surgically and those without any form of surgical intervention. The surgical group included 244 fractures (221 patients) that, either clinically or radiographically, demonstrated evidence of impingment or incarceration of the extraocular tissue, displacement of orbital contents, and/or comminution or malposition of the fracture segments. The type of surgical approach varied with the operator and the nature of the injury and included direct exploration of the orbital floor through an infratarsal incision alone in 151 instances. Alloplastic or autogenous implants were used for added support or to bridge osseous defects when a portion of the orbital floor was missing. Gelfilm, silastic, and bone from the anterior wall of the maxillary sinus was used in the treatment of 48, 33, and 4 fractures, respectively. A transantral approach in combination with an infratarsal incision was employed for evaluation and stabilization of comminuted fractures in 41 instances and in 36 of these an antral dressing was placed at the time of surgery

Table 3. Types of Fractures Involving the Orbital Floor

Pure Blow-out Fracture
Tripod-Zygoma with Linear Orbital Floor Fracture
Tripod-Zygoma with Comminuted Orbital Floor Fracture
LeFort II and III Mid-Facial Fracture
Medial Maxillary Fracture

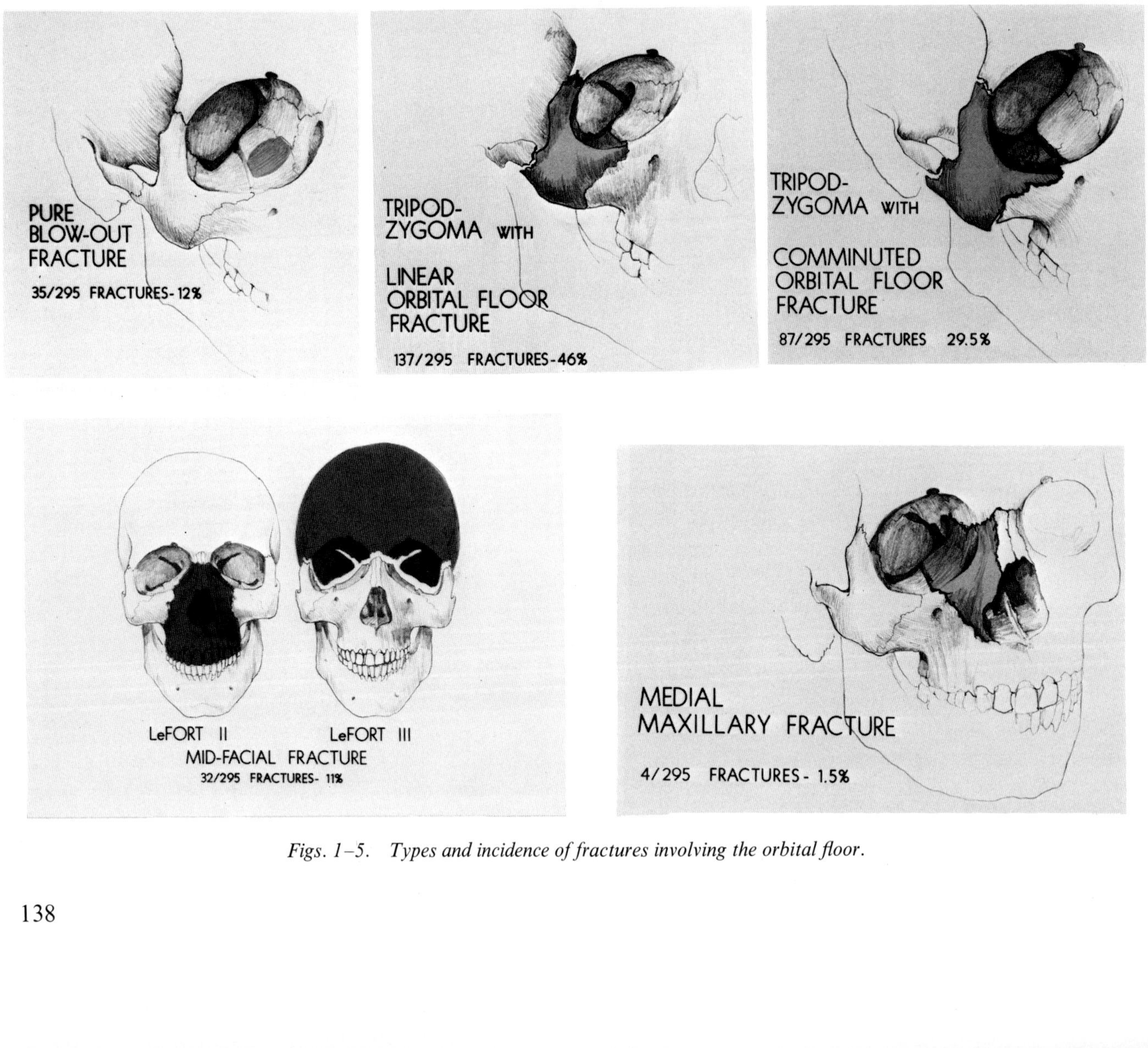

Figs. 1–5. Types and incidence of fractures involving the orbital floor.

(Table 4). Fifty-one fractures were managed without surgery. On the basis of clinical and radiographic evaluation, 20 of these were nondisplaced and there were no associated ocular symptoms. The remaining 31 fractures were felt to have significant displacement or entrapment but had no surgical therapy for one of the following reasons: physician judgment (6), refusal of surgery (4), bad surgical risk (9), concomitant ocular injury (11), and fetal risk (1).

Table 4. Methods of Repair of Orbital Floor Fractures

Orbital Floor Exploration	192/244—79%
Infraorbital Approach	151/244—62%
Infraorbital and Transantral Approach	41/244—17%
Implants	85/244—35%
Antral Dressing	36/244—15%

Patients with associated ocular injury make up a small but important group. Ocular injury occurred in 6.8 percent of the fractures and ranged from maccular edema to rupture of the globe requiring enucleation (Table 5). A thorough ophthalmological evaluation was performed on every patient and is felt to be an essential step in the treatment of all patients with orbital or periorbital trauma.

Table 5. Ocular Injuries Associated with Orbital Floor Fractures

Injuries to Globe	20/295—6.8%
Retinal Edema	
Hyphema	
Corneal Laceration	
Globe Rupture	
Retinal Detachment	
Lens Dislocation	
Iritis	

Results

Follow-up examinations were directed toward changes in visual acuity, diplopia, enophthlmos, unsightly scarring, infection, and implant rejection. Satisfactory results were obtained in all but 25 fractures giving an overall complication rate of 8.5 percent.

No follow-up complications were associated with the 20 nondisplaced fractures. Of the 31 fractures felt to have significant comminution and/or .displacement but in which nonsurgical management was employed, 8 had persistent diplopia and one developed enophthalmos which was cosmetically and functionally significant for a complication incidence of 29 percent (9/31). Of the 244 fractures which were treated surgically, 2 were associated with significant enophthalmos, three developed wound infections, implants were rejected in two instances, and 9 patients had persistent postoperative diplopia for an overall complication rate of 6.6 percent (16/244). In each case of wound infection the antrum had been dressed. Silastic rejection occurred in one patient and gelfilm rejection also occurred in one. Cosmetically unacceptable scarring was associated with two of the wound infections and both implant extrusions. There were twelve cases of transient postoperative diplopia and seven instances of transient lid edema. In no case was there any demonstrable loss of visual acuity secondary to the operative procedure (Table 6).

Table 6. Incidence of Complications and Long Term Sequelae

Overall	25/295— 8.5%
Surgical	16/244— 6.5%
Nonsurgical	9/51 —17.6%
*Nonsurgical	9/31 —29%

Discussion

A management technique which achieved optimal functional and cosmetic results while minimizing undesirable sequelae is the goal of every physician who cares for the facially injured patient. Ideally, no patient who has suffered from a traumatized orbital floor should have long term sequelae such as diplopia, enophthalmos, unsightly scarring, and decreased visual acuity. Diagnosis of orbital floor fracture is achieved by clinical and radiographical means. The history of trauma followed by periorbital edema, ecchymosis, and diplopia alert the clinician to the possibility of orbital floor fracture. Physical findings including hypesthesia in the distribution of the infraorbital projection of the fifth cranial nerve, enophthalmos, decreased ocular mobility, periorbital emphysema, palpable fracture, and positive forced duction test.[2,3,12–14] Radiographical findings on conventional radiographs and tomograms include soft tissue emphysema, opacified maxillary sinus, bombbay sign (convex hemisphere of tissue prolapsed through the orbital floor), and irregularity, displacement, or fragmentation of the orbital floor.[3,15,16] The size of the orbital floor defect is not necessarily directly related to the signs and symptoms.[17]

Up to 25 percent of patients with orbital floor fractures have serious ocular injuries (retinal edema, hyphema, corneal laceration, retinal detachment, globe rupture, lens dislocation) necessitating thorough ophthalmological evaluation prior to instituting any surgical therapy. Diplopia is probably the most common long term sequelae of orbital floor fractures and usually is the result of herniation of the periorbital contents, especially the inferior rectus and inferior oblique muscles, through a dehiscence in the orbital floor.[3,10,18] Early post injury diplopia may be secondary to edema and alone is not a satisfactory indication for orbital floor exploration. Residual diplopia has been reported in up to 50 percent of cases regardless of the mode of therapy; however, this high incidence may be reduced by early exploration and repair the defect.[3,10,12,13,18–20] In our series, of the 31 patients felt to have bony or soft tissue displacement and periorbital incarceration, but in whom nonsurgical management was elected, 8 or 25 percent (8/31) had persistent diplopia. Of the 244 patients with similar findings which were treated surgically only 9 had persistent postoperative diplopia (4 percent).

Perhaps more serious but less common than diplopia is enophthalmos, a cosmetic and functional sequelae of orbital floor fracture. It usually results from displacement, atrophy, scarring or fibrosis with subsequent decrease in the volume of the orbital contents. Undue delay in the treatment of orbital floor fractures with displacement or dehiscence leads to increased atrophy and fibrosis. The late treatment of enophthalmos is difficult and discouraging.[3,6,9–11,20,21]

Of the 31 fractures in which indications for surgical intervention were present but in which nonsurgical management was elected, significant enophthalmos occurred in one case (3 percent). Of the 244 orbital floor fractures which underwent surgical reduction, two cases (1 percent) of significant enophthalmos occurred. Enophthalmos which becomes a cosmetic or functional handicap appears to be uncommon.[12,19]

Loss of vision following any surgical procedure is a dread complication. Case reports of monocular blindness following open reduction of orbital floor fractures have appeared in the recent literature. Nicholson and Guzak in 1971 reported a series of 72 patients who underwent repair of orbital floor fractures at the Massachusetts Eye and Ear Infirmary in which 6 suffered postoperative loss of vision.[22–24] Other large series, however, do not report loss of vision with exploration of the orbital floor.[4,8,12,19]

Postoperative complications of lesser consequence include infection, extrusion of implant material, and unsightly scarring. Rankow and Megnogna, (1975) and Hightower (1971) report large series of orbital floor explorations for reduction of fracture without infection or unsightly scarring.[12,19] Implants must be chemically inert, cause no inflammation, not physically altered by tissue fluid, able to be sterilized and shaped into any form, resist mechanical strains, noncarcinogenic, and nonallergenic. When these criteria are met, extrusion appears to be an unusual consequence of their implanatation.[25] Rankow and Megnoga, (1975), Browning, (1970) and Abrahams, (1966) report 70, 58, and 12 cases, respectively, of orbital floor implant without extrusion.[12,26,27] Emory, (1972) however, reports infection and implant extrusion to represent postoperative complications in 10 percent of 190 blowout fractures treated surgically.[8]

Of 192 fractures involving orbital floor exploration analyzed in this retrospective study 85 had implants and 36 had antral dressing. There was no incidence of postoperative decrease in visual acuity. Three cases (1.5 percent) had postoperative wound infection associated with antral dressing, 2 of which had cosmetically unpleasant scarring. There were two instances (1 percent) of implant extrusion both of which had subsequent cosmetically unpleasant scarring. Infraorbital nerve hypesthesia appeared to be a sequelae of the injury rather than a postoperative complication.

Surgical intervention was recommended in all but six cases of orbital floor fractures in this series with findings of incarceration of periorbital tissue, comminution of the orbital floor, or displacement of periorbital tissue or bony fragments in which no concomitant contraindications to surgery were present. The six exceptions were managed by another service and nonoperative intervention was elected by the attending physician. If open reduction was elected, the infraorbital approach was used because of better visability and better control of the reduction. In spite of occasionally associated infection, a transantral approach with antral dressing was felt indicated where comminution, displacement, and entrapment made reduction and stabilization from above difficult. Implants were employed when comminution and bony defects left the integrity of the reduced orbital floor in question. Optimum results were obtained if exploration was undertaken within of two weeks of injury. Unusual instances of postoperative infection and implant extrusion resulting in cosmetically unpleasant scarring may occur. The surgeon must be mindful of the possibility of decrease postoperative visual acuity. However, this complication may be largely avoided by cautious, minimally traumatic surgical dissection accompanied by careful hemostasis.

References

1. MacKenzie W: Traite Pratique Des Maladies Desyeux. Trad. Laugier Et Richelot, Paris, 1844, pp 7
2. Patterson RW Jr, Tsujimura JK: Early detection and treatment of blowout fracture of the orbit, Amer Ophthal 53:841–45, 1962
3. Reeh J, Tsujimura JK: Early detection and treatment of blowout fracture of the orbit, Amer J Ophthal 62:79–82, 1966
4. McCoy FJ et al: An analysis of facial fractures and their complications, Plast Reconstr Surg 29:381–91, 1962
5. Putterman AM et al: Nonsurgical management of blowout fractures of the orbital floor, Amer J Ophthal 77:232–39, 1974
6. Kroll M, Wolper J: Orbital blowout fractures, Amer J Ophthal 64:1169–72, 1967
7. Goren SB et al: Blowout fractures of the orbital floor, Amer J Ophthal 61:893–5, 1966
8. Emery JM et al: Management of orbital floor fractures, Amer J Ophthal 74:299–306, 1972
9. Hopkins R: Fractures of the zygomatic complex. Ann Royal Coll Surgeons England, 48:403–413, 1971
10. Converse JM et al: Orbital blowout fractures. A two year survey, Plast Reconstr Surg 39:22–36, 1967
11. Rougier J: Late surgical treatment of orbital fractures. from fractures of the orbit. Ed Bleeker GM, Lyle TK, pp 177–187. The Williams and Wilkins Co., Baltimore, 1970
12. Rankow RM, Megnagna FV: Surgical treatment of orbital floor fractures, Arch Otolaryngol 101:19–22, 1975
13. Greenwald HS Jr et al: A review of 128 patients with orbital fractures, Amer J Ophthal 78:655–664, 1974
14. Smith B, Regan WF: Blowout fracture of the orbit, Amer J Ophthal 44:733–9, 1957
15. James AE: Blowout fracture of the orbit, Postgrad Med 42:61–4, 1967
16. Zesmore J et al: Roentgen diagnosis of blowout fractures of the orbit, Amer J Roentgen, 87:1009–18, 1962
17. Converse JM et al: Late treatment of blowout fracture of the floor of the orbit, Plast Reconstr Surg 28:183–191, 1961
18. Emery JM et al: Orbital floor fractures: long-term followup of cases with and without surgical repair, Trans Amer Acad Ophthal Otolaryngol 75:802–11, 1971
19. Hightower DR et al: Current concepts in the treatment of fractures of the orbit, The Laryngoscope 81:725, 1971
20. Smith B, Converse, JM: Early treatment of orbital floor fractures, Trans Amer Acad Ophthal Otolaryngol 61:602–7, 1957
21. Pfeiffer RL: Traumatic enophthalmos, Arch Ophthal 30:718–26, 1943
22. Gordon S, Macrae H: Monocular blindness as a complication of the surgical treatment of a malar fracture, Plast Reconstr Surg 6:228–32, 1950
23. Penn J, Epstein E: Complication following late manipulation of impacted fracture of the malar bone, Brit J Plast Surg 6:65, 1953
24. Nicholson DH, Guzak SV Jr: Loss of vision after repair of orbital floor fractures, Trans Amer Acad Ophthal Otolaryngol 75:1402, 1971
25. Shannon GM: Enophthalmos: foreign implants. From the proceedings of the second international symposium on plastic and reconstructive surgery of the eye and adenexa. Ed Smith B, Converse JM, 446–8. The C. V. Mosby Company, Saint Louis, 1967
26. Browning CW: Alloplasts in reconstruction of the orbit, 189–200. From fractures of the orbit. Ed Bleeker GM, Lyle TK. The Williams and Wilkins Company, Baltimore, 1970
27. Abrahams IW: Repair of orbital floor defects with premolded plastic implant. Arch Ophthal 75:510–12, 1966

Antral Packing and Orbital Floor Fractures

Howard K. Gelman, Emanuel M. Skolnik, and
William R. Janzen, Chicago, Ill.

Orbital floor fractures is an area of head and neck surgery where individual preferences in surgical indications and choice of surgical technique vary considerably. Ocular injury and blindness following repair of orbital floor fractures have been reported with many surgical techniques. Blindness and/or ocular injury have been reported after eyelid incision approach to the orbital floor with and without implants and after Caldwell-Luc antrostomy approach.[1–4]

We reported one patient with a comminuted orbital floor fracture in whom an overinflated maxillary antral balloon used to splint the fracture caused a reversible but potentially dangerous elevation of ocular tension. This raised a question. If this is not an isolated case of an antral balloon causing elevated ocular tension, how can we avoid ocular injury using maxillary packing in the repair of orbital floor fractures while attaining good functional and cosmetic results?

All patients with orbital floor fractures admitted to the otolaryngology service of the University of Illinois Eye and Ear Infirmary were studied. Orbital floor fractures were either pure blowout fractures, part of zygomatic complex fractures, or LeFort II or III fractures.

The surgical technique was decided by the surgeon. All patients in whom maxillary antral balloons or packing were used in the surgical repair are recorded here. Preoperative ophthalmological evaluation was performed to identify preexisting eye disease or ocular trauma. Intraoperative ocular tensions were measured during inflation of the antral balloon or during antral gauze packing and postoperatively. If the intraoperative ocular tension was increased, this was used as a gauge of the adequacy of floor repair. The following are the results of our study.

Of the twelve patients with orbital floor fractures in whom intraoperative ocular tensions were studied (Fig. 1), five had increased ocular tension following antral packing of the orbital floor fracture. In most of these, the amount of antral packing used was that amount thought by the surgeon to adequately splint the orbital floor. On all patients the ocular tension reverted back to normal after decreasing the antral pack.

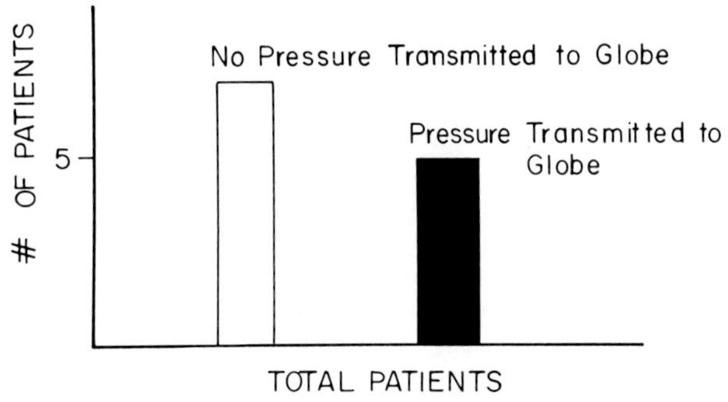

Fig. 1. Total patients.

Of the five patients in whom the antral pack caused an increase of ocular tension (Fig. 2) four had comminuted orbital floors clinically appraised by the surgeon. In one patient, the ocular tension was raised by the antral balloon, even though the

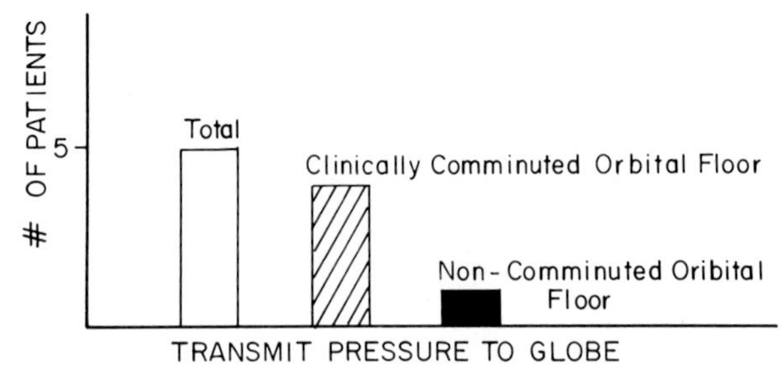

Fig. 2. Patients who transmit pressure to the globe.

surgeon evaluated the orbital floor not to be comminuted.

All patients, in whom the orbital floor was appraised to be comminuted (Fig. 3), antral pressure was transmitted to the globe. In only one of the patients with clinically noncomminuted orbital floors (Fig. 4) was there increased ocular tension with antral packing.

Both antral balloons and gauze were used to support the orbital floor (Fig. 5) and both were found to increase the ocular tension across the fractured orbital floor.

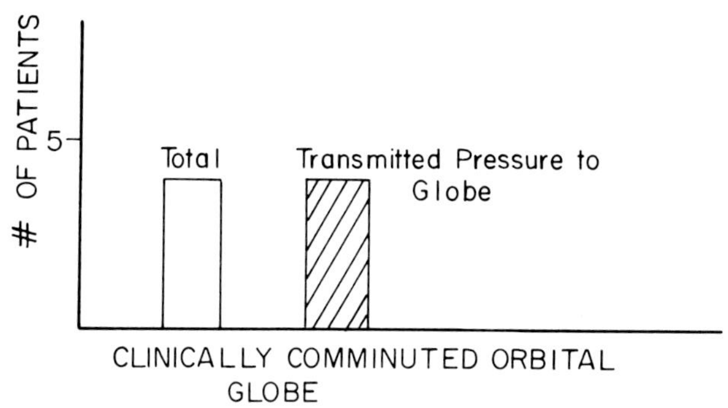

Fig. 3. Patients with comminuted orbital floors.

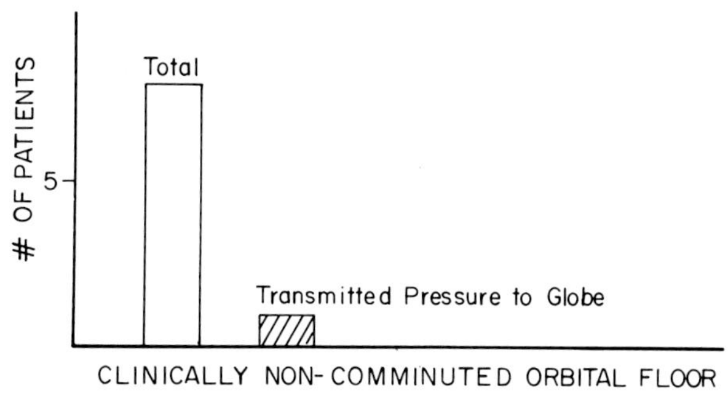

Fig. 4. Patients with noncomminuted orbital floors.

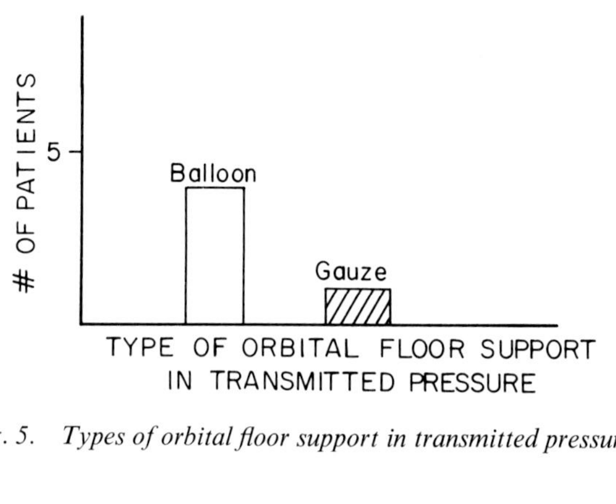

Fig. 5. Types of orbital floor support in transmitted pressure.

To summarize these findings, in patients with *comminuted* orbital floor fractures, whether clinically apparent or not, gauze or balloons used in the maxillary antrum to support the orbital floor can cause the ocular tension to be elevated to a potentially dangerous but reversible level.

We have attempted to use this increase in ocular tensions as a gauge to adequacy of orbital floor repair.

After reduction of other bony fragments in a zygomatic complex fracture, LeFort fracture, or in a blowout fracture, and after forced traction test to assure that the inferior rectus or inferior oblique muscle is free, an antral balloon is placed via a naso-antral window and slowly inflated with saline. Frequent ocular tensions are taken using a Shiotz tonometer until a rise in ocular tension is noted. If an increase of ocular tension is noted, saline is withdrawn at 1 cc intervals until the ocular tension again is normal, as in Figure 6. A forced traction test is again performed. The antral balloon is left for 10 days.

VOLUME CC	OCULAR TENSION mmHg
3	16
4	16
5	16
6	16
7	40
6	20

Fig. 6. Antral balloon volume/ocular tension relationship.

In the immediate postoperative period, the patient is observed frequently for any ocular pain, vision loss and ocular tension increase.

Figure 7 is the frontal tomogram of a patient with a blowout fracture of the orbital floor. Via a Caldwell-Luc maxillary antrostomy a Foley catheter was placed in the antrum and brought out via a

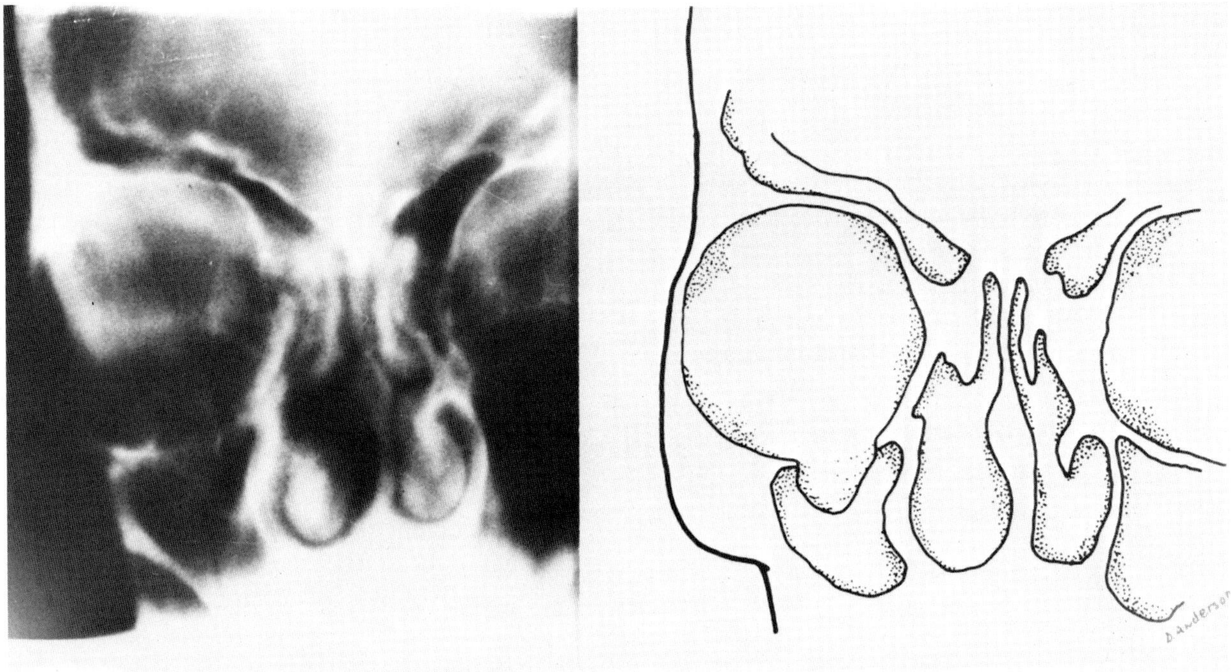

Fig. 7. Preoperative frontal tomogram showing fracture of the orbital floor.

naso-antral window. After testing for muscle entrapment and reducing the fracture fragments, the balloon was inflated with hypaque until just increasing the ocular tension and then removing fluid until ocular tension became normal. Figure 8 is a frontal tomogram with the hypaque fluid balloon in place splinting the orbital floor. Figure 9 is several weeks postoperative showing the repair of

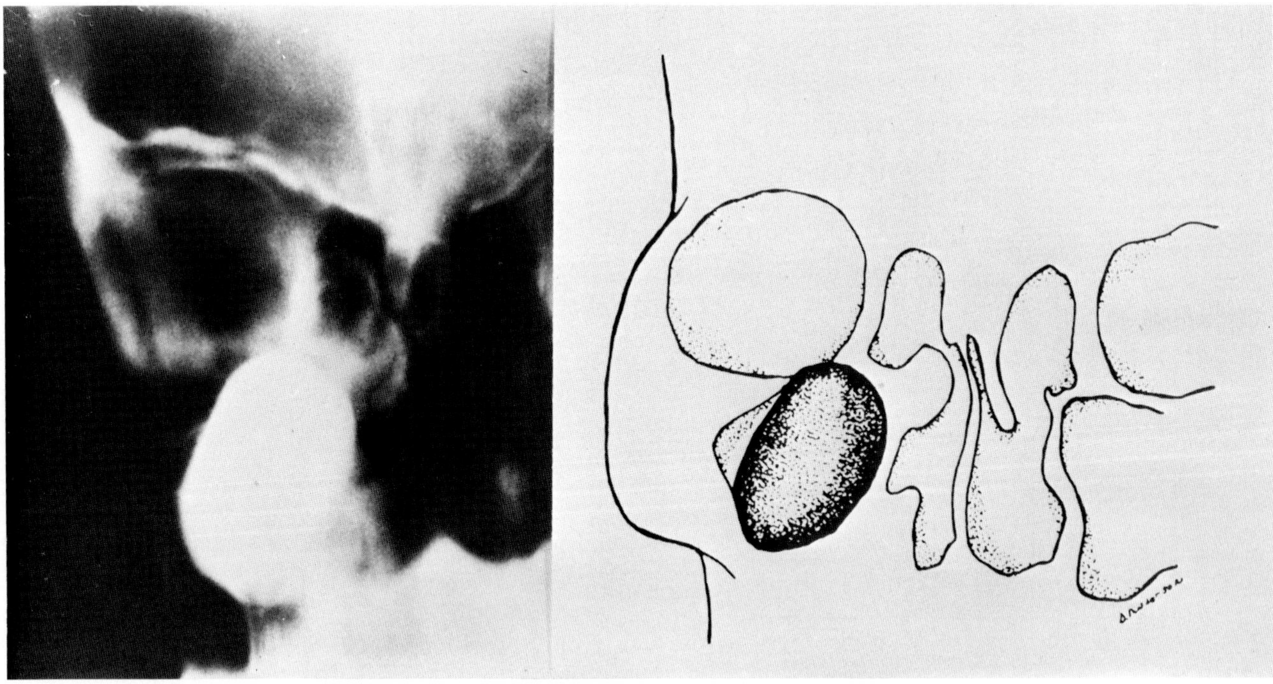

Fig. 8. Post reduction frontal tomogram with hypaque filled antral balloon.

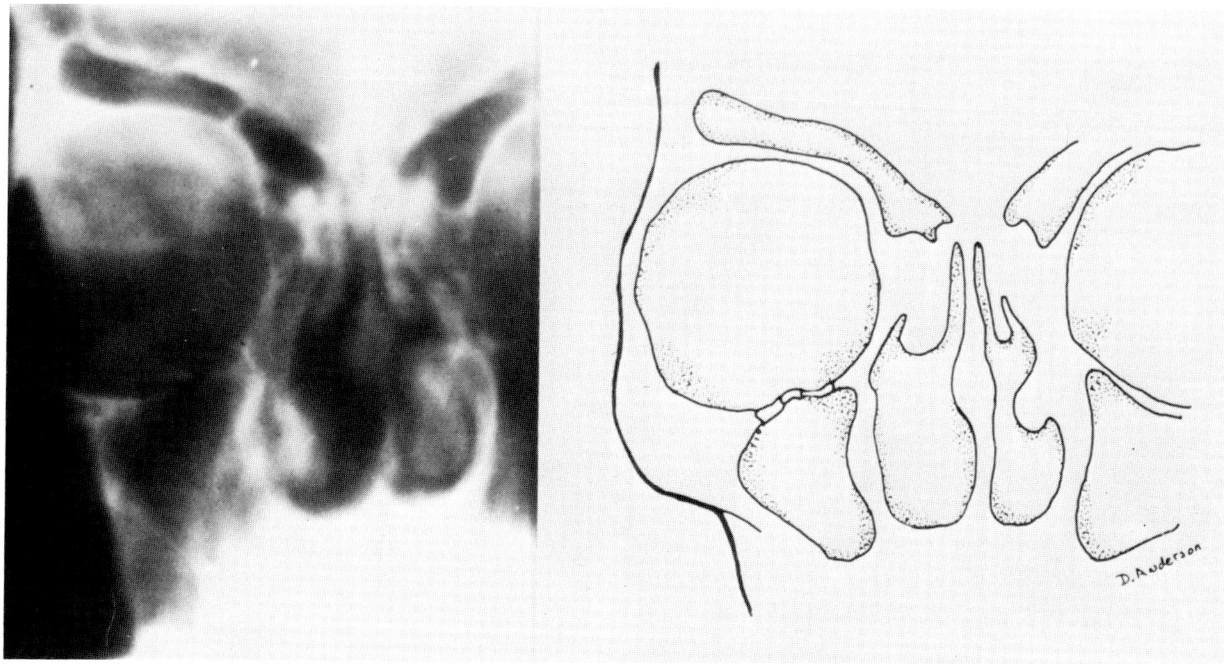

Fig. 9. Two months post reduction frontal tomogram.

the orbital floor. The cosmetic and functional results were excellent.

With a relatively small number of patients we can not say that this technique is the answer in avoiding ocular injury from orbital floor fracture repairs. But what can be stated with some assurance is that if maxillary packing is being used in reduction or splinting of the orbital floor, care must be taken to avoid causing ocular tension increases and possible ocular injury. This may be achieved by intraoperative Shiotz ocular tension measurements and close postoperative observation.

References

1. Emery JM, Huff JD, Justice J: Central retinal artery occlusion after blow-out fracture repair. Amer J Ophthalmol 78:538–540, 1974
2. Gelman HK, Janzen WR, Skolnik EM: Ocular tension following use of an antral balloon. Arch Otolaryngol 99:449–450, 1974
3. Nicholson DH, Guzak SV: Visual loss complicating repair of orbital floor fractures. Arch Ophthalmology 86:369, 1971
4. Slack WJ: Blindness of the repair of a fracture of the floor of the orbit. Minn Med 57:958–60, 1974

Entropion Repair—A Simplified Approach

Marvin L. Kwitko, Montreal, Canada

When multiple procedures are described for a specific condition, then it has to be concluded that none are considered to be entirely satisfactory. So it is with the treatment of entropion.

The procedure to be described here is based on the opinion that many cases of entropion occur when the tarsal plate becomes lax and loses its rigidity. When this happens the least amount of excess contraction of the orbicularis muscle will cause an infolding of the eyelid with all of the subsequent complications (Fig. 1A).

This procedure consists of excising a triangular wedge of conjunctiva-tarsal plate halfway along the length of the eyelid (Fig. 1B), while hemostasis is obtained with a large chalazion clamp. The surgeon must be careful to avoid the lid margin, otherwise as unsightly notch will occur. The base of the triangular wedge is 5 to 8 mm in length depending on the severity of the entropion and is located close to the lower margin of the tarsal plate. The sutures (three 4–0 plain catgut) are inserted through the entire thickness of the conjunctiva-tarsal plate edge while the clamp is still in place and tied once with a double tie. It is best to bury the knots to avoid a possible corneal abrasion. As the clamp is slowly released the sutures are pulled up and tied with a second and third single tie. This maneuver results in a minimum of bleeding. The removal of the wedge of tarsus strengthens the tarsal plate in such a way as to give added rigidity. The immediate result (Fig. 1C) is a moderately high vertical tarsal plate buckle which persists for two to three weeks in the postoperative period (Fig. 1D) but slowly flattens (Fig. 1E) until a satisfactory cosmetic result is obtained (Fig. 1F). This usually takes three to four weeks.

After surgery the eye is dressed with antibiotic ointment and a pressure dressing which is removed the following day. If tissue swelling persists, then a pressure dressing is reapplied. The patient is seen daily while the dressing is on. In the usual case pressure is required for only the first 24 hr, after which the patient applies antibiotic ointment to the eyelid four times a day for five days.

This has been the operation of choice for me since 1963. In a series of the first one hundred cases performed the following complications were noted: (1) Three cases of corneal abrasion due to exposure of the catgut knots. These knots are now all buried. The corneal abrasions responded to conservative therapy of patching of the eye; (2) one case of acute glaucoma due to pupil dilation under the eyepatch. A peripheral iridectomy was performed which cured the patient; (3) Three cases of recurrence of the entropion. The same operation was repeated in an adjacent portion of the tarsal plate which caused a cure in all three cases.

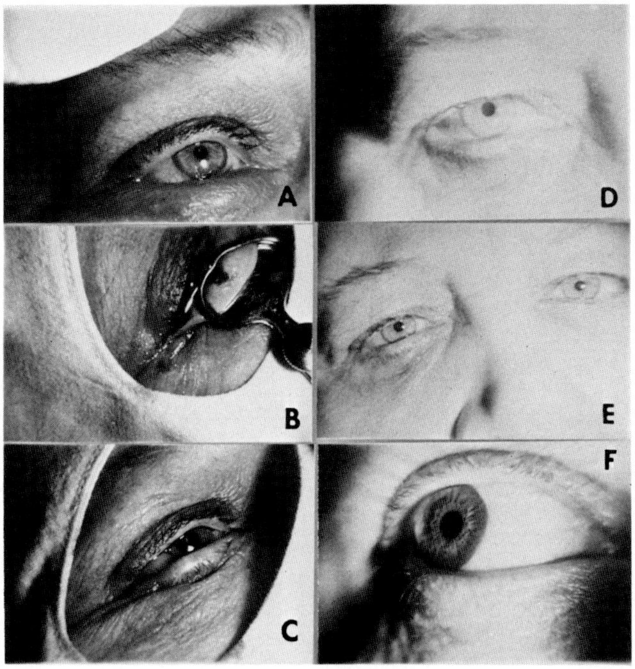

Fig. 1. (A) A typical case of entropion based on a loss of rigidity of the tarsal plate. (B) Large chalazion clamp is applied and tightened. Using a Bard-Parker No. 11 or No. 15 blade, a wedge of conjunctiva-tarsal plate is removed. The base is 5 to 8 mm in length, depending on the severity and persistence of the entropion, and is placed close to the lower margin of the tarsal plate. The eyelid margin is avoided at the apex of the triangle. At this stage three 4–0 plain catgut sutures are inserted (taking in the full thickness of the conjunctiva-tarsal plate edge) and tied loosely with a double tie. As the clamp is slowly released the sutures are pulled tight. The double tie keeps the edges of the tarsal plate approximated while second and third ties are made. This maneuver of releasing the clamp slowly while tying the sutures results in a minimum of bleeding. (C) The appearance of a moderately high vertical buckle of tarsal plate immediately after surgery. (D) Ten days after surgery. (E) 18 days after surgery. The buckle is beginning to flatten. (F) One month after surgery. The buckle has flattened completely, and a good cosmetic result is obtained.

In essence this is a modified version of the techniques of Fox[1] and Muller.[2] The only differences lies in the assumption that some cases of entropion are based on laxity of the tarsal plate, and the surgical procedure is directed here.

Summary

A simplified procedure is presented for the treatment of entropion due to laxity of the tarsal plate.

This method could be carried out as an office procedure by any surgeon who is already set up to do a chalazion operation,[3] since the instrumentation is similar except for the closing sutures.

References

1. Fox SA: Ophthalmic Plastic Surgery, 3rd ed, New York, Grune & Stratton, Inc. 1963, pp 247–248
2. Muller L: Ein new operations-methode zur heilung des entopuim Spacticum Klin Mbl. Auquenheilk 69:288, 1922
3. Kwitko ML: A simplified treatment for entropion Arch. Ophthal. 72:64, 1964

Management of Patients with Essential Blepharospasm

Charles Z. Weingarten Evanston, Illinois and Allen M. Putterman Chicago, Illinois

Essential blepharospasm is a bilateral, spasmodic, involuntary closure of the eyelids, the cause of which remains obscure (Fig. 1). Chronic and progressive, it occurs equally among men and women between the ages of 45 and 75. Spasm can involve other areas supplied by the facial nerve such as the lower part of the face and the musculus platysma and is absent completely during sleep. It variably progresses to a point where some affected patients become so severely handicapped that they are afraid to work, drive, or do minor tasks for fear of temporary blindness, which could endanger their lives. This often results in severe depression and social isolation of the patient.

Henderson speculated that a disturbance of the motor inhibitory system somewhere above the level of the facial nucleus was the cause of essential blepharospasm.[1] Possible sites of involvement include the reticular formation, basal ganglia, or more likely the 4-S area of the cerebral cortex or its descending pathways.

Emotional distress seems to make this condition worse. Casatanares suggested a psychogenic component, in which a conversion reaction becomes established along organic pathways.[2] However, the results of treatment with psychotherapy or tranquilizers or both have been disappointing.[3]

Various drugs have been used to treat essential blepharospasm including trihexyphenidyl hydrochloride (Artane), diphenylhydantoin (Dilantin), levodopa, haloperidol, and deanol, but for the most part they have been relatively ineffective.[3] Amantodine hydrochloride (Symmetrel), and meprobamate (Miltown) have successfully decreased the symptoms in several of our patients to the point where they were satisfied and declined surgery. A therapeutic trial with one or more of these drugs is indicated preoperatively.

Most effective therapeutic modalities involve either manipulation of the peripheral facial nerve or the eyelids. The oldest treatment is alcohol injection along the course of the facial nerve supplying the orbicularis oculi muscle.[4] However, relief of symptoms is temporary at best. The same can be said regarding procedures involving resection of major portions of the orbicularis oculi muscle.[3,5]

Putterman and Urist[6] demonstrated that suspending the eyelids from the frontalis muscle

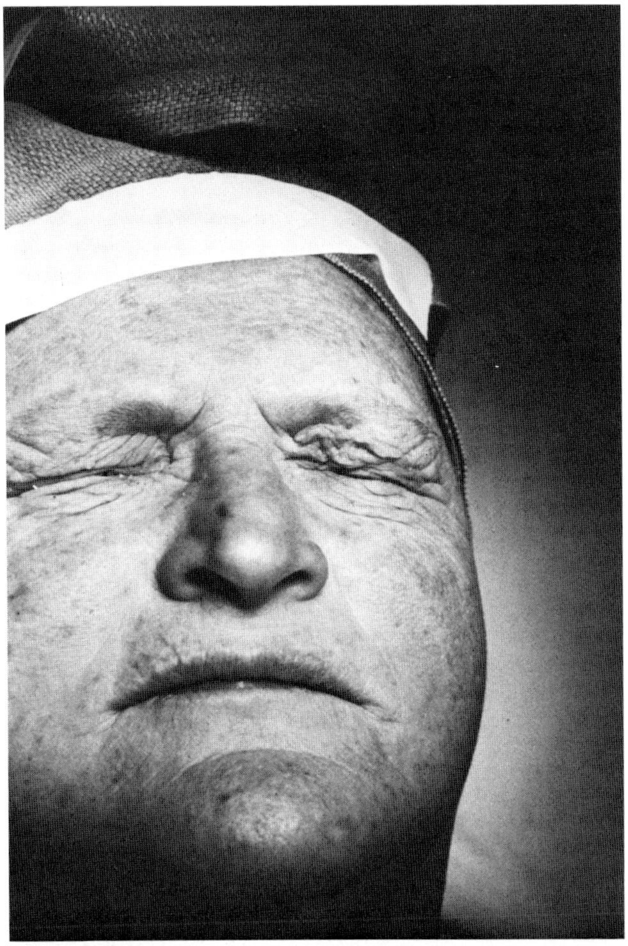

Fig. 1. Patient with severe visually handicapping essential blepharospasm.

(frontalis sling procedure) allows some patients to raise their eyelids during blepharospasm and also decreases the frequency and intensity of the spasm. It is recommended for those patients who attempt to break the blephrospasm by raising their eyebrows and desire relief of their visual handicap by a relatively innocuous procedure but are willing to accept some sensation of the tic.

Direct exposure and avulsion of the facial nerve peripherally has been popularized by Gurdjian[7] and Reynolds[3] as an effective means of treating essential blepharospasm. Reynolds's technique requires an incision 2 cm anterior to the ear, which is cosmetically objectionable, and identifying branches of the facial nerve at this level is technically difficult. Coleman first proposed an incision closer to and paralleling the preauricular line which Henderson utilized in at least one case.[1] We have used a modification of this parotidectomy-type approach to the facial nerve. Proximal exposure of the facial nerve just after it exits the stylomastoid foramen facilitates identification of the facial nerve and its branches.[8] It also allows direct stimulation of the facial nerve trunk to confirm complete removal of all involved branches at surgery and provides a cosmetically acceptable scar.[8]

To minimize disability without compromising successful control of the blepharospasm, selective avulsion of all branches, including the buccal, is performed, while the marginal branch supplying the lower lip is preserved. Removal of the buccal branch prevents residual blepharospasm in most patients.[9]

Significant postsurgical morbidity results from facial paralysis despite marginal branch preservation. A modified rhytidectomy with removal of redundant facial skin performed at the same time as neurectomy minimizes the postoperative cosmetic deformity. Many patients will still require secondary reconstructive procedures involving the periorbital structures, i.e., eyebrows and eyelids.

Surgical Technique

We have performed selective facial nerve avulsion on nine women and one man, ranging in age from 48 to 75, to control intractable and incapacitating essential blepharospasm (Table 1). Patient preparation included a detailed explanation of the procedure and resultant facial paralysis. Preoperative neurologic consultation and ophthalmologic evaluation are essential to discover preexisting problems that may become manifest postoperatively, i.e., incipient ectropion.

If desired, one can demonstrate the effects of facial paralysis to the patient by injecting the nerve trunk area with local anesthetic. This will cause a transient, complete paralysis. The patient should be reassured that lower lip function will be retained after surgery.

The surgical technique of selective facial neurectomy utilizes the standard approach to the facial nerve trunk via a preauricular incision. The branches of the nerve are identified and avulsed as described by Reynolds.[3] We have performed a

Table 1. Essential Blepharospasm Treated with Facial Neurectomy[a]

Case	Sex	Age Years	Months Free of Visually Handicapping Blepharospasm	Partial Unilateral Recurrence	Facial Paralysis	Ectropion	Eyebrow Ptosis	Exposure Keratopathy	Dermatochalasis	Other
1	F	69	54	+ (after 28 mo)	++	+	+++	+	+++	—
2	F	61	47	—	+	—	+	+	+	Buccal branche branches spared
3	F	71	46	+ (after 22 mo)	++	+	+	+	+++	Required buccal branch avulsion 24 hr postoperatively
4	F	58	25	—	+	—	+	+	+	Neck and choking spasm persist
5	F	64	17	+ (immediate)	++	—	+	+	+	—
6	F	68	14	—	++	—	+	+	+++	Resolution of preoperative entropion after neurectomy
7	F	75	10	—	+ (Rhydidectomy performed)	++	+++	+	+	—
8	F	55	6	—	++	—	+	+	+++	—
9	F	76	4	—	+ (Rhytidectomy performed)	—	+	+	+++	Accentuation of bilateral preoperative blepharoptosis
10	M	48	2	—	++	—	+++	+	+	—

[a] KEY: +, mild; ++, moderate; +++, severe; −, none.

primary modified rhytidectomy, or removal of redundant skin, on the last several patients in this series to reduce postoperative facial sagging. The required modification of the incision and technique is minimal. Both sides are operated at one session with the patient under general anesthesia. Muscle relaxants must be avoided during the procedure in order to use the nerve stimulator effectively.

The preauricular incision (Fig. 2) extends superiorly into the temporoparietal area and inferiorly is carried around the earlobe retroauricularly. Limited undermining of the skin flap is performed, as most of the lift required is in the upper two-thirds of the face. This may eliminate the need for cervical extension of the incision.

The posterior margin of the parotid gland is then mobilized from the root of the zygoma and cartilagenous ear canal. Inferior extension is carried to the anterior border of the sternocleidomastoid muscle, and the gland is reflected from the anterolateral surface of the mastoid. Firm, fibrous bands paralleling the tympanomastoid suture line become apparent and are divided.

The tragal cartilage is followed medially to its narrowest point and the bony vaginal process identified. By blunt dissection, tissues are spread parallel to the facial nerve (Fig. 3). The nerve trunk is located approximately 1 cm medial to the bony vaginal process just after it exits the stylomastoid foramen and enters the posterior surface of the parotid gland surrounded by fat and glandular elements. Following the main trunk peripherally

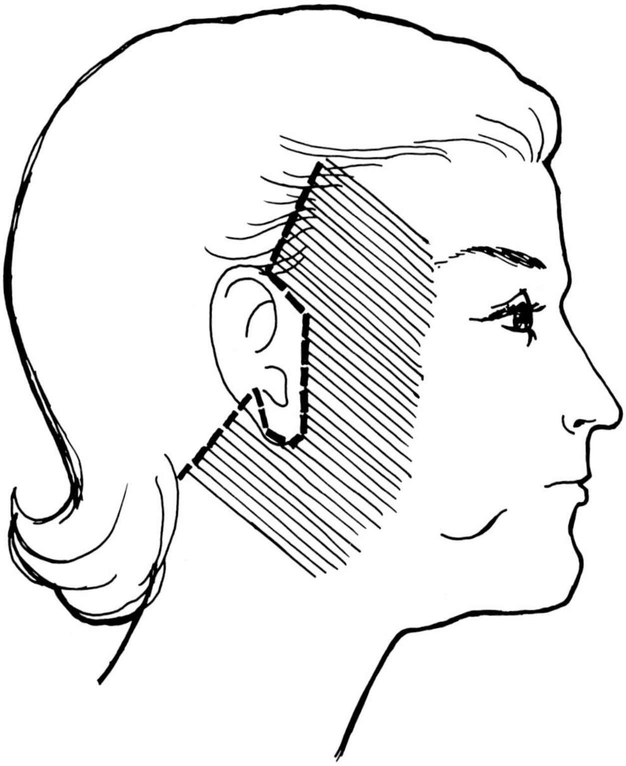

Fig. 2. Dotted line indicates incision line for facial neurectomy combined with rhydidectomy. Shaded area demonstrates extent of skin flap.

and dissecting off the superficial parotid gland exposes the parotid plexus. Once the pes anserinus is identified, each branch is followed distally in a similar manner for 2 or 3 cm, and the gland is reflected anteriorly.

The branches are avulsed one at a time beginning superiorly (Fig. 4). A fine hemostat grasps the nerve and divides it from the main trunk. Steady traction is applied as the nerve is rolled onto the hemostat. With care a 3- to 4-cm section of nerve can be removed. All branches down to and including the buccal division are taken. If the branching pattern is such that the buccal and marginal branches are combined into a lower division, dissection of the buccal portion can be facilitated by the use of the operating microscope and more distal exposure of the nerve.

The nerve stimulator is then applied to the main trunk and by observation as well as palpation the surgeon can determine if all branches have been completely severed, down to and including those supplying innervation to the upper lip (Fig. 5). Symmetric denervation should be performed to render the paralysis less obvious postoperatively.

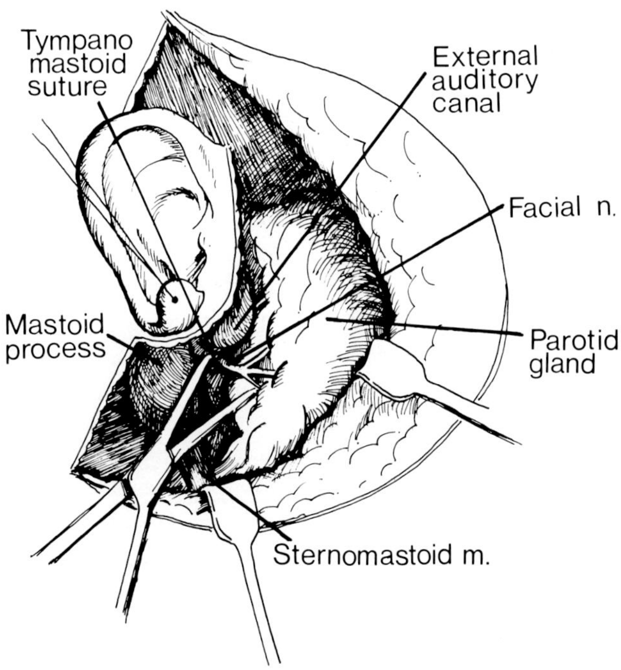

Fig. 3. Isolation of facial nerve and branches.

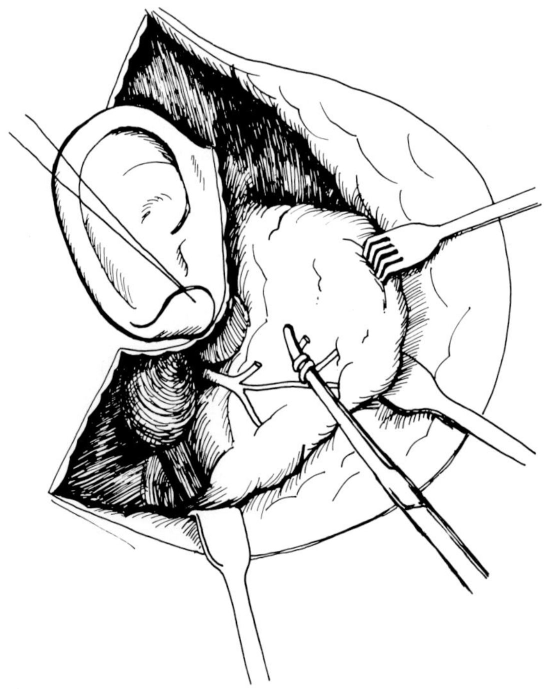

Fig. 4. Avulsion of facial nerve branches involved in blepharospasm by rolling cut branch around hemostat.

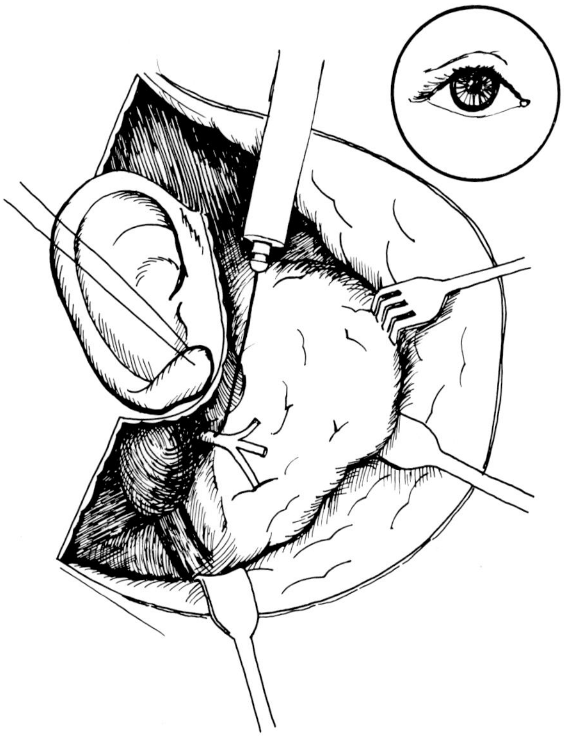

Fig. 5. Nerve stimulation of facial nerve trunk after avulsion of all branches except mandibular. Lack of blepharospasm and upper lip spasm indicates complete removal of involved branches.

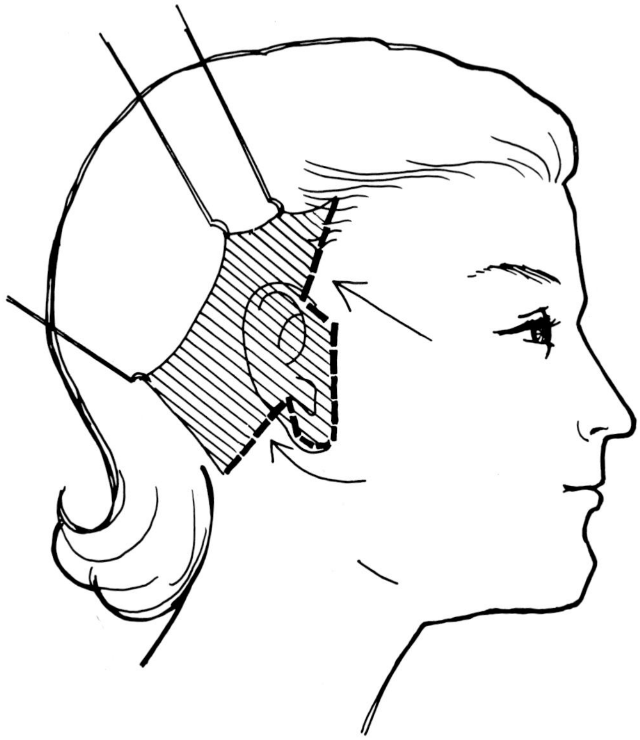

Fig. 6. Excision of redundant facial skin decreases postoperative facial sagging.

The skin flap is handled as in rhytidectomy (Fig. 6). Plication of the subcutaneous tissue may be performed. Flaps are retracted upward and backward, and redundant skin is excised. The temporal portion of the flap is anchored to the temporalis fascia, and the upper and postauricular incision are closed under moderate tension. The preauricular portion is approximated without tension. Drains are placed inferiorly and removed in 48 hr.

Results

Complete or adequate relief from blepharospasm has been attained in each patient. All the patients except one (Case 2) ultimately required avulsion of the buccal branch along with the zygomatic and temporal to provide relief of the blepharospasm. Preservation of this branch in one patient (Case 3) resulted in persistent spasm and required its avulsion 24 hr postoperatively. In Case 5, in whom the buccal branch was partially removed on one side and completely on the other, residual blepharospasm persisted on the side of incomplete avulsion.

Two patients who initially were completely relieved of the blepharospasm developed partial unilateral recurrences 22 and 28 months postoperatively (Cases 1 and 3). In these cases the blepharospasm has been minimal, not visually handicapping, and has remained stable for two years or more since recurrence. Case 4 had undergone bilateral neurectomy by Reynolds's technique one year prior to the development of unilateral recurrent spasm associated with bizarre cervical and choking spasm. A repeat selective facial neurectomy eliminated her blepharospasm but did not relieve the neck and choking symptoms.

Upper facial paralysis resulted in facial sagging and rhytid formation to some degree in all patients. The symmetric nature of the facial deformity associated with bilateral deneration renders it somewhat less obvious than unilateral facial palsy. Removal of redundant skin at the time of neurectomy significantly reduced this deformity in Cases 7 and 9. This technique was also particularly helpful in reducing the postoperative asymmetry following unilateral selective facial neurectomy performed on a patient suffering from hemifacial spasm.

All patients have had decreased blinking, lagophthalmos, with secondary exposure keratopathy, and ocular irritation. This has been easily controlled in all patients with artificial tears, administered from three times a day to once a week.

Several of the patients with eyebrow ptosis and secondary upper eyelid dermatochalasis have required surgery to improve their cosmetic appearance. In Cases 1 and 7, bilateral brow lifts were performed and five patients (Cases 1, 3, 6, 8, and 9) had excision of excessive upper eyelid skin.

Case 9 had a bilateral blepharoptosis preoperatively and lifted her eyelids by raising her eyebrows between spasms. Postoperatively the blepharospasm was entirely corrected, but the patient's visual symptoms increased due to her inability to elevate her eyebrows and therefore her eyelids. This was easily treated with a bilateral blepharoptosis procedure.

Paralytic ectropion of the lower eyelid occurred in three patients (Cases 1, 3, and 7). Case 1 was corrected by a bilateral medial tarsorrhapy while excision of excessive skin combined with horizontal shortening of the lower eyelid was performed on the other two.

Auricular anesthesia occurred almost uniformly as a result of interruption of the greater auricular nerve during surgery. This has not been bothersome and has allowed for painless suture removal.

Discussion

Essential blepharospasm reportedly occurs with equal frequency among men and women.[3,9] However, women predominate in the group of patients we treated as well as in the series reported by Reynolds[3] (Table 1).

The occurrence of associated dysfunction of one or more cranial nerves has been noted in at least one of our patients (Case 4). Reynolds also noted this phenomenon.[3] It may reflect a more diffuse disorder of the motor inhibitory system as noted previously.

The reported incidence of delayed recurrence of blepharospasm ranges from 0 to 50 percent.[8–10] This probably relates to the extent of removal of the buccal branch of the facial nerve. Distal avulsion is necessary to remove the small anastamotic fibers between branches that can bypass the resected portion of the nerve.[9] Two of our patients experienced minimal delayed recurrence of symptoms (Cases 1 and 3). In addition, one patient had residual unilateral blepharospasm immediately postoperatively which was attributed to incomplete unilateral removal of the buccal branch of the facial nerve (Case 5).

The ultimate disability and deformity resulting from selective facial neurectomy varies greatly. However, most patients are so gratified to be able to resume normal activity that the loss of mimetic function is seldom considered a problem. Many patients require secondary procedures on the eyelids or eyebrows to correct functional problems. From the aesthetic point of view, a significant number desire secondary reconstructive procedures of the face, eyebrows, and eyelids. The performance of a primary removal of redundant skin, or modified rhytidectomy, at the time of neurectomy minimizes the development of facial rhytids and gross sagging postoperatively.

Acknowledgements

We thank Jane Phillips for the medical illustrations. Figures 3–5 were drawn after illustrations by Sander Heilig and William Schwartz.

References

1. Henderson JW: Essential blepharospasm. Trans Am Ophthalmol Soc 54:453–520, 1956
2. Castanares S: Blepharospasm: A new approach to treatment. Plast Reconstr Surg 51:248–253, 1973
3. Reynolds DH, Smith JL, Walsh TJ: Differential section of the facial nerve for blepharospasm. Trans Am Acad Ophthalmol Otolaryngol 71:656–664, 1967
4. Harris W, Wright AD: Treatment of chronic facial spasm; by alcohol injection; by nerve anastomosis. Lancet 1:657–662, 1932

5. Fox SA: Relief of intractable blepharospasm: A preliminary report. Am J Ophthalmol 34:1351–1356, 1951
6. Putterman AM, Urist MJ: Treatment of essential blepharospasm with frontalis sling. Arch Ophthmol 88:278–281, 1973
7. Gurdjian ES, Williams HW: The surgical treatment of intractable cases of blepharospasm. JAMA 91:2053–2056, 1928
8. Putterman AM, Friedman B: Isolation of the facial nerve trunk in the treatment of essential blepharospasm. Ophthalmic Surg 3:60–65, 1972
9. McCabe BF: Management of hyperfunction of the facial nerve. Ann Otolaryngol 79:252–258, 1970
10. Mustarde JC, Jones LT, Callahan A: Ophthalmic plastic surgery—up-to-date. Birmingham, Aesuculapius Publishing Co., 1970, p 109

Auricle

Surgery of the External Ear (Panel)

R. Meyer and U.K. Kesselring:

Total or Subtotal Reconstruction of the Auricle

In cases of microtia or of traumatic destruction of the auricle we proceed to total or subtotal reconstruction in four or five stages. We have used for a long time our modification of the method of White, Rubin, and Walden[2] which consisted in placing a rib cartilage transplant beneath the skin in the area of the missing ear while at the same time a rectangular flap was being rolled back in the occipito-parietal region. The resulting defect was covered with a split skin graft. Four to six weeks later the flap was unrolled and, in continuity with the whole grafted piece of skin, brought forward in order to cover the posterior side of the raised skin cartilage structure.

More recently we have adopted the procedure of Tanzer[3–5] with or without combination of the temporal flap of Dufourmentel[6] to rebuild the helix contour (see Case 2). The position of the rudimentary lobule is changed, bringing it into an almost horizontal position by a Z-plasty procedure. In rare traumatic cases with total avulsion the lobule has to be reconstructed too and this we achieve also in the first session according to the well-known technique of Gavello[1] (Case 1). In the same first session we insert a rib cartilage graft from the contralateral thorax side in a subcutaneous pocket where it is held in place by mattress sutures.

If the helix of the opposite ear is developed as a roll we use for imitating that shape in the neo-auricle the temporal bipedicle flap of Dufourmentel[6] which is prepared in this first session still.

A subcutaneous strip of connective tissue enveloping the temporal artery is formed as a bipedicle flap. While Dufourmentel[6] covers its raw surface with a split skin graft we use a full-thickness graft taken from the inguinal region. Inserted along the border of the reconstructed auricle during the third stage, this very slender and well vascularized skin flap provides a quite natural look of the pinna.

At a second stage some 6 weeks later the skin-soft tissue-cartilage construction is elevated from the mastoid bone and the resulting defect covered with a split-thickness skin graft. Occasionally we perform some minor cartilage rearrangements or additions at that time.

As a third step the concha and the tragus are reconstructed. For the former we use a composite graft from the other ear and the latter is shaped out of a small folded local skin flap. It is at this moment that the above-mentioned roll can be brought down to the auricle in order to emphasize the helix where it is desirable.

In particular cases, for instance in the first brachial arch syndrome, the implantation border of the hair bearing skin appears at a too low and too anterior level. In a preliminary operative stage we then have to extend the skin area which is reserved for the implantation of the neo-auricle. This displacement of the border of the hair bearing skin is effected by rolling it backward and by covering the resulting raw surface with a full skin graft.

In cases of avulsion of the external ear and destruction of the surrounding skin area we have to resort to the use of a distant flap to carry to the auricular region a neo-pinna which has been prefabricated at the thorax or in the supraclavicular fossa.

Reconstruction of the Upper and Median Part of the External Ear

Loss of the upper part of the auricle which is practically always of traumatic origin can be repaired by using partially the procedure of Tanzer. In these particular cases in which the remaining skin area surrounding the auricular loss is scarred, the additional temporal flap of Dufourmentel[6] is especially indicated. For that purpose we envelope

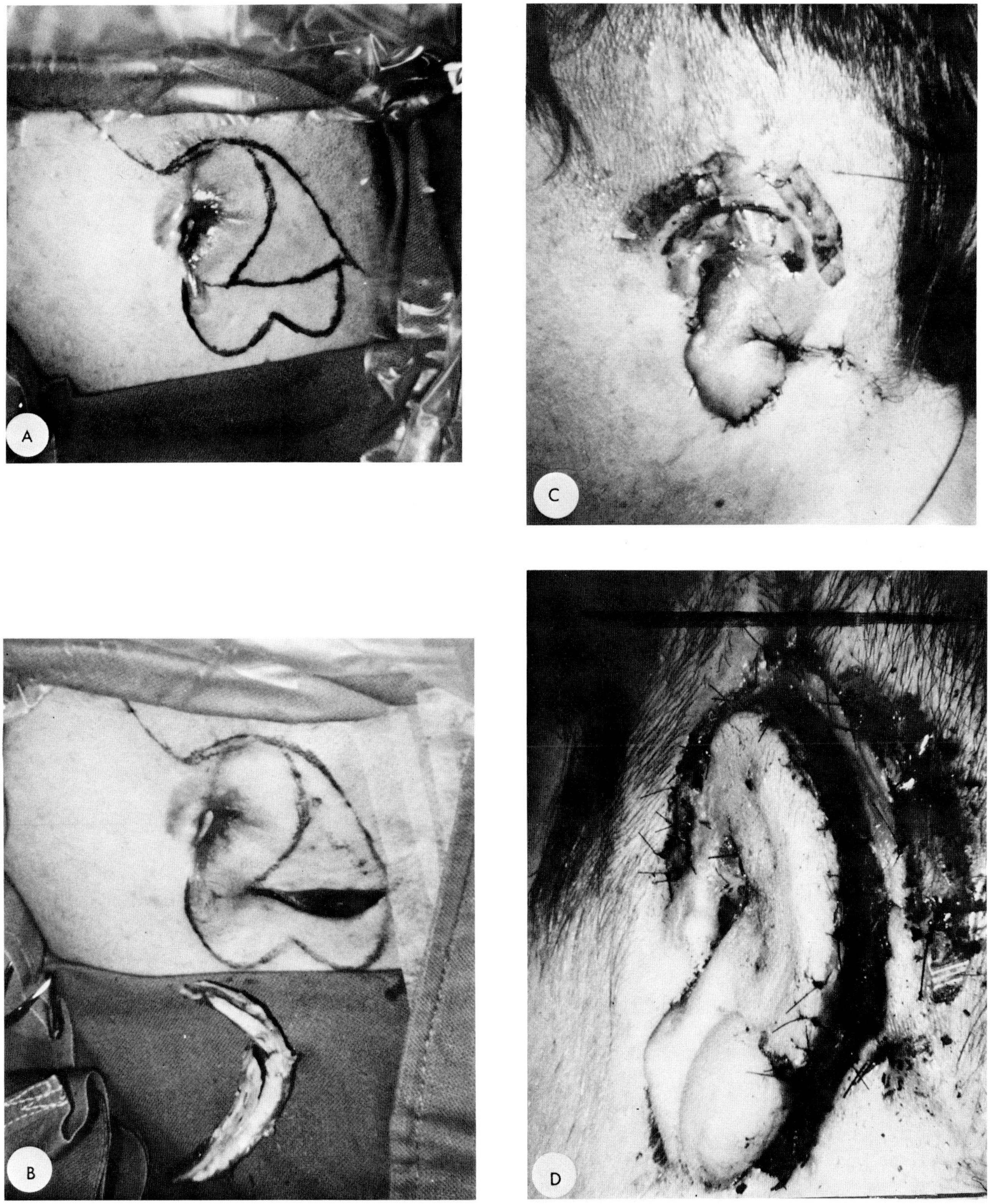

Case 1. Total ear loss in car accident. Here it is necessary to reconstruct the lobule too which we achieved with a Gavello flap (A). The cartilage graft is carved from rib cartilage which we take from the contralateral side and through a horizontal incision in the mastoid region the skin has been elevated to permit the introduction of the cartilage structure (B,C). In a second stage the neo-auricle is detached and the posterior side lined with a full thickness skin graft (D). At the same time the helix is accentuated and the cavum conchae reconstructed with a composite graft from the other ear. The result after 3 sessions (E).

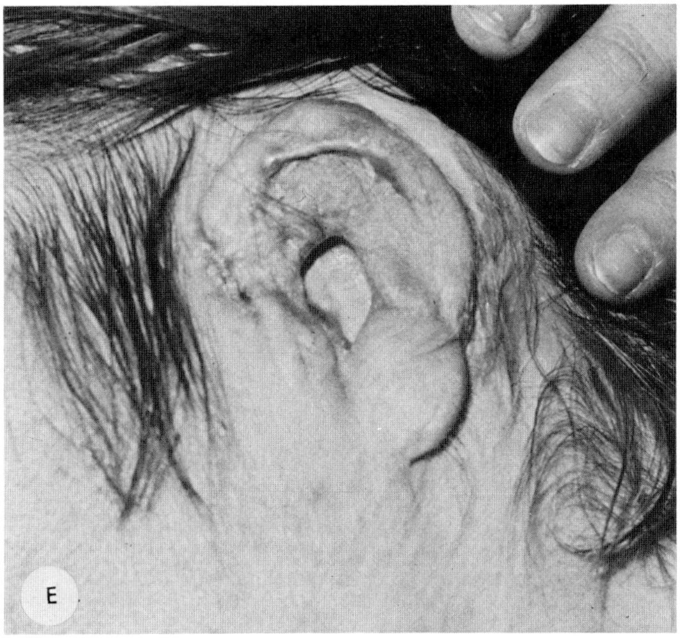

Case 1. (Continued) The result after 3 sessions (E).

the artery bearing bipedicle flap with a full thickness skin graft as we described it in total and subtotal ear reconstruction. In Case 2 it is sutured along the reconstructed part of the auricle.

For the repair of medial loss of the pinna we insert if possible composite grafts of the opposite ear using in addition the postauricular skin. For the reconstruction of the scapha and helix we have modified the methods of Dieffenbach,[7] Converse,[8] and Cronin[9] using postauricular skin flaps which are reinforced by autogenous cartilage grafts.

Depending on the dimension and site of the defect we can use the postauricular skin which in a first session has been underlaid with rib cartilage. In Case 3 the hair bearing skin was pulled back and rolled up, the cartilage graft was inserted into a deep subcutaneous pocket while the raw area was covered with a full thickness graft. In a further operation the postauricular skin was unrolled, the helix reconstructed from the prepared cartilage-skin structure and the posterior side of the auricle covered with a graft.

If there is enough hairless postauricular skin available, the rib cartilage is again placed beneath this skin and the whole is brought up into the defect as a composite flap in a later session (Case 4). Here too the resulting raw area is covered with split skin.

An alternative source of transplant material is the opposite ear where we can take a composite graft of retroauricular skin and conchal cartilage to replace the missing part of the mutilated ear (Case 5).

For the reconstruction of the middle sector of the pinna (Case 6) we have developed a method using a free composite graft from the other ear that is sutured beneath a flap of retroauricular skin which has been sewn into the defect. In a second session only the postauricular flap has to be severed and the auricle is freed with the segmental reconstruction achieved.

After tumor ablation in the concha we fill the central ear defect by infra- or postauricular island flaps: A flap of the needed size is marked inferiorly to the ear. To gain skin length in order to be able to move this flap upwards and posteriorly into the defect, we proceed in the same manner as for a facelift.

Correction of too Large Prominent Ears

In macrotia the site and dimension of the hyperplasia has to be defined. Usually a large auricle is combined with a prominent pinna, quite often we also find a disproportioned lobule. Thus

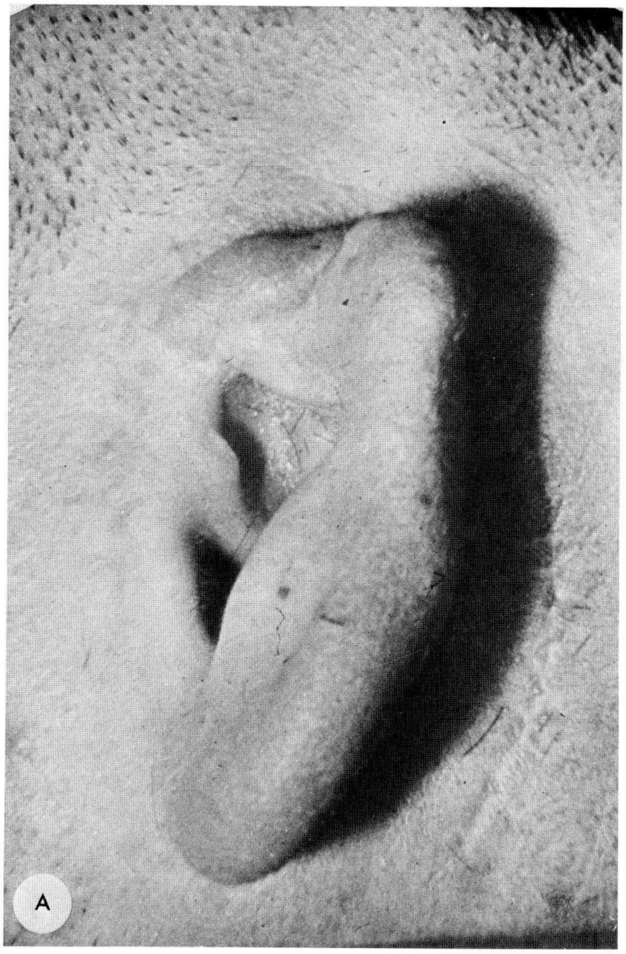

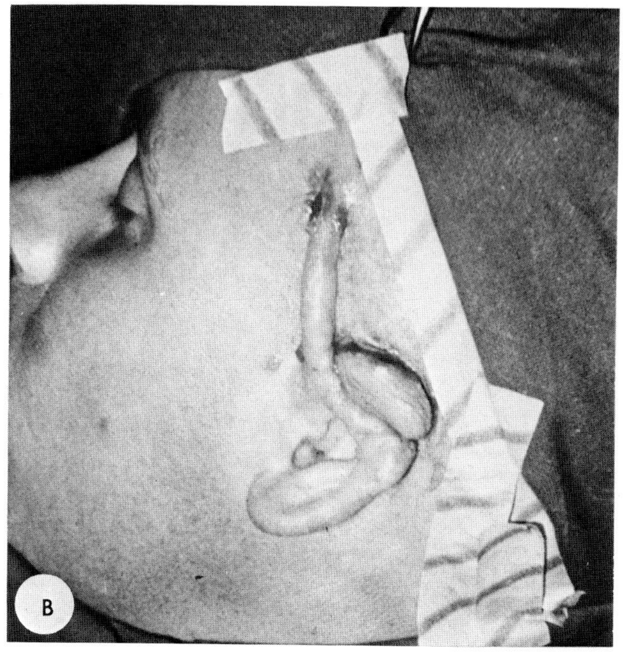

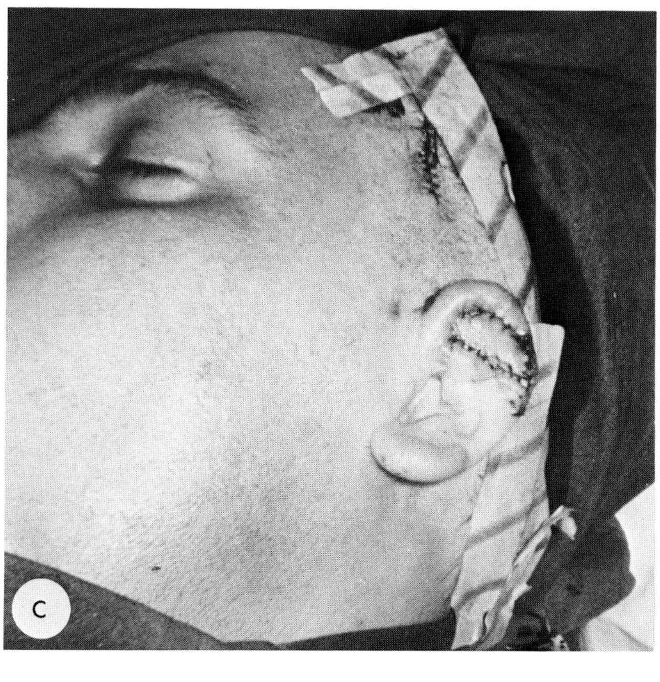

Case 2. (A) The defect to be repaired. (B) A composite graft from the other ear has been used for the reconstruction and in the same first stage a modified Dufourmentel flap has been prepared. Here just before the second intervention where (C) The tubed flap is sutured around the composite graft.

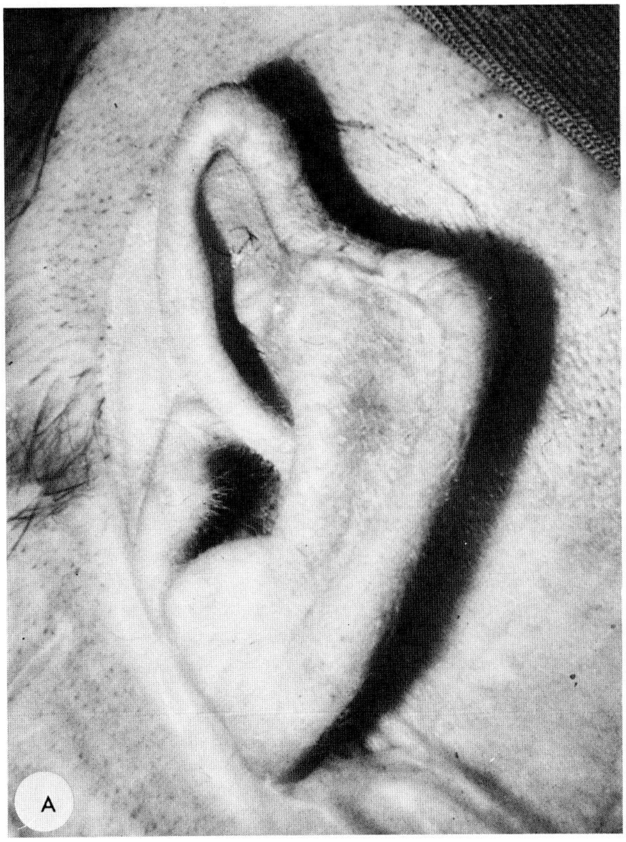

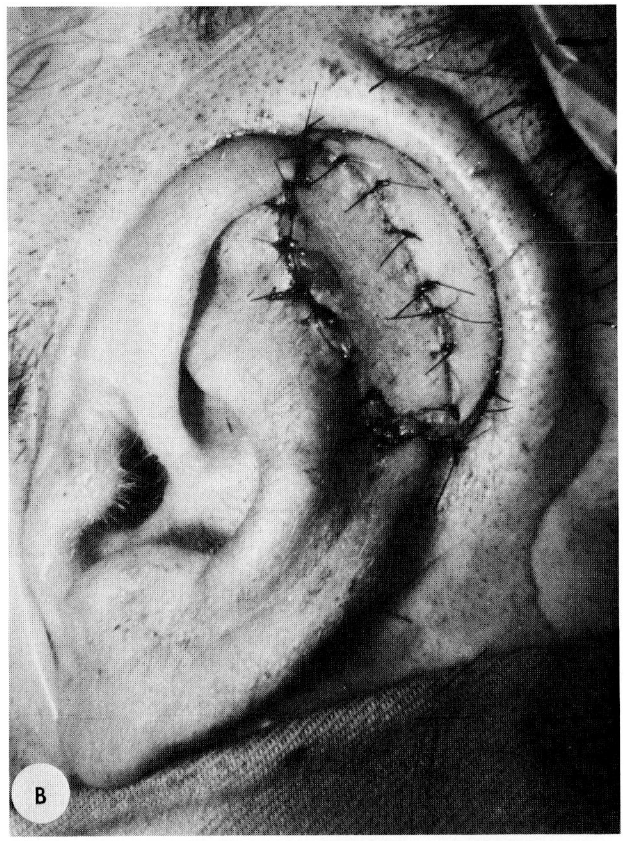

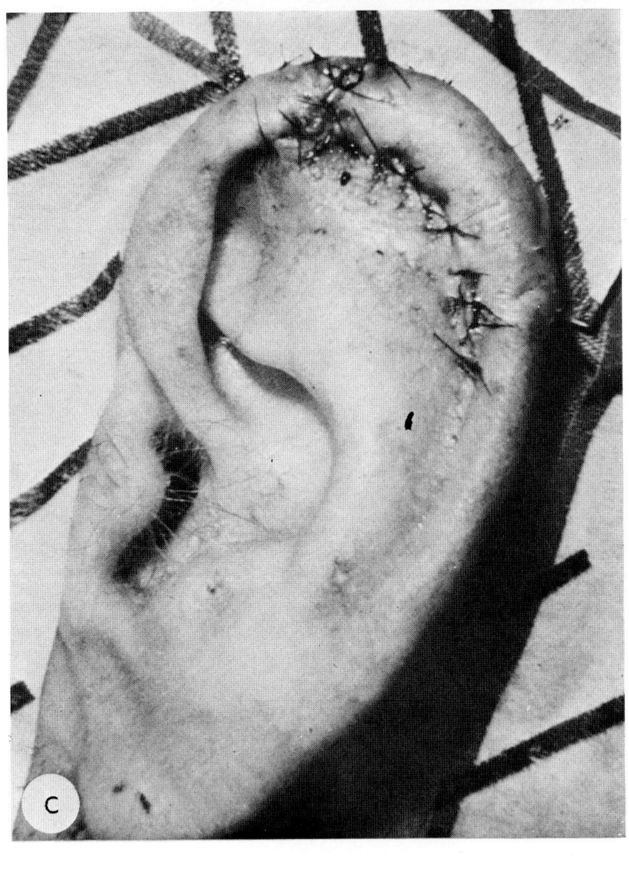

Case 3. (A) The defect and the marking on the hairbearing skin where it is to be rolled back. (B) The roll and the skin graft in place. (C) The result at the end of the second operation.

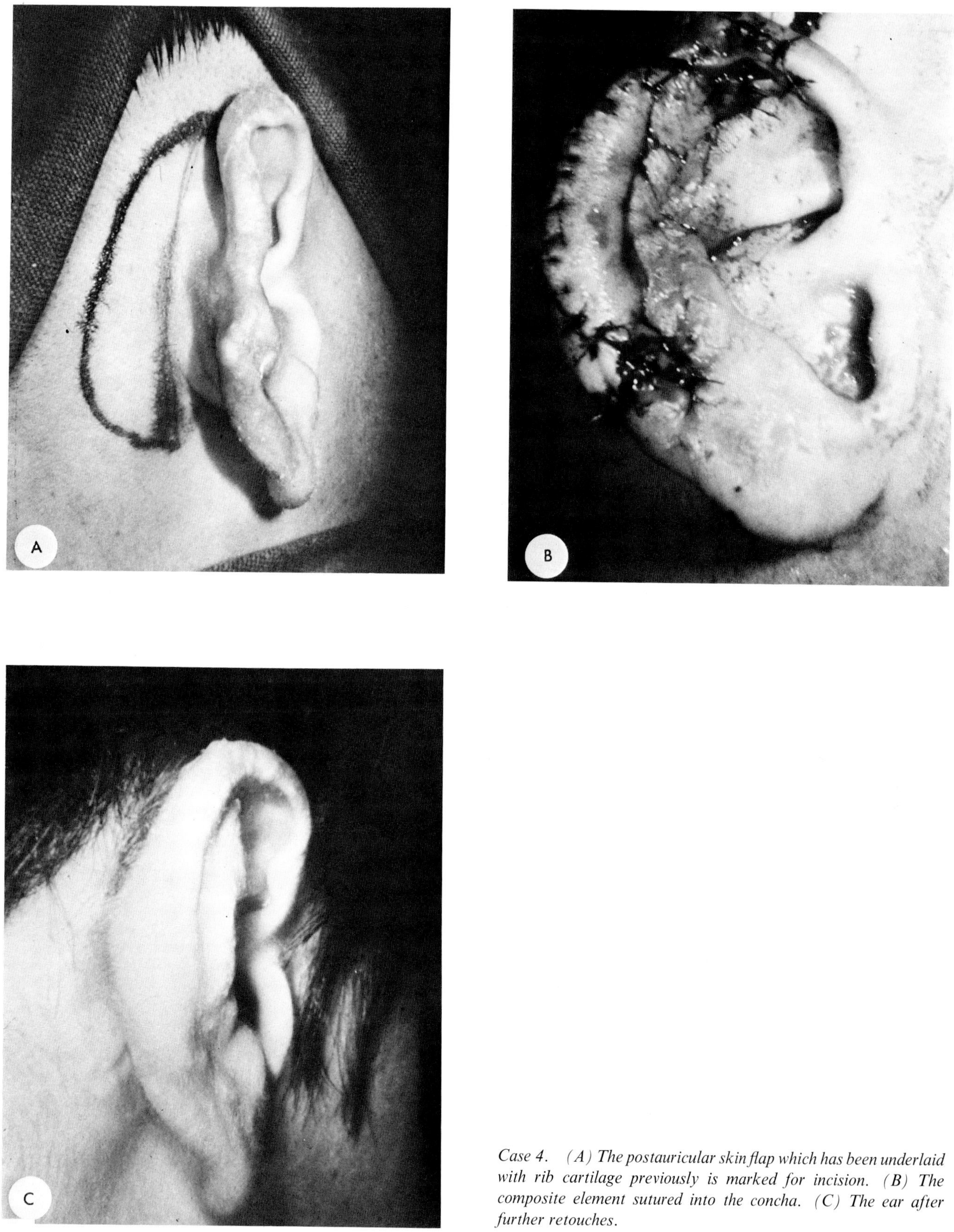

Case 4. (A) The postauricular skin flap which has been underlaid with rib cartilage previously is marked for incision. (B) The composite element sutured into the concha. (C) The ear after further retouches.

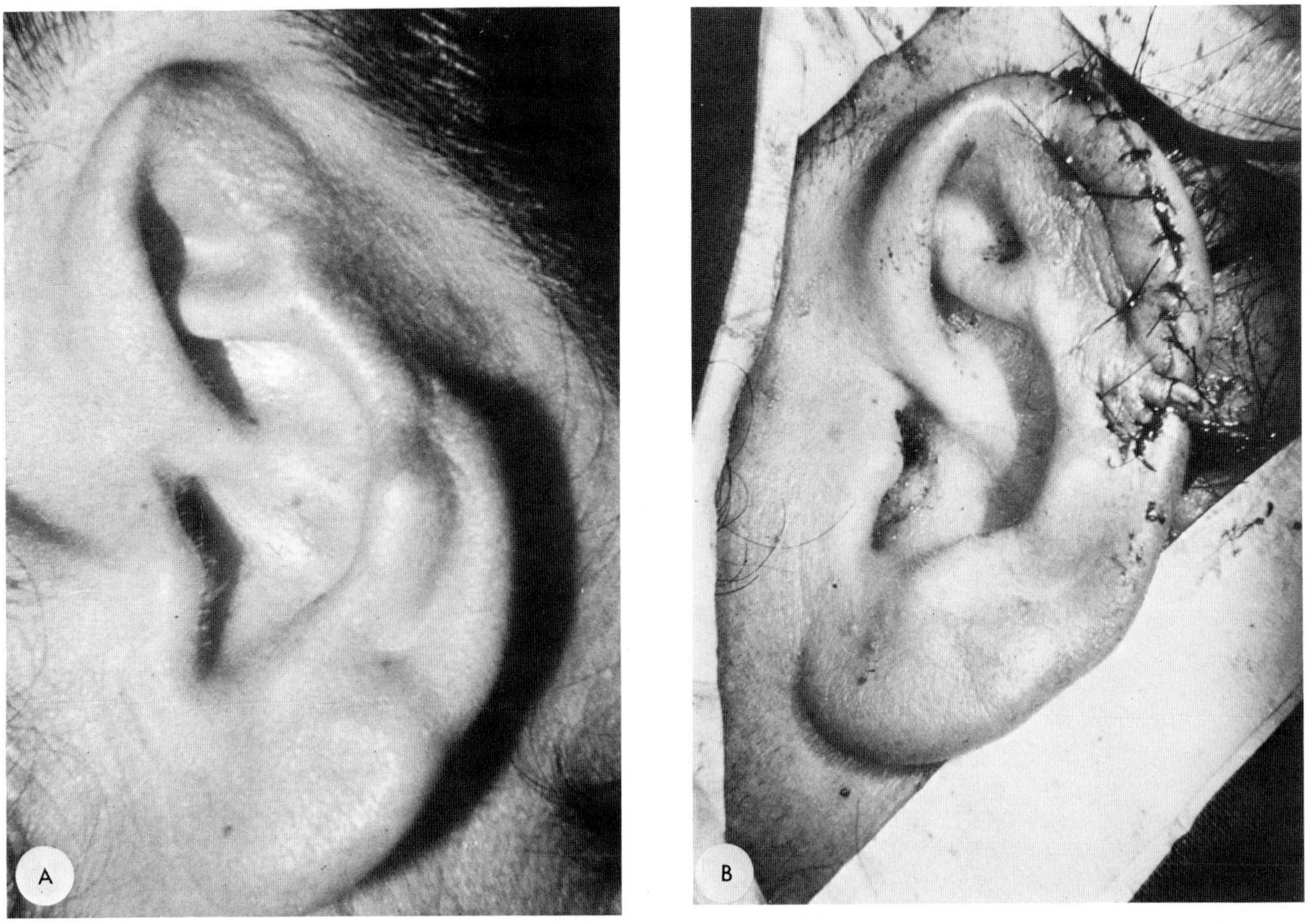

Case 5. (A,B) A reconstruction by means of a composite graft from the other ear.

it is desirable to correct these three deficiencies in one and the same operation.

For many years we used the method of Gersuny[1] for reduction of the auricle but we have now adopted a personal technique resecting the crus helicis together with a part of the scapha and rotating the helix along the new outer border of the scapha and around the cymba in order to shorten the circumference of the whole pinna. The skin of the posterior aspect of the ear is partially dissected and adapted to the new shape, eventually reduced by wedge resection in the postauricular fold. If necessary the ear lobe is reduced by marginal resection and the concha by semilunar shaped resection towards the anthelix (Case 7).

The anthelix and the remnant of the scapha are folded in order to reduce the prominence of the ear and held in position by posterior sutures after the cartilage has been cross-hatched and if necessary by mattress sutures which are placed at the fold between antitragus and anthelix.

References

1. Meyer R, Sieber H: Konstruktive und rekonstruktive Chirurgie des Ohres. Handbuch der Plastischen Chirurgie, Band 2, Beitrag 38, 1–62. E Gohrbandt, J Gabka, A Berndorfer. Walter de Gruyter & Co, Berlin-New York, 1973
2. White MF, Rubin LR, Walden RH: Total ear reconstruction. A three stage procedure with special reference to the scalp roll. Plast Reconstr Surg 18: 117, 1956
3. Tanzer RC: Total reconstruction of the external ear. Plast Reconstr Surg 23: 1, 1959
4. Tanzer RC: Total reconstruction of the auricle. Trans Internat Soc Plast Surg 2. Congress. Williams & Wilkins, 350, 1960
5. Tanzer RC: An analysis of ear reconstruction. Plast Reconstr Surg 31: 1, 1963
6. Dufourmentel C: La greffe cutanée libre tubulée. Nouvel artifice technique pour la réflection de l'hélix au cours de la reconstruction du pavillon de l'oreille. Ann chir plast 4: 311, 1959
7. Dieffenbach JF: Die operative Chirurgie. FA Brockhaus, Leipzig, 1845
8. Converse JM: Reconstruction of the external ear. Plast Reconstr Surg 55: 148, 1950
9. Cronin TD: One stage reconstruction of the helix: two improved methods. Plast Reconstr Surg 9: 547, 1952

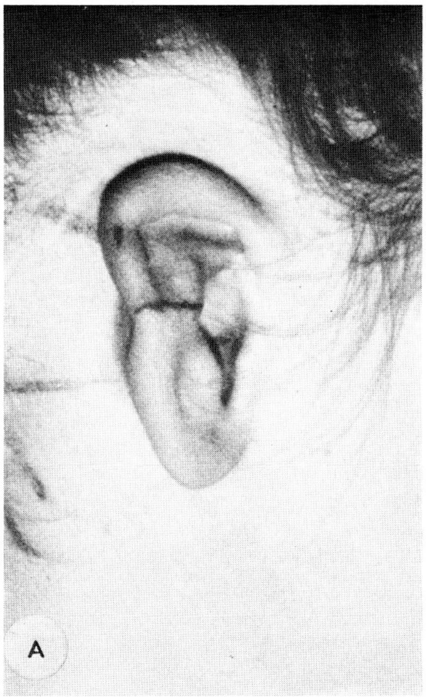

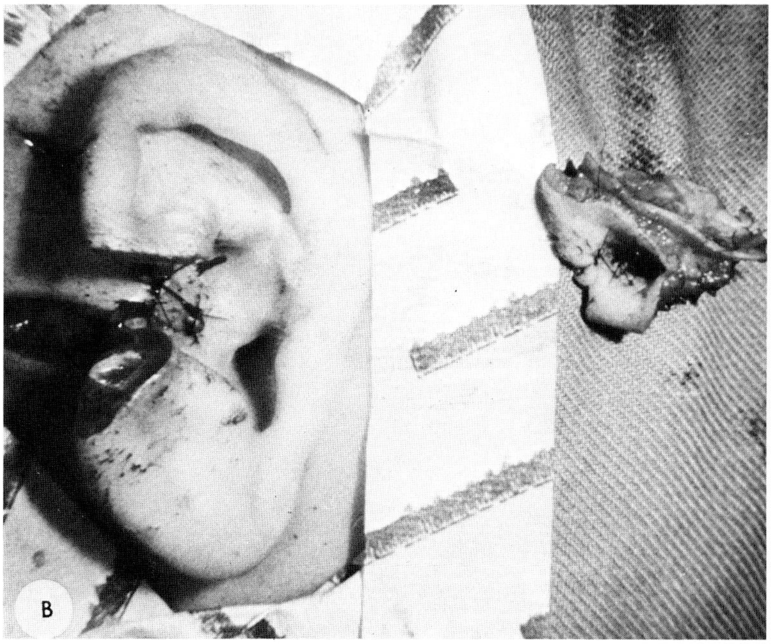

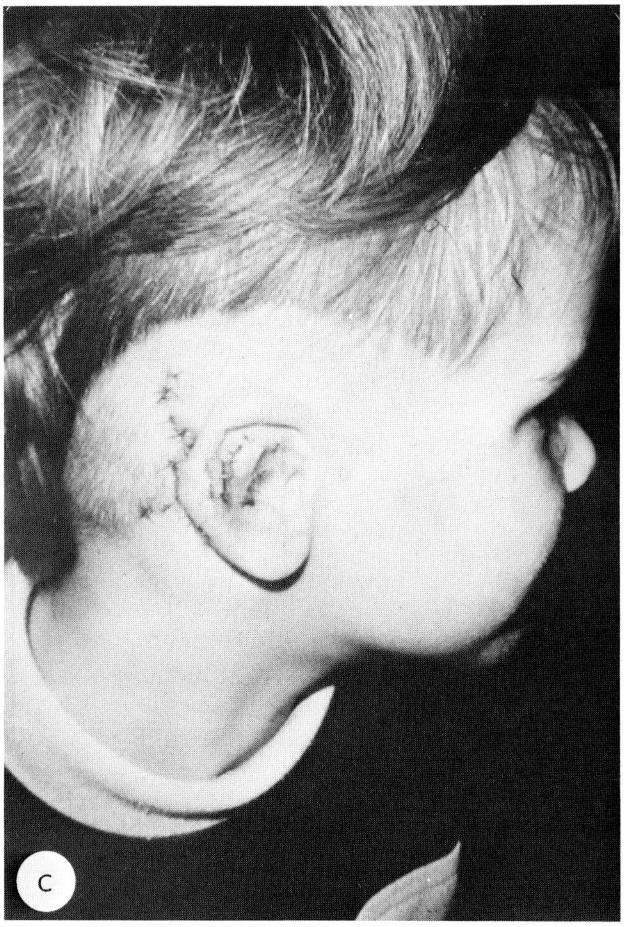

Case 6. (A) At the site of the defect in the middle part of the pinna the ear is split (B) to give room for the tubed composite graft which is partially covered with retroauricular skin (C).

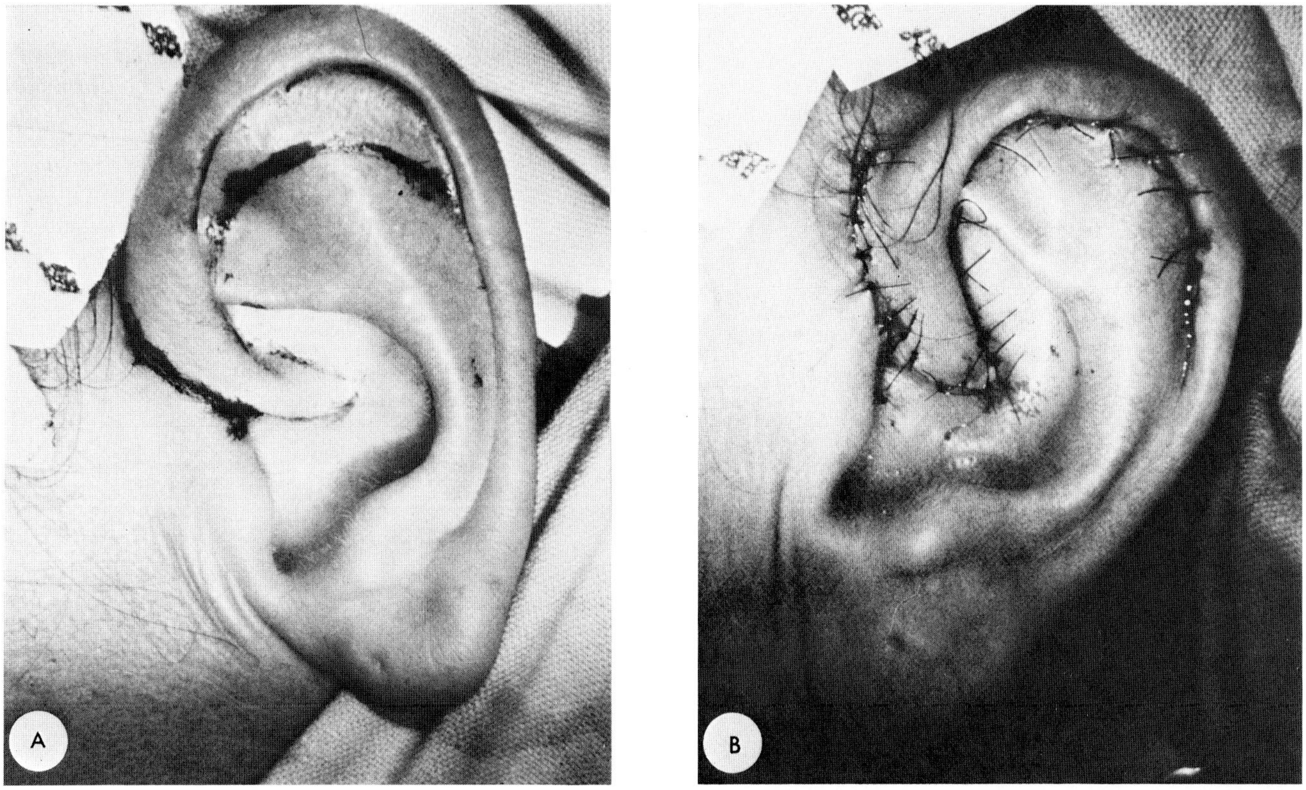

Case 7. Explications see text.

Gary J. Weitzel and Eugene N. Myers:

The causes of stenosis of the external auditory meatus are varied. Infection, trauma, or surgical manipulation in the area are the usual primary factors in its development. Resection of the stenotic area necessitates a reconstructive attempt for adequate functioning of the orifice as a conduit for sound waves and for access in examination of the eardrum and normal cleansing of the external auditory meatus. Resection of benign or malignant neoplasms also creates a defect requiring reconstruction. Presented in this paper is a review of surgical techniques which have shown some success in dealing with these problems.

The nature of the underlying problem dictates to a large extent what type of approach can be successfully attempted. The extent of the local resection may be minimal when it results from infection or minor trauma. It may be substantial when it results from major trauma or neoplasm. Stenosis of the entire external auditory meatus down to the tympanic annulus makes repair difficult using conservative measures. Often modified radical mastoidectomy is required. This is usually the case when fibrous and bony obliteration of the external auditory canal is found.

Reconstruction of the external auditory meatus will be discussed in this paper only. Intracanal lesions will not be considered as a separate entity. The primary purpose of the paper will be to discuss various plastic surgical procedures which have proven useful for reconstructing the external auditory meatus. External auditory meatal stenosis resulting from infection (chronic external otitis) is usually a part of complete canal stenosis. Stenting and/or split-thickness skin grafting after excision of the scar tissue has been reported by Conley, Beales, and Marlowe.[3,4,8] These are variations on the theme of removing scar tissue from the local area and either allowing the process of re-epithelialization to take place or to place split-thickness skin in the area which is then held in place by a stent. Beales has simply excised apposing strips of skin and underlying cartilage from the external auditory canal in a longitudinal fashion and afterward placed a bivalved plastic (acrylic) prosthesis for maintenance of patency in the canal until re-epithelialization takes place. The prosthesis in this instance must be kept in place for approximately three months. Marlowe uses silicon rubber tubing as stenting with split-thickness skin grafting after removal of the fibrous scar tissue from the canal via a postauricular approach. The posterior bony canal wall in this instance can be enlarged by drilling.

Conley reports that with traumatic injuries to the external canal a fibrous and bony obliteration of the canal may result. Modified radical mastoidectomy is usually necessary for repair in such cases. This he does through an endaural incision. Four weeks after the procedure with the occurrence of a layer of healthy granulation tissue, a split-thickness skin graft is then placed.

Although procedures of this sort yield favorable results in some instances, they have no predictability of success. When no tissue is grafted or split-thickness skin grafts are utilized for repair after resection for chronic stenosing external otitis the major problem is re-stenosis of the canal. The problem of secondary (postoperative) stenosis also occurs following resection of growths from the area of the external auditory meatus. Contraction of the graft during the healing phase is the rule with split-thickness skin grafting. Almost invariably there is diminution in the size of the lumen. Reconstruction with full-thickness skin provides a more satisfactory solution since this tissue retains its characteristics when transferred from another location to the site of repair. Free full-thickness grafts might take but their viability is compromised without an intact blood supply. Denuded canal wall cartilage and bone does not provide an adequate vascular bed for nourishment of this tissue. Tissue is best transferred using local flaps which retain their original blood supply. Several of these which have been used successfully will be discussed in detail in this paper.

Periauricular transposition flaps overall seem to be most feasible for reconstructing the external auditory meatus. These can be used in conjunction with endaural or postauricular mastoidectomy procedures. Restructuring the external auditory meatus after resection of scar tissue or neoplasm is best accomplished using these methods. Beale, Stewart, Stallings, and Sessions have outlined the design of four basic flaps in the region of the ear.[2] These are anterior flaps which are superiorly and inferiorly based and postauricular flaps which are superiorly and inferiorly based. These flaps have respective advantages and disadvantages with their use.

The preauricular superiorly based pedicle flap can best be used for defects in the anterior or superior quadrant of the external auditory meatus. The flap although not based as a pedicle on a named arterial blood supply probably receives some direct feeders from the superficial temporal artery. Collateral circulation from the postauricular and scalp vessels also provides a retrograde blood supply to this flap. Care must be taken not to remove too much subcutaneous tissue from the flap and thereby compromise the blood supply by destroying the subdermal plexus of vessels. The advantages of this flap are: (1) properly fashioned it has a strong blood supply; (2) in the female it is not hair bearing; and (3) primary closure leaves an inconspicuous linear preauricular scar. Its disadvantages are: (1) it can be used only for anterior or superior defects in the external auditory meatus; and (2) its venous drainage may be compromised since it is superiorly based which may result in poor perfusion and oxygenation.

The inferiorly based preauricular flap can be used for repair of defects in the inferior or anterior external auditory meatus. This has a more direct blood supply from branches of the superficial temporal and posterior facial artery. The donor site, after transfer of the flap with wide undermining of the surrounding skin, may be closed primarily, or full-thickness skin from behind the ear or elsewhere may be grafted to the donor site for good matching of color and skin texture.

Postauricular flaps either superiorly or inferiorly based are less conspicuous because of placement behind the pinna and beneath the hair. The inferiorly based postauricular flap which derives its blood supply from the postauricular branch of the occipital artery has a good predictability for success.

It can be used for reconstituting the posterior external auditory meatus and by a technique reported by Owens the anterior half of the meatus also. This flap can be combined with a postaural incision and mastoidectomy with relative ease. It is tunneled through a surgically created defect in the concha to fit it into the defect in the external auditory meatus. The distal two-thirds of the flap may be defatted and the proximal one third of the flap may be de-epithelialized. The epithelial shave allows immediate closure of the conchal defect by sewing the postauricular skin to this area of the flap. An ellipse of conchal cartilage often must be removed to prevent strangulation of the flap. The end of the flap is laid into the canal wall defect and the edges are sutured to the margins of excision in the meatus and concha. The postauricular defect is undermined and closed down to the base of the pedicle using a V-Y or straight line reapproximation. A split-thickness skin graft may also be used to resurface the defect. The hairline should not be distorted in an attempt at primary closure.

The superiorly based postauricular flap as with the superiorly based preauricular flap has a blood supply less substantially based than the inferior one and has less favorable venous drainage. However, the postauricular collateral circulation is extensive and provides adequate feeding. This flap if designed close to the curve of the concha posteriorly has two good features. (1) Its anterior border is the same as the usual postauricular incision for mastoidectomy. (2) It is almost hairless. Overall, it has the proper thickness with the right amount of subcutaneous tissue, to allow ease of placement into the surgical defect. Its major drawback is a dog-ear which results at its base once it is transposed anteriorly into the defect and sewn into place. This requires a second procedure for revision if the patient so desires.

A procedure designed by Owens is specifically used for closing defects in the external auditory meatus following resection of small neoplasms.[9] The meatal lesion is excised widely including underlying cartilage if necessary to obtain adequate margins of resection. Posteriorly in the external auditory meatus the skin of the external auditory canal and that overlying the cartilage of the concha are undermined, pulled together, and sutured to cover exposed cartilage. The anterior repair is made as follows:

(A) A postauricular inferiorly based pedicle flap is designed and an incision through the substance of the pinna is made to allow placement of the flap into the anterior edge of the surgical defect.
(B) The pedicle is left in place for two weeks.
(C) The pedicle is then sectioned in a manner to provide tissue for insertion into the ear canal anteriorly to complete the reconstruction of the surgical defect. The main part of the pedicle is then replaced postauricularly.

A modification of this technique is reported by Gingrass and Pickrell who raise a flap from the posterior surface of the ear. The advantage of this flap is its relative thinness. The transposed tissue, therefore, contains less bulk and resembles the excised conchal skin more closely. The flap after placement for two weeks is sectioned postauricularly and the defect behind the ear is then closed over.

Summary

Methods by which repair of the external auditory meatus has been successful have been discussed in detail with their relative merits and deficiencies. A rational design for the repair of surgically corrected defects has been presented. The relative merit of local flaps used in reconstruction over split-thickness skin grafting has been discussed.

References

1. Anthony WP: A method of meatoplasty. Laryngoscope, 84:1118–1121, 1974
2. Beal DD, Stewart KC, Stallinger JO, Sessions DG: Meatoplasty transposition flaps. Laryngoscope, 82:404–407, 1972
3. Beales PH: Atresia of the external auditory meatus. Arch Otolaryngol 100:209–211, 1974
4. Conley JP: Atresia of the external auditory canal occurring in the military service. Arch Otol 43:613–622, 1946
5. Eichel BS, Simonton KM: Stenosis of the external auditory meatus secondary to chronic external otitis treated by a simplified surgical method: report of a case. Laryngoscope 75:16–21, 1965
6. Gingrass RP, Pickrell KL: Technique for closure of conchal and external auditory canal defects. Plast Reconstr Surg 41:568–571, 1968

7. Heron TG, Dreyer A: External auditory meatal plasty. Arch Otolaryngol 87:41–43, 1968
8. Marlowe FI: Acquired atresia of the external auditory canal. Arch Otolaryngol 96:380–383, 1972
9. Owens N: An effective method for closing defects of the external auditory canal. Plast Reconstr Surg 23:381–387, 1959
10. Paparella MM, Kurkjian JM: Surgical treatment for chronic stenosing external otitis. Laryngoscope, 76:232–245, 1966
11. Shea JJ: Enlarging the ear canal in intact wall tympanoplasty. Laryngoscope, 82:884–890, 1922
12. Steffensen WH: A method of correcting atresia of the ear canal. Plast Reconstr Surg 1:329–331, 1946

Perichonditis and Chondritis of the Ear

Richard A. Martin, Anthony J. Yonkers, Omaha, Neb. and C.T. Yarington, Jr., Seattle, Wash.

Infection of the external ear usually takes a benign course and with treatment will heal without difficulty. However, when the perichondrium is involved, there is danger of infection of the underlying cartilage resulting in loss of structure and sometimes devastating deformity.

The difference between perichondritis and chondritis may be obvious, yet separating the two in the literature may be difficult. Perichondritis and chondritis both present as a painful red, warm swelling on the ear and may present as late as a month after the original insult which may be in the form of hematoma, burn, laceration, or pressure from improperly placed retractor during ear surgery. The organisms are invariably either pseudomonas or mixture of pseudomonas or staphylococcus aureus.[1–4] The treatments advocated are similar; that is, either surgical excision,[1,3] or drains with antibiotic and enzyme irrigation.[2,4] Perichondritis is discussed in the literature in regard to postoperative complications of the burned ear. Technically, the term perichondritis suggests that the cartilage has not yet been invaded. Preservation of structure would be more likely, assuming the infection were controlled. The term chondritis assumes destruction of cartilage and some structural damage would be inevitable.

Department of Otolaryngology and Maxillo-Facial Surgery, University of Nebraska Medical Center, Omaha, Nebraska

Indeed, this seems to be the case. Most cases of perichondritis following operations result from an attempt to create an adequate meatoplasty. This kind of infection is quite amenable to wide surgical excision which allows the removal of the diseased cartilage in the area of the choncha without disturbing the helix or antihelix thereby preserving structure of the ear. Stroud[1] in his discription stresses the importance of adequate margins in excision of the infected cartilage (Fig. 1). Strictly speaking, his discussion concerns chondritis as well as perichondritis. Wanamaker[2] in his discription of the treatment of perichondritis, describes the placement of No. 190 polyethylene tubes on each side of the infected cartilage with the installation of antibiotics (Fig. 2). Both of these techniques have apparently gained satisfactory results in the treatment of perichondritis. Chondritis of the burned ear follows a somewhat more aggressive course than perichondritis (or chondritis of other types of injury). The incidence is much higher, ranging from 20 percent to as high as 50 percent. The original burn may only have been a second degree burn without actual exposure of cartilage and the presentation may be as late as six weeks after burn. Once established, the infection tends to spread rather rapidly through the cartilage and despite adequate therapy may result in a deformed ear. The most popular treatment for chondritis following burns is essentially the same as described by

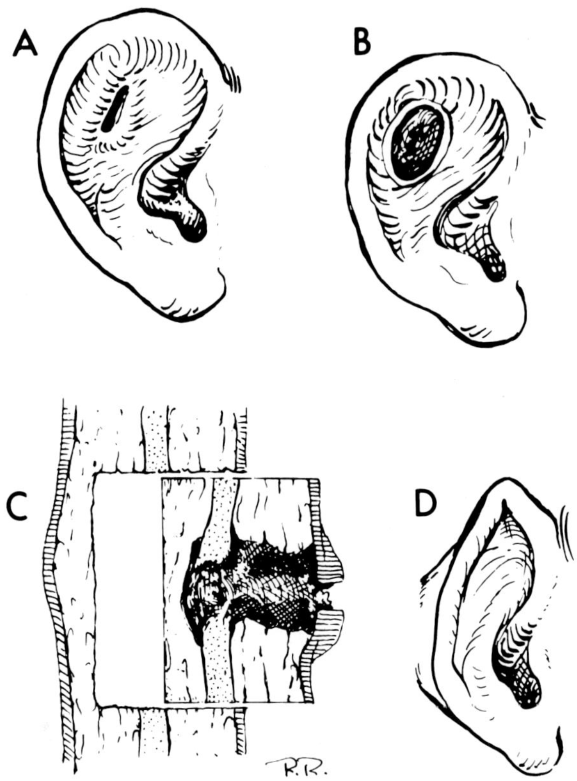

Fig. 1. Using this method the abscess is widely excised and dissection should be carried out to include what appears to be healthy cartilage. If any infected cartilage is left recurrence is inevitable.

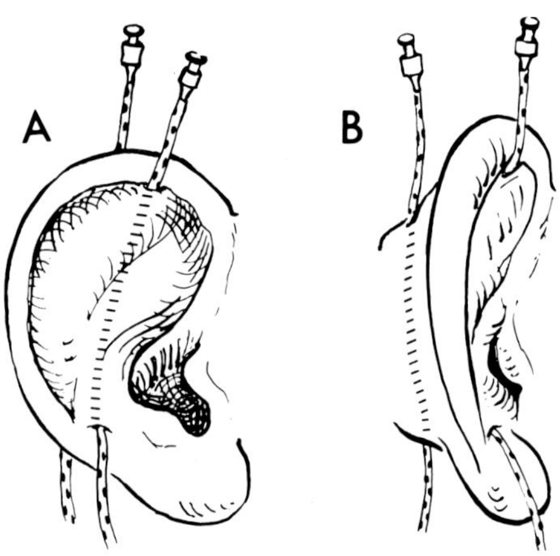

Fig. 2. Drains are placed anterior and posterior to the infected cartilage through which solutions of polymyxin or colistin can be irrigated. As many as three on each side of the infected cartilage can be placed. Wanamaker describes incisions in a step ladder pattern through the skin to enhance the drainage. This set-up could allow for continuous or intermittent instillation of antihelix and enzyme. This is the method advised by us in place of total chondrectomy or when debridement is going to mean destruction of the antihelix.

Stroud in which the abscess and all necrotic cartilage is widely excised. Dowling[3] describes a bivalving technique when the infection is extensive and total chondrectomy is required (Fig. 3). The problems associated with this treatment are best presented by these representative cases.

Case No. 1

A 42-year-old welder sustained second degree burns to his face, ears, neck and back in a dust explosion in a grain elevator on August 26, 1973. He received penicillin by mouth for the first six days, saline soaks were applied to his face and sulfamylon to his abdomen. He did well and was discharged on September 17. On the 25th of September, one month later, the patient presented with marked erythema and swelling bilaterally in the superior portion of the antihelix. Wide excision of the skin and underlying cartilages was carried out and colistin soaked dressings were applied four times a day. The culture grew Pseudomonas. The patient was discharged with dressing changes at home but returned on the 4th of October with purulent drainage and pain bilaterally. A second debridement was carried out and on the right ear it was necessary to remove a portion of the helix. He was again treated with colistin soaked dressing with a graft planned when it was felt certain that the ears were free of infection. The patient however discontinued his dressings. As a result, the posterior skin collapsed over the granulating bed. By October 30th both ears were healed, free of infection, but with resulting deformity (Figs. 4 and 5).

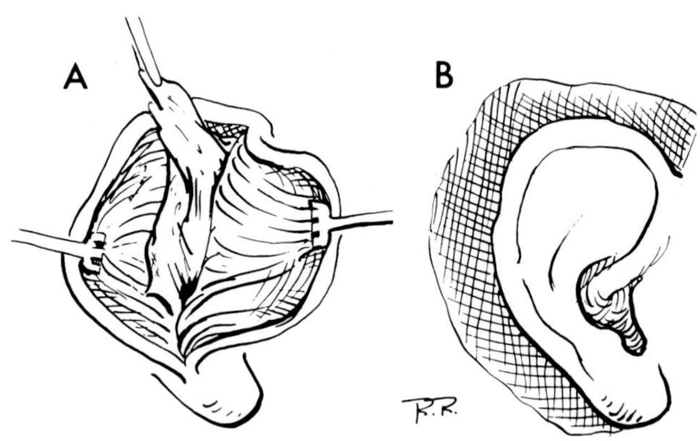

Fig. 3. In this method structural component of the ear is lost, and deformity is inevitable.

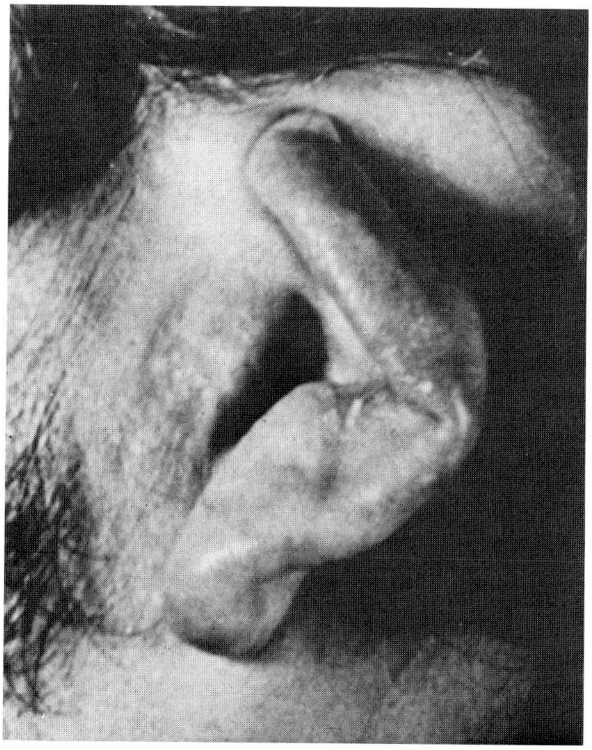

Fig. 4. After two debridements collapse from lack of helical support resulted in a lop ear.

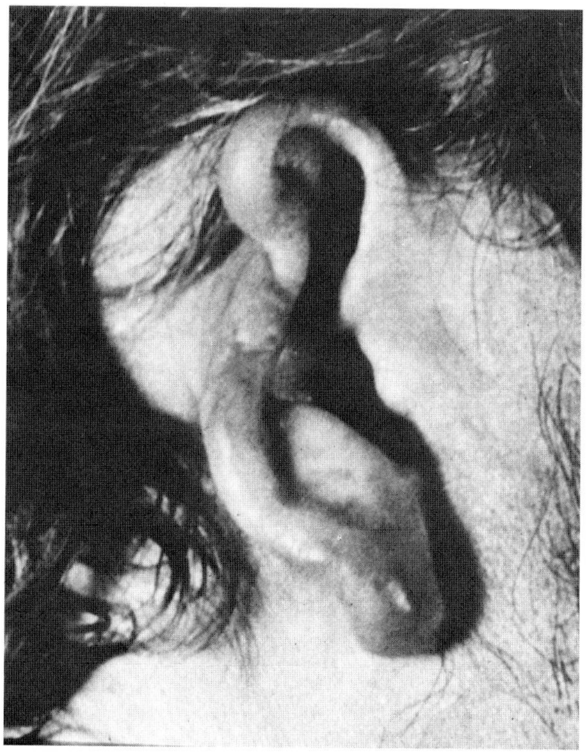

Fig. 5. The right ear similarly collapsed with the resultant deformity.

Comment

Sulfamylon has been shown to be effective in the prevention of perichondritis and could well have been used here. This patient's original infection involved the majority of the antihelix and an attempt to preserve the helix resulted in recurrence of infection and the need for the second debridement with the sacrifice of the helix.

Case No. 2

A second welder was burned in the same dust explosion as the previous patient and presented at approximately the same time. The left ear was initially treated by the referring physician by incision and drainage. No drain was placed. Two days later the patient presented to us with involvement of the majority of the antihelix. An attempt was made to treat this as an early perichondritis leaving the helix intact but within a week a bivalve technique was necessary with removal of the majority of the cartilage. At the time of the second debridement of the left ear, the right ear developed a small area of swelling and tenderness in the antihelix. This was treated with wide excision with the helix left intact. The culture grew Pseudomonas and *Staph. aureus* and again was treated with colistin soaked dressings. The ears were both healed by October 30th but the left ear was severely deformed (Figs. 6–7). This patient presented originally with a hearing loss and was found to have a 3 mm central perforation and otitis media.

Comment

This patient was inadequately treated initially, then treated with inadequate debridement. His otitis media with perforation points out the importance of a thorough initial examination. The results of the right ear emphasizes the importance of early recognition and treatment.

Case No. 3

A 36-year-old black male sustained second and third degree burns to the right ear, face, and arms

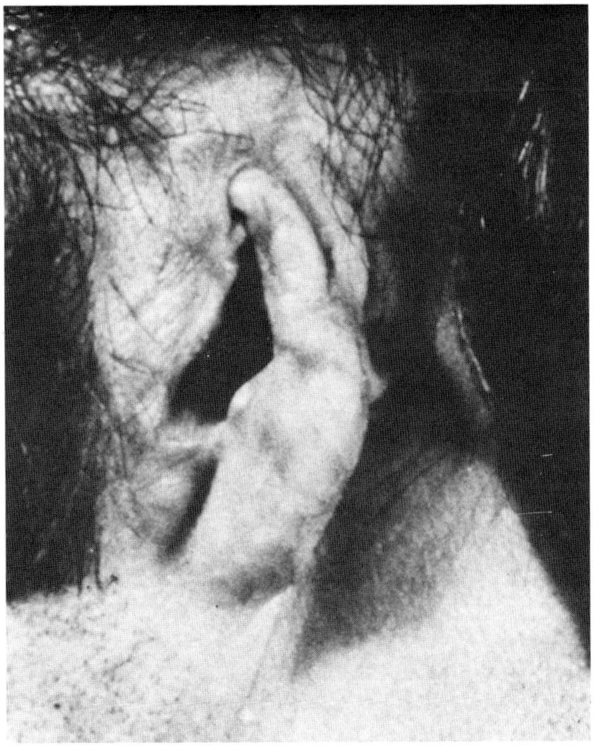

Fig. 6. The bivalve technique for total cartilagenous involvement resulted in almost total loss of ear above the lobe.

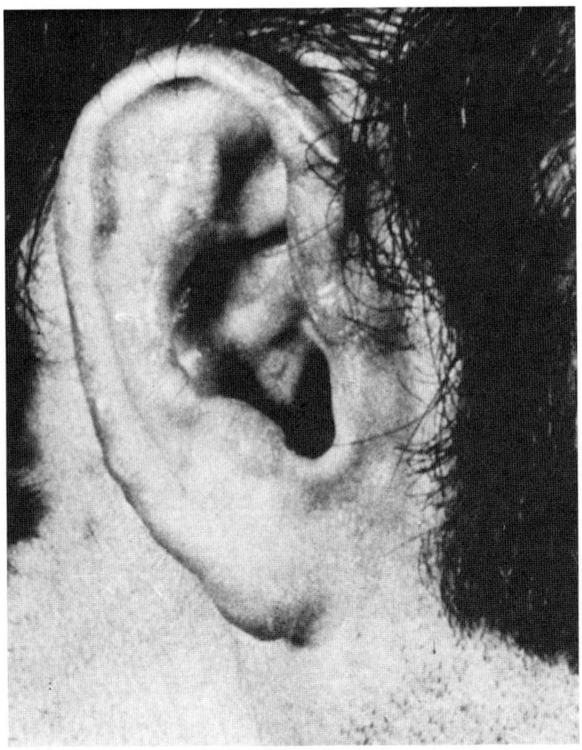

Fig. 7. The area of the superior cruz of the antihelix was treated early by debridement and structural components were preserved.

from scalding water on June 26, 1973. The patient was treated with saline soaks and antibiotics and presented seven weeks after the burn, the face and neck completely healed, the skin overlying the ear intact, but red, swollen, and markedly tender (Figs. 8 and 9). The entire ear was involved and was treated with a bivalve technique. Again, pseudomonas was cultured and colistin soaked dressings were applied. Ten days later a repeat debridement was necessary and at the time involvement of the external auditory canal necessitated removal of the diseased cartilage. This ear healed following prolonged therapy, but the patient was left with a marked deformity. Patient did not allow follow-up photos and threatened suit over the end results.

Comment

This case required total removal of the cartilage of the ear and still a recurrence of infection of the external canal occurred which required a second debridement. The combined blood loss from the two procedures was over a unit which from a more debilitated patient could mean the need for replacement. This man's reaction to the end result em-

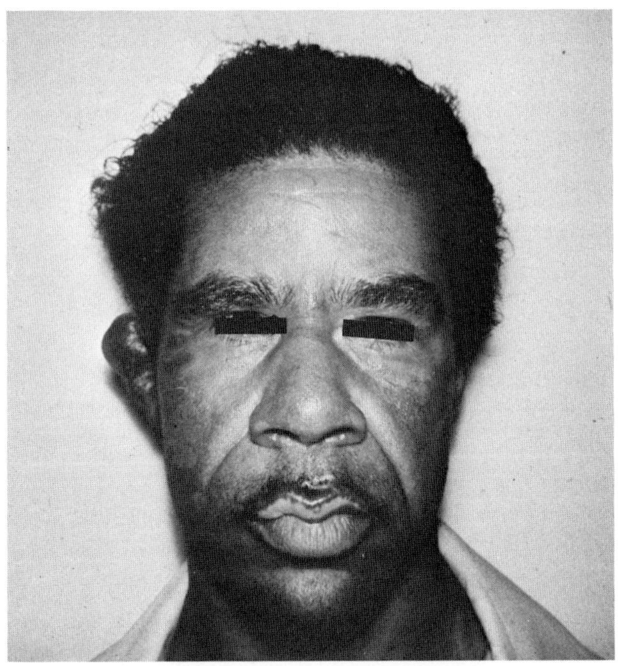

Fig. 8. Demonstrating abscess formation beneath intact skin on the pinna.

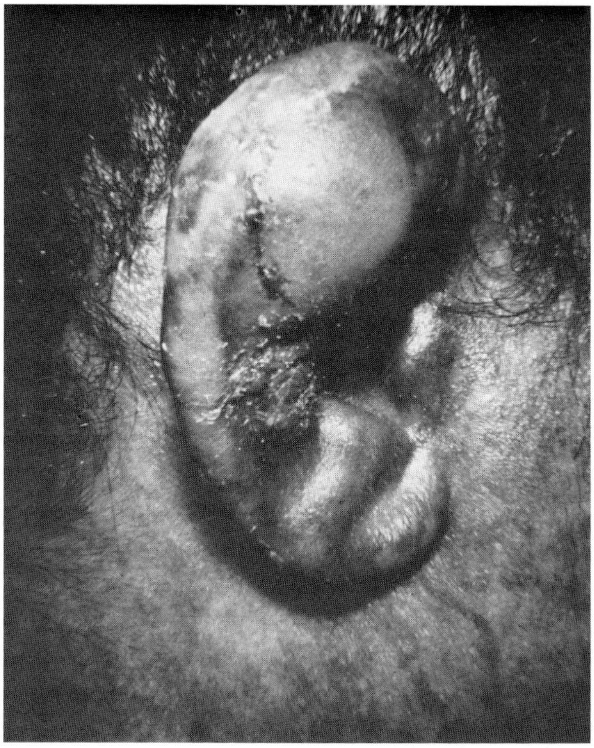

Fig. 9. Demonstrating abscess formation beneath intact skin on the pinna.

phasizes the importance of stressing initially the probability of deformity.

Discussion

Presented here are three men, all seen by the same physicians over a three month time period. All men had sustained first and second degree burns to the head and neck with second degree burns to five out of six ears. None had third degree burns to the ears. All were well on their way to healing from their burns elsewhere when pain and swelling was noted on their ears. All had initial swelling on the antihelix where cartilage is thick and skin is thin and all required debridements under general anesthesia due to the ineffectiveness of local or regional block of the enflamed area. All cultured pseudomonas or staph aureus. These cases point out rather dramatically the importance of early diagnosis and management. By the time these patients were treated, involvement of the helix was inevitable. If the swelling is noted early and involves only the antihelix or concha, adequate excision can be carried out without destruction of the helix and with minimal deformity. If the helix is included in the excision or the infection, deformity is inevitable.

Microscopically, the skin overlying the infected cartilage shows marked and pseudoepitheliomatous appearance and hyperplasia. Beneath the dermal layer lies the subcutaneous tissue which is characterized by edema and many white cells. The cartilage demonstrates a lack of lacunae and those that do exist show evidence of injury. Toward the center of the abscess, masses of phagocytes and PMN's are seen digesting the injured cartilage. (Fig. 10A–D). The possibility of autodigestion has been considered before. The lack of bacteria, the intact skin and the evidence of sick or dead cartilage would support this possibility, with infection being an opportunistic event. The drains themselves would prevent any pressure build-up beneath the intact skin.

Apfelburg[5] recently published a series of five cases with chondritis treated with installation of gentamycin or neomycin and polymyxin B, and added hyaluronidase as a spreading factor. His results are comparatively satisfactory.

It would seem that particularly when the cartilage is involved to the extent that debridement is going to necessitate total chondrectomy, treatment with drains in combination with antibiotics and enzymes would have a better chance of preserving the ear. If tubes such as Wanamaker has described were inserted, continuous or intermittent installation of antibiotics and enzymes could be carried out. Hyaluronidase, streptokinase or streptodornase would act to prevent skin from sealing over the cartilage and loculation of infection. It would seem that this form of treatment would avoid the need for general anesthesia, excessive blood loss and the possibility of a second debridement.

In summary, although there are many similarities between the infection of cartilage following surgical procedures or mechanical trauma and the chondritis following burns, there seems to be a significant difference in the incidence and aggressiveness of chondritis of the burned ear. Steps to be taken in prevention of chondritis following the burn would include daily washings with surgical soap solutions, and close inspection of eschars for signs of purulent drainage and the use of sulfamylon or 5 percent silver nitrate solution.[6,7] The hair should

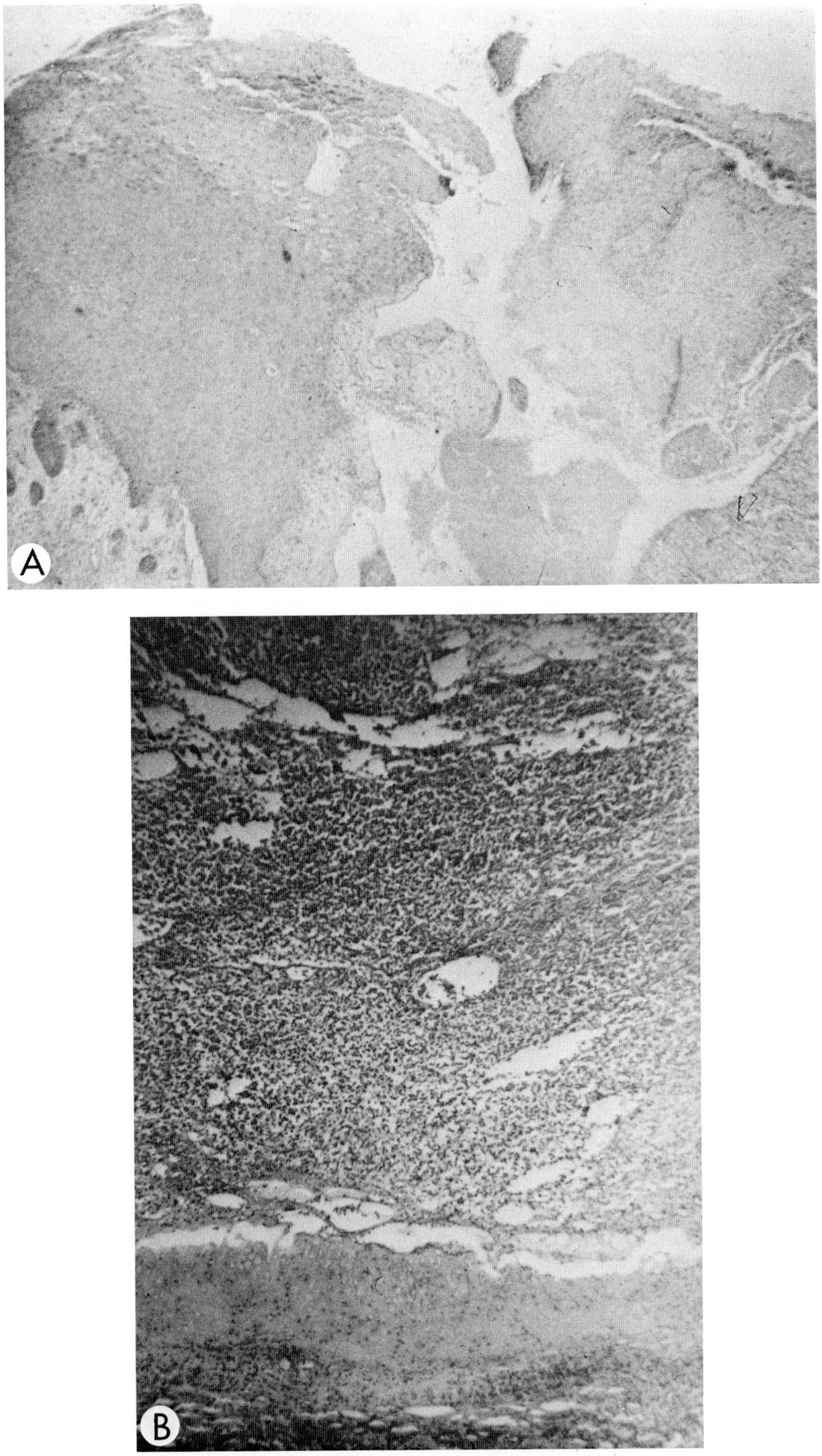

Fig. 10. *(A) Marked hyperplasia of the dermal layers with a pseudoepitheliomatous appearance. Many PMNs are seen in the underlying tissue. (B) Demonstrates the massive invasion of PMNs in the subcutaneous layer, the damaged perichondrium and the lack of normal lacunac in cartilage.*

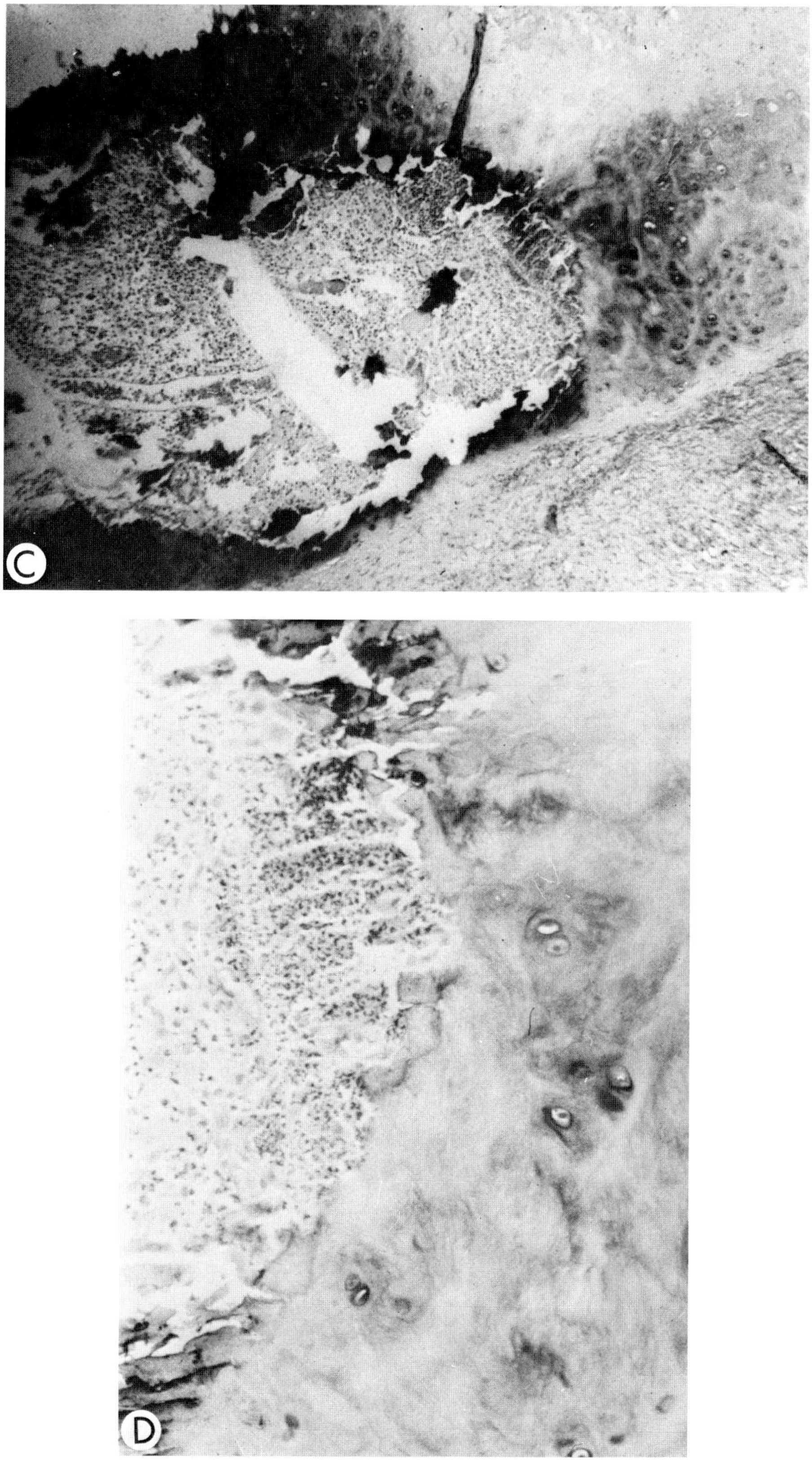

Fig. 10. (C) Displays the destruction of cartilage by masses of phagocytes and the destroyed and thickened perichondrium. (D) A higher powered view of the destruction of dead cartilage by PMNs Note the empty lacunae and general lack of cartilage cells.

be cut short to avoid matting in the eschar, and donut shaped pillows should be used to protect the ear. The use of oral antibiotics by themselves are probably ineffective, because of the incidence of pseudomonas and the lack of blood supply to the cartilage. Chondritis once it develops is a devastating complication and it should be explained to the patient from the beginning the possibility of deformity despite aggressive therapy. Early in the treatment of chondritis, wide excision is indicated when the structure of the ear can be left intact. However, when debridement means sacrifice of the helix or structural component of the ear, then insertion of drains with antibiotic and enzyme irrigation should be considered as the alternative method.

References

1. Stroud MH: A simple treatment for suppurative perichondritis. Laryngoscope 73:556–563, 1963
2. Wanamaker HH: Suppurative perichondritis of the auricle. Trans AA00 76:1289–1291, 1972
3. Dowling JA, Foley FD, Moncrief JA: Chondritis of the burned ear. Plast Reconstr Surg 42:115–122, 1968
4. Stevenson EW: Bacillus pyocyaneus perichondritis of the ear. Laryngoscope 74:255, 1964
5. Apfelberg DP, Waisbren BA, Masters FW, Robinson DW: Treatment of chondritis in the burned ear by the local instillation of antibiotics. Plast Reconstr Surg 53:179–183, 1974
6. Moyer CA, Brentano L, Gravers DL, Marjraf HW, Monafa WW: Treatment of large human burns with 0.5% silver nitrate solution. Arch Surg 90:812–867, 1965
7. Grant DA, Finley ML, Coers CR: Early management of the burned ear. Plast Reconstr Surg 44:161–165, 1969

The Reconstruction of the Human Auricle as in Animal Experiments

Felix Nagel, Germany

The construction or reconstruction of an external ear is one of the most difficult tasks facing plastic and reconstructive surgery today. On examining the external ear closely, it soon becomes obvious which difficulties have to be overcome when copying such a somplicated form in flesh and blood. These very difficulties are the reason why plastic surgery has only been able to produce a rather unsatisfactory solution to the problem up to now. After consulting international literature on the subject we reach the conclusion that only a few surgeons such as Tanzer[4] and Converse,[2] to name two of the most successful, have managed to produce an acceptable, but by no means ideal, auricle. The majority of surgeons engaged in plastic surgery, therefore, refuse to attempt to reconstruct the external ear because of the great length of time and the large number of individual operations necessary which, even today, still lead to comparatively dissatisfying results in general.

To track down the reasons why all the known techniques have more or less failed as yet, we have studied the problem through a long and extensive series of experiments on animals; our aim being to develop a method of reconstruction which (a) results in a normal-looking resemblance of the human ear; (b) enables us to produce an auricle in any individual or desired form.

As is known the auricle is made up of two components: the cartilage framework, which is also responsible for the shape of the external ear, and the relatively thin skin as coverage. If we are to construct an auricle of natural appearance, these two components, cartilage and skin, must be matched perfectly and become one, i.e., they must complement and assimilate each other and in no way hinder each other in the moulding of the ear.

We gained this knowledge by reason of the initial failures in our experiments. Through this unfortunate experience we learned that it is not possible to produce an ideally formed auricle if the skin has to fit a pre-prepared frame no matter how precisely such a frame is carved or moulded and how exactly the postoperative bandaging is performed. The results of our first experiments resembled those we know from various publications on this subject; that is to say they were, at best, similar to the human ear.

In techniques practiced up to now the moulding of the frame played the decisive role and the skin had to be fitted around this framework as best it could. The whole operation, therefore, was concentrated on the fine moulding of the frame. However, the appearance of an external ear is not judged by the construction of the frame, which is invisible anyway, but whether or not the external appearance is that of a human ear. In other words, the skin should first be moulded to the shape of an auricle and the frame then fitted to this prepared form.

The realization of this idea was the subject of further experiments on animals and we have developed a method which we find satisfactory and which is described as follows.

Skin, being flexible and elastic, is a particularly favourable tissue for copying complicated formations. We can prove that skin can be formed into an auricle in an almost ideal way if it is adapted to a negative plastic model of an external ear. We chose Paladon, as used in dentures, as the most suitable material for our mold. A minute adaptation is achieved by suction through the usage of a suction chamber on the outside of the model, the model being extremely well perforated to enable us to exert sufficient suction on the skin to pull it firmly into the form. (See Figure 1.) If the skin flap from the back of a test animal, in our case an albino rabbit, is sucked into such a negative model, the skin fits in with the elevations and depressions of the model thus itself producing an auricle formed according to the curves of the negative model (Fig. 2). Our task is now to maintain this achieved form even when suction has been removed.

From tests made by Peer[3] and based on Young's[5] experiments we know that if chips of cartilage are placed in a perforated form which is then implanted into living tissue, the chopped cartilage becomes a flexible plate made up of many

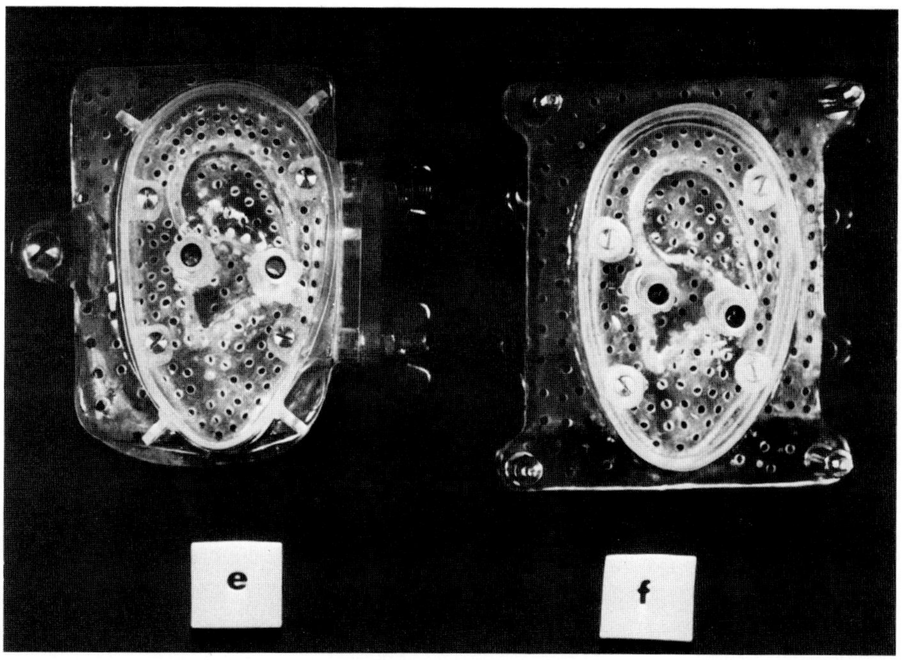

Fig. 1. Two variations of the negative models made of Paladon. The large holes in the centre are the nipples for the suction tubes.

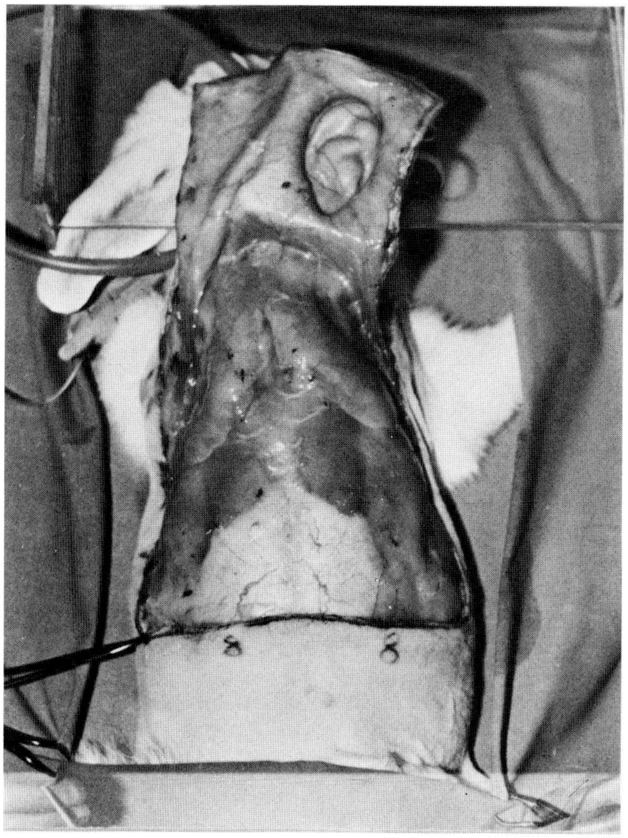

Fig. 2. *This shows a part of the elevated skin flap sucked into the negative form.*

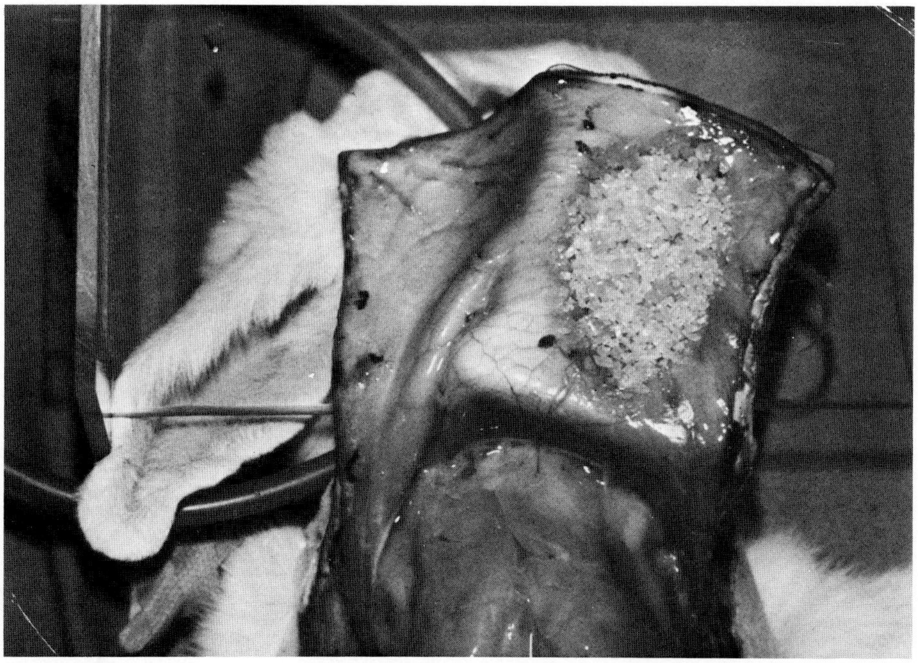

Fig. 3. *The ear after filling the skin mould with silastic chips. Suction tubes have not yet been removed.*

pieces of cartilage which can now be formed into any shape wished. Through normal processes fibrous tissue grows through the perforations and around the chips in the form thus joining them together with a membrane of tissue. This is exactly what was needed for our experiments.

Because of the lack of sufficient cartilage in a rabbit we used Silastic chips for our purposes. These chips were then filled into the inside of the sucked-in skin (Fig. 3). The remaining flap of skin was laid over the chips and the wound and a second plastic mould, this time representing the retro-auricle side of the ear, was placed on top. The two plastic plates forming the model were then screwed together. Extreme care was taken to prevent a stoppage of the capillary flow by inserting springs between the plates to ensure a continuously even pressure of about 8.5 Torr on the surface of the skin flap (Figs. 4 and 5). The whole construction was then attached to the back of the rabbit in such a way as to enable healing to follow uninterrupted. The plastic moulds now had to fulfill their second task, namely to fix the skin in the form desired by the operation and to enable a controlled scarring process to follow and not to leave it to pure chance.

In our experiments the model was left on the skin flap for 4–10 weeks before removal (Fig. 6). This early removal was necessary because of the resumption of fur growth which led to increased pressure on the tissue causing skin necrosis. As we know from Blake's[1] experiments, however, this space of time is inadequate for good scarring. A period of five months would be ideal. Less than five months means you must reckon with a certain flattening of the postoperative form as the cartilage chips and the connective tissue have not knitted sufficiently.

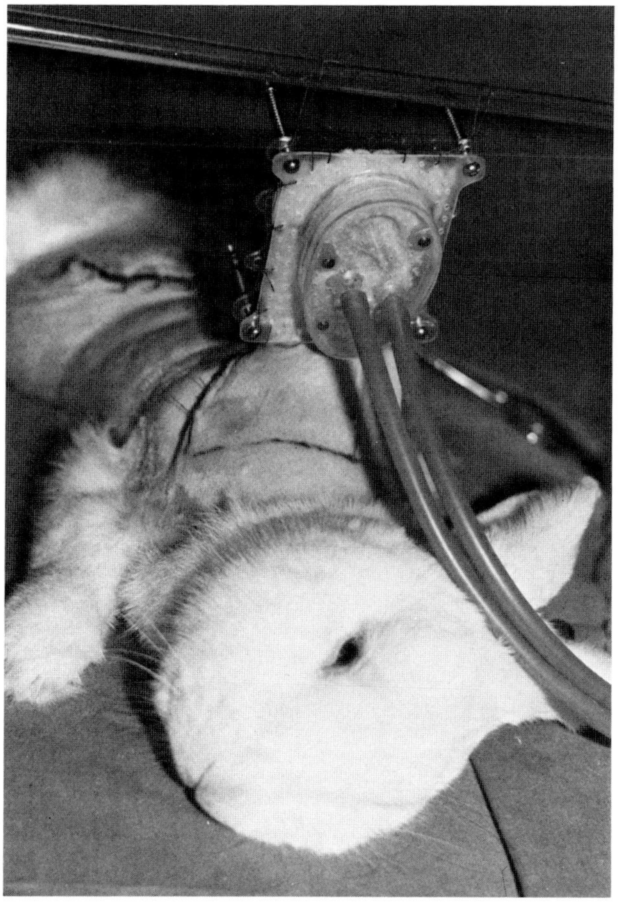

Fig. 4. The model after the remaining skin has been placed over the wound and the two plastic moulds screwed together.

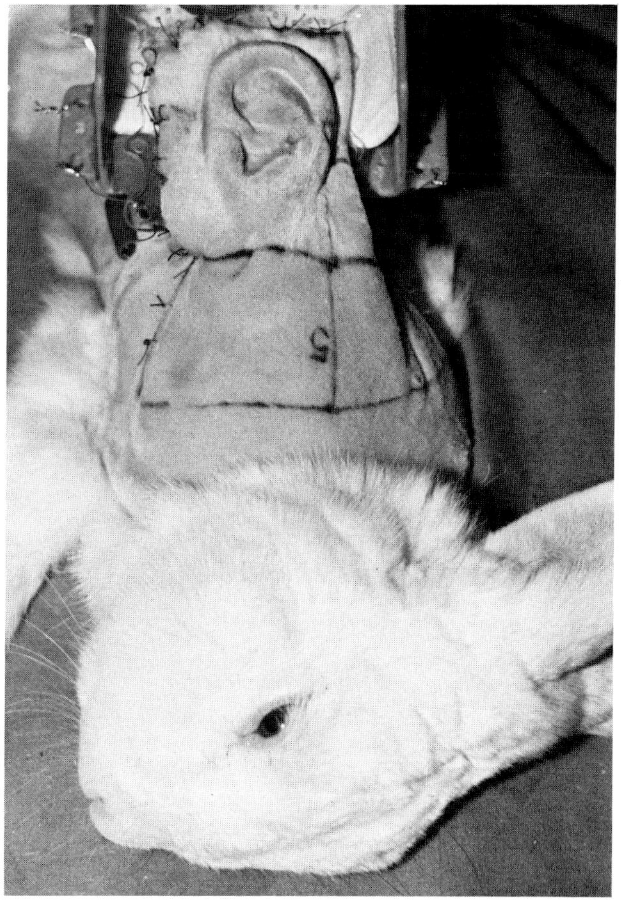

Fig. 5. Here the model was removed for demonstrational purposes to show the impression immediately after the operation.

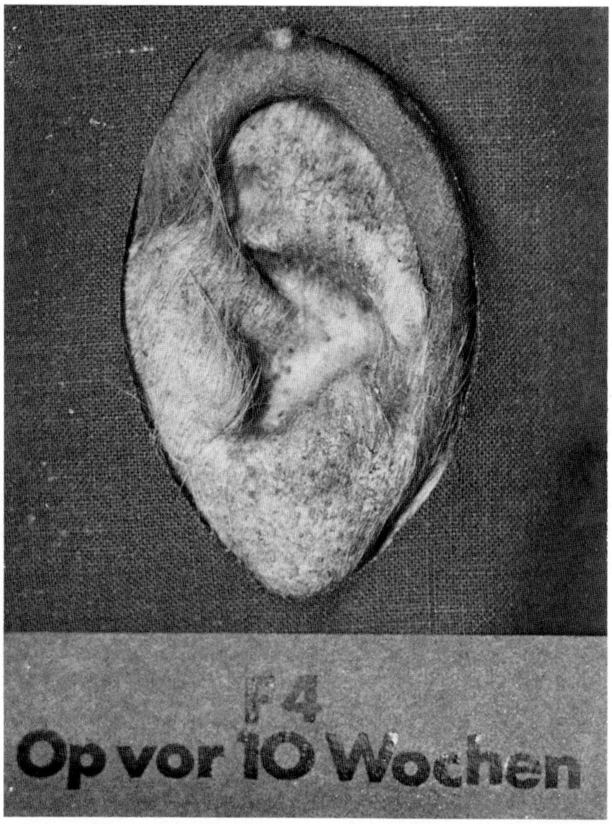

Fig. 6. This shows the state of the ear on removal of the moulds 10 weeks after the operation.

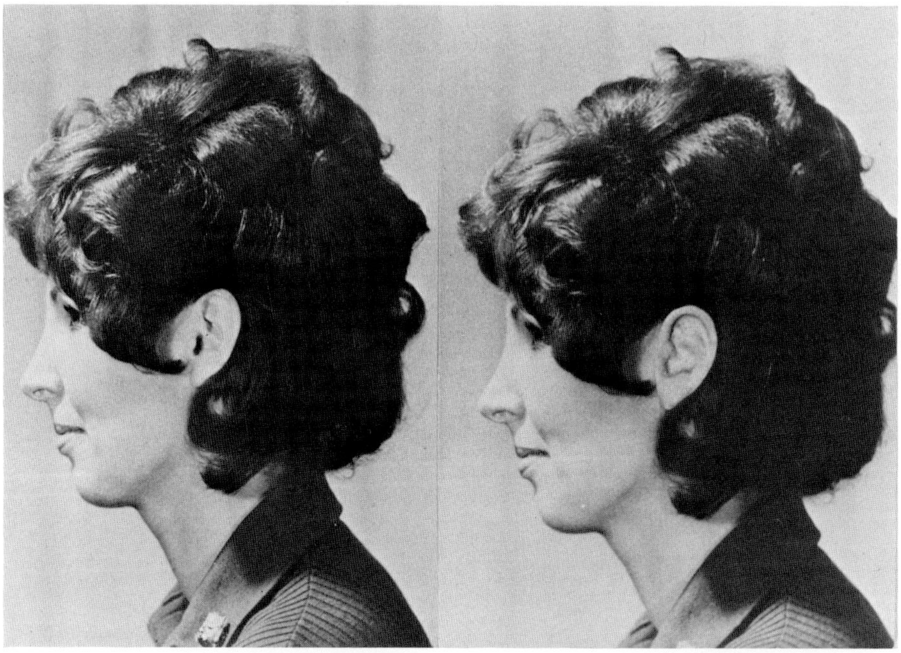

Fig. 7. Here we see the results of one of our experiments with rabbit skin. On the left the ear used as a model, on the right a photolayout of the reconstructed ear.

As our final illustration (Fig. 7) shows, left, the original ear; right, a layout showing the ear reconstructed in rabbit skin, it is not only possible to achieve the fine structure of the human auricle with this method, but also any form of ear desired.

In summing up we come to the conclusion that although the problem of transplanting the reconstructed ear to its final position and the creation of an acoustic duct is far from trivial, we believe this new method is a great step towards a natural-looking reconstruction of the auricle.

References

1. Blake HE: Prefabricated autogenous ear cartilages. Brit J Plast Surg 1:220,1949
2. Converse JM: Reconstruction of the auricle—Part I Plast Reconstr Surg 22:150, 1958; Reconstruction of the auricle—Part II Plast Reconstr Surg 22:230, 1958
3. Peer LA: Reconstruction of the auricle with diced cartilage grafts in a vitallium ear mold. Plast Reconstr Surg 3:653, 1948
4. Tanzer RC: Total reconstruction of the external ear. Plast Reconstr Surg 23:1, 1959
5. Young F: Autogenous cartilage grafts. Surgery 10:7, 1941

Microtia Reconstruction

Burton F. Jaffe, Boston, Mass.

Microtia refers to a small pinna, while aural atresia refers to the absent external auditory canal. This is an uncommon congenital anomaly and the incidence has been reported as 1:10,000 to 1:20,000 newborn births.

My interest in congenital microtia began in 1966 when I was at the Public Health Service Hospital in Gallup, New Mexico. A statistical survey of Navajos with microtia was started because an apparently large number of these Navajo patients with congenital microtia was seen in the Otorhinolaryngology Clinic. In Navajos under the age of 21, 55 were identified with microtia in a population of 60,000. The newborn incidence was 1:1200. This high incidence may be due to the genetic factor of inbreeding.

This paper will discuss the concepts and techniques in repairing congenital microtia.

Timing of Surgery

The length of the pinna reaches adult size by about age six or seven years. Fukuda[1] obtained data in 148 cases and found the following: at ages five to six the pinna averaged 5.5 cm in length, at age eight the pinna averaged 6.0 cm in length, at age nine the pinna averaged over 6.0 cm in length.

If one operates before age six, the reconstructed pinna should be a little longer than its mate. However, better cooperation is obtained in children between 6 and 10 years of age. After age 10, the damaging psychological aspects of the unrepaired malformed ear are often permanent and these adolescent patients often tend to be overly critical of the result which is, in the best of hands, less than perfect.

Strict attention to fine detail is essential in this operation. Many technical points pointed out by others (Tanzer,[2,3] Cronin,[4] and Converse[5]) have been incorporated into this paper.

Preparation for Surgery

Protection for the operated ear should be provided by a rigid ear frame secured to the head by straps. The orthopedic prosthetic department can measure, make, and adjust this ear guard in advance so it is available immediately postoperatively.

Trauma from pressure on the reconstructed pinna may cause flattening of the helical rim and this complication can be minimized.

A phisohex wash the night before surgery may diminish the bacterial count and prevent a serious post operative problem, the infected framework. A betadine scrub and prep is given. Local infiltration with 0.5 percent Xylocaine and 1:200,000 adrenalin is given to balloon out the tissues while providing some hemostasis without sacrificing blood supply leading to necrosis of the skin cover.

An aperture steridrape is placed. The proper level is marked and the axis is selected to be slightly oblique with the top of the pinna positioned slightly posteriorly. Excellent details given by Tanzer[2] and Converse[5] to achieve this will not be repeated.

Stage I

Level of Pinna Reconstruction

The top of the reconstructed pinna should be at the same level as the top of the univolved pinna. Often this means that hairbearing skin will cover the upper part of the framework. When small hairy areas are involved, electrolysis or removal of hair follicles may be used at a later time to remove the hairs. When large hairy areas are involved, a scalp roll works well[6]; the adjacent cephalic scalp is rolled superiorly and the defect filled with a full thickness skin graft from the opposite post auricular sulcus. Later, when the pinna is elevated from the scalp, the scalp roll is released and lowered to its earlier level behind the pinna.

Incision and Rotation of Lobule

Figure 1 demonstrates some of the principles of rotation of the lobule. The basic concept is to handle the tissues very delicately and sometimes lengthen the pinna while rotating the lobule. The lobule can be lengthened by making the vertical incision lower than the pinna and joining it to a horizontal incision. The length of the lobule used will become the width across the lower pinna, and this should measure about half of the height or about 3.0 cm. This incisions are made close to the lobule so that a thick subcutaneous tissue can be used for closure. The skin of the lobule is then rotated and the lower edge sewn horizontally.

The cartilage of the upper unused remnant is removed and may be banked in an abdominal pocket for later use to increase projection of the reconstructed pinna from the side of the head or to be used for making a tragal cartilage. Any cartilage in the tragal area is preserved for a normal cosmetic result.

Creation of Framework Pocket

The incision is then carried to but not through the mastoid periosteum and the temporalis fascia, and the skin is undermined at this level for the framework placement. The anterior inferior portion of the mastoid skin which will be adjacent to the vertical and horizontal lobule incisions must be undermined deeply or not at all to prevent necrosis with subsequent fistulae. The pocket should be large enough to accommodate a cartilage or silastic frame without tension and a trial placement is advised at this time. The subcutaneous soft tissue

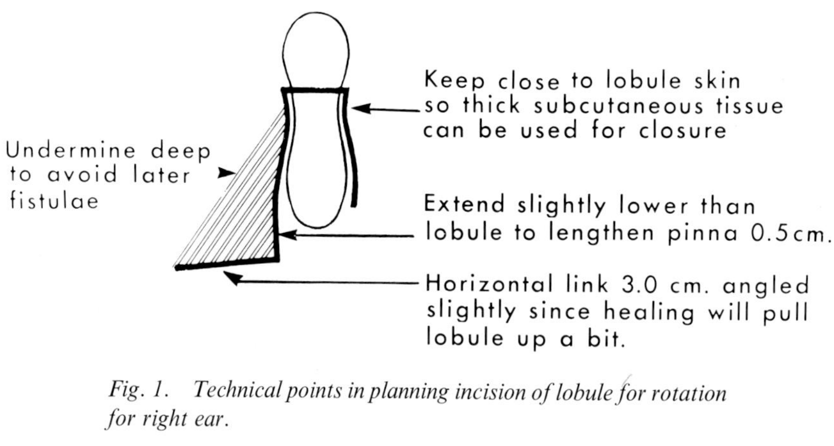

Fig. 1. Technical points in planning incision of lobule for rotation for right ear.

in the region of the conchal bowl is excised down to periosteum and sometimes the mastoid bone is drilled out to obtain a more pleasing cosmetic result simulating the normal concavity of the concha and ear canal region.

Insertion of Hemovac Drain

The needle point is placed within the pocket and pierces the skin well below the lobule or about 2 in. below the lobule so that closure of the tract will occur when the tubing is withdrawn. Using this technique, no air will dissect up the tract to separate the close approximation of skin to framework. The subcutaneous tube is cut about $2\frac{1}{2}$ in. long and placed into the conchal bowl area. Wall suction is immediately applied and is maintained until the end of the operation, and for two to three days thereafter.

Choice of Framework

Silastic and autologous rib cartilage are the two most common frameworks for usage today.

In most surgeon's hands the percent of rejected silastic frames is far higher than cartilaginous frames. Better success with silastic occurs when it is completely bonded to the dacron mesh to allow for firm fixation and to prevent migration and exposure.

Recently a technique was described by Brent for obtaining and carving an autogenous rib cartilage even in a five-year-old child.[7] After the rib is obtained, a pocket is made in the abdominal skin and the child is awakened. The surgeon then carves the cartilage in the sterile operating room, and when completed, places it in the abdominal pocket and closes it with previously placed sutures. In the second stage the rib cartilage can be removed (with no alteration in shape) and placed in the location of the new pinna.

Insertion of Framework

Any frame is inserted with provisions that it is not covered with taut skin and that it is tilted slightly posteriorly at its upper edge.

Closure of Incision

The frequent occurrence of fistulae at the suture line should alert one to the need for a precise closure, and it must be air tight so the suction works well. An excellent contour of the pinna should now be present (Fig. 2).

Dressing

Multiple small cotton pieces soaked with mineral oil make an excellent dressing. A mastoid dressing will keep the cotton pledgets in good position. One should inspect the lobule a few hours postoperatively to make certain excessive pressure does not occur.

Postoperative Care

Antibiotics are started immediately. On the first post operative day the dressing is removed and the preformed ear guard is placed. The hemovac is removed after 48 hr or when the drainage is zero for 24 hr, whichever is longer. Betadine ointment on the wound provides antibacterial effect and seals the incision for better suction.

If erythema of the skin occurs, a scalp vein needle is inserted subcutaneously at a position cephalic to the frame, and an antibiotic drip is run continuously until the erythema improves. Neomycin has been suggested, but it is ototoxic and

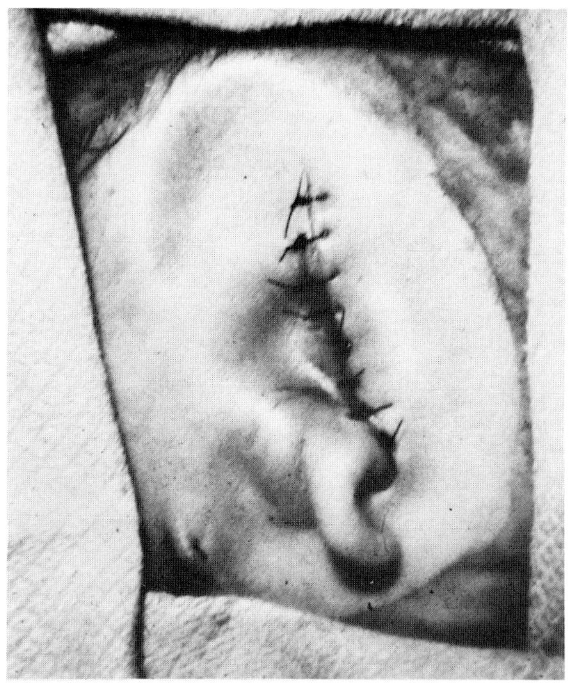

Fig. 2. Photograph showing excellent contour relief achieved with hemovac suction tubing. (The lobule in this case was rotated in the second stage.)

could be most disastrous for the opposite "normal" hearing ear.

Stage II

After three to six months when the skin is well healed, Stage II is begun. An incision is made 3 mm beyond the ridge of the pinna (Fig. 3). If hair is present on the helical rim, it may be depilated by removing the hair follicles from the subcutaneous tissue. A Telfa pattern is made and two elliptical pieces of full thickness skin are obtained from the inner aspect of the arm. These grafts are sewn in the denuded post auricular area, leaving the sutures long for a tie-over bolster. This bolster is left for three weeks to give good projection to the pinna. (A split thickness skin graft may be used, but might contract to give less projection of the pinna.)

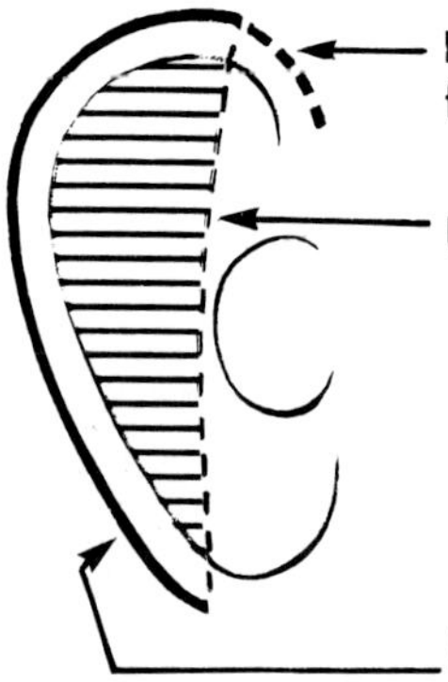

Fig. 3. Technical points in planning incision for elevation of pinna.

Subsequent Stages

These are needed to improve minor cosmetic areas, such as increasing the projection, or adjusting the helical crus.

Other Staging Sequences

It is possible to rotate the lobule in the first stage, insert the framework in the second stage, and elevate the pinna from the side of the head in the third stage.

One may also insert the framework in the first stage, and both rotate the lobule and elevate the pinna from the side of the head in the second stage (Fig. 4).

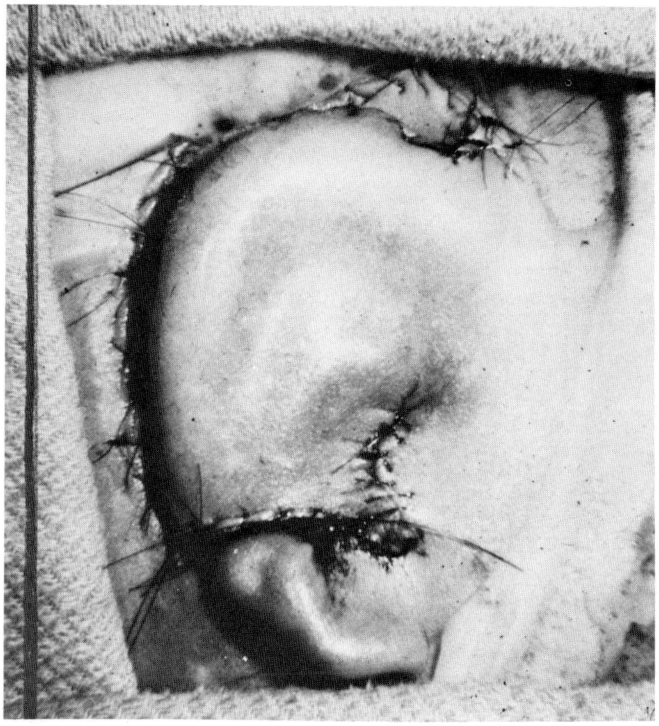

Fig. 4. Photograph showing a staging sequence where the second stage consists of rotation of lobule and elevation of pinna from side of head with placement of full thickness skin grafts.

Complications

Loss of Contour

This occurs from hematomas, infections, and repeated elevations of skin in the region of the pinna.

Hematoma

This occurs when meticulous hemostasis is not achieved. It may lead to increased fibrosis with loss of contour. Even worse, the hematoma becomes the key factor in postoperative infections.

Early Local Infection

These must be dealt with aggressively, since delay in therapy will lead to exposure of graft and mandatory removal. Early therapy consists of systemic antibiotics based on a smear of aspirated material and may be modified when a culture and sensitivity is available. In addition, a subcutaneous scalp needle may be placed above the reconstruction site and an appropriate antibiotic dripped in slowly. If overwhelming or uncontrollable infection occurs, implant removal is required so dense fibrosis will be prevented. Later reinsertion of the frame may be possible.

Exposure of the Implant

This may occur for many reasons. Excess skin tension must be avoided by making the recipient graft pocket large enough so that exposure through a dehiscent suture line or over a prominent part of the implant will not occur. Postoperative trauma can be avoided with an ear guard, although late occurring trauma will give exposure in an occasional patient. Infection alone is a major cause of exposure and the steps listed above can be followed. If exposure occurs and the infectious component controlled, local advancement of skin or rotation flaps are utilized to cover the implant, and small portions of the graft can be trimmed off.

Seroma

A seroma will almost always develop, but hemovac suction should prevent these. Once the hemovac is removed late occurring seromas are treated with frequent needle aspiration.

Discussion

Silastic versus Cartilage

Silastic frameworks, although providing a uniformly reliable pinna contour to work with and although easier for the surgeon to prepare than cartilage grafts, are more likely to be exposed and subsequently removed (Table 1). Cronin[4] in 1968 reported on 19 microtic patients and 11 of traumatic origin. In the microtia patients the exposures in 3/9 occurred when no dacron mesh was used, but only 1/11 exposed silastic frames occurred if a D-116 tricot dacron mesh was sutured over the helix of the frame. Altogether five out of 30 silastic frames were removed. Later 4/4 were successfully reimplanted.

Table 1. The Incidence of Failures in Using Silicone Framework for Microtia Repair.

Silicone Ear Implants for Microtia		
	Number of Fistulae or Exposure	Number Removed
CRONIN	WITH DACRON 1/11	0
	WITHOUT DACRON 3/9	0
OHMORI	WITH DACRON 22/116	11 (9.5%)
WRAY	WITH DACRON 0	
	WITHOUT DACRON 13/16	13 (81%)

Ohmori et al[8] in 1974 reported on 116 microtia patients with a failure rate of 9.5 percent (22/116). He analyzed the rate of fistula and most occurred at the site of the incision for the rotation of the lobule (Fig. 5).

Wray and Hoopes[9] in 1973 reported that 13/16 were removed but none of these frames had a dacron mesh cover. Eleven were removed after exposure and two were removed due to infection. Exposure occurred from one week to four years postoperatively.

In my own personal series with silicone partially covered with a dacron mesh four out of seven had to be removed. We also advocate a rib cartilage graft.

In summary, no remark could be more appropriate than the one written by Dr. Tanzer,[10] "This recital of pitfalls in ear reconstruction should by no means dampen the enthusiasm of the surgeon who accepts the challenges of this intriguing facet of plastic surgery. Careful planning, strict adherence to the fundamentals of successful wound healing, close postoperative supervision, and quick, decisive action in the event of the unexpected complications are the guidelines to a satisfying and rewarding experience in the restoration of damaged or hypoplastic auricles."

References

1. Fukuda O: The microtic ear: survey of 180 cases in 10 years. Plast Reconstr Surg 53:458–463, 1974
2. Tanzer RC: Total reconstruction of the external ear. Plast Reconstr Surg 23:1, 1959
3. Tanzer RC: Total reconstruction of the auricle. Plast Reconstr Surg 47:523–533, 1971
4. Cronin T, Greenberg R, Brauer R: Follow-up study of silastic frame for reconstruction of external ear. Plast Reconstr Surg 42:522–529, 1968

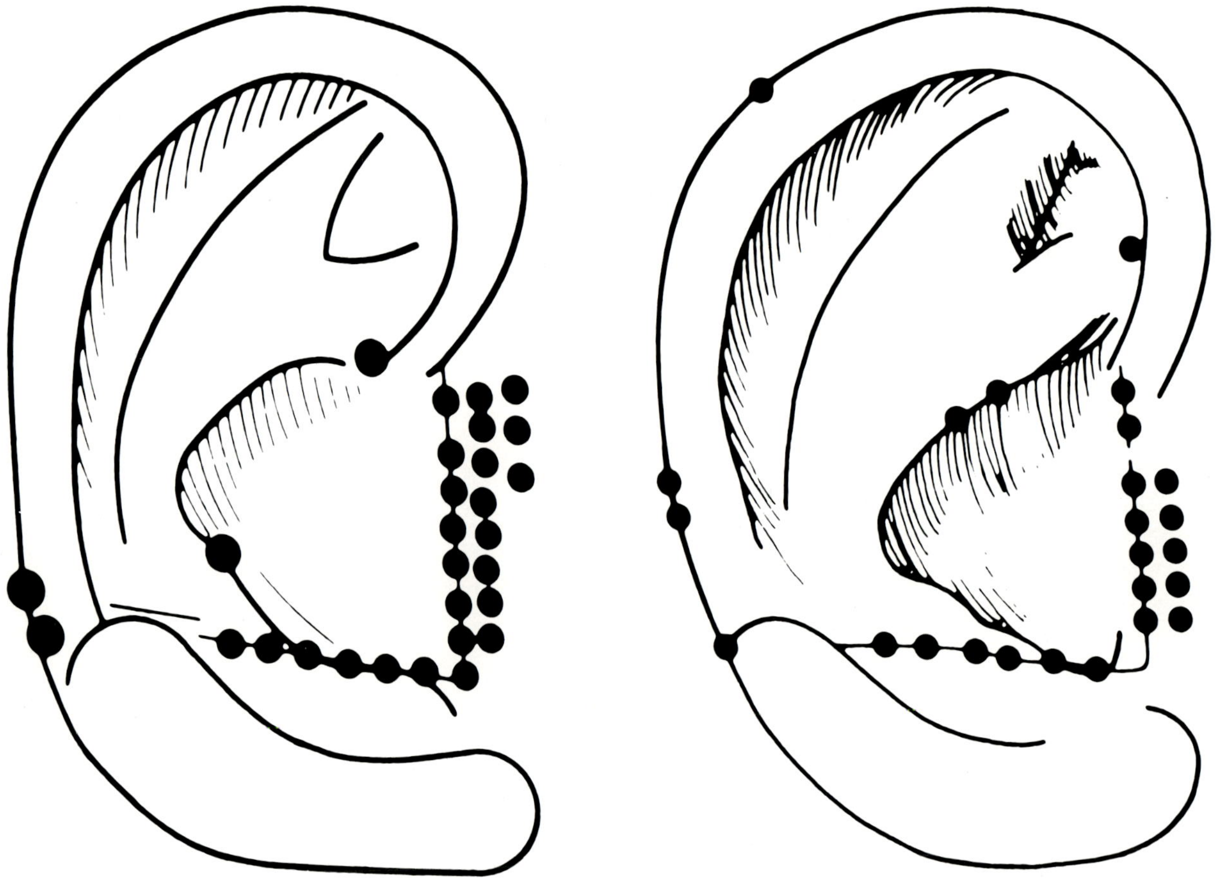

Fig. 5. Results of study by Ohmori showing (left) the location of fistulae before elevation and (right) the location of fistulae after elevation.

5. Converse JM: Construction of the auricle in unilateral congenital microtia. Trans Amer Acad Ophth Otol 72:995, 1968
6. Burdach J: Reconstruction of microtia auricle in a four-stage operation. Trans Amer Acad Ophth Otol 73:340, 1974
7. Brent B: Ear reconstruction with an expansile framework of autogenous rib cartilage. Plast Reconstr Surg 53:619–628, 1974
8. Ohmori S, Matsumoto K, Nakai H: Follow-up study on reconstruction of microtia with a silicone framework. Plast Reconstr Surg 53:555–562, 1974
9. Wray R, Hoopes J: Silastic frameworks in total reconstruction of the auricle. Brit J Plast Surg 26:296–297, 1973
10. Goldwyn R: *The unfavorable result in plastic surgery*. Little, Brown and Company Publishers, Boston, Mass, 1972, 156

Minor Surgery of the External Ear

Albert L. Roper, Norfolk, Virginia

The basic convoluted structure of the ear which presents such obstacles to otic reconstruction in cases of loss or atresia, serves conversely to hide the minor defects encountered in less extensive surgical procedures. Whereas symmetry of the nose or eyes is of paramount importance, asymmetry of the ears is seldom noted, providing relative protuberance is maintained, and the essentials of structure are present. These essentials are a full helix, or smooth helical rim, a lobule, and absence of obvious disruption of smooth lines. Fairly major differences in helical size, depth of post auricular sulcus, and inequality of antihelical folds can be accepted as long as a general "ear-like" appearance is preserved.

General Principles and Materials

Most procedures on the external ear may be accomplished under local anesthesia in a clinic or surgicentre setting.

Anesthesia is accomplished using 1 or 2 percent xylocaine with 1:100,000 epinephrine, available in 1.8 cc carpules, and administered by dental syringe with a 27 gauge needle.

Sutures are predominantly 4–0 nylon for non-visible cutaneous closures, and 5–0 nylon for visible cutaneous closures. Although silk is slightly easier to use, I feel that it is more reactive. I have used 4–0 and 5–0 mersilene for subcutaneous and cartilage sutures, however I am using more Dexon where approximation is needed without the requirement for prolonged strength (as in cartilage remoulding).

Hemostasis may be by ligature or electrocoagulation.

Bandages are avoided, but when necessary are made of moulded cotton impregnated with mineral oil and are removed in 24 hr. Ice packs are not employed.

All suture lines are meticulously cleaned with hydrogen peroxide every 4 to 6 hr, until no crusts are formed. A continuous application of neosporin or bacitracin ointment (not cream, preferably ophthalmic) is maintained until complete skin healing is attained, usually about two weeks.

Antibiotics (Penicillin, Erythromycin, or Tetracycline) are frequently administered orally for ten days.

Helical Wedges (Fig. 1)

Small lesions of the helix and antihelix, near the rim, may be removed by simple "pie-wedge" excision and primary closure. Lesions requiring larger wedges (more than one centimeter of rim removed) may require the further removal of hemi-cresents on either side of the wedge to prevent abnormal folding of the helix. Although the resultant helix is smaller, this is not usually noticeable unless one ear is quite protuberant. (One might consider otoplasty or reduction of the opposite ear if necessary.) These crescents may be well hidden in the natural contours of the ear, and are an excellent aid in preventing jagged deformities of the antihelix and crura.

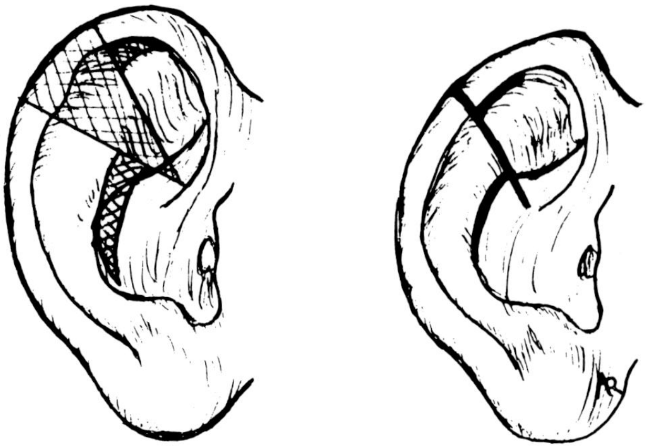

Fig. 1. Excision of full-thickness crescents adjacent to wedge resections prevent deformities of relative protuberance. The incision lines can be hidden in the conchaland antihelical folds.

Defects of the Helix

Trauma may result in loss of the helical cartilage or erosive lesions may require surgical removal. *Small* defects may be well covered by a full thickness free graft from the postauricular sulcus.

Larger defects may require a posterior advancement flap (Fig. 2). The anterior suture line should be hidden under the rim anteriorly if possible. The free end of the flap is sutured upon itself to create a delicate rim. Posterior lateral triangles may be excised in the postauricular sulcus or at the hairline to aid in advancing the flap.

Traumatic loss of the superior helix may be corrected by suturing the open defect into a periauricular pocket, and delaying the final reconstruction for six weeks (Fig. 3).

Periauricular tissues may then be employed to fashion a new helix. Small grafts of cartilage may

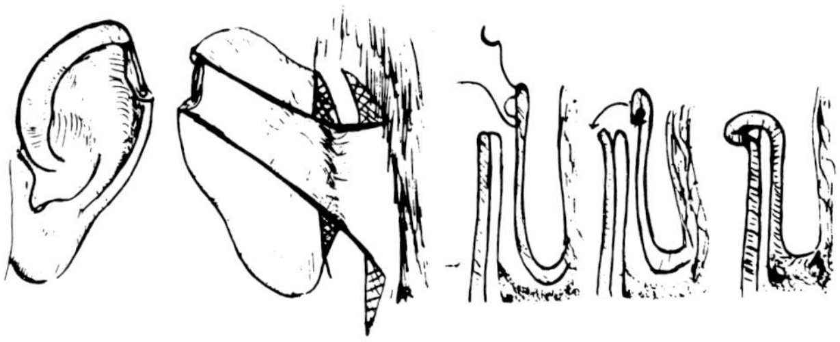

Fig. 2. Posterior Advancement. A delicate rim is formed by folding the tip of the flap onto itself, and hiding the scar under the rim.

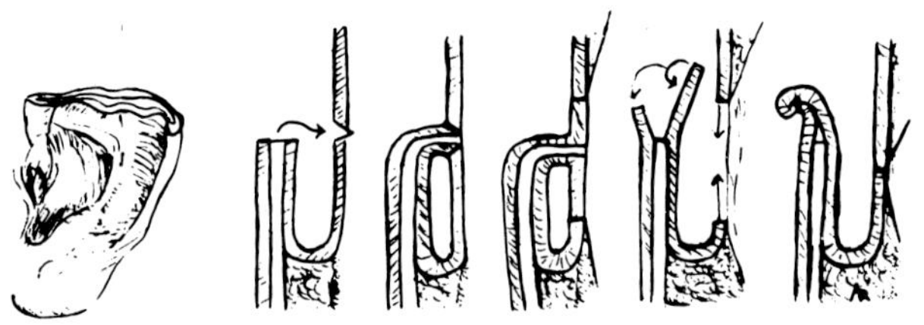

Fig. 3. Delayed reconstruction. The tissue obtained from the periauricular area may be supplemented with free cartilage slivers. Cresents (see Fig. 1) may also be removed to effect an easier closure, and as a source of cartilage. Depitiation may be required on larger flaps.

be slipped into sub-cutaneous pockets to add support.

Losses such as this are frequently infected, and may be several days old when first presented. Human bites must always be considered as infected.

Portions of the auricle, even if completely severed, should be reattached primarily when possible, and handled in the same way as a free graft. A two-layer closure of skin and cartilage is sufficient. Perichondrial sutures are seldom necessary for fragments of less than one-third of the auricle.

Tunnel Flaps (Fig. 4)

Lesions involving the skin and cartilage of the concha may be suitable for reconstruction by a tunnel flap from the postauricular area. A cutaneous strip must be removed from the flap for subcutaneous approximation of the midportion of the flap as it passes through the auricle. Manipulation of the flap is made easier if sutures are placed at the free corners, rather than the traditional skin hooks.

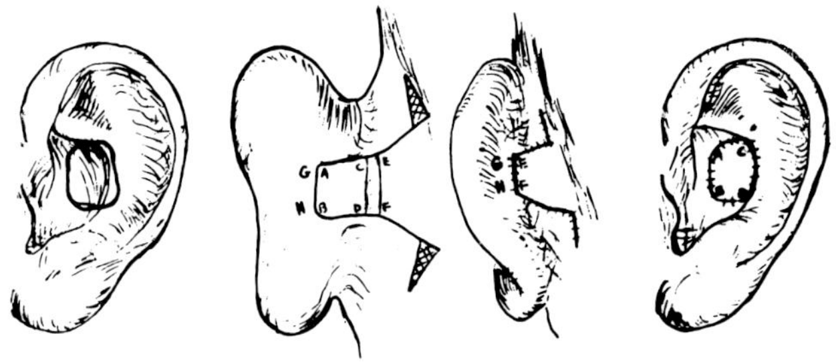

Fig. 4. Cutaneous tissue is removed CD–EF to provide a non-squamous strip as the flap passes through the auricle. Note that AB lies posteriorly on the back of the auricle, but anteriorly on the front of the auricle.

Miscellaneous

Adequate excision of lesions must never be compromised in order to effect a particular repair. The primary purpose of excising malignancies must be eradication of the disease. Incisional biopsies may be employed if the clinical appearance is questionable. Occasionally large portions of the auricle require removal. If possible enough tissue should be left to support a prosthetic auricle. If the external canal is involved, fairly extensive advancement flaps may be required for closure of the defect and maintenance of the external meatus.

Cartilaginous nodules, frequently associated with secondary pressure ulcers require only simple exposure through incisions conforming to the natural lines of the auricle. The excess cartilage may then be shaved with a fine blade, and the skin closed primarily. Microscopically these lesions show changes of chondrodermatitis nodularis chronicus helicus (Winkler's Disease).

Summary

The correction of traumatic and surgical defects of the auricle cannot be prescribed in "cookbook" terms. It is necessary for the surgeon to familiarize himself with many alternate approaches to a particular problem in order to chose one which is most applicable to a particular situation. Wedges, tunnel flaps, delayed pedicles, and advancements should make up a comfortable part of his repertoire. Basic principles of auricular surgery and technique should be familiar, as well as clinical recognition of lesions and conditions affecting the external ear.

Mandible

Cleft Lip and Palate (Panel)

Charles Krause:

There have been tremendous advances in the management of cleft lip and palate patients during the past 100 years. A multidisciplinary approach to the problem has evolved, stressing the effect of surgery upon function and facial growth in addition to the esthetic result.

Dr. Stuteville stressed the importance of a multidiscipline team approach to cleft management, including a pediatrician, social worker, speech pathologist, plastic surgeon, otolaryngologist, prosthodontist, and orthodontist. In addition to providing care for the cleft children, such a team is able to support and counsel the parents effectively. Dr. Stuteville advocated a modification of the Millard lip repair. He performs this when the child has reached 10 weeks of age, 10 g of hemoglobin and 10 pounds in weight. Palatoplasty is performed after eruption of the first deciduous molars, at 18 to 24 months of age.

Dr. Wynn discussed and illustrated his technique of lateral osteotomy cleft palate repair. By advancing each palatal shelf medially with mucoperiosteum remaining attached, he feels that retardation of maxillary growth is prevented. Incisions are made bilaterally through mucoperiosteum, beginning at the maxillary tuberosity and extending just medial to the alveolar process anteriorly. An osteotomy is made along this line through palatal bone but not the nasal mucoperiosteum. The palatal shelf with attached oral mucoperiosteum is then shifted to the midline bilaterally. The nasal cavity is not entered into as the soft tissue on the nasal side stretches over the gap produced. The margins of the cleft are incised and sutured in one layer. After utilizing this technique for about 25 years, Dr. Wynn has noted no retardation of maxillary growth directly related to the palate surgery. Any growth problems result from labial muscle action in the associated repaired cleft lip patient, or those who have had to have anterior mucoperiosteal elevation techniques for further closure. The good speech results which 92 percent of his patients achieve compare favorably with other methods, and good hearing results are also obtained.

Dr. Yules discussed the evaluation of speech in postoperative palatoplasty patients to determine which will require a secondary procedure. He utilizes two methods to ascertain the need for a secondary procedure:

(1) Air study—a respirometer is utilized to measure the amount of air leak present.
(2) Roentgenography—lateral views
  (a) at rest
  (b) phonating ("quack" or "hiss")

Based upon the findings in these studies, the following results may be anticipated:

(1) Greater than 1 cm gap on x-ray or 1800 cc air leak—results are so poor with any method of secondary correction that he recommends a dental obturator.
(2) Less than 1 cm gap and 1000 to 1800 cc air leak—would do pushback palatoplasty and superiorly based pharyngeal flap. Good speech results may be expected in 70 percent.
(3) Less than 1 cm gap and 300 to 1000 cc air leak—would do pushback and superiorly based pharyngeal flap. Good speech should be obtained in 80 percent.
(4) Less than 1 cm gap and less than 200 cc air leak—these patients will be able to learn good speech, so no surgical procedures are necessary.

Dr. Yules does not always perform an adenoidectomy prior to pharyngeal flap surgery, but many of his patients require the pharyngeal flap because an adenoidectomy was done in a patient with an unsuspected submucous cleft of the palate.

Dr. Farrior discussed surgical correction of the cleft lip nasal deformity. He stressed the importance of correcting the functional as well as esthetic deformity. The cleft lip nasal deformity remains extremely difficult to correct surgically because this embryologic abnormality includes a deficiency of mesodermal derivatives. The surgical procedure must be patterned after the needs of each individual patient since each varies considerably in the type and extent of deformity. Underdevelopment of the maxilla requires placement of onlay iliac bone grafts beneath the alar base. Both lower lateral cartilages must be delivered and their lateral crura dissected from the underlying vestibular skin. The soft tissue of the nose is dissected and shifted to a symmetrical position. The nasal septum is straightened utilizing standard techniques. The problems faced in bilateral cleft lip nasal deformity are not just doubled, but are compounded. Methods of lengthening the columella and reshaping the nose were described.

In response to a question, Dr. Farrior stated that he would in general await full facial growth before doing extensive corrective surgery on the nasal septum. He did not feel such surgery would have much effect on speech. He also pointed out that a pharyngeal flap may cover pathology developing in the nasopharynx such as chronic adenoiditis or nasopharyngeal angiofibroma.

Problem Fractures of the Mandible

Gordon W. Summers, Portland, Oreg.

The classification and management of mandibular fractures has been presented in numerous articles and textbooks. Most authors discuss the management of these facialbone injuries in rather general terms and little attention is often given to some of the specific fractures or combinations of fractures that can be difficult to treat. An in-depth analysis of certain specific situations can be quite helpful in understanding the pathophysiology of such injuries and hopefully aid in preventing undesirable long term sequallae and deformities. The purpose of this paper is to present several problem situations with suggested methods of management.

The Unstable Symphysis Fracture Combined with a Unilateral Subcondylar Fracture

The symphysis consists of the anterior region of the mandible between vertical lines passing just distal to the canine tooth of each side. Most fractures in this region are oblique and only rarely occur through the midline. Unfavorable muscular pull produces displacement of the fracture segments and separation with instability results. Since most of these fractures involve only a single fracture line, good stabilization can generally be achieved with open reduction and the application of direct interosseous wires or insertion of a metal pin. Injury or fracture in the anterior mandibular region is often associated with a subcondylar fracture on one or both sides. Intermaxillary fixation with reestablishment of preinjury occlusion generally completes the treatment in these fractures.

Extensive comminution of the symphysis into multiple small bony fragments occurs with a crushing type of injury or one of a greater degree of violence. Disruption and compounding into the oral cavity further complicates this type of fracture into one which may not be securely stabilized by open reduction and interosseous wiring techniques, intramedullary pin fixation or even metal plate fixation. Such a fracture when combined with a unilateral subcondylar fracture sets the stage for pathologic twisting or rotation of the mandibular body. The long term effect or final result may be a malocclusion which may not be obvious to the casual observer. Due to the strong unbalanced muscular forces acting on the mandibular body and the rather slow healing of the symphysis fragments, this malocclusion may even worsen for a period of time after the intermaxillary fixation is discontinued.

Report of a Case

A 17-year-old female was struck by a car while riding her bicycle. Clinical and x-ray findings revealed a 3 cm chin laceration, a severely comminuted compound symphysis fracture, loss of one mandibular incisor and near avulsion of the remaining 3 incisor teeth, and a displaced left subcondylar fracture. The remaining teeth were in good condition and her occlusion had previously been normal having completed orthodontic therapy. There were no other injuries noted. Immediate surgical repair was carried out and the symphysis fracture explored through the laceration.

Because of the comminution of most of the symphysis into multiple small bony fragments, direct interosseous wiring and the use of a Kirschner wire did not provide stability and were abandoned. The laceration was repaired, arch bars applied, the loose teeth stabilized and intermaxillary fixation instituted with a normal occlusal relationship being achieved. She was discharged four days later to be followed in the office. Normal occlusion was maintained and the intermaxillary fixation was discontinued after 5 weeks. One week later, occlusion was normal, however almost t weeks later an open bite had developed in the right bicuspid-cuspid region and the right mandibular body appeared to be rotating or "twisting" such that the lingual mandibular cusps were displaced inferiorly. Intermaxillary fixation was reapplied with a split bar on the lower arch. The open bite closed up promptly and normal occlusion was again established. Fixation was continued for an additional 5 weeks, then discontinued. The symphysis appeared to be firmly healed and her occlusion then remained stable.

The major muscular forces acting on the mandibular ramus and body are depicted in Figure 1A. With the above combination of fractures resultant

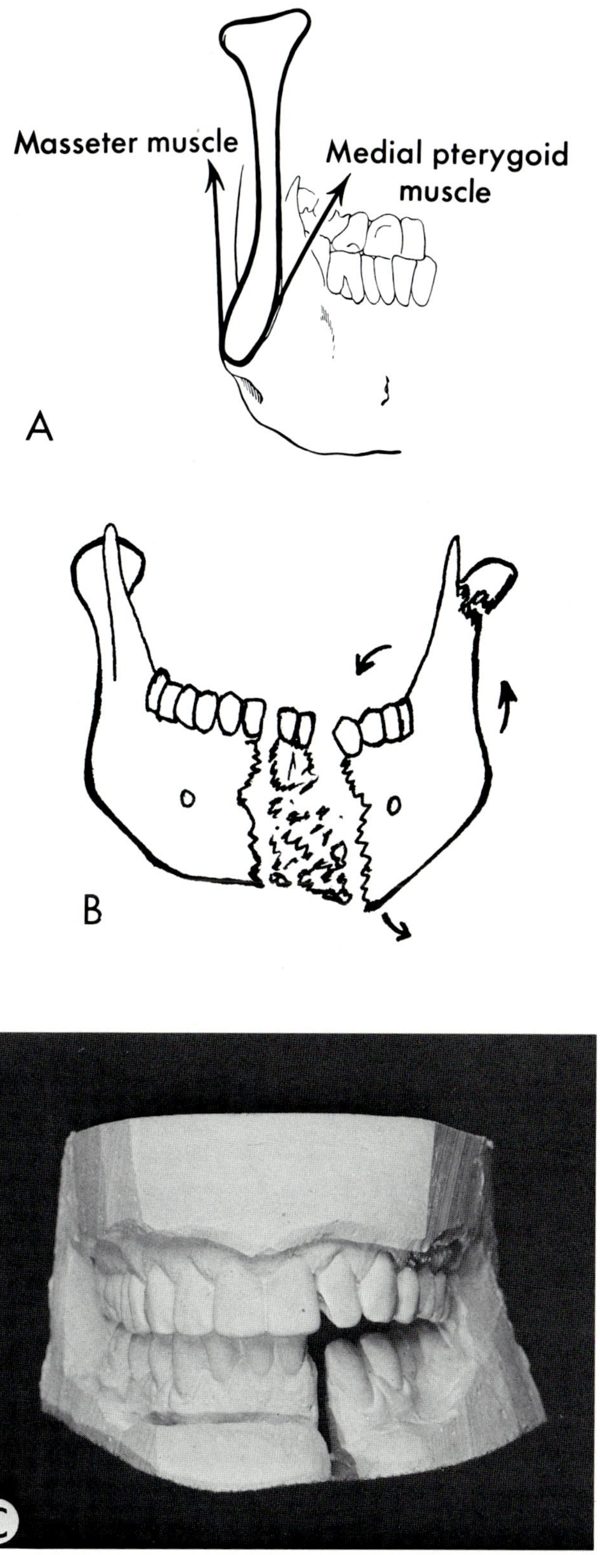

Fig. 1. (A) Major muscular forces affecting the mandibular ramus and body. (B) Rotation or twisting effect on mandibular ramus and body. (C) Models demonstrating malocclusion resulting from "twisting" of hemi-mandible.

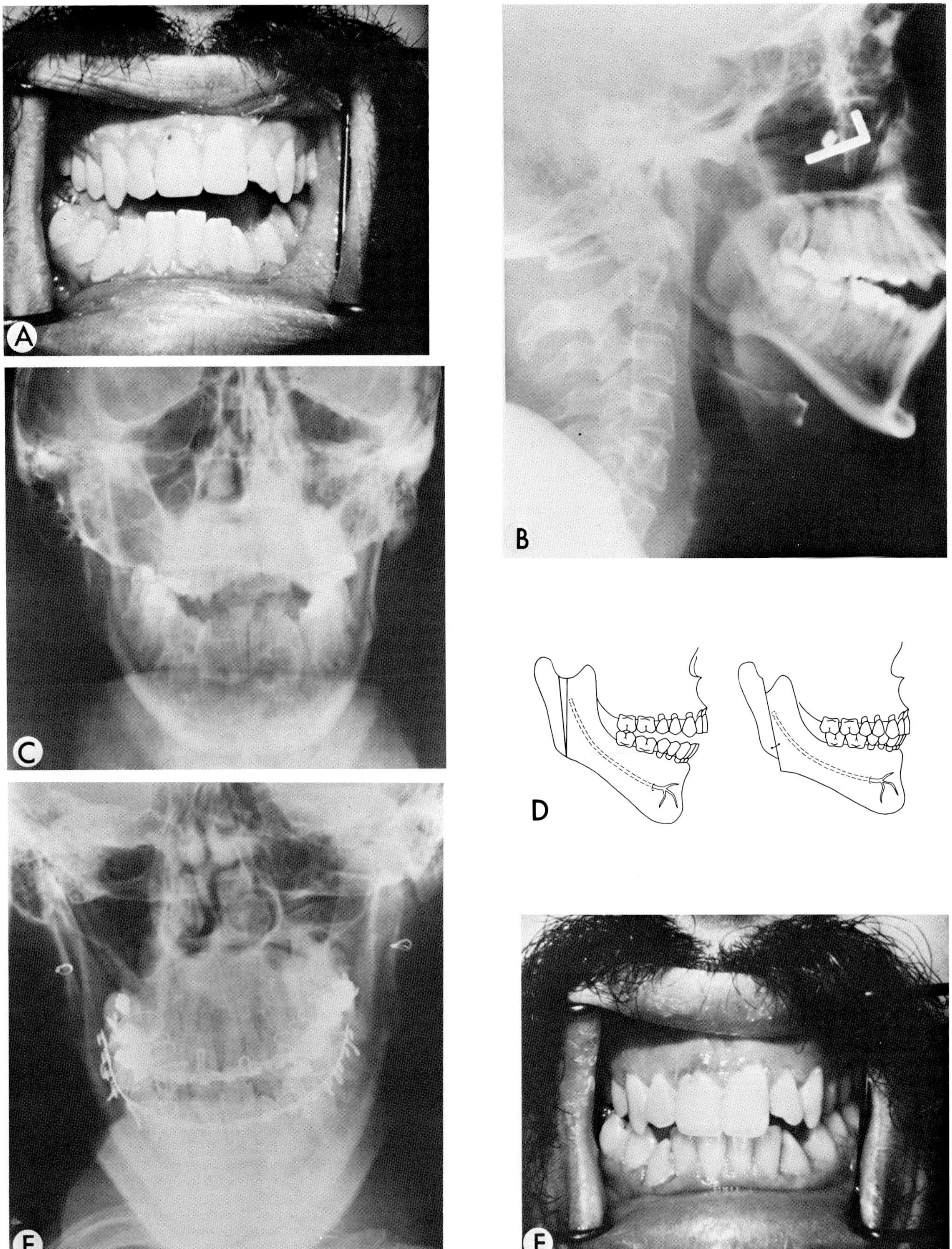
A
B
C
D
E
F

muscular forces tend to rotate or twist the mandibular fragment using the posterior molar tooth as a fulcrum. The masseter is stronger than the medial pterygoid and the mylohyoid-supra hyoid muscle pull adds further downward and rotational displacement to the mandibular body (Figure 1B). It would appear that multiple symphysis bone fragments tend to heal slowly and maximum stabilization may require a somewhat longer period of time than that usually utilized for intermaxillary fixation. Thus considerable potential for this muscular displacement may exist for several weeks after what is ordinarily considered an adequate period of fixation. If one does not observe this type of fracture patient for several weeks after the fixation is removed, a unilateral open bite malocclusion can easily develop and be overlooked (Figure 1C). Simple reapplication of intermaxillary traction may adequately correct the deformity when detected early and was effective in the patient presented. Subsequent orthodontic therapy may be necessary if this delayed malocclusion goes undetected and firm healing is established.

Alternative or additional procedures may be indicated as part of the initial treatment in a patient with this combination of fractures. Initial open reduction of the subcondylar fracture would eliminate this rotatory effect exerted by the strong masseter muscle and thus prevent the delayed malocclusion. However, it is generally recognized that most subcondylar fractures are quite adequately treated in a conservative manner. Fabrication of a cast metal or acrylic appliance applied either as a lingual or occlusal splint with circumferential wires would also help stabilize the severely comminuted symphysis. Perhaps more important is the recognition that such a potential for a delayed malocclusion exists in patients with this combination of fractures. Only with careful observation and management, can superior results be achieved in reestablishing the patients normal preinjury occlusion.

Unrecognized Bilateral Condylar Process Fractures

The region of the condylar process includes the neck or subcondylar area and the articular head or condyle of the mandible. The majority of fractures in this region are satisfactorily managed by conservative closed reduction techniques. Bilateral displaced condylar process fractures produce a characteristic anterior open bite deformity due to unbalanced muscular forces. Occasionally such fractures may go unrecognized and an undesirable occlusal dysfunction results. The delayed correction of this deformity depends somewhat on the period of delay involved, precise level of the fractures, status of fracture healing and degree of displacement of the fragments.

Report of a Case

A 27-year-old male was admitted following a motor vehicle accident with multiple injuries including a head injury, rib and chest contusions and fractures of the left hip, femur and tibia. Emergency reduction and stabilization of the lower extremity fractures was carried out and the patient was kept in the intensive care unit for about 11 days. The patient was critically ill during this period with complications including fat embolization, respiratory distress with hypoxia, acute psychosis and disorientation. His condition improved somewhat and by the 13th day of hospitalization, definitive left hip surgery was carried out. His mental status continued to improve and about 6 weeks after admission he complained that he could not occlude his teeth, or chew normally. He was seen in consultation and an anterior open bite deformity, shift to the right with opening, and reduced lateral movements were noted. Occlusal contact was present only on the posterior molar teeth (Figure 2A).

Fig. 2. (A) Anterior open bite deformity from untreated bilateral condylar process fractures. (B) Lateral radiograph of anterior open bite deformity. (C) Radiograph of anterior open bite deformity. (D) Vertical osteotomy technique to close anterior open bite deformity. (E) Postoperative radiograph after correction of open bite deformity. (F) Postoperative occlusion.

Optimum radiographic studies were difficult because of the patients complicated traction devices, however bilateral high intracapsular fractures with overriding of the fragments were demonstrated (Figure 2B, C).

The patient was taken to surgery where jaw motion and function was assessed under general nasal endotracheal anesthesia. The fractures appeared to be firmly fixed in the foreshortened position. Through bilateral submandibular incisions, both mandibular rami were exposed and vertical osteotomies made from the sigmoid notch to the angle on each side (Figure 2D). This allowed the distal mandible to rotate closing the anterior open bite and reestablishing a satisfactory occlusal position. Each ramus was stabilized in the new position with direct interosseous wiring and arch bars with intermaxillary fixation were placed (Figure 2E). Fixation was removed after 7 weeks. Followup exam at 6 months revealed maintainance of satisfactory occlusal relationship with good mandibular function (Figure 2F).

Condylar process fractures occur at several levels ranging from the base of the condylar process at or below the level of the sigmoid notch to high fractures through the condyle completely within the joint capsule. Intracapsular fractures or those above the level of the insertion of the lateral pterygoid muscle usually do not result in much displacement. Fractures below the insertion of the lateral pterygoid muscle usually exhibit medial and downward displacement of the condylar fragment due to the pull of this muscle. In bilateral fractures the fragments overlap and premature contact occurs on the posterior teeth. This characteristic anterior open bite deformity is the result of the strong masseter-medial pterygoid contraction with upward displacement of the ramus.

Unrecognised bilateral condylar process fractures diagnosed within the early stages of bone healing can be treated satisfactorily with intermaxillary traction which should realign the fragments in most instances. This should always be tried perhaps even up to several weeks post injury. If a normal preinjury occlusion cannot be reestablished, then other surgical procedures are necessary.

Attempted reopening of high subcondylar fractures or condylar fractures within the joint capsule would appear to promote excessive scarring and eventual undesirable limitation of temporomandibular joint motion. Even condylar process fractures treated conservatively will occasionally have late ankylosis and restricted motion as a final result. Low subcondylar fractures through the base of the condylar process could certainly be approached surgically and reopened without undue risk of subsequent joint ankylosis.

Bilateral condylar process fractures that have healed in the malaligned position then will require a surgical position to realign the mandible for satisfactory occlusion and function. Resection of both condyles and substitution of autogenous bone grafts or alloplastic implants is a possible method of treatment but would seem to be less desirable than osteotomies to realign the mandible.

Bilateral osteotomies in the body of the mandible will close the anterior open bite deformity and is a well recognized method of repositioning the anterior mandible. Vertical osteotomies in the ramus, commonly employed in the treatment of prognathic mandible deformities, were used in this patient. Vertical osteotomies are easily performed, well stablized with direct interosseious wires, and heal well. In this patient with high condylar process fractures that were firmly healed, the mandibular repositioning resulted in satisfactory occlusion without further compromising temporomandibular joint function.

Several alternative methods of treating delayed bilateral condylar process fractures have been discussed. Vertical osteotomies in the mandibular ramus can be sound effective method depending on the circumstances of the specific case.

Total TM Joint Reconstruction (Following Resection of Rhabdomyosarcoma of the Ear)[†]

John Kelly, Lennard T. Swanson, and
Burton F. Jaffe, Boston, Mass.

Introduction

The case presented here is unique in that the patient required reconstruction of the entire temporomandibular joint. The clinical situation dictating removal of the entire joint complex will be presented as well as the technique for total TMJ reconstruction which has not been described previously. Both the glenoid fossa and the proximal mandible were synthetically reconstructed, and the functional and cosmetic results were good.

Case Report

M. D. was a $4\frac{1}{2}$-year-old female with a two week.history of a right earache. One week prior to admission a mass in the ear canal was biopsied and revealed an embryonal rhabdomyosarcoma. On 6/30/70 she was admitted to the Children's Hospital Medical Center for evaluation. A red, friable, granular tumor was filling the right ear canal. No neck masses were palpated. The rest of the physical examination including cranial nerves and cerebellar testing was normal. Tomography and arteriography revealed that the tumor was localized to the temporal bone. Radiation theraphy (6000R) and a course of chemotherapy including vincristine and actinomycin D were given. Five months after initial therapy the tumor was again seen in the ear canal. At this time she heard a soft to moderate whisper in the right ear, the Rinne was negative, and the Weber was referred to the right ear. On 1/19/71 a biopsy revealed rhabdomyosarcoma and exploration of the middle ear revealed bony erosion anteriorly in the mesotympanum and erosion inferiorly in the hypotympanum. En bloc resection was considered to encircle the area involved. On 1/29/71 an en bloc resection of the total temporal bone, TM joint and ascending mandible and pterygoid muscles was performed (Fig. 1). She developed a CSF leak that was repaired on 2/5/71. Two weeks

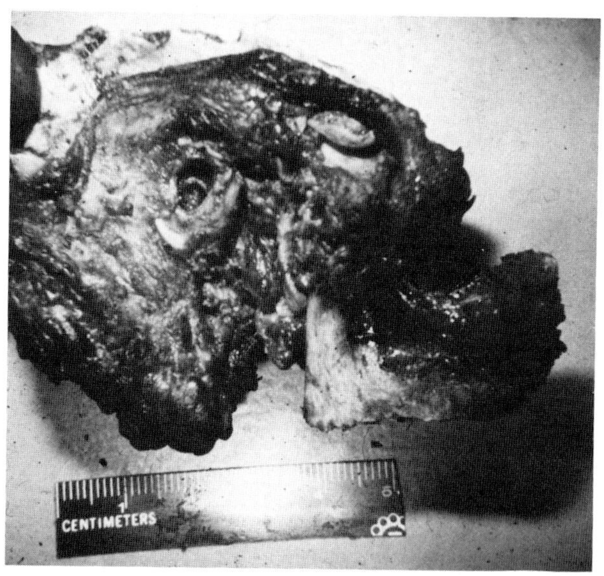

Fig. 1. Photograph of en-bloc resected specimen revealing ascending mandible, TM joint, and temporal bone with the external canal in the center.

[†] We wish to thank Leslie Silverstein (572 Pleasant Street, Brockton) for allowing us to present his patient. We wish to acknowledge the Jimmy Fund Staff, especially Norman Jaffe, for their excellent therapeutic and supportive care given to the patient. We also want to express our appreciation to John Shillito, neurosurgeon, for participating in the intracranial surgery, and for his advice in the postoperative care.

post operatively she was well healed and discharged home (Fig. 2). In May 1972 she fell while playing and suffered a puncture wound in the right preauricular area very close to unprotected dura. She was admitted and observed but no meningitis or CSF leak occurred. This wound healed uneventfully, but led to the decision that cranioplasty for protection of the dura should now be undertaken in an active child. It was also decided to reconstruct the mandicular condyle and glenoid fossa at the same time in order to intercept further dental malocclusion and to achieve partial cosmetic correction of the depression along the right side of her face. She entered the hospital in July 1972 without any evidence of local or metastatic tumor 24 months after the initial diagnosis and 18 months after her major temporal bone resection.

Design of Total TM Joint Prosthesis

The prosthesis had to include a replacement for the ascending mandible, the condyle of the mandible, and the glenoid fossa of the temporal bone. Since all of the temporal bone had been removed it was also necessary to consider this unit as attaching in some way to the cranioplasty designed to protect her posterior and middle cranial fossa.

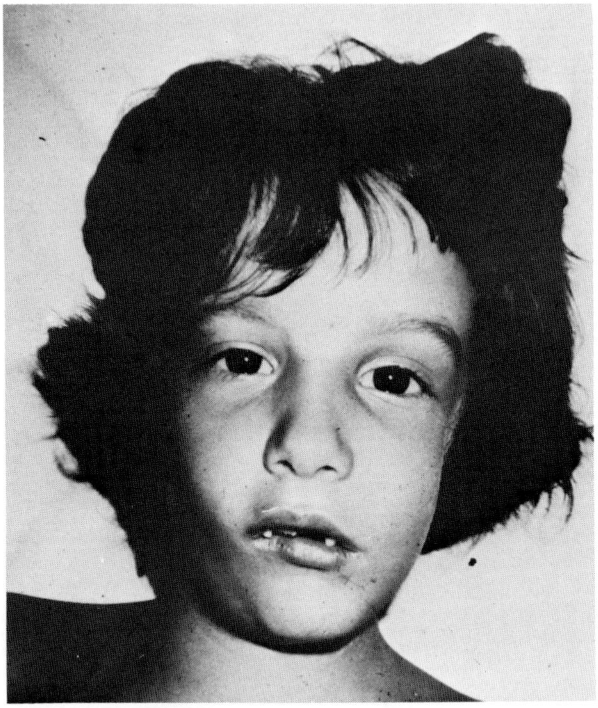

Fig. 2. Post operative right temporal bone, TM joint and ascending ramus resection revealing asymmetry of face.

To provide these functional components two units were necessary—a *silastic mandible* for the condyle and an *acrylic cap* to fit over the condyle to serve as a *glenoid fossa* (Fig. 3). This allowed for the multiplicity of motions characteristic of the TM joint.

The silastic mandibular prosthesis[1] was fabricated preoperatively based on radiographic measurements and checked against the patient for three dimensional contour. Preoperative radiographs showed absence of the right temporal bone and ascending ramus of the mandible. The condyle but no coronoid process was included in the prosthesis. A groove was made in the horizontal portion of the silastic mandible to accept the lower border of the existing mandibular body to facilitate fixation.

The *glenoid fossa* was made by placing uncured acrylic into a small glass cup. As the acrylic became pasty, the silastic condylar portion of the prosthesis was pushed into the paste and moved through the range of motion that was appropriate to simulate the normal range of motion of the functioning condyle. After the acrylic was hardened, it was possible to rotate the condyle 90° and pop it both in and out of the acrylic cap. The "pop-out," "pop-in" articular fossa was designed to allow for reinsertion of a longer silastic mandible (but with a

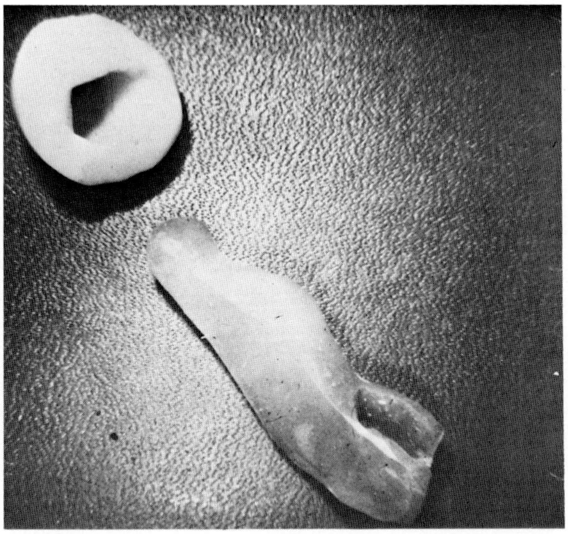

Fig. 3. This shows the two components of the totally reconstructed TM joint—the acrylic "glenoid fossa" cap and the silastic mandible with condyle.

similar sized "condyle") when increased mandibular length would be required based on the continued growth of the uninvolved side. A duplicate second acrylic cap was made to serve as a future template for this purpose. It was anticipated that on two occasions in the future a longer silastic mandible would be needed to provide symmetry.

Operation

The original preauricular incision was utilized to gain access to the proximal end of the mandible and to the temporal area. After identification of the middle and posterior cranial fossa dura and the surrounding bony landmarks, a doughy mixture of self-curing methylmethacrylate (Simplex P. Howmedica) was molded in place to the desired contour. After the material had undergone the initial setting reaction it was removed from the temporal area and allowed to complete its exothermic curing reaction outside the operative field.[2,3] Then the acrylic temporal cranioplasty was trimmed, smoothed, and a niche was drilled out for the second prosthesis. This temporal acrylic prosthesis was fixed in place by means of interosseous wires to the frontal, parietal, and occipital bones. A smaller amount of acrylic was molded by the head of the silastic condyle to form a "glenoid fossa" as previously described. The silastic prosthesis was then secured to the mandible with two laterally placed Vitallium screws and a circumandibular wire, made necessary when a short inferior screw could not be placed adequately. Finally, with the patient's teeth held in occlusion, the acrylic glenoid fossa was placed over the silastic condyle and both rested in the previously planned niche in the temporal acrylic (Fig. 4). While held in the desired position, the two acrylic pieces were luted together with a fresh mix of acrylic (Fig. 5). Tissues were then closed in layers and dead space was avoided. Meticulous control of bleeding was maintained and no drains were used. The postoperative period was uneventful. Her cosmetic result was satisfactory (Fig. 6). The stability of the silastic to mandible fixation was adequate as determined by palpation. She ate food on the second postoperative day and went home on the sixth postoperative day.

TM Joint Function

Preoperatively she was able to bring her teeth into proper occlusion, but the jaw deviated sharply

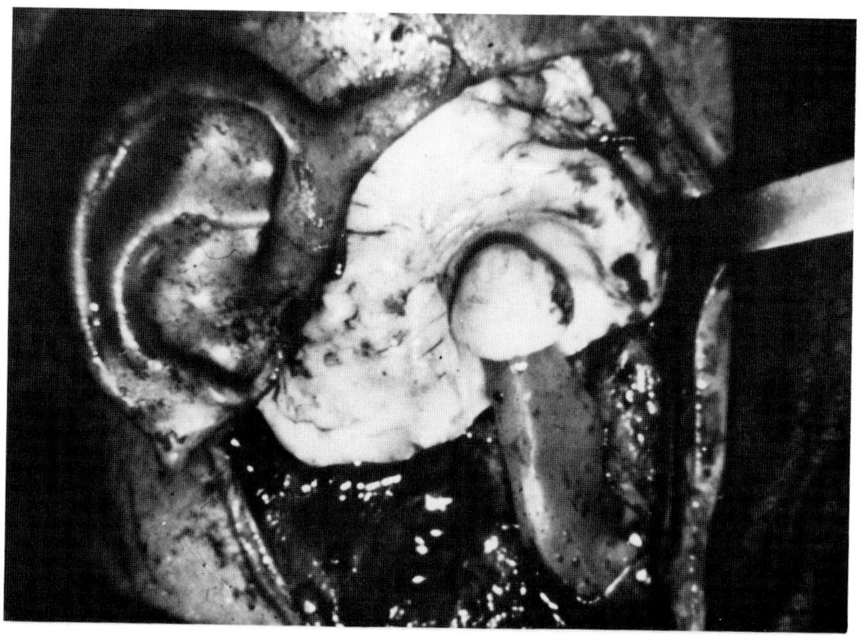

Fig. 4. Intra-operative photograph shows the acrylic temporal prosthesis with a groove for the "TM joint," the acrylic cap, and the silastic mandible already screwed and wired to the horizontal body of the mandible.

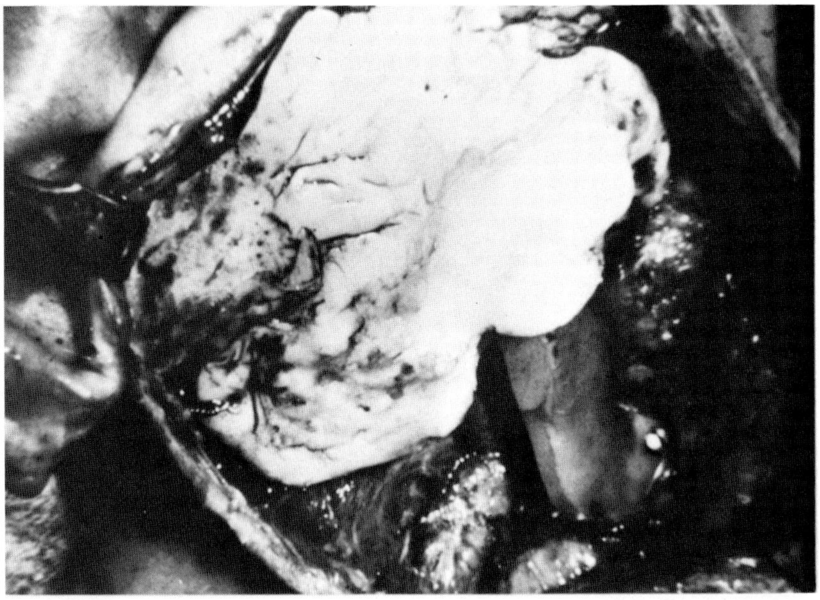

Fig. 5. Intra-operative photograph after cranioplasty and acrylic cap were luted together with a fresh mix of acrylic.

to the right on opening because of the unopposed action of the left external pterygoid muscle. In the early postoperative time her mandible deviated slightly to the right on opening, but her occlusion and range of motion were good.

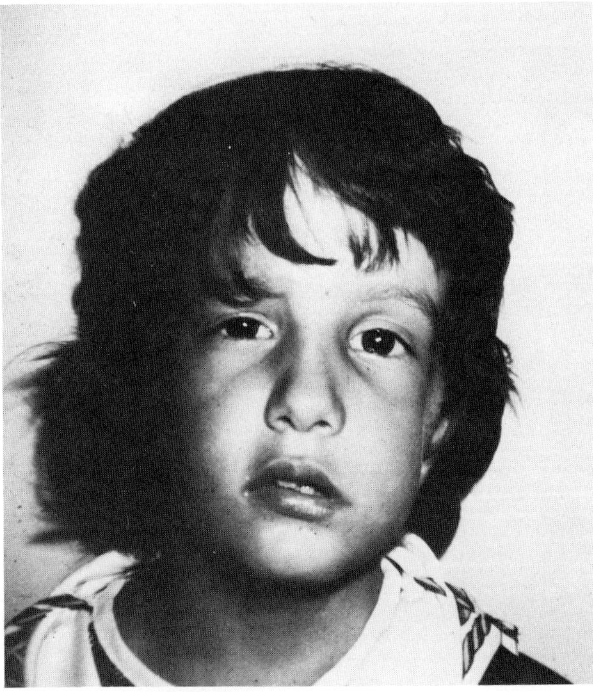

Fig. 6. Excellent facial cosmetic result following reconstruction of mandible and TM joint.

When evaluated two weeks later, her mandibular function was good with minimal deviation on opening; the wound was well healed.

Discussion

The primary objective in this reconstruction effort was the protection of the dura and cranial contents in the area of the previous temporal bone resection. The use of acrylic for cranioplasty is well documented[4] and even recommended in preference to bone in most situations.[5]

A secondary goal in this procedure was the reconstitution of the contour and function of the temporomandibular joint and the mandible. In a patient of this age, a graft with potential for growth would have been most desirable, but in the absence of a temporal bone and zygomatic arch, the use of metatarsal,[6] rib,[7] or sternoclavicular[8–10] grafts were not possible. Furthermore, the viability of the homologous sternoclavicular joint graft depends on revascularization via attachment of the external pterygoid muscle to the joint capsule,[10] but this muscle was also absent in this case. Hence, a biologically inert material was selected as the replacement for the mandible. The acrylic condyle of Hahn and Corgill[11] was not used because of the probable abrasive action between such an acrylic condyle and the acrylic temporal prosthesis, leading either to direct failure or to indirect failure secondary to tissue reaction to minute abraded fragments of acrylic.[2] A silastic mandible implant articulated with an acrylic glenoid fossa seemed to offer the most favorable solution in terms of their compatibility with the tissues and with each other. In addition, any necessary adjustments in the size or shape of the silastic prosthesis could be readily made at the time of operation.

This reconstruction procedure achieved both of these stated goals; namely, protection of the dura, and functioning and cosmetic reconstruction of the mandible and temporomandibular joint.

In July 1973 recurrent tumor developed in the right temporal area. The entire prosthetic device (cranioplasty and TMJ and mandible) was removed and cryosurgery was performed to destroy the tumor. The patient did well for about one year when another recurrence occurred and this was again treated with cryosurgery. In December 1974 she died of intracranial spread of tumor. This has been the ultimate fate of almost all children with rhabdomyosarcoma of the middle ear.[12]

It had been anticipated that at least two additional grafts to the mandible would have been necessary to keep up with the continued growth of the unaffected left side of her mandible. One such replacement would have been made at the conclusion of her adolescent growth spurt and another would have been performed after condylar growth had ceased. A duplicate of the acrylic cap and silastic prosthesis was retained so that future replacements could have been precisely fitted to the already constructed acrylic glenoid fossa.

Summary

The reconstruction of the temporal bone and glenoid fossa with methylmethacrylate and the reconstruction of an articulating mandibular ramus and condyle with silastic in a 6½-year-old girl is described. The procedure was undertaken 18 months after resection of these structures for treatment of embryonal rhabdomyosarcoma of the middle ear. In summary, this operation achieved protective, functional, and aesthetic restoration. The design of the total TMJ prosthesis allowed for future reconstructive changes to harmonize with the anticipated growth of the opposite mandible. The TMJ functioned well for one year until removal and the child subsequently died 4½ years after original diagnosis.

References

1. Leake D, Murray J, Hakal M, Swanson L: Custom fabrication for mandibular reconstruction. Oral Surg, Oral Medicine, Oral Path 33:879, June, 1972
2. Bloch B, Hastings GW: Plastics in Surgery, Thomas Publishing Company, Springfield, MA, 1962
3. Dowson D, Wright V: Lubrication, friction and wear of total hip replacements, in Total Hip Replacement, Jayson, M., Ed., Philadelphia, J. P. Lippincott Company, 1971
4. Woolf JI, Walker AE: Cranioplasty. International Abstracts of Surgery. 81:1, 1945
5. Leivy DM, Tovi D: Autogenous bone cranioplasty. Acta Chir Scand 136:385, 1970
6. Dingman RO, Grabb WC: Reconstruction of both mandibular condyles with metatarsal bone grafts. Plast Reconstr Surg 34:441, 1964
7. Robinson M: Congenital absence of the ramus of the mandible. J Oral Surg 28:302, 1970
8. Snyder CC, Levine GA, Dingman DL: Trial of a sternoclavicular whole joint graft as a substitute for the temporomandibular joint. Plast Reconstr Surg 48:447, 1971
9. McDowell F, Ohlwiler D: Mandibular resection and replacement. Int Abstr Surg 115:103, 1962
10. Hunsuck EE: Autogenous grafts for replacing temporomandibular joints and mandibular condyles in Rhesus monkeys. J Oral Surg 27:167, 1969
11. Hahn GW, Corgill DA: Surgical implant replacement of the fractured displaced mandibular condyle. J Oral Surg 28:898, 1970
12. Jaffe BF, Fox J, Batsakis J: Rhabdomyosarcoma of the middle ear and mastoid. Cancer 27:29, 1971

Dental Occlusion and Arch Relationship in Segmental Resection of the Mandible

Mohamed A. Aramany and Eugene N. Myers, Pittsburg, Pa.

Radical surgery for cancer of the oral cavity frequently requires resection involving the mandible, floor of the mouth, tongue, and soft palate. This extensive loss of tissues often impairs the related functions. Patients following these surgical procedures have problems with mastication, deglutition, and speech, compounded in some instances, with drooling. Mandibular deviation due to loss of structure, scarring and altered muscle function results in facial asymmetry and malocclusion. This prevents the patient from ever chewing normally.

Normal occlusion where the posterior natural teeth interdigitate is lost and the teeth on the remaining segment occlude lingual to the maxillary teeth. In the edentulous patient, the residual ridge on the unoperated side deviates medially and superiorly. This situation is awkward for the construction of dentures and frustrates the efforts for maxillofacial rehabilitation.[1-3]

Definition

Although there is an effort in the literature[1] to classify mandibular resection, we have found that the most important factor to be considered is whether the continuity of the mandible is preserved or not. Marginal resection denotes the loss of alveolar bone sparing the inferior border whereas the term segmental resection refers to the loss of continuity of the body or the ramus. Marginal resection does not result in malocclusion.

The best method of rehabilitation is to restore the continuity of the mandible either by autogenous bone graft or alloplastic material which will facilitate the intraoral prosthetic reconstruction.[4] This effort as a primary reconstructive effort at the time of surgery is frequently unsuccessful due to contamination by saliva with infection or poor healing in radiated tissues.

Functional Impairment

Impairment of function in patients undergoing mandibulectomy varies in degree depending upon the extent of the surgical resection, structures involved, rehabilitative procedures and the mental attitude of the patient and his (or her) capability to adjust and cooperate in the rehabilitative process.

The speech problem may be related to a soft palate defect, scarring of oral structures and restriction of tongue mobility. This will affect the various valving mechanisms essential for both articulation and voice quality. Mastication and deglutition are impaired as a result of alteration in temporo-mandibular joint function and disruption of the neuromuscular system which controls the masticatory apparatus. Restricted tongue motility, difficulty in swallowing, absence of the vestibular sulcus, scarring or paralysis of the lower lip as well as loss of sensory awareness impairs the patients ability to control salivary secretion which leads to drooling. The prosthetic rehabilitation is complicated by loss of part of the denture bearing areas, mandibular deviation, and loss of occlusal contact with the opposing teeth.

Rationale

One of the vexing problems during intraoral prosthetic restoration for patients who have had mandibulectomy is the establishment of the mandibular position in relation to the maxillary arch. The mandible tends to deviate medially and superiorly to a greater degree in the edentulous patient where a segment of the mandible is resected and the defect is not restored than in a patient who undergoes the same procedure but who still has posterior teeth in good occlusion. It is generally accepted that there are fewer problems with rehabilitation of partially edentulous patients than with those who are completely edentulous.

Preservation of the presurgical alignment of the remaining mandibular structure is a logical goal toward facilitating the rehabilitation of mandibulectomy patients, especially those who are edentulous. The Head and Neck Team of the Department of Otolaryngology, University of Pittsburgh, embarked on a project to reduce the degree of deviation in both the dentulous and edentulous patients by immediate immobilization of the mandible after segmental resection of the mandible.

The patients are seen by the Maxillofacial Prosthetic Center before the surgery. Records are obtained for each patient including dental casts and jaw relation records where the mandible is related to the maxillary cast in normal relationship before the surgery. For the dentulous patients, the interdigitation of the teeth was accepted as centric position. In the edentulous patients, the patient's dentures were used as a base for the construction of modified Gunning splints.[5] In the edentulous patients who are not using dentures, a modified complete denture technique was used to construct the splints. In the latter group it was expected that more problems will be encountered after surgery, if the reason for not using dentures previously was the patient's attitude toward the dentures.

Surgical Procedure

The patients included in this original group are homogeneous only in that each one had cancer, and resections were carried out for the purpose of irradicating this disease. The lesions included in the treatment of this group were those primarily in the retromolar trigone, the posterior aspect of the lower gum, and in the posterior aspect of the oral tongue and tonsil area. These included both squamous cell carcinomas and mucoepidermoid carcinoma.

There were two patients in this group who had previously received a full course of radiation therapy. These were failures at radiation therapy, and local resection was carried out to resect residual disease. These patients were both treated by upper neck dissection, partial mandibulectomy, and rehabilitation of the resected site with a split-thickness skin graft. There were no difficulties with healing in these patients.

The remainder of the group of patients were those who were treated by primary surgery. Some of these patients had resection of their primary tumors and segmental mandibulectomy in continuity with radical neck dissections. There were several patients treated primarily who had localized resections with upper neck dissections, but not radical neck dissections.

Three patients in this group were treated by primary split-thickness skin graft; two of them were radiated patients. Approximately half of the remaining patients in this group had reconstruction with deltopectoral flap to rehabilitate the resected area. The remainder of the patients had primary closure of the resected site just utilizing local tissues. No forehead flaps, tongue flaps or intentional oral stomas were utilized in this group of patients.

Review of Cases

To illustrate the procedures used for treatment of these patients, two patients were selected and the procedure described in detail. The first patient is an edentulous patient, and the second patient is partially edentulous.

Patient No. 1

A 57-year-old patient was referred to our service with squamous cell carcinoma of the left alveolar ridge. The patient was seen by the surgeon and the prosthodontist, and the procedure of fixation and surgery was planned. The patient's history revealed that he had lost all his teeth fifteen years ago and had dentures made but was never able to get used to them. This indicated that the patient would be difficult as far as adaptation to the mandibular resection appliance is concerned after the completion of the treatment. The procedure was explained to the patient, and the need for his cooperation to adjust to his prosthesis was stressed.

The dental records were made and impressions were made of the maxillary and mandibular arches. The patient's dentures were not available so we proceeded, while the patient was still in the hospital, to mount the casts in their proper relationship. The relationship was made in wax rims and these wax rims were transformed into modified Gunning Splints (Figs. 1–3). A tracheotomy was carried out under local anesthesia and general anesthesthesia induced. A curved incision over the upper neck was carried out anteriorly, and the lower lip split in the midline. A segment of mandible was resected from the mental foramen to a point just inferior to the mandibular condyle. Following an upper neck dissection, the primary tumor was removed along with a portion of buccal mucosa, retromolar trigone, soft palate tonsil and the segment of mandible. A split thickness skin graft was used to dress the defect and was maintained in position using a bolus of Xeroform gauze and tie over silk sutures. The remainder of the wound was closed in layers and a cuffed tracheotomy tube inserted; the maxillary splint was fixed by suspension to the zygomatic arch and wiring to the nasal spine, and the mandible splint by circumferential wiring (Fig. 4). A small gap in the splints was left in the anterior region to facilitate feeding. Ten days later the intermaxillary wiring was opened and the packing was removed

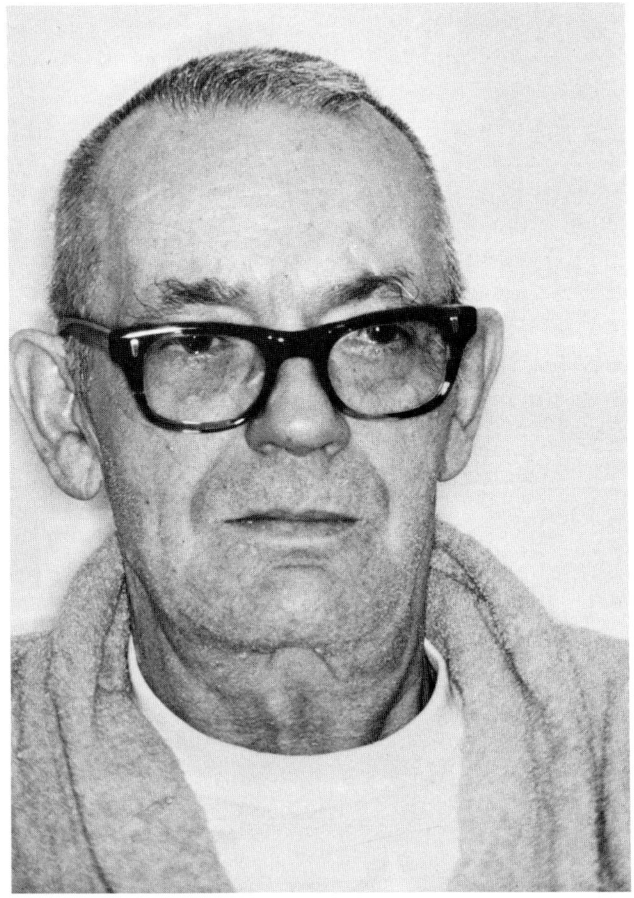

Fig. 1. Face view before surgery.

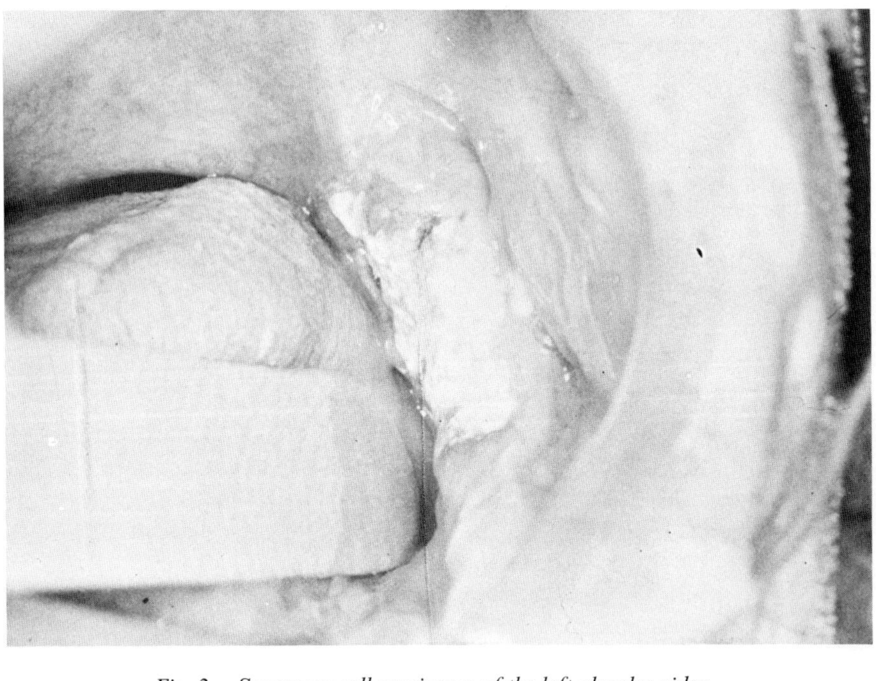

Fig. 2. Squamous cell carcinoma of the left alveolar ridge.

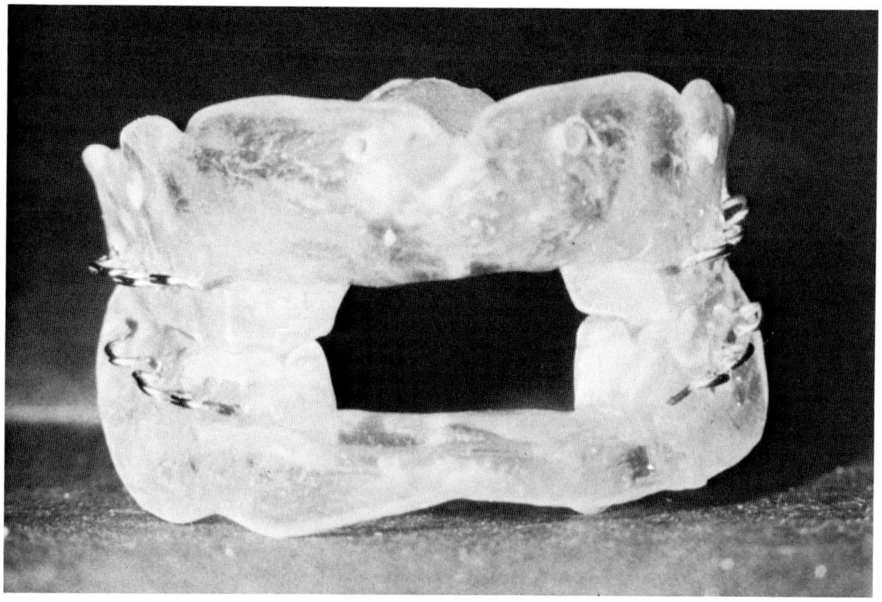

Fig. 3. Modified Gunning Splints completed before surgery.

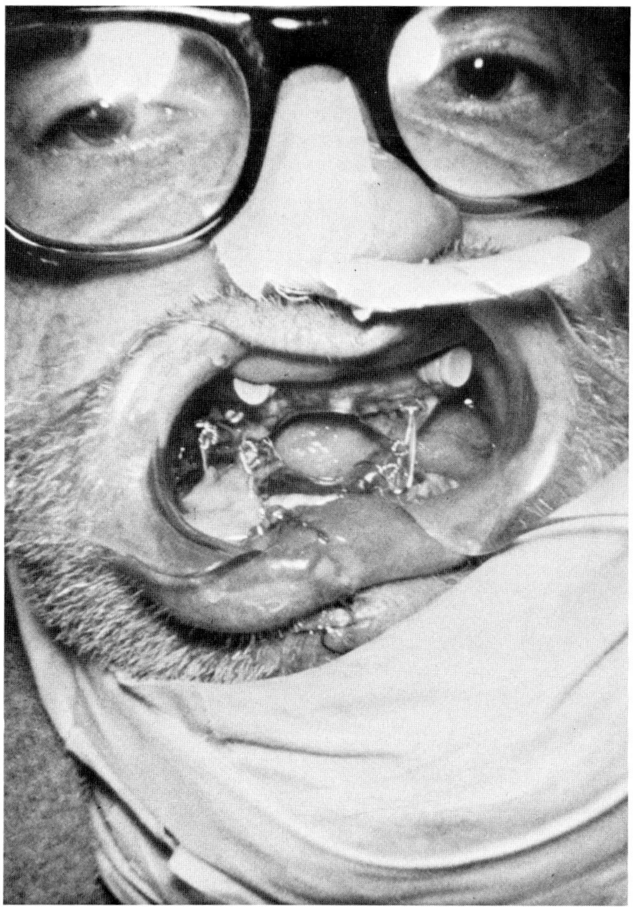

Fig. 4. Mandibular resection completed, surgical splint wired and intermaxillary wiring.

and then the patient was rewired again for an additional four weeks. The patient complained at the time of problems associated with intermaxillary fixation, and we decided at that time to open the intermaxillary wiring and leave the splints in place so they could guide the mandibular fragments into occlusion (Figs. 5–7). Two weeks later (seven weeks since the splints were made) the splints were removed and they were relined with the temporary relining material and reinserted for the patient to use and maintain the memory of the original position. The splints were utilized as a guide to construct complete upper and a section of the lower denture using the same occlusal relationship that was obtained before surgery (Fig. 8). The patient could get into occlusion although he started from a deviated position in the wide open position (Fig. 9). After the first six months, we noticed that the mandible deviated slightly to the extent that the patient could not get the teeth into occlusion. A ramp was then constructed on the maxillary denture on the normal side. This helped in starting the occlusion from this deviated position so that as he reached the final closure the teeth come into occlusion (Figs. 10–12).

Patient No. 2

A 51-year-old male had a mucoepidermoid carcinoma of the lower gum on the left side. The

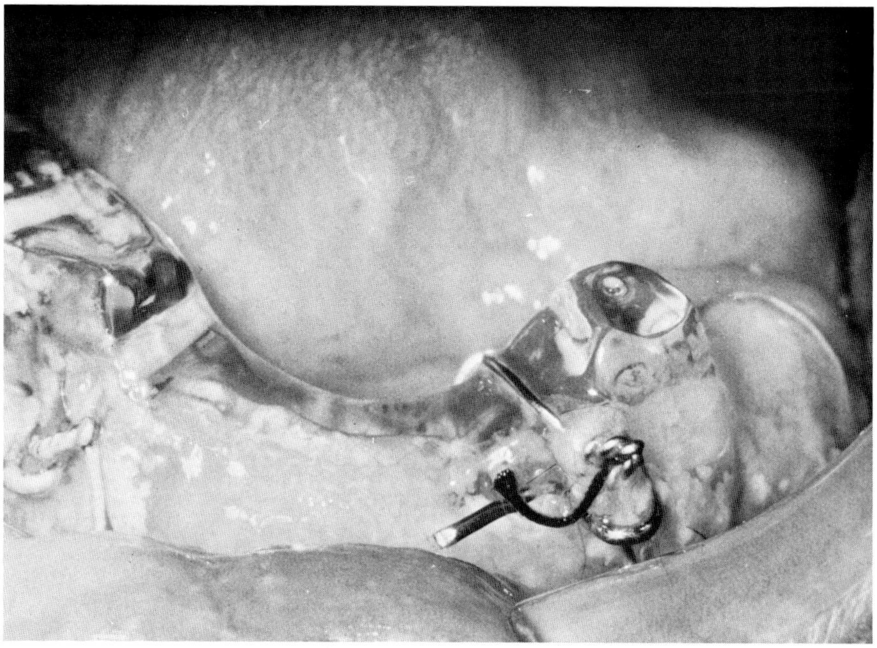

Fig. 5. The intermaxillary wiring was removed 5 weeks after surgery and splints left wired in position for 2 weeks so the patient could identify centric position.

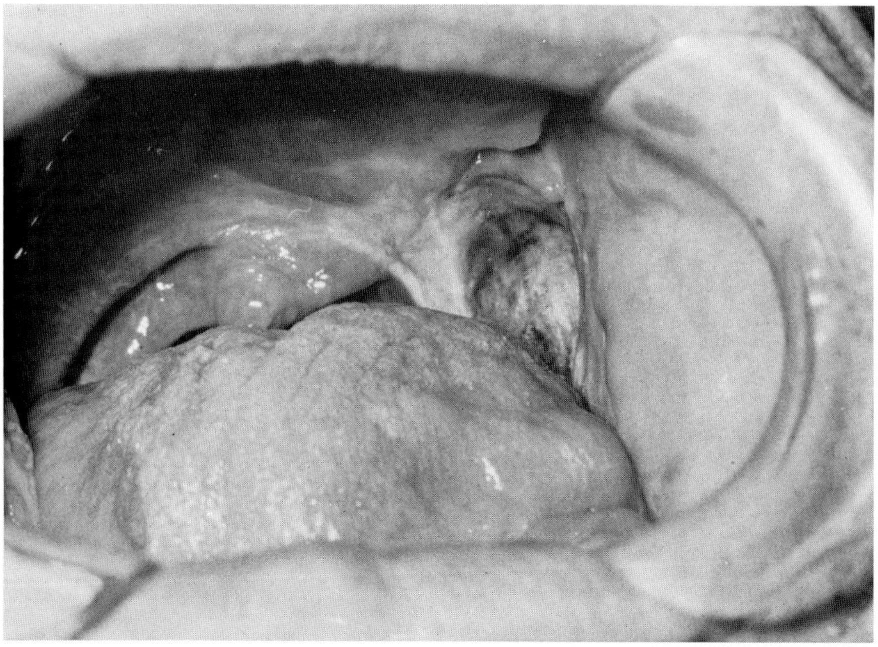

Fig. 6. Splints removed 7 weeks after surgery. Splints were relined and inserted as a temporary prosthesis during fabrication of dentures. Note skin graft rehabilitating area of surgical resection.

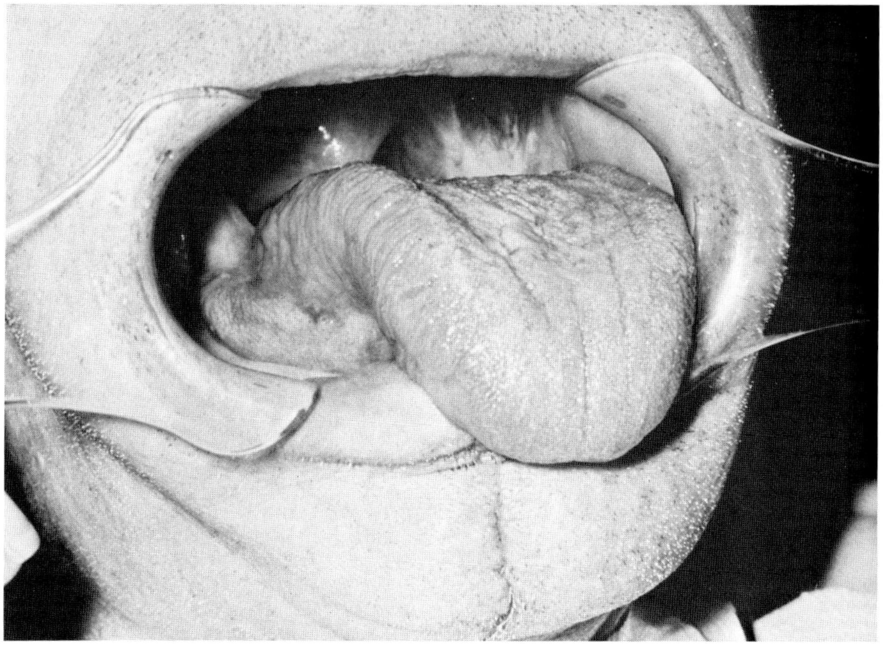

Fig. 7. Patient maintained full range of tonnage movements after surgery.

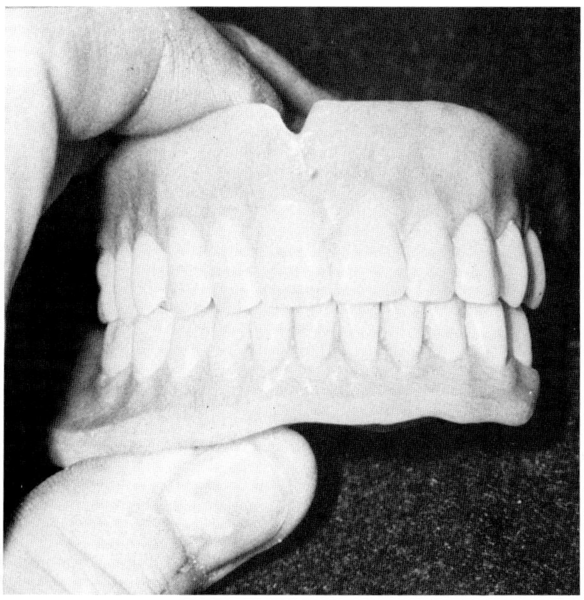

Fig. 8. The dentures were constructed duplicating the centric relationship the patient had before surgery.

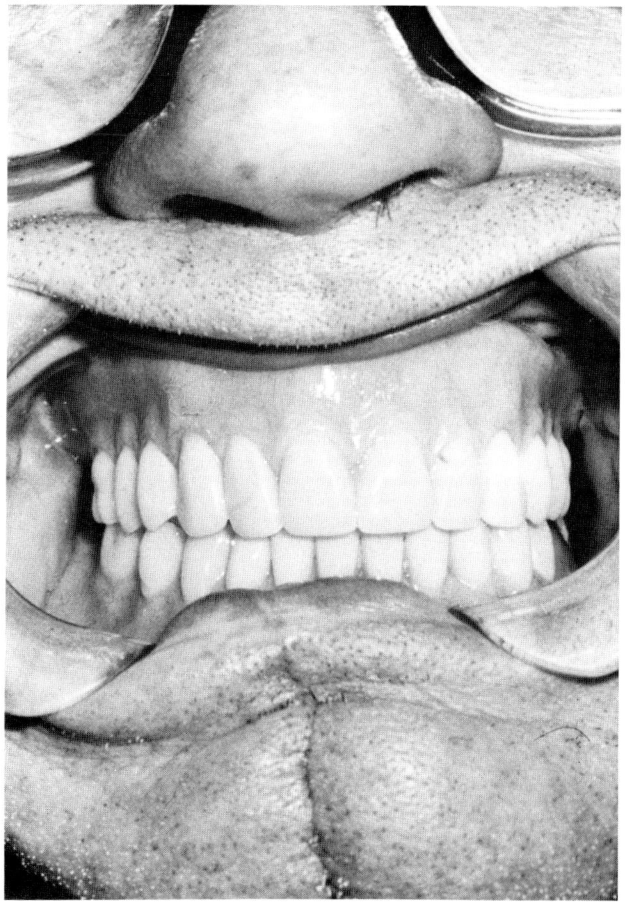

Fig. 9. The patient closing in centric position with no difficulty.

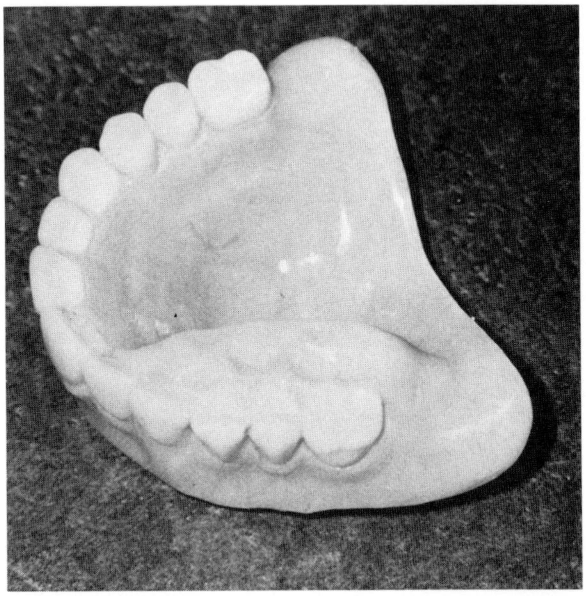

Fig. 10. One year later a ramp was added to maxillary denture to overcome slight mandibular deviation.

patient was seen before surgery (Figs. 13–15) for records and dental impressions. A unilateral mandibular splint to restore the missing lower teeth and arch band were used over the natural maxillary teeth. Surgery on December 16, 1974, included tracheotomy, left upper neck dissection, partial mandibulectomy, and excision of lower gum and tonsil. The area of resection was dressed with a split-thickness skin graft. Before the patient left the operating room, the mandibular surgical splint was wired in place, and elastic was used for intermaxillary fixation (Figs. 16–18).

The patient was readmitted on December 12, 1974, and the wiring was removed. The mandibular splint was used by the patient without wiring. Clasp retention was effective. The patient was able to close in centric position (Figs. 19–21). The patient was instructed to use his mandibular partial denture one month later (Fig. 22). At that time he still closed in centric position with conscious effort. Slight deviation was noted on a follow-up visit and a guiding plane was used by the patient for five weeks (Figs. 23–25) after which the centric position was reestablished and the patient started using his original denture. He is using his original denture without the guiding plane at present.

Discussion

The Maxillofacial Department has seen forty patients with mandibular resection over the past two years. The surgical interventions in this population varied greatly, and were carried out by different surgeons. A variety of surgical reconstructive procedures were used. We noticed in our series that the degree of mandibular deviation was greater

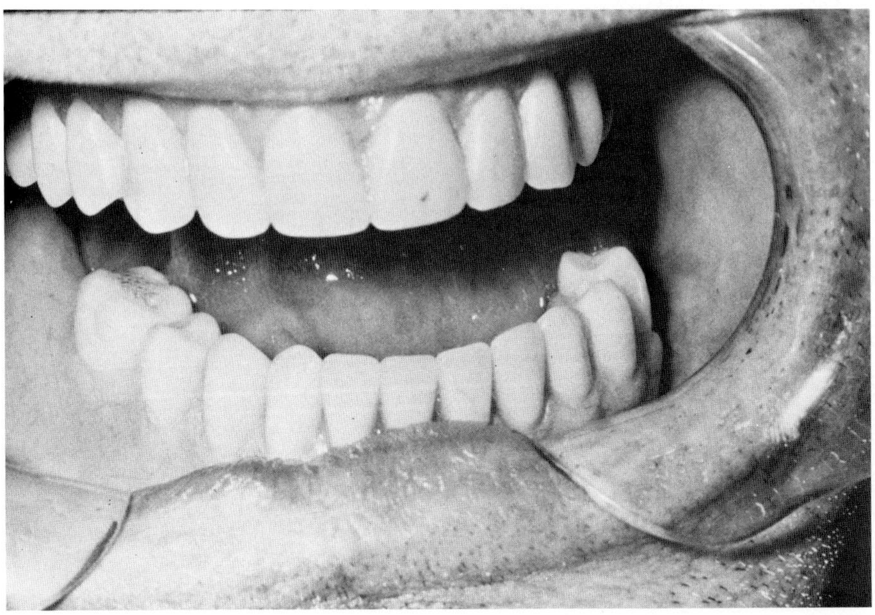

Fig. 11. The patient in open position with the modified denture in place.

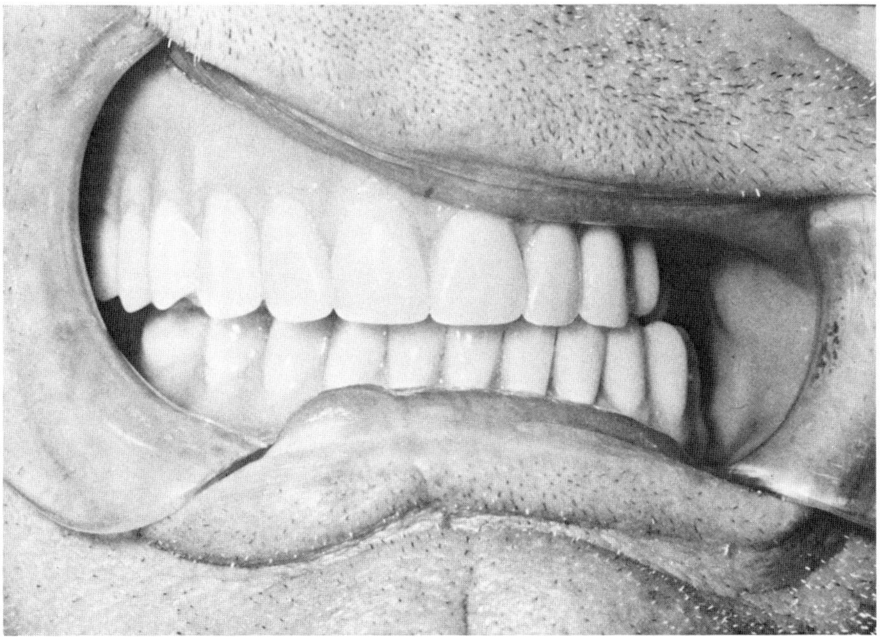

Fig. 12. Initial tooth contact in deviated position before patient gets into terminal occlusion. When he is in the terminal centric position the dentures interdigitate as in Figure 9.

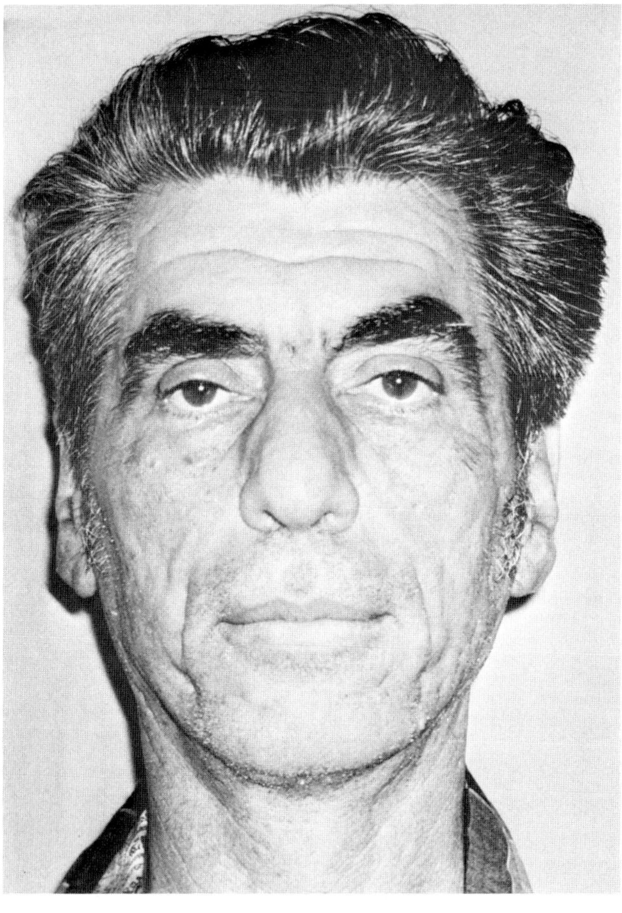

Fig. 13. Face view before surgery.

in the edentulous population than in the partially edentulous patients. The reason for this may be due to the effect of the intercuspation of the remaining dentition which reinforces the memory of the mandibular position through the proprioceptive nerve endings in the periodontal membrane of these teeth.

We found in our experience in treating the edentulous patients that the construction of dentures for this group is very difficult. We felt that this was due to the deviation of the remaining mandible. The greater the deviation the more difficult the prosthetic rehabilitation becomes. A protocol for immobilization of the remaining mandibular segment resulted from these observations and was instituted both for the edentulous and for partially edentulous patients.

Over the past 15 months, twelve patients came under this protocol; seven were completely edentulous and five were partially edentulous. The immobilization of the mandible was maintained for a period of five to seven weeks. The intermaxillary wiring or elastics were then removed and the patient was encouraged to use the splints for an additional two weeks to keep the same relationship. The splints were removed after the two weeks and they were relined with a temporary resilient material. The patient wore these while the definitive prosthesis was constructed. The packing was removed in those patients requiring skin grafts within

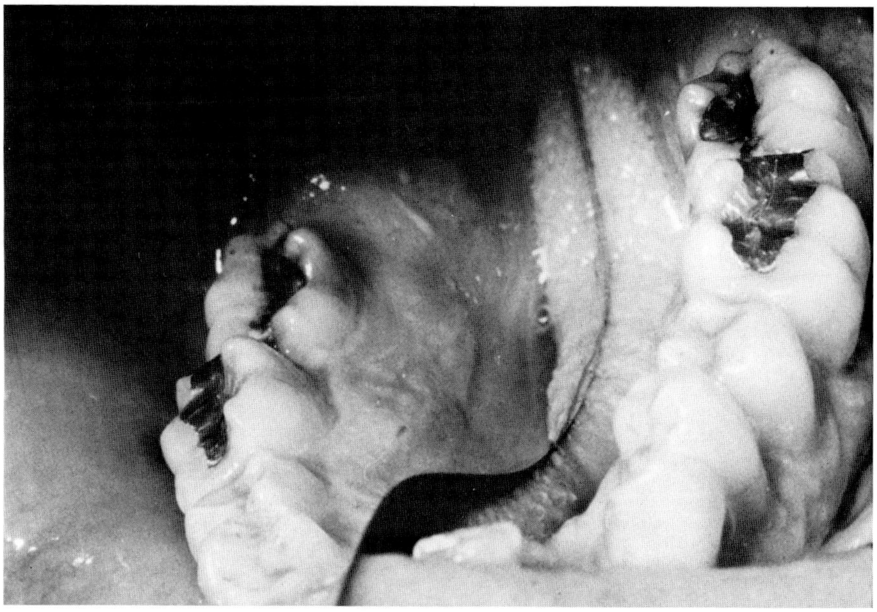

Fig. 14. Mucoepidermoid carcinoma of the left alveolar ridge.

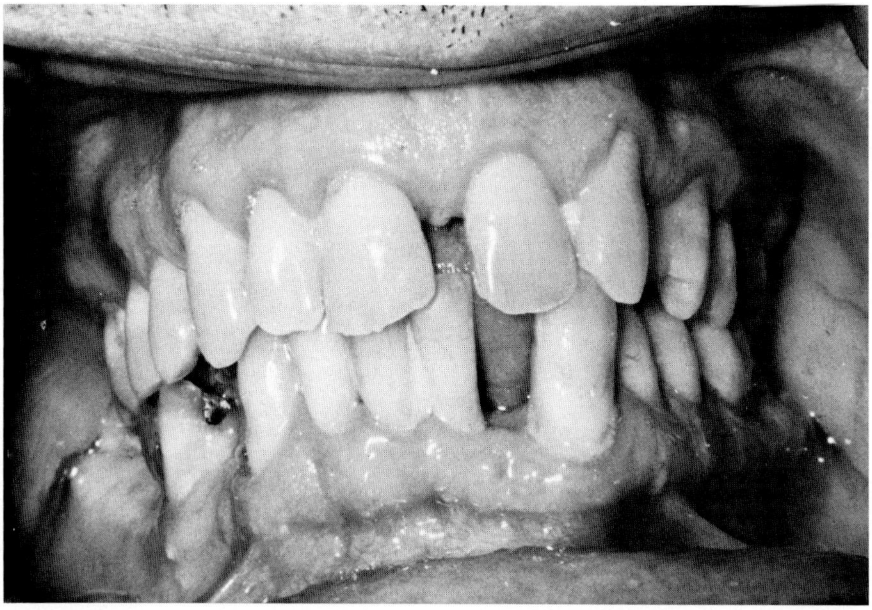

Fig. 15. Centric occlusion of teeth before surgery.

ten days after the surgery by removing the intermaxillary wiring or elastics and then rewiring the splints.

Our immediate reaction and observation reinforced the contention that the degree of deviation observed over this period was much less than the deviation observed in the patient who never had wiring. All of these patients maintained the same centric relationship of the remaining dentition or the original dentures after the treatment. Two of the edentulous patients could not maintain the exact relationship, and a ramp was constructed on the maxillary denture to guide the mandible into position. The patient can function with this denture (Fig. 10). Among the five partially edentulous patients who went through the protocol, one showed deviation. We then incorporated guiding ramp onto the mandibular denture to maintain the intercuspal relationship. The patient, after using the guiding plane for a period of time, was able to utilize

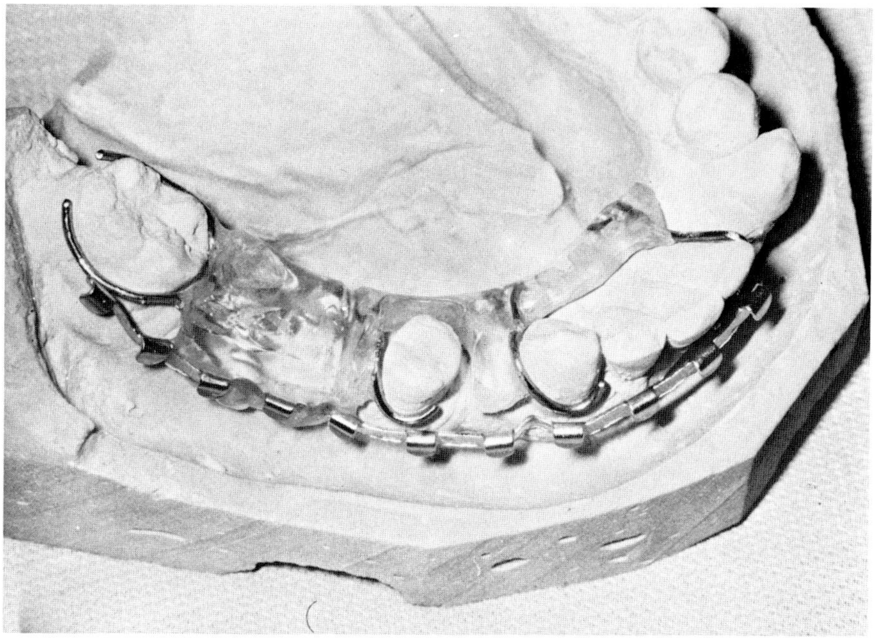

Fig. 16. Partial mandibular splint on lower cast. Note clasps to be used for retention after removal of wiring.

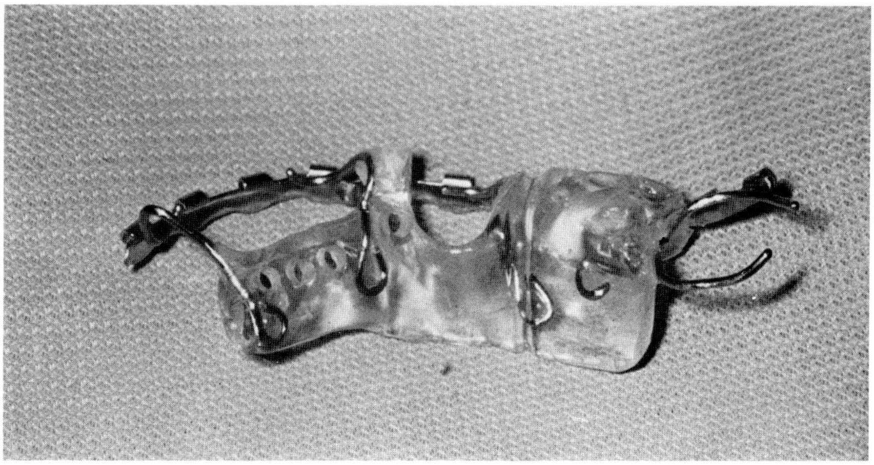

Fig. 17. Mandibular splint ready for fixation. Note holes drilled for wires to pass through.

his original partial denture without the guiding plane.

Our philosophy now in treating patients following mandibular resection in the completely edentulous patient is to wire them immediately after surgery and maintain the fixation for a period of six weeks, then encourage the patient to use the mandible immediately afterwards with a temporary prosthesis until the definitive prosthesis is constructed. If the patient can maintain the original relationship, artificial teeth 33° cusp high are utilized, so that the patient can identify the position. If the patient deviates off the centric relation, we use flat plane teeth with a guiding ramp so that the patient can have a starting contact point and then he can slide into centric.

The partially edentulous patients are treated with intermaxillary wiring utilizing arch bars and elastics or wires. This is instituted immediately after the surgery, and the patient is encouraged to use his natural dentition immediately after the wiring is removed. If we notice any deviation in the original position, we insert a guiding plane until the patient can return back to the intercuspal posi-

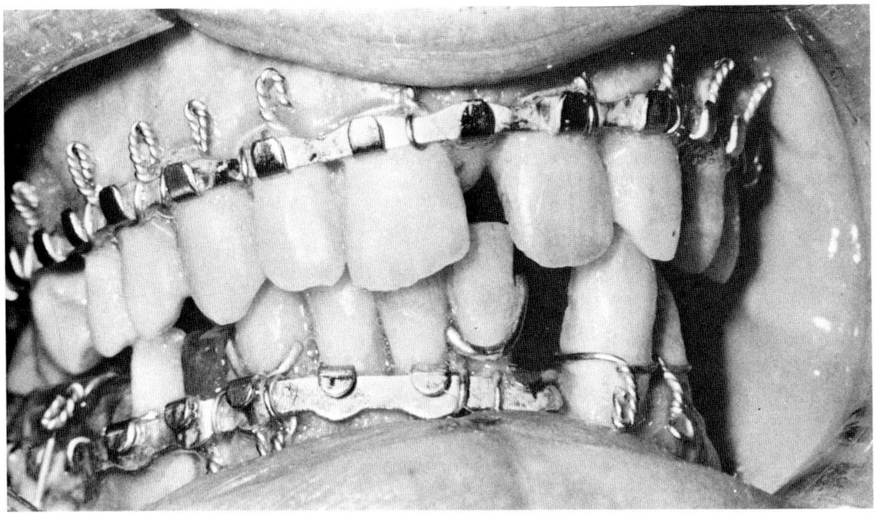

Fig. 18. Arch band wired to maxillary teeth and the circumferential wiring of mandibular splint completed. Elastic bands were used for intermaxillary fixation.

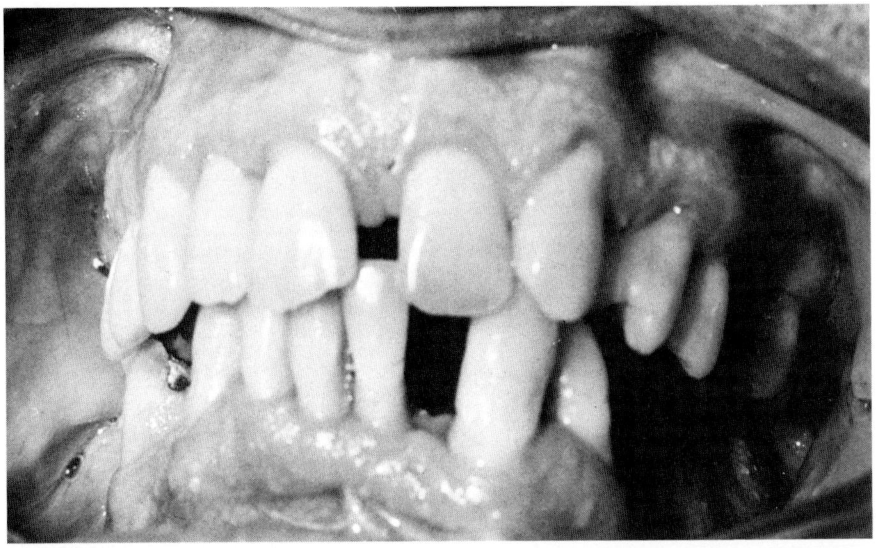

Fig. 19. The wiring was removed 6 weeks after surgery, and the patient could bring teeth into intercuspal position with ease.

tion. The guiding plane may be used after a period of a few months if we notice the same deviation to reoccur.

The intermaxillary wiring helped to alleviate the problem of deviation to a great extent. We do not feel, however, that this is the ideal type of rehabilitation of these patients, and we maintain that restoring the continuity of the mandible is the best form of treatment when possible.

Summary

This report concerns twelve patients who were treated with immediate intermaxillary fixation after segmental resection of the mandible to irradicate cancerous lesions. Mandibular resection usually produces problems in surgical and prosthetic reconstruction. The idea of using intermaxillary fixation during the first six weeks postsurgically is to reduce

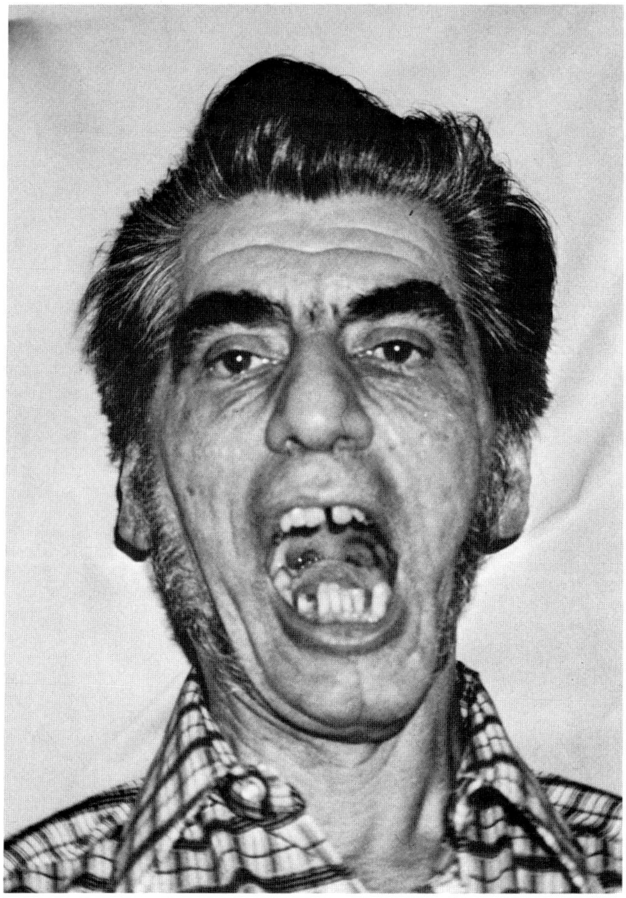

Fig. 20. On extreme opening of the mandible, deviation is noted.

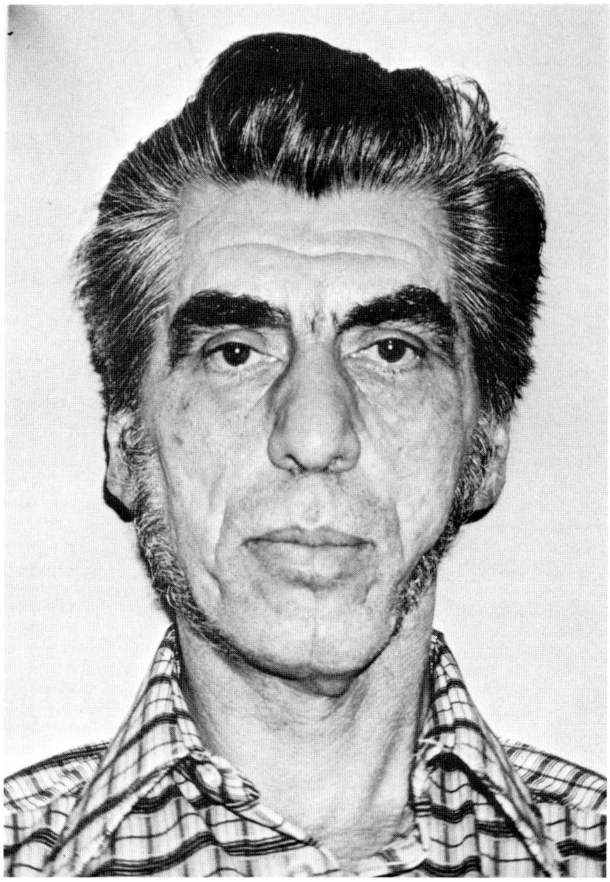

Fig. 21. In closed position, facial symmetry is obtained.

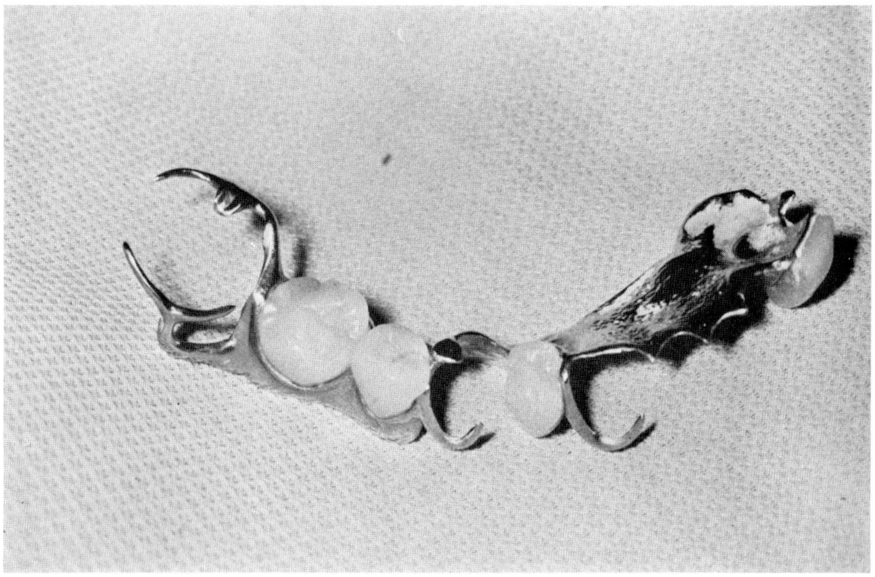

Fig. 22. The partial denture the patient used before surgery was used one month later with no alteration.

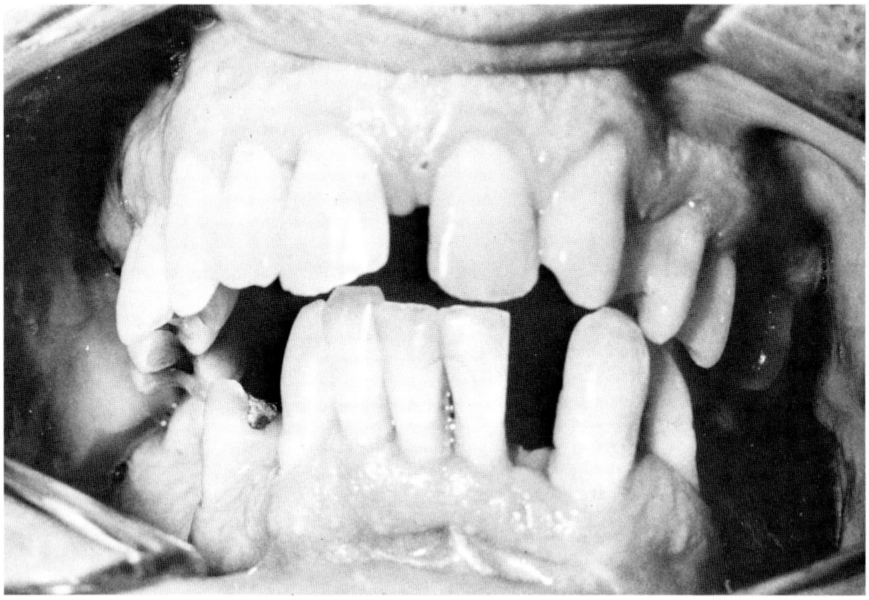

Fig. 23. Deviation was noted 3 months after surgery.

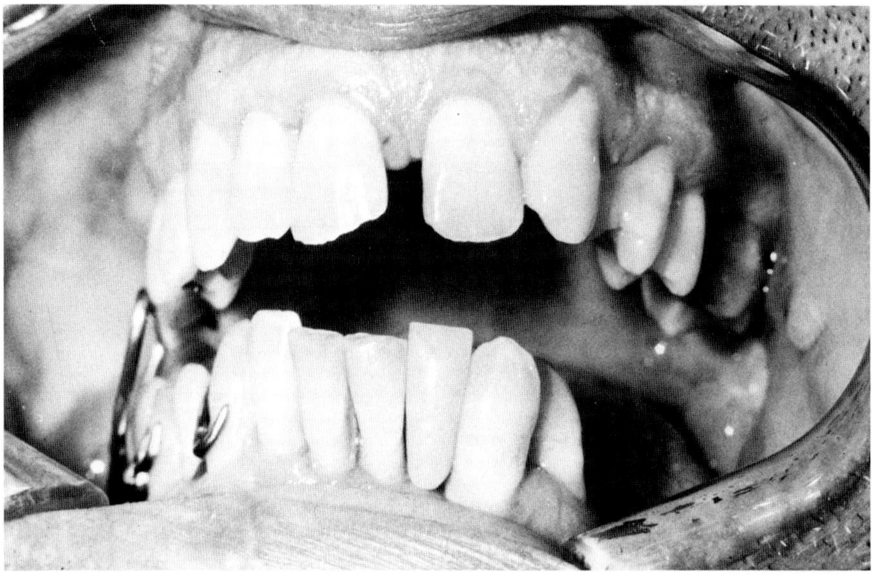

Fig. 24. Guiding plane prosthesis used for 5 weeks by the patient. The initial contact of the plane with the maxillary teeth.

the degree of expected deviation. The results of this work indicated that the mandibular deviation was reduced or eliminated. In mandibular resection for edentulous patients, the original dentures that the patient used were used postsurgically with slight modification or no modification at all. The dentulous patients showed a lesser degree of deviation with fixation and with encouragement of early functional movement of the mandible. Some of the patients of the latter group needed the use of guiding appliances during the postsurgical period to get the mandible back to the centric position. Edentulous patients who deviated slightly were fitted with maxillary ramp which guided the mandibular segment after the initial contact into the proper centric relation.

References

1. Cantor R, Curtis TA: Prosthetic management of edentulous mandibulectomy patients. Part I. Anatomic and physiologic considerations. J Prosth Dent 25:446–457, 1971

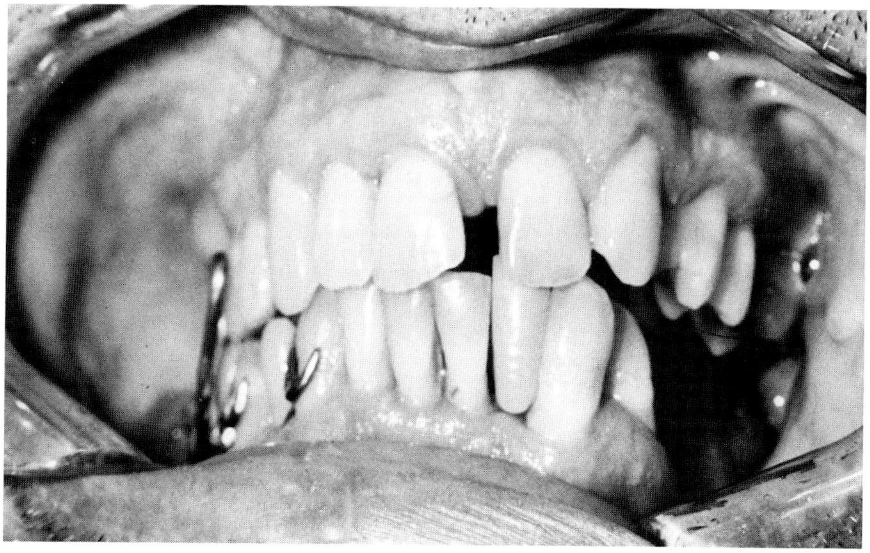

Fig. 25. Terminal centric position with guiding plane in place. Five weeks later the patient returned to the use of his denture and discarded the guiding plane.

2. Cantor R, Curtis TA: Prosthetic management of edentulous mandibulectomy patients. Part II. Clinical considerations. J Prosth Dent 25:546–555, 1971
3. Cantor R, Curtis TA: Prosthetic management of edentulous mandibulectomy patients. Part III. Clinical evaluation. J Prosth Dent 25:670–678, 1971
4. Aramany MA: Replacement of missing or defective organs. In Sassouni V, Sotereanos G: Diagnosis and Treatment of Dentofacial Abnormalities. Springfield, IL, Charles C Thomas, 1974
5. Aramany MA: New trends in construction of splints. J Prosth Dent 23:88–95, 1970

Proplast Chin Augmentation

Michael L. Merrin, Morey L. Parkes, and Frank M. Kamer, Los Angeles, California

Introduction

The importance of chin prominence in the overall aesthetic evaluation of the facial profile is now well accepted.[1–3] One of the most common chin abnormalities encountered in facial surgery is that of the recessed mentum without significant malocclusion. This relative deformity tends to overemphasize a normal nose and exaggerate an already large nose, contributing to an unattractive "bird-like" appearance.[4] Chin augmentation has been done for many years using several techniques and a variety of implant materials.[3,5]

The surgery is performed by either the intraoral or the extraoral approach. We favor the extraoral approach. A major area of controversy exists as to whether the implant should be placed above or beneath the periosteum. The rationale for subperiosteal placement centers on the need for firm fixation of the implant. Robinson et al, have reported on post operative bone resorption in 12 of 14 acrylic and silastic chin implants placed in subperiosteal pockets.[6] The etiology of this bone resorption is hypothesized to be pressure and/or the hardness of the implant.[7] For this reason, in addition to greater ease of implant insertion, the supraperiosteal placement is advocated.

Implant materials for chin augmentation have run the entire gamut from homograft and banked cartilage and bone to ivory, various metals, paraffin, and most recently "the plastics".[3,5] Bone and cartilage, although well tolerated, have often proved less than satisfactory due to unpredictable resorption and the occasional necessity of an additional surgical procedure to procure the implant. The early alloplastic materials such as paraffin, ivory, gold, silver, etc. were discarded due to poor tissue tolerance.[5] In recent years, primary attention has been directed towards the use of newer plastic materials as alloplastic implants. These implants should fulfill certain criteria which include chemical inertness, stability, noncarcinogenicity and allergenicity, ease of sterilization, and the ability to be shaped. Nylon derivatives, polytetrafluoroethylene (Teflon), Dacron, acrylics and the silicone compounds have been among the most popular plastic implants. Proplast, a newer plastic derivative especially formulated for tissue implantation, is evaluated in this series of chin augmentations.

Description

Proplast is an extremely porous material made from Teflon fluorocarbon polymer and vitreous carbon fibers. It is approximately 80 percent porous allowing for rapid tissue ingrowth (Fig. 1). The material is a dark-grey in appearance and has a felt-like consistency. It is a relatively malleable substance and may be cut and shaped with a scalpel or sharp scissors. Animal studies have shown diffuse connective tissue infiltration rather than sequestration. This phenomenon is seen from 2 to 6 weeks after transplantation[8] (Fig. 2). If sepsis occurs, the Proplast does not adhere to the surrounding tissue. Further implant studies in oral surgery and cavity obliteration have shown excellent biocompatibility, the implants being surrounded and infiltrated by mature fibrous tissue.[9,10] Evidence of some tissue reaction is reflected in the presence of multinucleated giant cells.

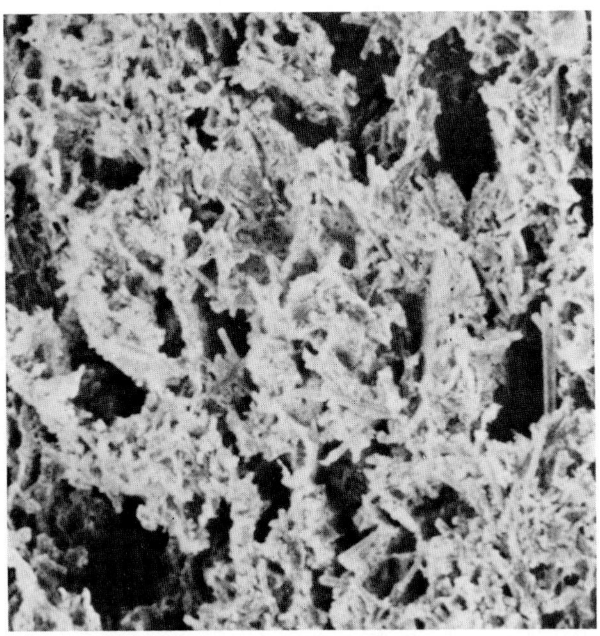

Fig. 1. Porous structure of Proplast (×50).

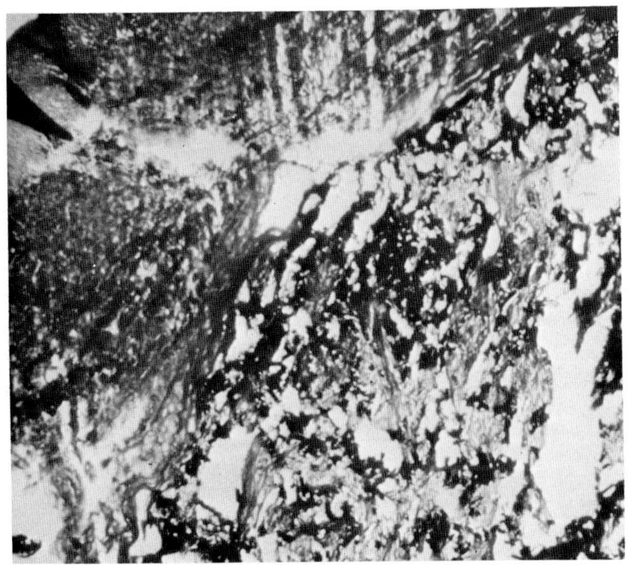

Fig. 2. Connective tissue ingrowth throughout implant. Dog mandible, six weeks (Masson, ×40).

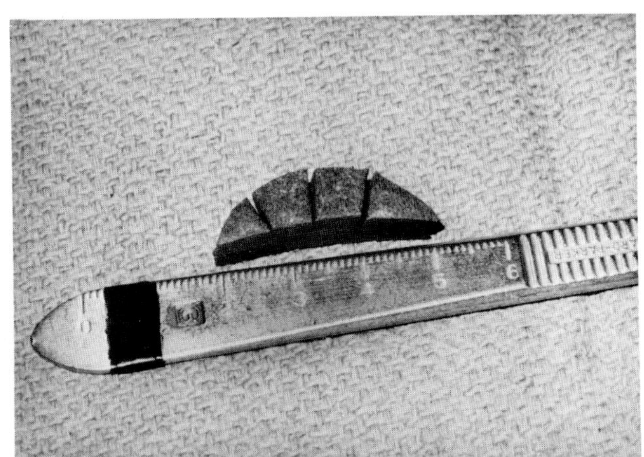

Fig. 3. Chin prosthesis is carved to correct size and shape and then sectioned into four pieces.

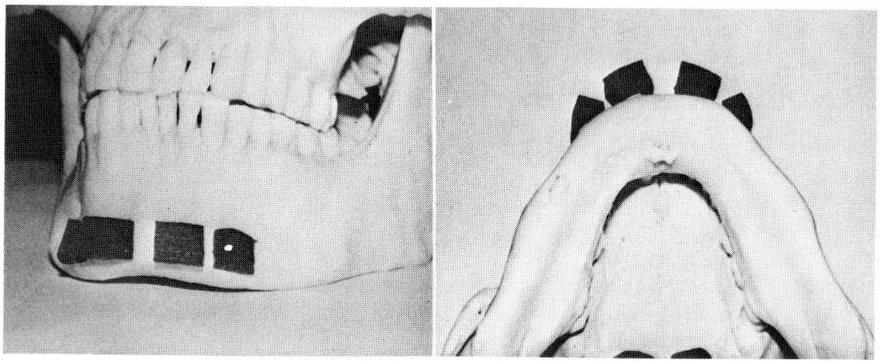

Fig. 4. Left, Proplast segments in position, AP view. Right, Submental view.

Methods and Materials

The objectives of this study were to: (1) determine if bone resorption occurs under Proplast implants: (2) evaluate the efficacy of the material as to shape, stability, ease of use, etc.; and (3) confirm the biocompatibility of Proplast. To this end, a protocol utilizing twenty successive chin augmentation cases was set up. All patients received AP and lateral radiographs of the mandible preoperatively and at six months. One year, and two year follow-up radiographs are scheduled. In addition, preoperative and six month postoperative determinations were made for CBC, PTT, calcium, phosphorus, and alkaline phosphatase. All available participants were clinically evaluated on a monthly basis for tenderness, erythema, edema, drainage, implant stability, and healing of the incision.

Surgical Technique

The Proplast is retained in its plastic shipping envelope until ready for use. It is steam autoclaved in the envelope in a routine fashion. The appropriate size (it is available in 6, 8, and 10 mm thicknesses) is chosen, and a suitable implant is carved at the surgical table with a #15 scalpel blade (Fig. 3). The surgeons gloves are rinsed to remove powder before handling the material.

Infiltration of the mental shelf, mental nerves, and the immediate submental area is carried out with 1 percent xylocaine and epinephrine 1:100,000. A submental incision 1 to 2 cm long is made in the first crease. A pocket is then fashioned, above the periosteum and below the mentalis muscle, just large enough to accomodate the sections of the implant. The median raphe may be left intact. Extensive dissection is avoided to minimize the possibility of implant shift in the crucial early stages.[7] Meticulous hemostasis is carried out with electrocautery. The previously shaped implant is now sectioned into four or more pieces which are soaked in autogenous blood. The lateral sections are placed first; then the medial ones are put into position (Fig. 4). The external chin is then molded until the exact desired effect is achieved. The incision is closed subcutaneously with a layer of 4–0 plain catgut while the skin is approximated with interrupted 6–0 nylon suture. A drain is not routinely used. A tape dressing is placed above and below the implant and all sutures are removed within seven days.

Results

Nineteen of the twenty chin implants have remained in place at the six month examination. One implant was removed after 4 months secondary to direct trauma and sepsis.* The successful implants all had a similar postoperative course. The

* The single implant that necessitated removal occurred in a 32-year-old male. Although moderate bleeding took place during his surgery, his postoperative course was uneventful until he suffered direct trauma to his chin about six weeks after surgery. There was subsequent erythema and tenderness for which the patient was placed on a ten day course of antibiotics. In spite of this, he developed intermittant drainage from the site of the incision. Three months after surgery, a small granuloma was noted at the incision, and *Staphylococcus aureus* was cultured from the drainage. The implant sections were easily removed one week later. The pieces of Proplast were not surrounded by a capsule nor was there any fibrous ingrowth. Healing took place rapidly after implant removal.

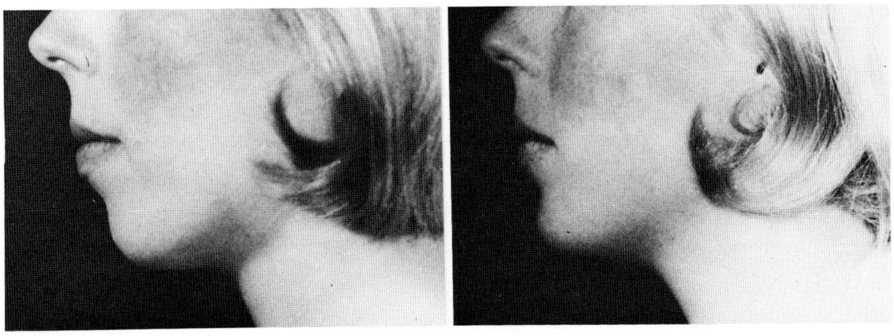

Fig. 5. Left, Preoperative view showing moderate chin recession. Right, Six month postoperative view of Proplast chin augmentation.

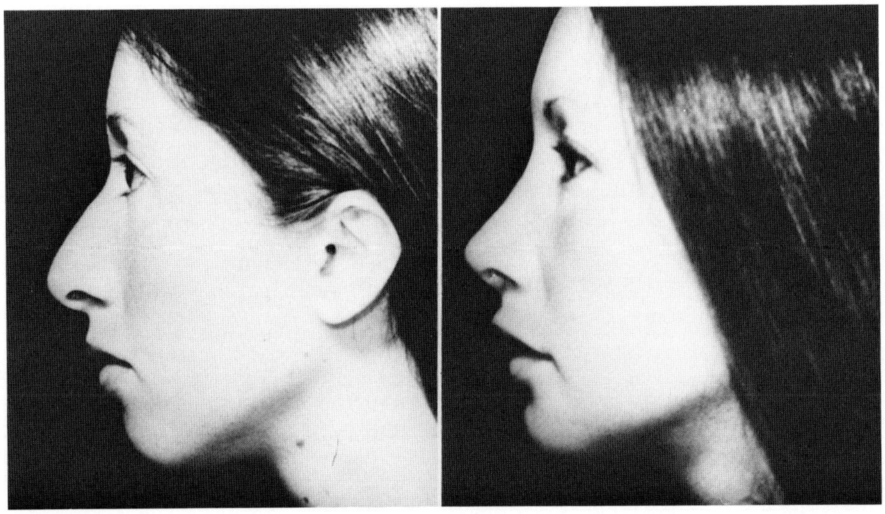

Fig. 6. Left, Preoperative view with combined chin and nasal deformities. Right, Six month postoperative view following combined Proplast chin augmentation and rhinoplasty.

first week is marked by mild to moderate edema, erythema, and/or ecchymosis. Tenderness at the site of the implant was the most common complaint during this early period. No drainage appeared at the incision in the successful implants. All edema, erythema, and ecchymosis disappeared by three weeks and tenderness was gone by six weeks. The implants became relatively fixed to the underlying hard structures between three and eight weeks. There was no subsequent shifting or shrinkage.

The six month examination revealed all nineteen successful implants to be stable and firmly fixed to surrounding tissue (Figs. 5 and 6). No skin adhesions were noted nor was the implant externally visible in any instance. Radiographs revealed no bony absorption in any of the twenty cases including the patient whose implant had to be removed. Serum laboratory studies showed no significant change from preoperative values.

Comment

Since completion of the original twenty procedures, over thirty additional Proplast chin augmentations have been performed without incident. Although the follow-up period is as yet still quite short, it is encouraging to note just one failure in over fifty procedures performed over the past year.

From this study, Proplast appears to offer several substantial advantages as an alloplastic material for chin augmentation. It is essentially nonreactive to human tissue. It is 80 percent porous and allows for rapid fibrous tissue invasion with subsequent fixation. It is relatively pliable for compatibility with soft tissue augmentation. It is easily trimmed and shaped, and can be readily steam autoclaved.

Mechanical compression of Proplast should be avoided, since collapse of some of the porosity will occur with a subsequent decrease in connective tissue ingrowth. Although the essential dark color of Proplast could be discerned if covered by only a thin layer of tissue (0.5 mm),[10] it has not been a problem in this procedure due to the thick covering of muscle and subcutaneous tissue.

Even the most well tolerated implant, if exposed to excessive trauma or sepsis, can be the site of an inflammatory response causing eventual extrusion.[5] Once exposed, implants in human tissue are almost always rejected. Slippage and movement must be prevented. It is well known that tolerance of alloplastic substances is much better in areas where mobility is restricted and ample tissue coverage is available.

The surgical technique advocated is well adapted towards the goal of implant fixation when used in conjunction with Proplast. The procedure requires only fifteen minutes operating time and is not technically difficult. The method of sectioning the implant takes advantage of the porous nature of Proplast by exposing a much greater surface area for tissue ingrowth and subsequent fixation. In addition, the multiple components can be easily arranged to compensate for any mandibular assymetry.

Conclusion

Proplast appears to be an ideal material for chin augmentation. It is well tolerated, pliable, easily shaped, and rapidly invaded and stabilized by host tissue. *Note:* Proplast supplied by Smith Kline Surgical Specialities.

References

1. Millard DR: Chin implants. Plast Reconstr Surg 13:70, 1954
2. Pitanguy I: Augmentation mentoplasty. Plast Reconstr Surg 42:460–464, 1968
3. Rish BB: Alloplastic materials in the creation of facial contour. Arch Otolaryngol 72:212–218, 1960
4. Parkes ML: Chin implants with a newer plastic compound. Arch Otolaryngol 75:429–436, 1962
5. Dickinson JT, Jaquiss GW: Alloplastic implants 1972. Otolaryngol Clin 5:3 481–500, 1972
6. Robinson M, Shuken R: Bone resorption under plastic chin implants. J Oral Surg 27:116–118, 1967
7. Parkes ML: Avoiding bone resorption under plastic chin implants. Arch Otolaryngol 98:100–101, 1973
8. Homsy CA, Caine JE, Kessler FB, Anderson MS, King JW: Porous implant systems for prosthesis stabilization. Clin Orthop 89:220–235, 1972
9. Kent JN, Homsy CA, Gross BD, Hinds EC: Pilot studies of a porous implant in dentistry and oral surgery. J Oral Surg 30:608–616, 1972
10. Janeke JB, Komorn RM, Cohn AM: Proplast in cavity obliteration and soft tissue augmentation. Otolaryngol 100:24–27, 1974

Chronic Ear Disease in Adult Patients with Unrepaired Cleft Palate*

Charles J. Krause, Iowa City, Iowa and Ward B. Litton, Moline, Ill.

A high incidence of middle ear disease in patients with cleft of the palate has been noted and studied for nearly 100 years. Yet many facets of this relationship remain poorly understood. Delineation and control of the etiologic factors involved should result in more effective prevention of long term aural pathology.

It is well documented that middle-ear effusion is common in infants with cleft palate.[1,2] The

* This study was financed in part by the Cleft Palate Research Grant (# DE-00853) at the University of Iowa.

somewhat lower incidence of middle ear pathology noted in older children[3–5] has been attributed by some authors to surgical closure of the palatal cleft. Severeid's study suggests that this decline in middle ear pathology may be related primarily to advancing age.[6]

Eustachian tube malfunction with failure of middle ear air pressure equilibration appears to be the primary cause of middle ear effusion.[7,8] This fluid may result in repeated bouts of acute suppurative otitis media and their sequelae: middle ear scarring and tympanic membrane perforation. It has been theorized that cleft palate patients may be particularly prone to eustachian tube malfunction prior to palatoplasty because of irritation about the pharyngeal openings due to food reflux,[9] and to the lack of a firm anchorage from which the tensor veli palatini muscle may function to open the eustachian tube.

The medial portion of the tensor palatini muscle opens the nasopharyngeal orifice of the eustachian tube. It arises from the lateral lamina of the tubal cartilage and forms a tendon which passes around the hamulus and inserts into the palatal aponeurosis and the posterior edge of the hard palate. Failure of midline fusion of the palatal aponeurosis might result in a lack of firm anchorage for the muscle and impair its very important function.

Holborow[10] is the leading advocate of this theory. He demonstrated that transection of the tensor palatini tendon in dogs resulted in impaired eustachian tube function. Odoi et al[11] found that middle ear effusion developed in 16 of 34 dogs undergoing palatal midline split. In an additional experiment, 43 dogs were subjected to a hamulotomy on one side and a sham operation on the other. Middle ear effusion developed in 31 of 43 ears on the side of the hamulotomy, and in only 4 of the 43 on the side of the sham operation.

Bluestone[8] found obstruction at the nasopharyngeal opening of the eustachian tube in all unrepaired cleft palate children studied. Though not all infants with repaired palates had normal function, most were able to open the tube to some degree.

This study was designed to ascertain the incidence of chronic middle ear pathology in cleft palate patients in whom a palatoplasty had never been performed. If an intact soft palate is important for normal eustachian tube function, one might anticipate a much higher incidence of chronic aural pathology in this group of patients than in similar groups of patients in whom palatoplasty was performed at an early age.

Description of Method

A total of 32 patients with unrepaired clefts of the palate were studied. The patients' ages ranged from 7 to 63. Eight of them were male and 24 were female. In most instances a decision had been made against palatoplasty because the clefts were felt to be too wide to close successfully. Three of the patients were unoperated because their parents had refused to allow surgery. All patients who had undergone surgery about the soft palate were excluded from the study. All patients wore dental obturators to improve their speech. Thirteen patients had complete clefts of the lip, alveolus and palate; 14 of the secondary palate; and 5 of the soft palate only.

Aural examination was performed on all patients by the two investigators. The absence of middle ear fluid was ascertained on the basis of tympanic membrane position and mobility. When there was a question whether middle ear fluid were present, myringotomy was performed and a ventilating tube inserted if fluid was found.

Routine audiometric testing was performed, including pure tone thresholds in all patients and speech reception thresholds when the pure tone testing indicated a hearing loss. The speech reception threshold was utilized to express hearing levels when available, and the average of pure tone thresholds at 500, 1000, and 2000 Hz when it was not. The audiometers were calibrated to ISO standards.

Results

Table 1 lists the findings noted on aural examination. The most common finding was that the tympanic membrane was judged to be entirely normal in appearance and mobility (31 ears). The next most common finding was that of tympanic

Table 1. Unoperated Cleft Palate Patients: Physical Findings on Aural Examination

	Number of Ears
Normal	31
Ventilating tube	1
Tympanic membrane scarred	17
Tympanosclerosis	3
Adhesive otitis media	3
Perforation	
Central	7
Marginal	2
Cholesteatoma	—
TOTAL	64

membrane scarring (17 ears). Perforations were present in 9 ears, with tympanosclerosis and adhesive otitis media each noted in 3 ears. Only one ear required a ventilating tube at the time of examination.

One patient had undergone previous aural surgery. A complete mastoidectomy had been performed for chronic suppuration, followed by a myringoplasty 2 years later. However, a persistent central perforation was present at the time of examination.

Table 2 lists the severity of hearing loss detected in the 64 ears examined. Normal hearing was the most common finding, with more than 40 dB loss detected in only 4 ears.

Table 2. Unoperated Cleft Palate Patients: Auditory Acuity

Air Conduction Threshold[a]	Number of Ears
Less than 10 dB	42
10 to 25 dB	15
25 to 40 dB	3
More than 40 dB	4
TOTAL	64

[a] ISO Standard.

In Table 3 the number of patients found to have a hearing loss of at least 25 dB in one or both ears is indicated. Such a hearing loss was present unilaterally in 5 patients and bilaterally in one patient.

Table 3. Unoperated Cleft Palate Patients: Incidence of Conductive Hearing Loss Greater Than 25 dB[a]

	Number of Subjects
Unilateral	5/32 (15.6%)
Bilateral	1/32 (3%)

[a] ISO Standard.

Discussion

Reports of middle ear pathology noted in cleft palate patients are frequently confusing in that authors fail to differentiate between middle ear effusion and other more permanent forms of pathology. In a review of the literature, Bluestone found a 50 percent incidence of conductive hearing loss in cleft palate patients "before the infant age group, and an equal, if not greater, degree of aural pathology".[8]

Though not all agree,[6,13] several authors[14–16] have reported less hearing loss in cleft palate children when palatoplasty was done early rather than late. On this basis they advocate early palatoplasty. We were interested in determining the incidence and types of middle ear pathology present in a group of patients in whom the palatal cleft had never been surgically closed.

Though 33 of the ears (52 percent) were found on aural examination to be abnormal in some way, in only 15 (23 percent) ears was this abnormality other than scarring of the tympanic membrane. Further, it is anticipated that the 9 ears in which perforations were present may be successfully reconstructed surgically.

The incidence of significant conductive hearing loss was somewhat lower than we anticipated. In 42 ears (66 percent) the hearing loss was less than 10 dB, and was less than 25 dB in an additional 15 ears (23 percent). In only 7 ears (11 percent) was a hearing loss greater than 25 dB detectable. No sensorineural hearing loss was detected other than mild high-frequency loss in the older patients.

In 1964, Graham[12] reported the otologic findings in a group of cleft patients followed at this institution. Middle ear effusion had been treated with myringotomy or adenoidectomy both before and after palatoplasty, but no transmyringeal ventilating tubes were placed. In 175 postpalatoplasty cleft patients more than 8 years of age, 28.5 percent were found to have a unilateral hearing loss greater than 15 dB ASA, and 9.7 percent to have such a loss bilaterally. He noted that after 6 years of age the degree of hearing loss tended to remain stable.

In 1972, Litton et al[9] reviewed the hearing acuity in 65 cleft palate children aged 8 to 10 followed at this institution. These children had been treated with transmyringeal ventilating tubes when middle ear effusions were noted on follow-up examination during childhood. The 23 percent incidence of hearing loss greater than 25 dB ISO unilaterally and 6 percent bilaterally was somewhat lower than that noted in the earlier study.

The incidence of significant hearing loss in this group of unrepaired cleft palate patients was actually somewhat lower than that noted in the two groups of repaired cleft palate patients reported above. A hearing loss greater than 25 dB ISO was detected unilaterally in 15.6 percent of these patients (5 of 32), and bilaterally in 3 percent (1 of 32). This difference in incidence was not statistically significant when compared to the other two groups.

Conclusions

Though the number of unoperated cleft palate patients studied was quite small, the incidence of significant middle ear pathology appears to be similar to that in postpalatoplasty patients. Whether or not palatoplasty does result in improved eustachian tube function during childhood, this appears to have little effect upon prevention of long term aural pathology. The fact that 75 percent of the ears studied were air-containing without ventilating tubes suggests that adequate eustachian tube function does commonly develop after 7 years of age even though the palatal cleft remains unrepaired.

References

1. Stool SE, Randall R: Unexpected ear disease in infants with cleft palate. Cleft Palate J 4:99–103, 1967
2. Paradise JL, Bluestone CD, Felder H: The universality of otitis media in 50 infants with cleft palate. Pediatrics 44:35–42, 1969
3. Bennett M, Ward RH, Tait CA: Otologic-audiologic study of cleft palate children. Laryngoscope 78:1011–1019, 1968
4. Graham MD, Lierle DM: Posterior pharyngeal flap palatoplasty and its relation to ear disease and hearing loss. Laryngoscope 72:1750–1755, 1962
5. Skolnik EM: Otologic evaluation of cleft palate patients. Laryngoscope 68:1908–1949, 1958
6. Severeid LR: A longitudinal study of the efficacy of adenoidectomy in children with cleft palate and secretory otitis media. Trans Am Acad Ophthalmol Otolaryngol 76:1319–1324, 1972
7. Holborow CA: The assessment of eustachian function. J Otolaryngo Soc Aug 2:18–20, 1969
8. Bluestone CD: Eustachian tube obstruction in the infant with cleft palate. Ann Otol, Rhinol, Laryngol 80: Suppl 2:1–30, 1971
9. Litton WB, Severeid LR, Tharp R: Cleft palate and otitis media. National conf on otitis media, Proc Glorig A and Gerwin K (eds), Springfield, Ill., Charles C Thomas, 1971
10. Holborow CA: Deafness associated with cleft palate. J Laryngo Otolaryng 76:762–773, 1962
11. Odoi H, Proud GO, Toledo PS: Effects of pterygoid hamulotomy upon eustachian tube function. Laryngoscope 81:1242–1244, 1971
12. Graham MD: A longitudinal study of ear disease and hearing loss in patients with cleft lips and palates. Ann Otol 73:34–47, 1964
13. Holmes EM, Reed GF: Hearing deafness in cleft palate patients. Arch Otolaryngo 62:620–624, 1955
14. Masters FW, Bingham HG, Robinson DW: The prevention and treatment of hearing loss in the cleft palate child. Plast Reconstr Surg 25:503–509, 1960
15. Aschan G: Hearing and nasal function correlated to postoperative speech in cleft palate patients with velopharyngoplasty. Acta Otolaryngo 61:371–379, 1966
16. Yules RB: Hearing in cleft palate patients. Arch Otolaryngo 91:319–323, 1970

Maxilla

Trauma and Fractures: Maxillofacial (Panel)

The panelists and their subtopics were introduced and opening remarks made about maxillofacial trauma.

Dr. Dickinson:

Maxillofacial trauma patients generally fit into three broad categories: (1) those in whom full reconstruction can be accomplished with initial treatment; (2) those in whom reconstruction is limited by the general condition of the patient; and (3) those in whom reconstruction is limited by the condition of local or regional tissues.

Dr. Bernstein:

Basic intermaxillary fixation techniques should be well known to the surgeon managing maxillofacial trauma. These include simple interarch wire ligatures, loop eyelet wires, continuous wiring techniques and various types of arch bars for patients with natural dentition. Acrylic splints are frequently necessary in edentulous and partially edentulous patients. The selected use of circumferential mandibular wires, pyriform aperture, zygomatic and frontal suspension wires is essential in the proper treatment of fracture patients. Fixation of a maxillary denture or splint to the maxilla using short K/wire pins is a very useful technique.

Mandibular body fractures in children are probably best managed with acrylic splints circumferentially wired to the mandible to avoid injury to developing tooth buds.

Dr. Casey:

The proper management of injured teeth can be very important in total patient care. Uncomplicated enamel fractures often do not require any treatment other than delayed dental restoration, however, exposed dentin may require a protective covering such as calcium hydroxide paste or zinc oxide cement. Complicated fractures through the pulp cavity require immediate pulp treatment for best results and eventually may necessitate root canal therapy. Teeth with root fractures below the gingival margin are probably best treated by extraction.

Permanent teeth that are completely extruded or avulsed out of the socket have traditionally been managed by immediate root canal filling, replacement and stabilization in the socket. Over 80 percent of such teeth demonstrate root resorption within 5 years. The current philosophy in management of avulsed teeth is to gently cleanse the tooth and replant it in the socket without a root canal filling.

It should be stabilized with suitable wire ligature techniques or acrylic splinting for several months. Root canal filling is delayed until pain, swelling, loss of vitality, discoloration or periapical x-ray changes develop. Progressive root resorption, ankylosis and loss of vitality eventually occur in most of these teeth, however, they may serve as useful dental units for many years before they are ultimately lost.

Clinically intact teeth in an alveolar process fracture have a guarded prognosis and will undergo pulp necrosis in about 75 percent of the cases. Root resorption and loss of marginal bone support will occasionally occur. These teeth should be managed expectantly with good stabilization.

The management of permanent teeth in fracture lines has always been somewhat controversial. Teeth in the fracture line reportedly lead to significant infection in 5 to 19 percent of cases. These teeth are subject to pulp necrosis, loss of marginal bone support, root resorption and ankylosis. It is generally recommended to maintain fracture line teeth when they are in good condition and when their presence helps stabilize the fracture.

Prophylactic antibiotic coverage is recommended in maxillomandibular fractures particularly when the fracture is compounded intraorally and teeth are present. A recent prospective study by Zallen and Curry (J Oral Surgery, June 1975) indicates that fracture site infection can be significantly reduced by the routine use of prophylactic antibiotics.

Dr. Bailey:

Condylar neck fractures in children are classified into two groups. First, there are those with minimal displacement in which good occlusion prevails and no lateral deviation occurs. The second group consist of those with moderate to severe displacement in which premature molar contact occurs along with chin deviation to the side of the fracture and loss of chin protrusion. Symptoms and findings in condylar neck fractures include subjective changes in occlusion, malocclusion, pain, restricted motion, chin deviation and tenderness to palpation over the condyle. Complications of condylar neck fractures in children include malocclusion, ankylosis or limited motion, pseudoarthrosis, arthritis, and mandibular growth disturbance.

There are three schools of thought regarding management of condylar neck fractures in children:

(1) no treatment with early motion recommended;
(2) conservative treatment with either intermaxillary fixation or splinting;
(3) open surgical reduction.

Most patients are managed with early motion or conservative treatment and open reduction is rarely necessary. The indications for open reduction have never been satisfactorily elucidated. There have been no large series of patients treated by open reduction with long term follow-up adequate to justify the use of open reduction.

Large series of cases have been reported with adequate follow-up and excellent experimental studies are in recent literature to support early mobilization and conservative treatment. The following conclusions have evolved:

(1) Over 93 percent of patients will have good to excellent results with less than 1 percent having a significantly poor result.
(2) Complete anatomic healing usually occurs with remodeling of dislocated condyles.
(3) Growth is not affected in most cases.
(4) There is no correlation between fracture severity and final outcome.
(5) Early mobilization does not hinder healing and may produce a better result.

Mandibular fractures in adults can be satisfactorily managed by conservative closed methods in the majority of cases. Some of the indications for open reduction include symphysis fractures, unfavorable body fractures posterior to the last tooth in the arch and those fractures not satisfactorily reduced or immobilized by intermaxillary fixation alone.

Dr. Kothary:

Delayed union of mandibular fractures is generally associated with persistent or chronic infection, presence of foreign bodies, inadequate immobilization and interference with blood supply as etiologic factors. Massive loss of bone in the initial traumatic event can be an obvious factor. Delayed union is more common in compound comminuted fractures. Osteomyelitis with sequestration of infected bone fragments can occur requiring proper antibiotic therapy and surgical debridement procedures. Non-union may be the eventual outcome and bone grafting will then become necessary. Bone grafting should be delayed until all wound sepsis has cleared. The graft should be placed in good contact with healthy mandible fragments and the surrounding soft tissue environment should be healthy. Strict immobilization is essential.

Delayed union of the maxilla is quite uncommon but is likewise related to persistent infection and inadequate immobilization.

Infections associated with jaw fractures must be treated vigorously and promptly for best results. Local wound care, meticulous oral hygiene, culture studies, appropriate antibiotic therapy and properly timed drainage or debridement procedures are all essential in preventing the undesired sequellae of osteomyelitis and non-union.

Dr. Dickinson:

Several cases with massive soft tissue injury and multiple fractures were presented and discussed by the panelists. Immediate regional flap placement to repair massive soft tissue defects should always be considered as an alternative to delayed repair.

Simplified Protocol for Management of Malar Fractures (Based on a 1200 Case 8-Year Experience)

Ronald S. Matsunaga, William Simpson, and Paul H. Toffel, Los Angeles, California

In the course of the years 1966 through 1973 the senior author, in his private practice, and the Maxillofacial and Plastic Reconstructive Division of the Department of Otolaryngology at the Los Angeles County/U.S.C. Medical Center, managed more than 1900 cases of major maxillofacial trauma. Approximately 1200 of these cases were malar fractures (Tables 1 and 2). Based on this experience, a simplified protocol of surgical management for reduction and fixation of malar fractures has been developed. It is presented as an alternative to current literature methods.

Table 1. Eight Year Major Maxillofacial Case Experience, 1966–1973.

Type Fracture	No. Cases	Percent
Malar	1176	61.1
Le Forte I, II, III and other Mid/Third Fractures	612	31.8
Mandibular Fractures	136	7.1
Total	1924	100.0

Table 2. Major Maxillofacial Cases Managed during Academic Year, 1973.

Type Fracture	No. Cases	Percent
Malar	147	62.0
Zygomatic Arch	6	2.5
Le Forte I	16	6.5
Le Forte II	24	10.0
Le Forte III	2	1.0
Nasofrontal Complex	23	9.5
Orbital Floor Blow-out	3	1.5
Mandibular	17	7.0
Total	238	100.0

Problems with Standard ORIF Method

The classic tripod body fracture is still the most common malar injury in our experience, paralleling the findings of Knight and North[1] in which 76 percent of malar fractures are of this type. The most common approach to these fractures in the current literature is the method in which direct incisions are made at the brow for the fronto-zygomatic fracture line and in the infraorbital region for the zygomatico-maxillary fracture line.[2–4] The fracture is reduced via levered elevation from the brow incision. Drill holes are made at the proximal and distal fragments around the fracture sites and direct interosseous wiring is performed.

For many years at the L.A. County/U.S.C. Medical Center tripod malar fractures were managed by this method, but two shortcomings were noted. First, the leverage which could be exerted upon the fracture fragment via the brow incision was sometimes inadequate for proper reduction. Using engineering leverage models, the leverage available via the brow incision was compared with that available via the Gillies type temporal approach.[5] It was found that the Gillies approach could develop three to fourfold greater mechanical advantage for reduction of the malar fragment than the brow technique. The second shortcoming was also an engineering point that others have related in the literature as a problem with nonfixated malar methods; that is the chronic tractive action of the masseter muscle which results in postoperative displacement of the zygoma.[2,6] This action seems also to apply to the standard interosseous wiring method, because in the period of healing the two-point rim fixation may be inadequate to stabilize the tripod malar fracture fragment against the tonic downward pull of the masseter muscle, especially if the thin lateral wall of the antrum has been badly damaged. Thus the wired fragment can still rotate in hinge fashion into the antrum, producing late postoperative flattening of the malar contour, in our experience.

There appeared to be a need for an alternative method of dealing with malar fractures which could overcome these defects of inadequate leverage for consistent reduction, and inadequate fixation against the chronic hinging rotatory forces of the musculature. A satisfactory method was developed over a two-year period by the senior author, and was introduced at the Los Angeles County/U.S.C. Medical Center in 1966.

The Internal Wire Pin Method

The alternative method was found in combining the Gillies approach to reduction with an Orthopedic internal wire pin fixation tailored to the specific mechanical requirements of the malar fracture. The use of the internal wire pin for facial fractures had been described before by J. B. Brown in 1952,[7] however, it was sought to secure a pinning method for routine use which would fixate the tripod malar fracture fragment eccentric to the axis of hinging forces previously described. The method meeting these requirements was worked out for the typical malar fracture, along with a protocol for dealing with contingencies of comminution, impaction, and orbital floor damage. A byproduct of the pinning method is that it remarkably simplifies the corrective surgery of the applicable cases, in that the usual brow and infraorbital incisions are eliminated, along with the concurrent drilling of fragments and placement of interosseous wires. The method is as follows:

A Gillies type temporal incision is made behind the hairline and deepened to the temporal fascia. A stout facial bone elevator is passed below the temporal fascia to the zygoma and the tripod fracture is disimpacted and reduced. The malar fracture fragment is held in reduction by digital pressure counterbalancing the leverage of the stout facial elevator. Once the reduction is properly obtained, as demonstrated by elimination of orbital rim step offs and palpably symmetrical malar eminences, a small nick is made in the skin over the lateral aspect of the greatest bulk of the malar bone. While taking cognizance of the plane of the orbit, and while the assistant maintains the reduction, the 1/8 in. to 3/16 in. caliber spear-point unthreaded Kirschner type wire pin is driven with bit and chuck transmalar, aiming obliquely through the antrum for a point on the hard palate approximately 2 cm posterior to the anterior nasal spine. This passage will anchor the tripod malar fragment eccentric to the usual axis of rotation, and thus it will not hinge and rotate into the antrum as a postoperative sequelae (Figs. 1–6). The wire pin is cut off flush with the skin and the skin is pulled over the pin. The Gillies incision is closed, concluding the procedure. The wire pin is left in place for fixation for six weeks,

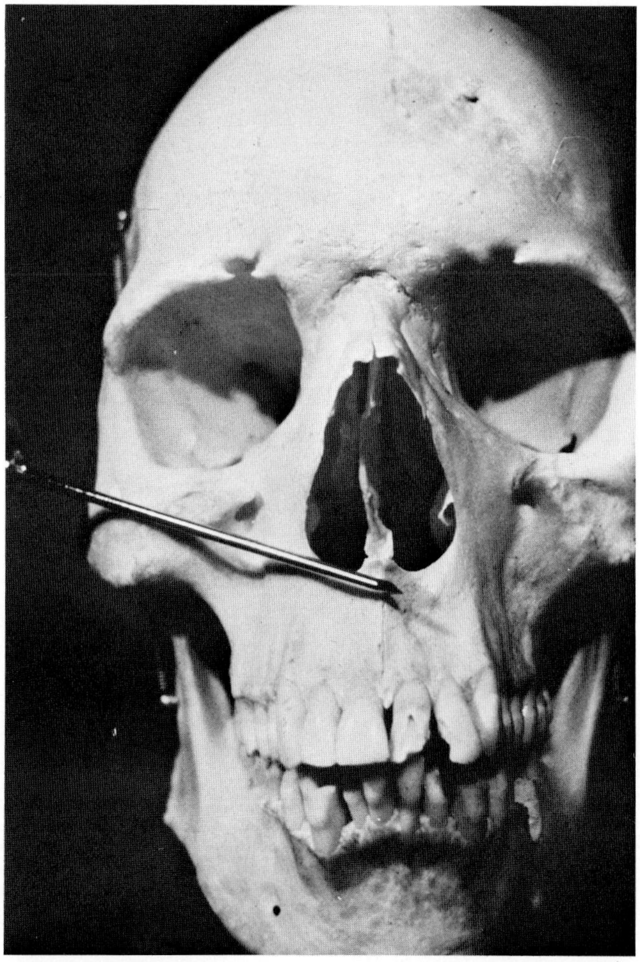

Fig. 1. Frontal view of skull demonstrating plane of passage of the internal wire pin for fixation of malar fracture.

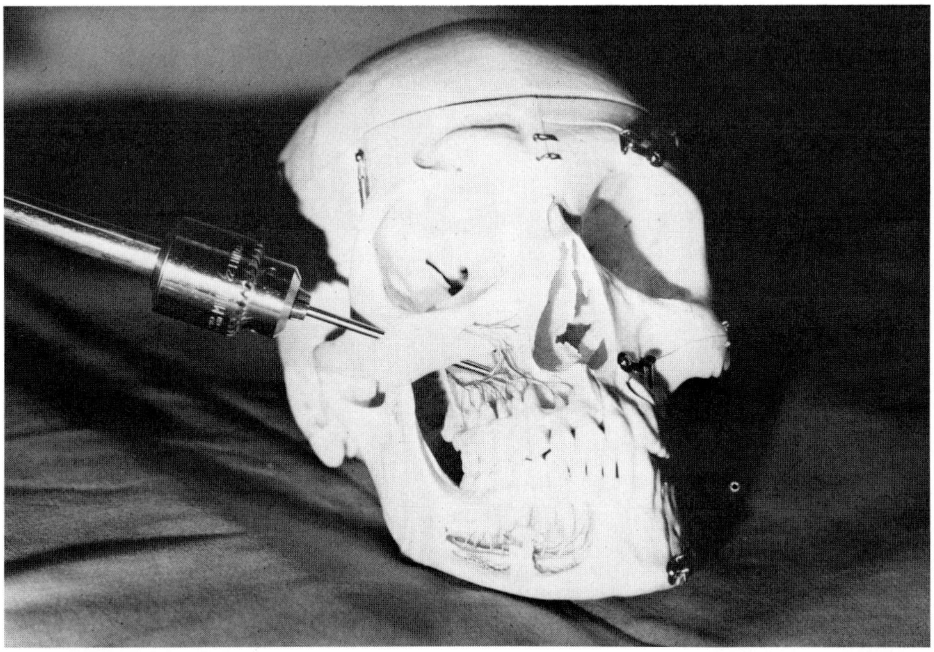

Fig. 2. A pinned prepared skull. Note antrum open to demonstrate typical trans-antral course of internal wire pin. Fixation is eccentric to usual axis of hinging rotation of malar fracture fragment. Pin has not caused significant tooth root problems in over 800 estimated cases.

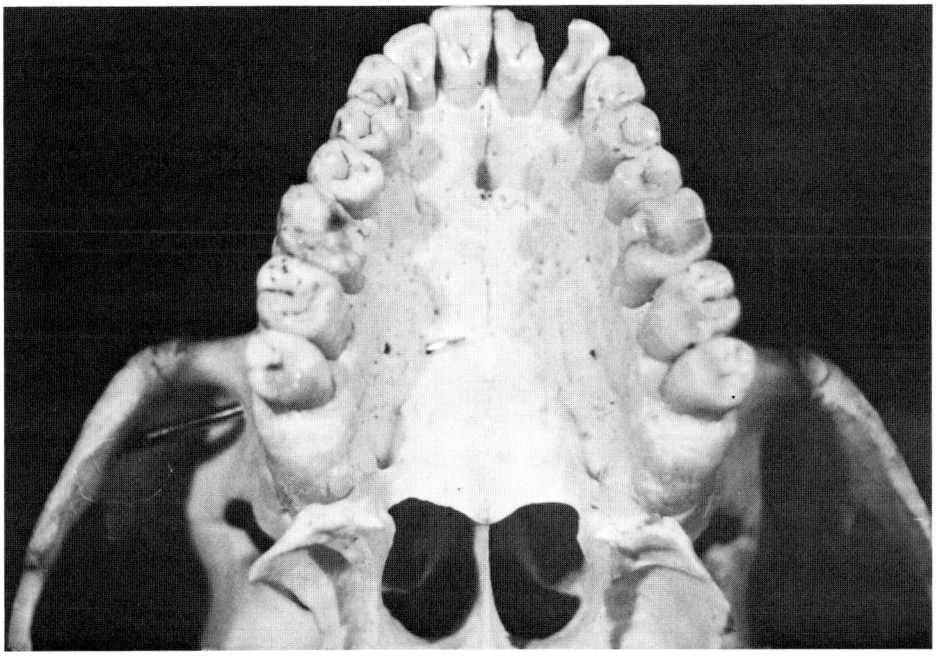

Fig. 3. Submental-vertex view demonstrating typical plane of passage of internal wire pin. Pin may pass into hard palate anywhere between roof of mouth and floor of nose.

then removed as an outpatient procedure by nicking over it under local anesthetic and removing it with a stout gripping instrument (Figs. 7–12).

It is found that the internal wire pin malar method takes 1/4 to 1/3 the operating time of the standard brow and infraorbital wiring approach, in the applicable cases, and it is felt that it has less associated intraoperative morbidity and complications. For example, the potentials for injury to the globe at drilling and wiring, or for postoperative ectropion of the lower lid, are eliminated. Intraoperative complications of the internal wire pin procedure involve overshooting the palate, with the pin passing into the nose, or undershooting the palate and passing the pin into the mouth. These are regularly checked for with use of headlight and

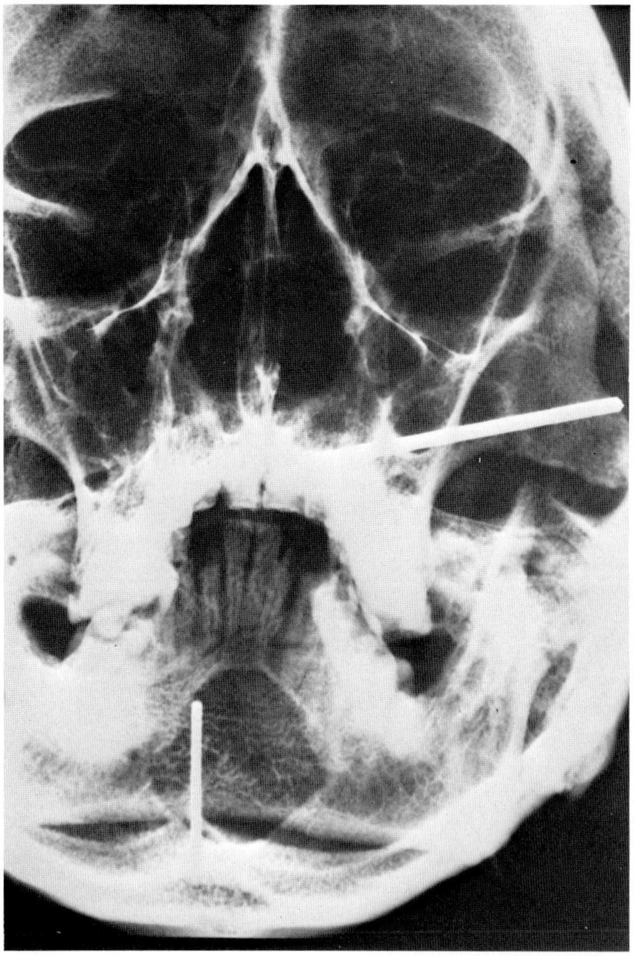

Fig. 4. Waters view facial radiograph demonstrating proper plane of passage of internal wire pin.

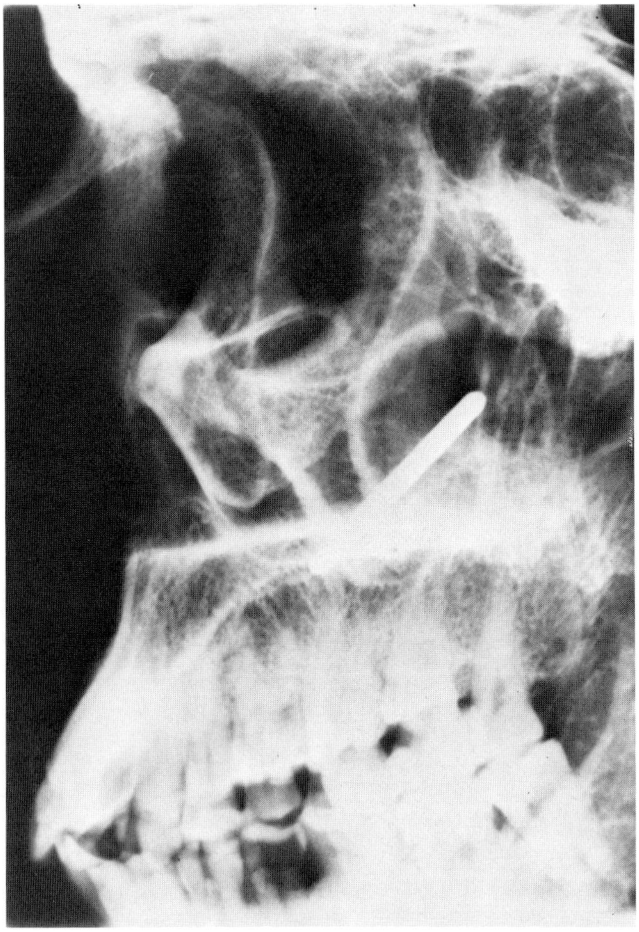

Fig. 5. Lateral view facial radiograph demonstrating plane of passage of internal wire pin. Pin should typically engage hard palate approximately two centimeters posterior to anterior nasal spine.

digital palpation at the conclusion of the procedure, and if found are corrected by backing out and redirecting the pin.

The internal wire pin malar technique was originally utilized in private practice, however, since it's introduction onto the Maxillofacial Service of our medical center, Residents have been able to learn the technique quickly with moderate intraoperative instruction from more experienced surgeons.

Protocol for Comminution, Orbital Floor Damage, and Impaction

As cited earlier by Knight and North[1] 76 percent of malar fractures are of the classic tripod type which in our hands lend themselves to the use of the internal wire pin technique. That leaves approximately 24 percent of cases for which contingency methods must be applied. Following are guidelines that we have used in dealing with these cases.

When moderate comminution of the malar fragment is present, the internal wire pin method may still be attempted and can often skewer the fragments successfully. However, when it is found that the fracture is not stable with the internal wire pin technique, or severe comminution is present, the next step of protocol is for the surgeon to perform the standard brow and infraorbital incisions and direct wire fragments as necessary. Furthermore, when ocular entrapment is present as demonstrated by extra ocular muscle testing and forced

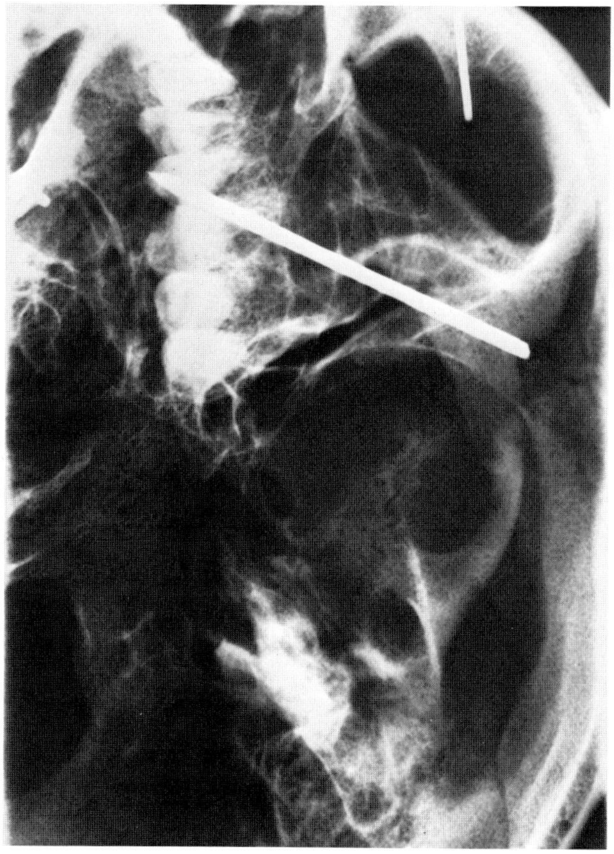

Fig. 6. Submental-vertex view radiograph demonstrating plane of passage of internal wire pin.

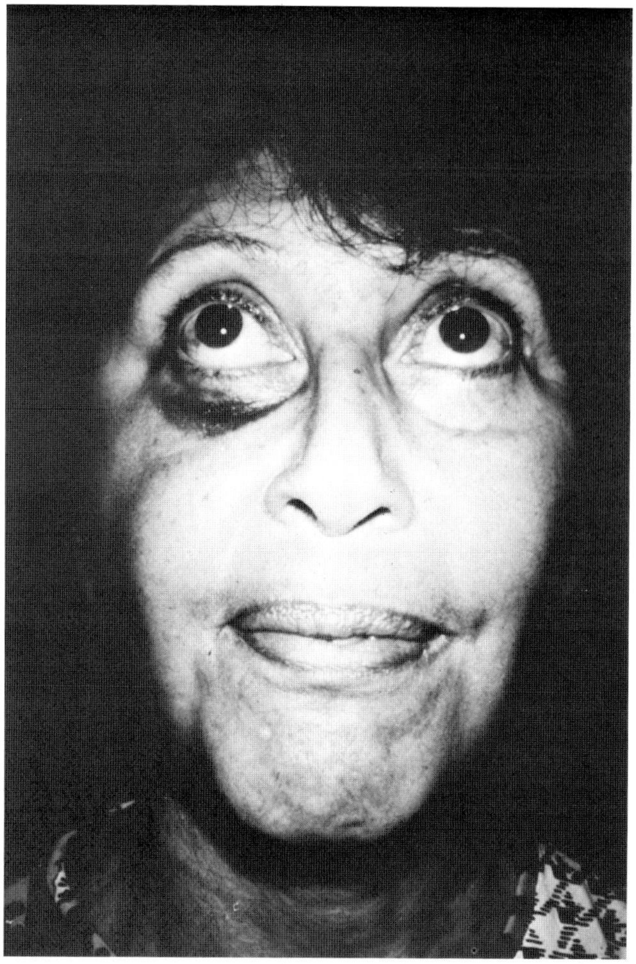

Fig. 7. Patient demonstrating marked flattening of right malar eminence secondary to tripod fracture.

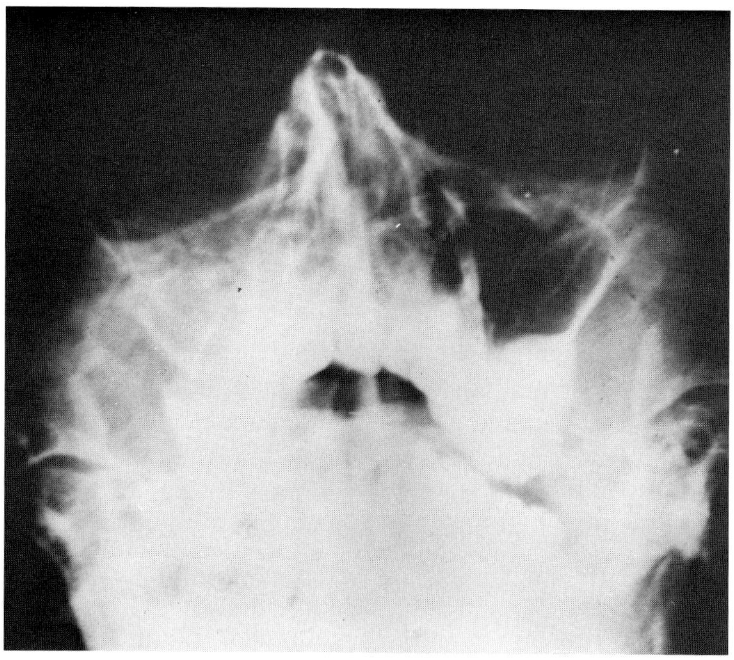

Fig. 8. Waters view radiograph of patient in Figure 7.

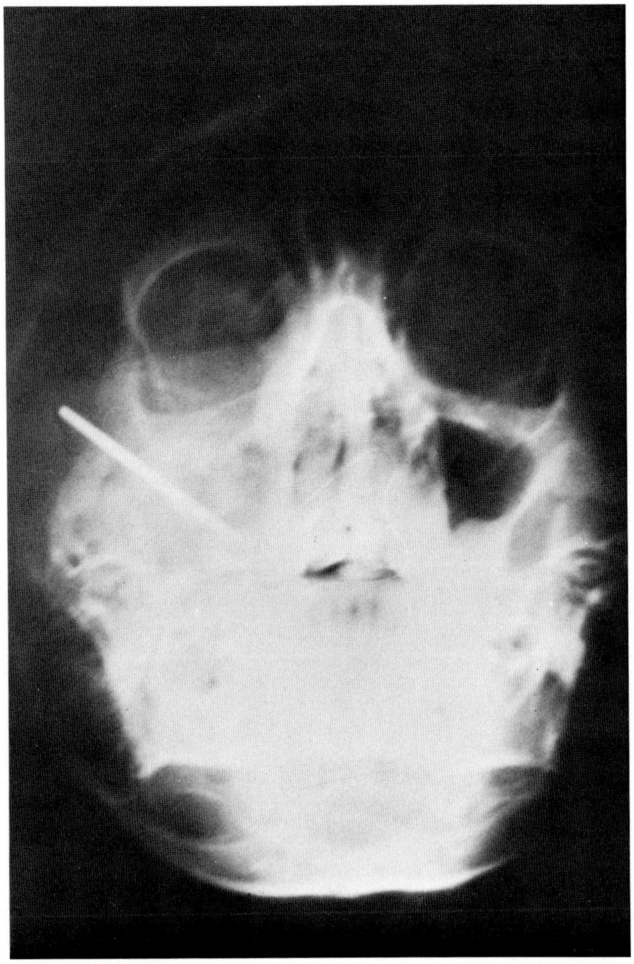

Fig. 9. Postoperative Waters view radiograph of patient in Figure 7. Note application of internal wire pin which has been cut off flush with skin.

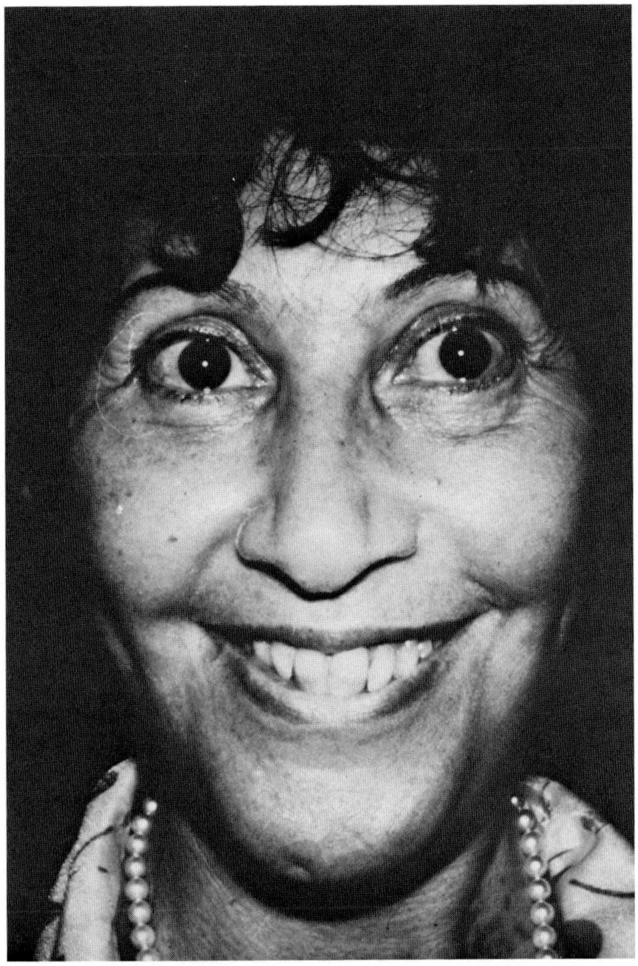

Fig. 10. Six week postoperative appearance of patient in Figure 7 after removal of internal wire pin.

ductions, confirmed preoperatively by our Ophthalmology collegues, exploration of the orbital floor via a subperiosteal approach is accomplished, with insertion of Silastic plastic sheeting as described by Freeman.[8]

When the rare "pulverized" type of malar communition is encountered, as that resulting from a violent high speed blow, we utilize the Caldwell-Luc approach to augment orbital floor exploration, and may pack the antrum.[2] If antral packing is done, however, we do not insert Silastic sheeting into the orbital floor, as we have found that the region may tolerate one or the other of these foreign bodies, but usually not both. Extrusion of the Silastic will occur.

When concurrent Le Forte type fractures are present in association with malar fractures, these are stabilized by intermaxillary fixation and Adams suspension wiring,[9] usually followed by pinning of the malar component.

An alternative situation requiring the judgement of the surgeon is that in which the malar fragment cannot be totally disimpacted into proper reduction. In this situation a transcutaneous wire or small bone screw is placed into the malar eminence and post-surgery a plaster head cap is fashioned for external rubber band traction to pull the fragment out at the appropriate vector.[10]

Application of Protocol

Using the above protocol, in the academic year 1973, in which 147 malar fractures were managed

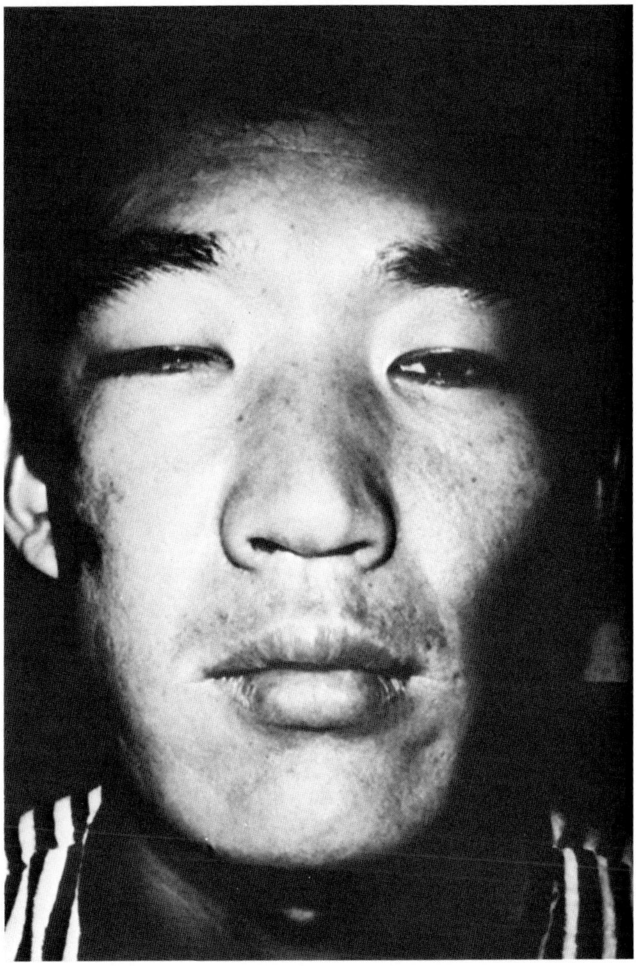

Fig. 11. A patient with extremely prominent malar eminences who sustained a right tripod fracture.

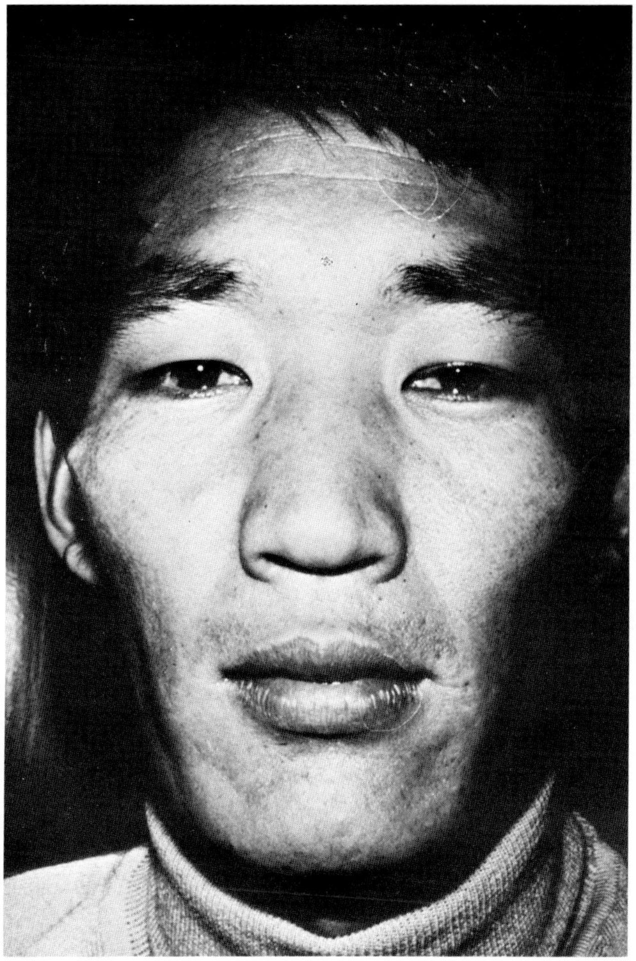

Fig. 12. Six week postoperative view of patient in Figure 11. Note tenting of internal wire pin under skin just prior to removal.

at our medical center, 73.0 percent were managed solely by the internal wire pin method, 7.0 percent by the interosseous wiring approach, 7.5 percent by headcap vector traction, and 12.5 percent were managed by various combinations of the foregoing methods. In addition 14.0 percent of the cases had associated orbital floor explorations with insertion of Silastic implants, and 2.5 percent had Caldwell-Lucs with antral packing. Overall, the internal wire pin was used in 84.0 percent of the malar procedures (Tables 3 and 4).

Acknowledgments

Our acknowledgements and sincere gratitude are due to Alden H. Miller, M.D., Chairman, Clay W. Whitaker, M.D., Director, and to the 32 Resident colleagues of the Department of Otolaryngology during the eight year span of the study.

Table 3. Breakdown of Type Malar Fixation Procedures Utilized during Academic Year, 1973.[a]

Type Fixation Procedure	No. Cases	Percent
Internal Wire Pin (sole appliance)	107	73.0
Interosseous Wiring	10	7.0
Headcap Vector Traction	11	7.5
Combinations of above Methods	19	12.5
Total	147	100.0

[a] Note: Internal Wire Pin was used in 123 or 84.0 percent of all malar procedures.

Table 4. Ancillary Procedures for Malar Fractures managed during Academic Year, 1973.

Type Ancillary Procedure	No. Cases (out of 147 total)	Percent
Orbital Floor Exploration with Silastic Implant	20	14.0
Caldwell-Luc with Antral Packing	3	2.5

References

1. Knight JS, North JF: The classification of malar fractures: An analysis of displacement as a guide to treatment. Brit J Plast Surg 13:325, 1961
2. Dingman RO: The management of facial injuries and fractures of facial bones., in Converse JM: Reconstructive Plastic Surgery. Philadelphia, WB Saunders Co., 1964
3. Dingman RO, Natvig P: Surgery of Facial Fractures; Philadelphia, WB Saunders Co., 1964
4. Kazanjian VH, Converse JM: The Surgical Treatment of Facial Injuries. Baltimore, Williams & Wilkins Co, 1974
5. Gillies HD, Kilner, TP, and Stone D: Fractures of the malar-zygomatic compound. Brit J Surg 14:651, 1927
6. Gillies HD, Millard DR: The Principles and Art of Plastic Surgery. Boston, Little, Brown and Co, 1957
7. Brown JB, Fryer MP, McDowell F: Internal wire-pin fixation for fractures of upper jaw, orbit, zygoma and severe facial crushes. Plast Reconstr Surg 9:276, 1952
8. Freeman BS: The direct approach to acute fractures of the zygomatic-maxillary complex and immediate prosthetic replacement of the orbital floor. Plast Reconstr Surg 29:587, 1962
9. Adams WM, Adams LH: Internal wire fixation of facial fractures; 15-year follow-up report. Am J Surg 92:12, 1956
10. Kazanjian VH: Treatment of automobile injuries of the face and jaws. J Am Dent A 20:757, 1933

Larynx and Trachea

Post-Laryngectomy Speech Rehabilitation (Panel)

Hitosi Iwai:

In the treatment of laryngeal cancer preservation of voice is one of the most important problems. At the present stage of cancer therapy, however the radiation and chemotherapy have their own limitation and cover only limited cases of laryngeal cancer. On the other hand, even with our best[4] effort for voice preservation about 30 percent of all laryngeal cancer cases were inappropriate for partial laryngectomy and total laryngectomy was inevitable.

Asai's laryngoplasty[1] seems to be an outstanding method of reproducing voice after a total extirpation of the larynx. The principle of his technique is to expire the air through a dermal tube into the hypopharynx and to produce sound at the small orifice of the dermal tube by the vibration the mucous membrane. With respect to Asai's laryngoplasty, we encountered several difficulties: namely, an aspiration of liquid into the trachea, a prolonged period for the completion of the reconstruction, and an nonuniformity of the quality of the reproduced voice.

In our clinic, a new larynx can successfully be reconstructed consecutively after total laryngectomy.[3] The main points of this reconstructive procedures are: (1) reconstruction of the resected posterior laryngeal wall; (2) resurfacing the severed inner aspect of the larynx using a hypopharyngeal pedicled mucous membrane flap; and (3) elevation of the reconstructed larynx toward the lingual basis. The postoperative voice was as good as in Asai's laryngoplasty. The aspiration was negligible as in the case undergoing subtotal laryngectomy.[2] This new surgery will be referred to as "primary laryngoplasty" and its outline will be shown herein.

The total laryngectomy and radical neck dissection are performed. The inner aspect of the laryngeal cavity immediately after this resection is similar to that after total laryngectomy but the lateral halves of the thyroid alae are preserved.

The first step of the reconstruction is the formation of the posterior laryngeal wall. The superior horns are used as the horizontal supporting frame of the posterior laryngeal wall. The superior horns of the both sides are fractured at the basis of their attachment to the thyroid laminae and are turned at right angle inward to touch their tips to each other (Fig. 1A).

In order to obtain an adequate width of the posterior wall, the tips of the superior horns are sutured end to end or side to side, depending on the length of the horns. Through the practice of this operation, it has been recognized that the best results in terms of voice production and degultition are obtained when the laryngeal opening is about 1 cm in diameter. The length of the sutured superior horns is adjusted to make a frame of 1 to 1.5 cm in width (Fig. 1B).

A pedicled 3 × 5 cm mucosal flap with its base down is formed in the lateral part of the hypopharyngeal wall.

The flap is rotated inferiorly and transpositioned toward the inner surface of the reconstructed laryngeal cavity, covering the posterior cartilaginous frame made of the superior horns. The tip of the rotated mucosal pedicled flap is sutured to the upper margin of the dissected subglottic mucosal linning (Fig. 1C).

The same manipulation is performed on the other side. Posteriorly the margins of the mucosal flaps are sutured together (Fig. 1D).

The anterior margins of the flaps are also closed by suturing to each other. With these procedures a new laryngeal mucosal cavity is formed which communicates downward with the trachea and opens upward to the pharyngeal cavity. The

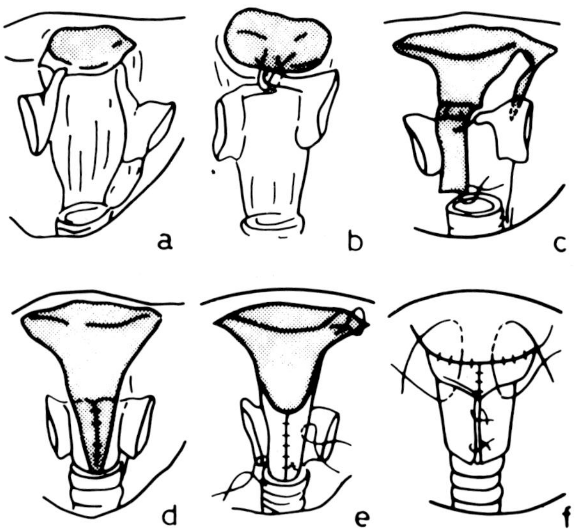

Fig. 1. The reconstructive procedures of the larynx. (a) Superior horns are fractured at their attachment to the thyroid alae. (b) Superior horns are turned inward and their tips are sutured together. (c) The hypopharyngeal mucosal flap is transpositioned toward the inner surface of the new larynx. (d) Posteriorly the margins of the mucosal flaps of the both sides are sutured together. (e) Anterior margins of the flaps are sutured. (f) Thyroid laminae are closed.

diameter of this cavity is approximately 1cm and the vertical length is about 3 cm (Fig. 1E).

The mucous membrance of the new larynx is stitched at several points to the inner surfaces of the remaining lateral halves of the thyroid laminae.

The thyroid laminae are finally sutured together in the midline. The anterior surface of the thyroid cartilage is reinforced with the perichondrium and the anterior cervical muscles (Fig. 1F).

The orifice to the reconstructed larynx opens closely to the lingual base.

By utterance, the contrast media is expired upwards and it vibrates at the level of the narrow slit of the laryngeal ostium.

In swallowing, the contrast media is pushed down by the lingual base and cleared in to the hypopharynx. The lingual base, instead of the epiglottis, touches to the reconstructed posterior laryngeal wall and closes the laryngeal opening.

The laryngoscopic picture reveals a close resemblance to the larynx after supraglottic horizontal partial laryngectomy (Fig. 2). Instead of the arytenoid portion of the normal larynx, the posterior laryngeal wall reconstructed from the superior horns separates the larynx from the hypopharynx.

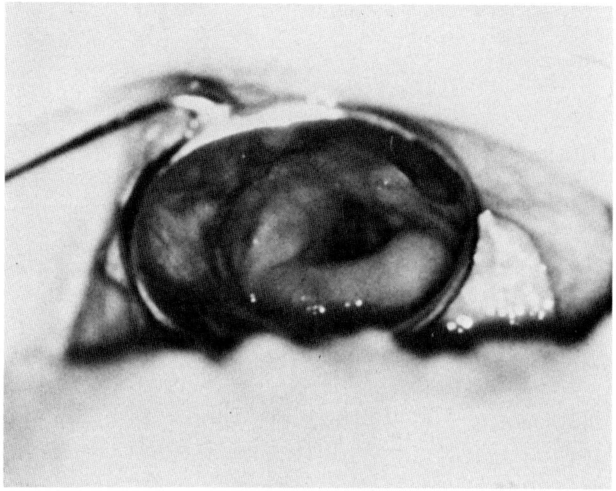

Fig. 2. The laryngoscopic picture of the adequately reconstructed larynx.

The laryngeal opening has a triangular form, the basis of which is about 1–1.5 cm in diameter. Because of the infolding of the rotated mucosal flap, the mucous membrane forms a narrow slit of about 0.7 cm in horizontal length closely below the level of the laryngeal opening. During phonation, vibration of the mucous membrane can be observed exactly at the level of this slit which is thought to be the new glottis.

Here is another example of the reconstructed larynx where the superior horns were sutured side to side to regulate the size of the laryngeal opening (Fig. 3).

The laryngeal opening of Figure 4, is cicatrically narrow because of the postoperative fistula formation.

Since it is expected that the quality of voice produced by a reconstructed larynx is directly related to the physical characteristics of such a larynx, it seems meaningful to study the physical properties of the laryngeal vibrator in each case. Although such physical characteristics of the larynx during phonatory actions are not easily measurable, some parameters can be assessed indirectly from some physiological measures such as air flow and air pressure. The glottal resistance is one of such physical indices of the larynx indirectly derived from the mean volume velocity and the mean subglottal pressure.[6] The values of the mean volume velocity during phonation, the subglottic pressure, and the glottal resistance are shown in Table 1. In

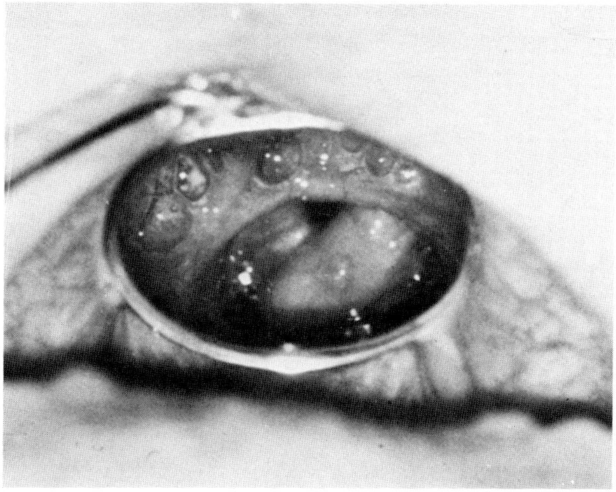

Fig. 3. The reconstructed larynx where the tips of the superior horns were sutured side to side to adjust the length of the posterior laryngeal wall.

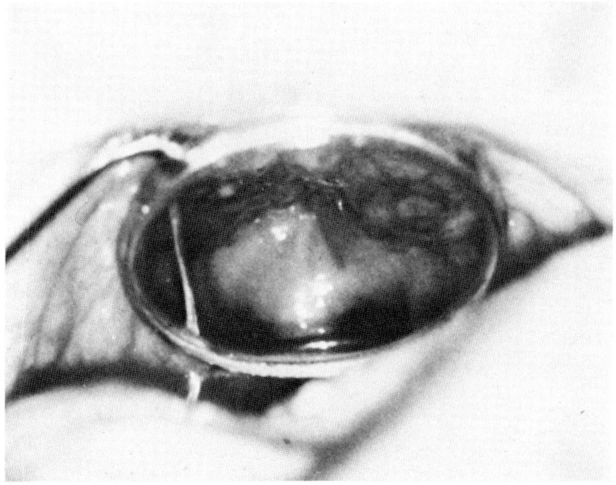

Fig. 4. The narrow opening of the reconstructed larynx as a result of a cicatric healing of the post-operative pharyngeal fistula.

Table 1. The mean volume velocity during phonation, the subglottic pressure and the glottal resistence of the patients undergone primary laryngoplasty and Asai's laryngoplasty

		Flow (cc/sec)	Pressure (cm H_2O)	Resistance (Ω)	Duration (sec)
A. Primary laryngoplasty					
1 T.M.	M.	315	33.7	107	3.4
	S.D.	67.5	1.1	21.5	0.6
2 K.B.	M.	169	30.3	177	1.6
	S.D.	55.5	3.7	82.6	0.4
3 I.K.	M.	86	37.4	435	2.3
	S.D.	16.8	3.4	128.2	0.5
4 O.S.	M.	57	30.4	638	2.5
	S.D.	14.0	4.7	71.0	0.3
B. Asai's laryngoplasty					
1 M.Y.	M.	200?	28.3	141?	2.5
	S.D.		3.4		0.4
2 N.I.	M.	150?	20.2	135?	0.8
	S.D.		3.4		0.1
C. Normal value					
	M.	100	10	100	>2.0
	S.D.				

the cases 1 and 2 the larynx was built adequately as shown in Figures 3 and 4. In cases 3 and 4, the laryngeal opening was narrow because of the cicatrical healing of the postoperative fistula.

The subglottic pressure was three times as high as the normal value. The cause of the high subglottic pressure may be explained by the fact that the new larynx is a narrow tube covered anteriorly by the thyroid lamina. During phonation, the laryngeal cavity can expand backward only where the mucous membrane touches to the hypopharynx.

Table 2. The articulation score in percent in the cases of hemilaryngectomy, subtotal pharyngolaryngectomy and primary laryngectomy

Case No.	u	o	a	e	i	mean
1 Primary laryngoplasty	76	92	100	100	56	85
2 Primary laryngoplasty	100	76	92	64	100	86
3 Asai's laryngoplasty	64	84	100	100	64	82
4 Subtotal laryngectomy	36	96	100	100	88	84
5 Subtotal laryngectomy	100	100	100	100	92	98
6 Subtotal pharyngolaryngectomy	32	96	100	100	28	71
7 Vertical hemilaryngectomy	80	100	100	100	76	91

In the case where the larynx was built adequately the glottal resistance was close to the value of normal subjects.

To give a sort of quantitative evaluation of speech quality, the results of the vowel listing test are summarized in Table 2. The mean articulation scores, which are shown in the right column, varied considerably from patient to patient.

Compared with the voice resulted from a various types of conservation surgeries such as vertical hemilaryngectomy, subtotal laryngectomy, and subtotal pharyngolaryngectomy,[5] it can be said that the reconstructive procedure presented here is one of the surgeries which can produce a usable voice after total removal of the larynx.

A negligible amount of the contrast media stays in the supraglottic space during the first phase of swallowing and is aspirated into trachea in the second phase of deglutition. This phenomenon is similar to the behavior observed after supraglottic horizontal partial laryngectomy in which case the epiglottis is removed and the vocal cords are facing to the pharyngeal cavity. Another chance of aspiration of liquid exists during the inspiration of the air after swallowing. Following the passage of the contrast media in to the hypopharynx, the lingual base returns upward and the patient inspires air though the tracheostoma. With the action of inspiration, the contrast media remaining in the pyriform sinus is sucked down into trachea through the laryngeal cavity. This type of aspiration is generally seen in patients having an open tracheostoma. These patients learn to avoid the aspiration by pushing the air upward to the glottis by themselves.

Based on our experiences in this operation it may be concluded that the primary laryngoplasty is one of the best procedures at present day in order to preserve vocal function without sacrificing the curability of surgery for the extended laryngeal malignancy.

References

1. Asai R: Asai's new voice production method. Substitution for human speech. Proc. VIII Int Congr Otorhinolaryngol Tokyo p 730, 1965
2. Iwai H: Subtotal laryngectomy. Arch klin exp Ohr-Nas-u Kehlk-Heilk 197:85, 1970
3. Ieai H: Limitation of conservation surgery in the carcinoma involvling the arytenoid. Can J Otolaryng (in press)
4. Iwai H: Primary Laryngoplasty. Arch Oto-Rhino-Laryng 206:1, 1973
5. Iwai H: Subtotal pharyngolaryngectomy: conservation surgery for carcinoma of sinus pyriformus extending toward the larynx. Arch Oto-Rhino-Laryng (in press)
6. Rothenbery M: The breath-stream dynamics of simple-released-plosive production. Bibl phonet (Basel) 6:1, 1968

Laryngeal Reinnervation: The Nerve-Muscle Pedicle Technique

Harvey M. Tucker, Cleveland, Ohio

Because the presently employed surgical procedures for the management of bilateral vocal cord paralysis[1–5] all sacrifice remaining voice at least to some degree in providing an acceptable airway, researchers have attempted to reinnervate the larynx by various means.[6–10] Those techniques which involve nerve anastomosis have generally yielded less than ideal return of function due to loss of nerve fiber population, neuroma formation and, most important, because of reinnervation of abductor motor units by abductor fibers and vice versa, resulting in dyssynergia and inappropriate vocal cord motion. Recent work[9,10] has shown that the problem of crossed reinnervation can be avoided by reinnervating only the posterior cricoary tenoid muscle. When successful, this approach provides good abduction and depends upon mass action and remaining tension in the cricothyroideus to return the cord to the paramedian or midline position. In at least one human case,[11] reimplantation of avulsed recurrent laryngeal nerves resulted in restoration of adequate abduction. The remaining problem with these proposed methods lies in their dependence on the use of the cut end of the phrenic, recurrent or portions of the vagus nerve itself as the source of reinnervation. Since the nerve to be used in each of these techniques is transected, retrograde degeneration must take place before regeneration and subsequent restoration of abduction can occur. Thus, there is usually a six to nine month delay between surgery and return of function of the vocal cord. Furthermore, the use of the phrenic nerve results in paralysis of the hemidiaphragm, which is not always well tolerated, particularly in older patients.

In an effort to overcome these problems, we developed the nerve-muscle pedicle technique for reinnervation in 1970. This procedure dealt with reinnervation of a transplanted canine larynx using a pedicle derived from the recipient animal's recurrent laryngeal nerve and a small portion of the laryngeal musculature from the point where the nerve entered the larynx.[12,13] Reinnervation was achieved within two to six weeks and at least fifty percent of normal cord function was restored in all animals. The rapidity of reinnervation was shown to be due to the need to wait only for sufficient healing to take place between the muscle of the pedicle and the recipient bed to allow propagation of a nerve impulse from the intact nerve. The delay and loss of nerve fiber population due to degeneration was avoided since the nerve itself was not cut. This technique was modified to permit its application to cases of bilateral vocal cord paralysis in 1972.[14] In this approach a nerve-muscle pedicle was fashioned from a branch of the ansa hypoglossi to one of the strap muscles and then transposed into an incision made in the posterior cricoarytenoid muscle. Inasmuch as the strap muscles are accessory muscles of respiration, which exhibit EMG activity during inspiration, this resulted in restoration of abduction, occurring spontaneously during inspiration within six weeks of the procedure. EMG confirmed synchronous nerve function and the dogs were able to tolerate transection of the remaining recurrent laryngeal nerve without the need for tracheotomy. In a later experiment[15] it was demonstrated that at least six months could elapse between denervation and successful reinnervation by this technique. Since the function of one strap muscle is readily expendable and since the nerve does not undergo degeneration in this procedure, both of the problems inherent in the techniques that involve implantation of cut ends of other cervical nerves are avoided. This operation is now being employed in human volunteers suffering from uncorrected bilateral vocal cord paralysis at The Upstate Medical Center on an experimental basis.

Indications and Contraindications

The procedure is indicated in patients with bilateral vocal cord paralysis in whom airway is inadequate for reasonable day-to-day exercise tolerance and in whom it is desirable to preserve remaining voice. It is necessary that at least one arytenoid cartilage be passively mobile. Therefore, previous unilateral, unsuccessful arytenoidectomy or arytenoid mobilization is not a contraindication to the procedure. Contraindications include: (1) bilateral arytenoid fixation, (2) neurologic or local conditions that interfere with normal nerve function of the ansa hypoglossi and its branches, (3) other uncorrectable stenoses or laryngotracheal injuries that preclude eventual decannulation, and (4) inability to tolerate the surgery on medical grounds. Length of time of paralysis is not, in itself, a contraindication to attempted reinnervation, as will be seen from our results.

Technique[16]

Suspension laryngoscopy is performed under light general anesthesia. After examination confirms bilateral nonfunction of the vocal cords, both arytenoids are palpated to ascertain that at least one is passively mobile. The laryngoscope is then removed and the neck prepared for sterile surgery. If both cords are passively mobile, the left side is used routinely. An oblique incision is made along the anterior border of the sternocleidomastoid muscle, through skin, subcutaneous fat and platysma muscle. The anterior border of the sternocleidomastoid muscle is mobilized and retracted to expose the anterior belly of the omohyoid muscle and the lateral surface of the jugular vein. The posterior limb of the ansa hypoglossi can be identified as it lies upon the jugular vein (Fig. 1). This is very carefully dissected inferiorly until both the anterior and posterior limbs and several branches are seen. Usually, the two most anteriorly placed branches innervate the anterior belly of the omohyoid muscle. When these structures have been identified and carefully mobilized a nerve tester is used to demonstrate contraction of the anterior belly of the omohyoid muscle. If for some reason this branch is unavailable, any other branch to the strap muscle will serve. Stay sutures of 5-0 or 6-0 nylon are placed in the muscle on either side of the point where the nerve enters. Using these as retractors, a block of muscle measuring approximately 3–4 mm square is cut from the omohyoid, containing the point of entry of the appropriate nerve branch (Fig. 2). Care is taken in mobilizing the pedicle not to injure the vasa nervorum, which are usually quite readily seen on the surface of the nerve. Once freed, the pedicle is laid gently back in place and protected with a wet sponge. The lateral border of the thyroid cartilage is identified, retracted, and the inferior constrictor muscle fibers are incised along it. This exposes the mucosa of the pyriform sinus, which is carefully reflected with a "peanut" dissector, thus exposing the posterolateral aspect of the cricoid lamina and the fibers of the posterior cricoarytenoid muscle. These fibers will be noted to pass from inferior and medial to superior and lateral. Using a knife, the fibers of this muscle are incised part way through so that they "pout" open somewhat. The previously prepared nerve-muscle pedicle is transposed into position and sutured into place using the nylon stay sutures (Fig. 3). An additional two or three fine nylon sutures can usually be added at this time. It has been possible in all cases done to date to reach the posterior cricoarytenoid muscle without tension on the pedicle. If necessary, the remaining inferior branches of the ansa hypoglossi to the other strap muscles could be severed to gain greater mobility of the pedicle. The larynx is allowed to rotate into its normal position and the sternocleidomastoid muscle is sutured into place after placement of a penrose drain. The skin incision is closed in the usual fashion. The drain is generally removed after 24–48 hr. No antibiotics are used and the patient may be fed the morning after surgery.

Results

This procedure has been performed, at the time of this writing, in ten patients, in whom follow-up is

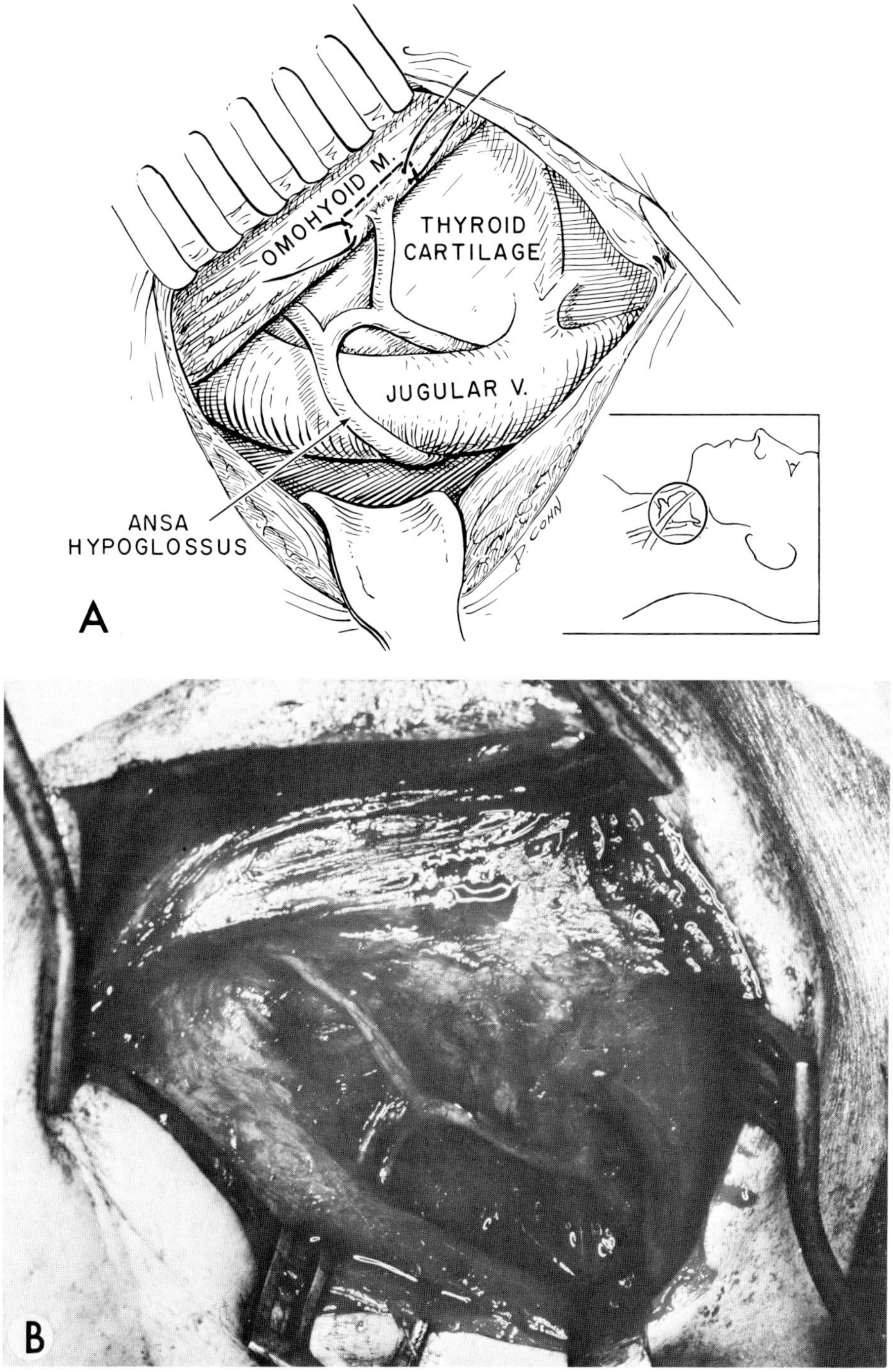

Fig. 1. A,B Ansa hypoglossi nerve exposed on surface of jugular vein.

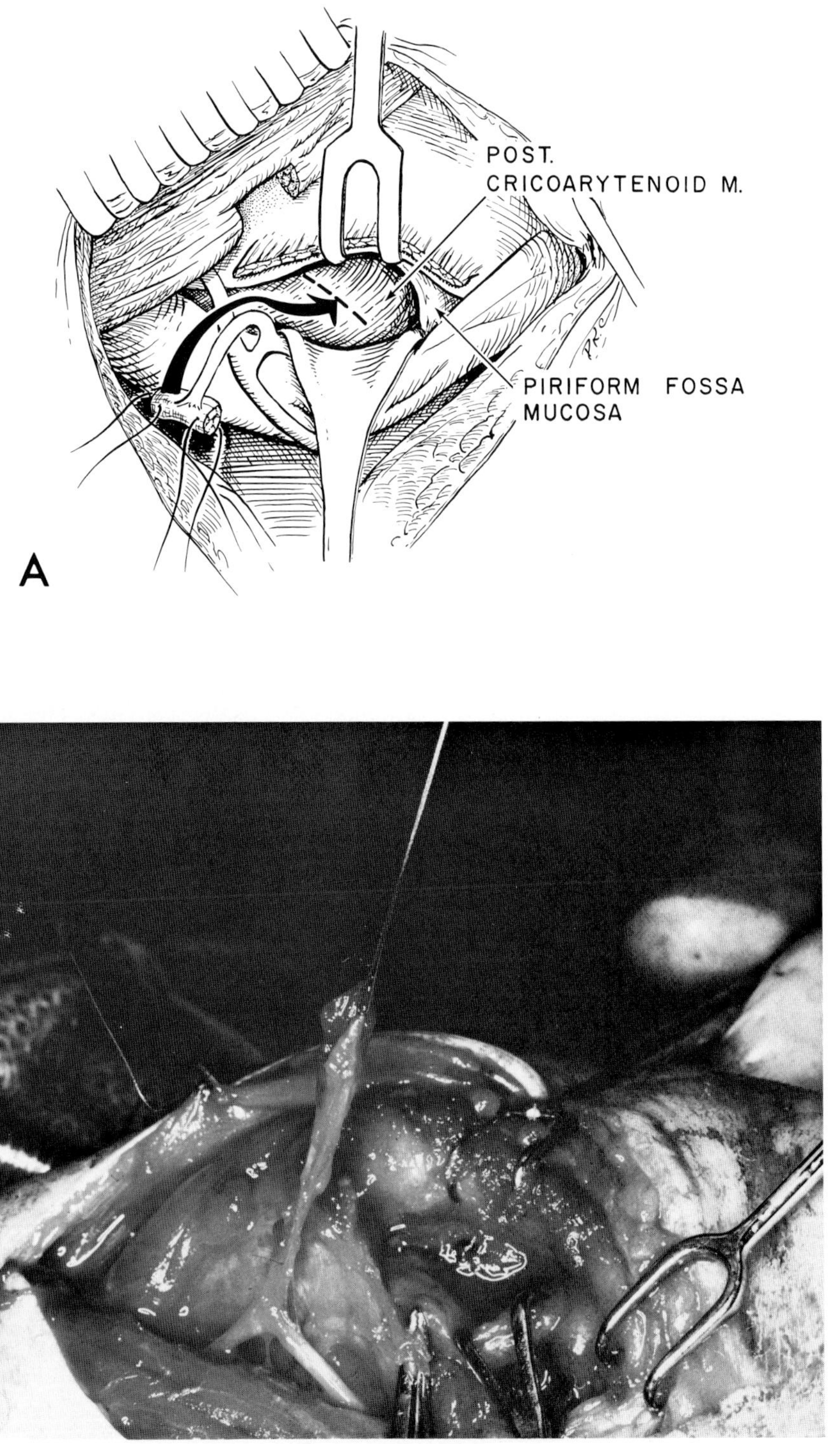

Fig. 2. A,B Nerve muscle pedicle prepared. Note nylon stay sutures.

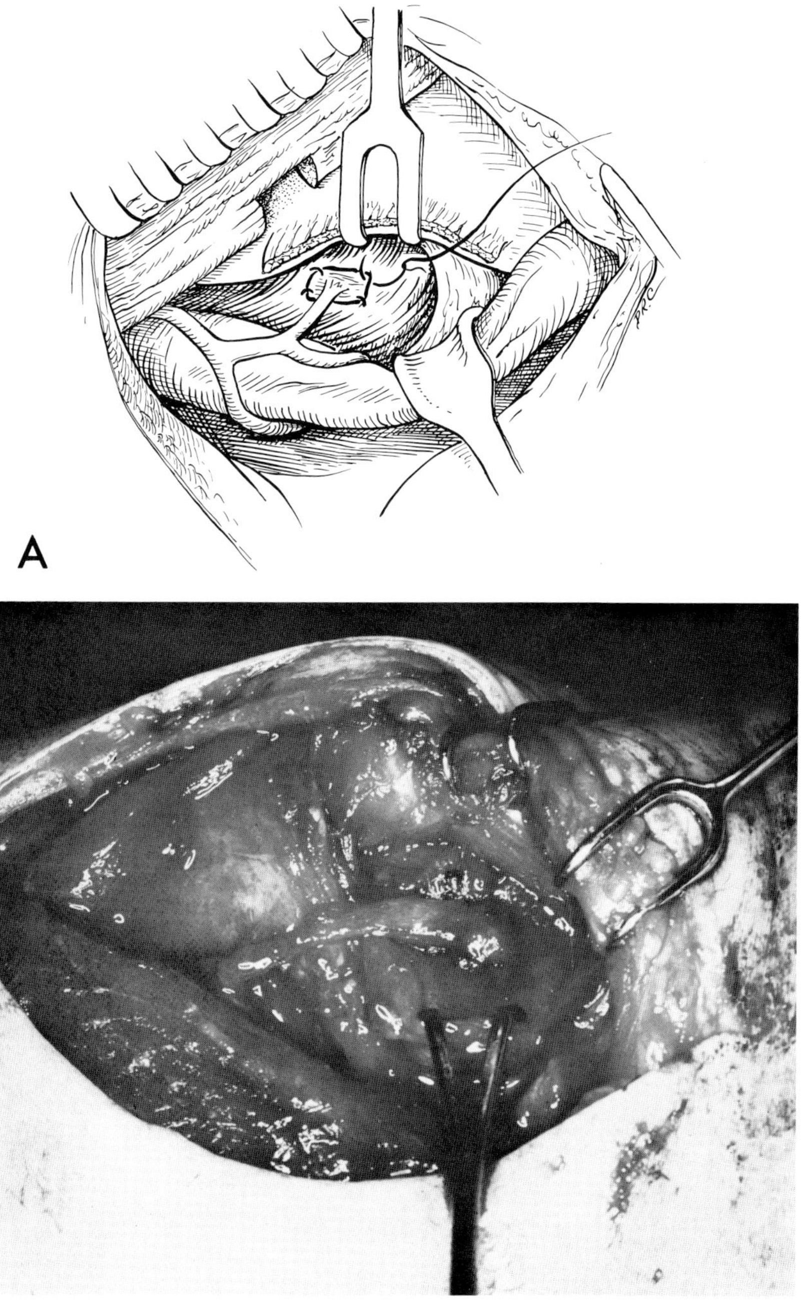

Fig. 3. A,B Nerve muscle pedicle sutured into posterior cricoarytenoid muscle.

of sufficient length in eight to evaluate success or failure. Length of paralysis varied from 7 months to 51 years. In all eight, active abduction of the reinnervated vocal cord has been restored within six to eight weeks of surgery (Table 1). In six of these, resultant airway has been adequate for daily activities without the need for tracheotomy and without further deterioration of voice from that which existed before the procedure. Of the remaining two, one has good vocal cord function but is still awaiting repair of a subglottic stenosis sustained in the same accident that produced the paralysis. In one patient who had been observed to have return of abduction such that he could tolerate a

Table 1. Human Laryngeal Reinnervation: The Nerve-Muscle Pedicle Technique

Patient number	Time paralyzed	Time to return of function postsurgery	Follow-up	Results initial	Results present
1	7 mo	6 weeks	3 yr	+	−
2	14 mo	8 weeks	2 yr	+	+
3	36 mo	8 weeks	2 yr	+	+
4	3.5 yr	6 weeks	1 yr	+	+
5	22 yr	8 weeks	10 mo	+	+
6	10 mo	8 weeks	6 mo	+	+
7	51 yr	8 weeks	4 mo	+	+
8	7 mo	6 weeks	4 mo	+	+

continually corked tracheotomy tube for over three months, a subsequent bout of influenza and pneumonia resulted in loss of cord function. At that point, an arytenoidectomy was performed via the same incision at the patient's request, without waiting for possible spontaneous return of function.

Discussion

Although the number of patients operated upon has been small, it would appear that this procedure can be applied successfully in most cases of bilateral vocal cord paralysis that now are managed either by arytenoidectomy or by permanent tracheotomy, without the need to accept either a poor airway or further deterioration of the remaining voice. In successful cases, it might even be possible to *improve* the voice with subsequent Teflon injections into the remaining paralyzed cord.

Because this technique does not result in fixation of the arytenoid and does not require manipulation of or further damage to the recurrent laryngeal nerves, it could be considered for immediate use in cases of bilateral paralysis due, for example, to trauma, since it would not interfere with subsequent spontaneous return of function, should such occur. On the other hand, length of time that paralysis has persisted does not appear to preclude attempting this procedure. Our results seem to bear out clinically the recent electron microscopic studies that indicate survival of significant numbers of viable muscle fibers even after prolonged paralysis.[17]

Conclusion

The nerve-muscle pedicle technique for reinnervation of paralyzed vocal cords has been successfully applied in humans. It appears to avoid most of the difficulties encountered in other approaches to this problem. It could be considered for immediate use in cases of bilateral vocal cord paralysis secondary to trauma.

References

1. King BT: A new and function-restoring operation for bilateral abductor cord paralysis. Preliminary report. JAMA 112:814–823, 1939
2. Woodman G: A modification of the extralaryngeal approach to arytenoidectomy for bilateral abductor paralysis. Arch Otol 43:63–65, 1946
3. Thornell W: Transoral intralaryngeal approach for arytenoidectomy in bilateral vocal cord paralysis with inadequate airway. Ann Otol 66:364–368, 1957
4. Montgomery W: Cricoarytenoid arthrodesis. Ann Otol 70:451–462, 1961
5. Loré JM: An atlas of head and neck surgery. Philadelphia, W. B. Saunders Company, 1962
6. Miehlke A: Rehabilitation of vocal cord paralysis. Arch Otol 100:431–441, 1974
7. Doyle PJ et al: Results of the surgical section and repair of the recurrent laryngeal nerve. Laryngoscope 77:1245–1254, 1967
8. Murakami Y, Kirchner JA: Vocal cord abduction by regenerated recurrent laryngeal nerve: An experimental study in the dog. Arch Otol 94:64–68, 1971
9. Taggart JP: Laryngeal reinnervation by phrenic nerve implantation in dogs. Laryngoscope 81:1330–1336, 1971

10. Fex S: Functional remobilization of vocal cords in cats with permanent recurrent laryngeal nerve paresis. Acta Otol 97:291, 1973
11. Miglets AW: Functional laryngeal abduction following reimplantation of the recurrent laryngeal nerves. Laryngoscope 84:1996–2005, 1974
12. Tucker HM, Harvey JE, Ogura JH: Vocal cord remobilization in the canine larynx. Arch Otol 92:530–533, 1970
13. Tucker HM, Ogura JH: Vocal cord remobilization in the canine larynx: An histological evaluation. Laryngoscope 81:1602–1606, 1971
14. Hengerer AS, Tucker HM: Restoration of abduction in the paralyzed canine larynx. Arch Otol 97:247–250, 1973
15. Lyons R, Tucker HM: Delayed restoration of abduction in the paralyzed canine vocal cord. Arch Otol 100:176–179, 1974
16. Tucker HM: Human laryngeal reinnervation. Laryngoscope, in press, 1975
17. Conley J, Hamaker RC, Donnenfeld H: Long-standing facial paralysis rehabilitation. Laryngoscope 84:2155–2162, 1974

Laryngoplasty for the Transsexual

Richard L. Goode, Donald Laub and
F. Mark Rafaty, Stanford, California

In recent years, a new area of plastic surgery interest has developed—surgical rehabilitation of the transsexual. These individuals have the physical characteristics of one sex, but the psychologic makeup of the other and wish to change gender. Surgical therapy is only part of the transformation process which includes extensive psychiatric evaluation, counseling and endocrine therapy.

Laryngoplasty, or thyroid cartilage shave, is part of the surgical transformation from male to female, since a prominent "Adam's apple," a male secondary sex characteristic, is disconcerting to these patients in their new female role. The psychological effect of reducing this structure is usually more significant than the anatomic change. This paper will describe a technique for removal of the thyroid cartilage prominence in transsexuals, based on experience in twelve cases.

Under local anesthesia, a horizontal incision 4-cm long is made either above or below the laryngeal prominence, ideally in a preexisting skin crease. The incision is carried down through the platysma and a skin flap elevated so the prominence is exposed. The investing layer of the deep cervical fascia is incised vertically in the midline; the paired sternohyoid muscles are separated and retracted laterally along with the thyrohyoid muscles. The thyroid cartilage is stabilized with a skin hook and the thyroid cartilage eminence shaved down using a large scalpel until a flat laryngeal profile is achieved (Fig. 1A, B). Cartilage excision is performed only in the upper one-half of the thyroid cartilage to avoid the vocal cords; care is taken to avoid entry into the larynx. After hemostasis is obtained, the sternohyoid muscles are closed in the midline with absorbable 4-0 sutures. The skin is closed with subcutaneous 5-0 chromic sutures and 6-0 nylon skin sutures. A pressure dressing is applied; drains are not routinely used. The patient is observed overnight for any signs of airway obstruction or hematoma. The skin sutures are removed five days later.

The only complication in this series was inadvertent entry into the vallecula in one case. The opening was closed with an absorbable chromic suture without further problem. No change in voice occurred in our series, but one case of persistent hoarseness following thyroid cartilage shave has been reported.

The procedure should be considered in male to female transformation surgery as part of a total transsexual rehabilitation program.

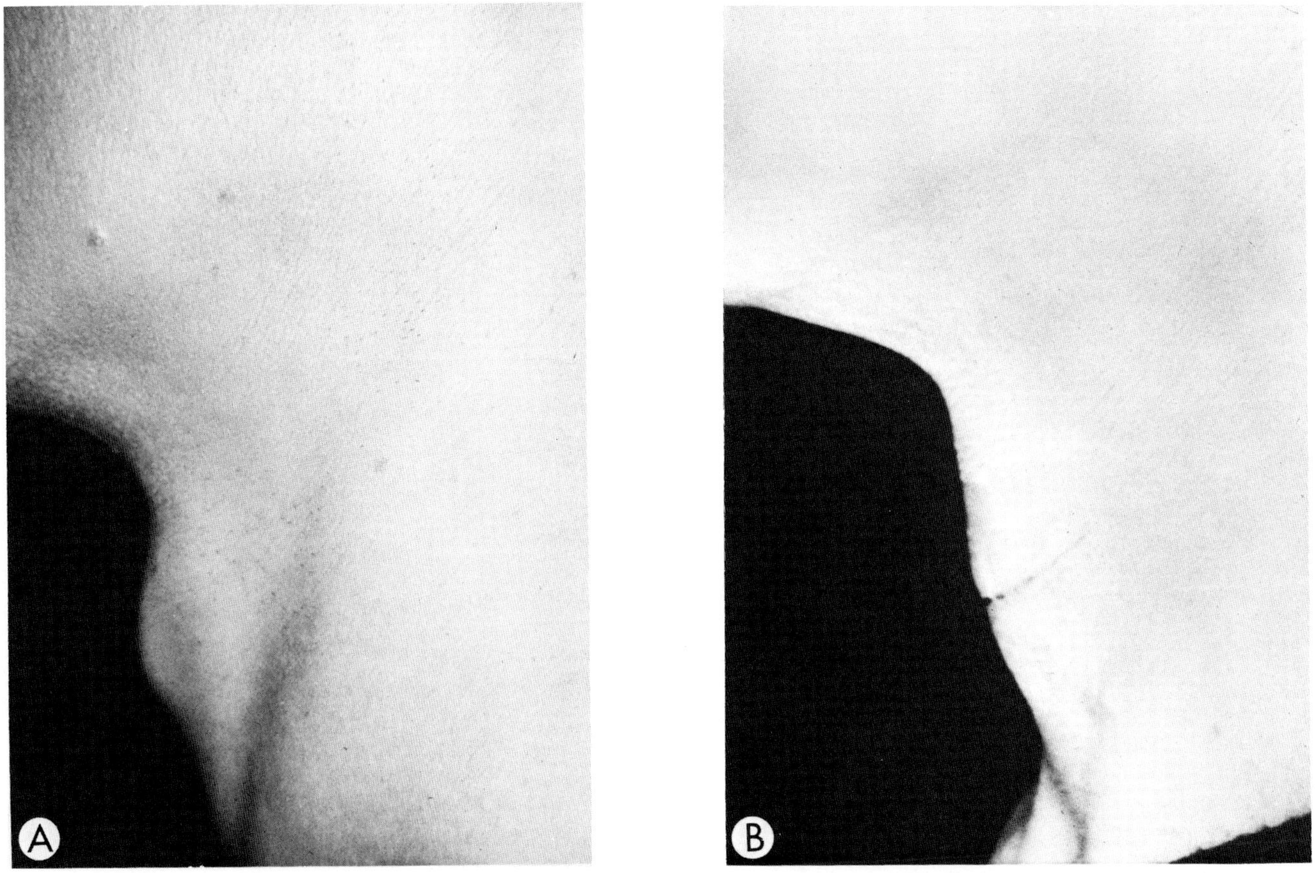

Fig. 1. *(A) A typical male Adam's apple. (B) The same patient, one week following surgery showing the new laryngeal profile.*

Plastic Surgery of the Trachea and of Head and Neck After Tumor Resection With Preliminary Report of Total Reconstruction of the Larynx

R. Meyer and U.K. Kesselring Lausanne, Switzerland

Plastic Surgery of the Trachea

Since 1959 we have developed seven procedures of surgical therapy which can be used besides the segmental resection and anastomoses. We began with a one-stage technique[1-3] consisting in the amplification of the mucus tube of the trachea by means of interposition of a spindle-shaped mucus graft at the posterior wall. Two pedicle flaps of the mucus membrane are previously dissected free from the fibrocartilaginous mantle on both sides of the trachea and pulled forward in order to leave posteriorly the elliptic raw surface to be covered by the graft. The bipedicle flaps are sutured together in the anterior median line. The external fibrocartilaginous tube has now to be adapted to the new calibre of the enlarged mucus tube and for this purpose we interpose a costal cartilage graft between the anterior borders of the opened fibrocartilaginous mantle (Fig. 1). We have operated on 34 patients with this technique by cervical approach with or without sternotomy and one at the level of the bifurcation through lateral thoracotomy in collaboration with thoracic surgeons.

A second method[4,5] which we use finds its indication in the laryngotracheal stenoses or in the more extensive tracheal stenoses with important loss of the mucus membrane. It concerns a two-stage procedure which can be applied only in the cervical part of the trachea. At the first stage we open to a maximum the stenotic segment and after having mobilized the lateral walls we perform a tracheopexy by means of percutaneous mattress sutures.

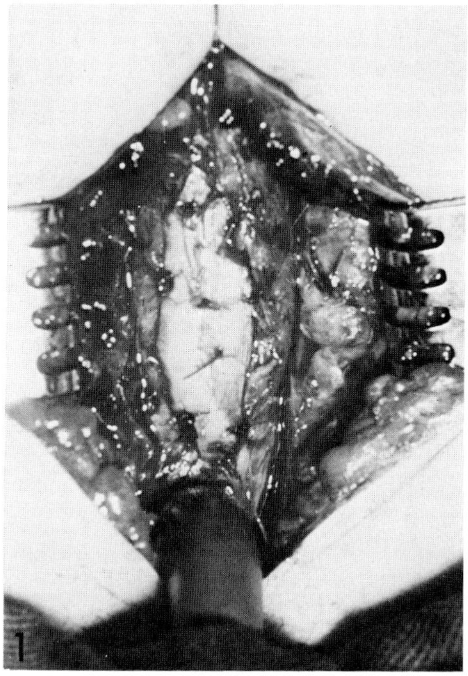
1

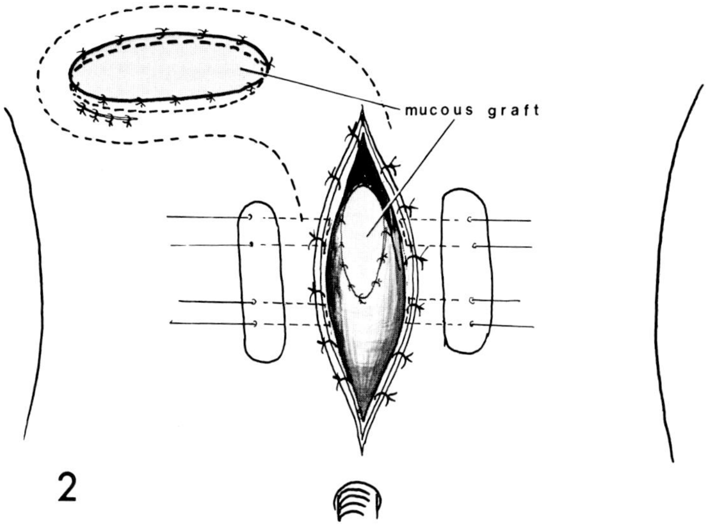

2

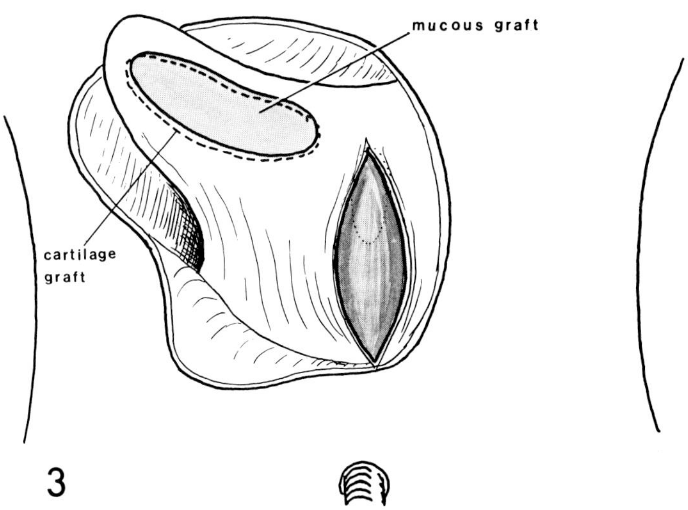

3

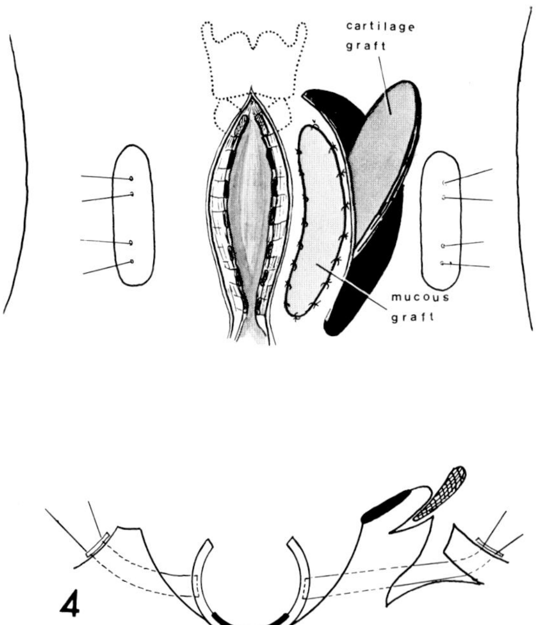

4

Figs. 1–4. See text.

The edge of the mucus membrane is then sutured to the skin border and if after resection of scarred tissue in the trachea a too extensive area of the tracheal or laryngotracheal wall remains raw, we have to cover it by a buccal mucosal flap. In the same session we prepare a direct flap on the adjacent cervical skin which will serve as cover for the open trachea. For this purpose we suture another rhombic mucus graft on a previously deepithelized skin area lateral to the tracheal gap at the level of its superior angle. In the same region we make a subcutaneous pocket where we insert a concave coffin-lid-shaped cartilage graft from the rib as support for the future covering flap (Fig. 2).

At the second stage the flap is outlined, being based at the proximal extremity of the open tracheal or laryngotracheal segment. It is cut in a way that incorporates the mucosal and the cartilage graft. A strip of skin around the mucosal flap is deepithelized and the flap is turned in order to cover the tracheal gap and the edges of the mucus graft are adapted with a few sutures to the borders of the tracheal mucosa (Fig. 3). Stiffened by the cartilage graft the new anterior wall cannot collapse. Even after the second operation we can again insert a splint which is then anchored through the tracheal wall and the skin.

In easier cases we prepare a similar composite flap in the zone adjacent to the tracheal window and close the opening like putting the lid on a box. This flap is usually prepared and brought down in a two-stage procedure as well as the formerly described. It can however even be raised and sutured in place in one stage in particular cases (Fig. 4).

It is easy to place a luminal splint into the trachea when it is still open. But when such an internal constriction or prolonged postoperative dilatation becomes necessary once the trachea is already closed surgically, the plastic tube has to be inserted with the aid of a bronchoscope and held in place with a Reverdin needle piercing through the skin and the trachea.

In cases where the tracheal wall collapsed or in cases of tracheomalacia for about ten years we have been using a method of extension of the lumen without opening the trachea. The technique consists in placing and fixing two or three concave cartilage grafts from the rib to the external wall of the trachea in order to effect a lateral or anterior tracheopexy.

More and more we combine this procedure with the use of an internal luminal splint. With these plastic surgical techniques we have actually at our disposal enough methods to face nearly every kind of tracheal or laryngotracheal stenoses which cannot be treated by segmental resection and end-to-end-anastomosis.

In tumor cases or in cases of circumscript prominence we have to cut out a round or elliptic full thickness piece of the wall of the trachea. Then the method of choice is to fill the parietal defect with a composite graft of mucosa and cartilage from the whole cartilaginous nasal septum according to Wilflingseder.[6] The mucoperichondrium of one side of the septum is left intact in order to avoid a septal perforation. The composite graft is sutured to the borders of the tracheal gap in two layers and covered externally with a muscle flap of the neighbourhood (Fig. 5). With these different procedures we can manage practically all stenoses in the cervical segment of the trachea where treatment by resection and end-to-end anastomosis fails.

Plastic Surgery of Head and Neck after Tumor Resection

Extensive carcinomas of the oral cavity are mainly treated by composite operations. Many superradical ablative procedures as well as immediate or delayed methods of repair have been used for intraoral malignancy involving the different structures of the mouth.

These malignant growths are sometimes difficult to define in an anatomical classification since they invade frequently multiple sites by direct extension. Carcinoma of the tongue may extend to the floor of the mouth and by further growth reach the gingiva, the alveolus of the mandible and the mucosa of the jaw. Reconstructive surgery after extensive "en bloc" ablation of the involved structures (partial or total glossectomy with hemimandibulectomy and neck dissection) is complex and usually requires more than one intervention. Concerning the functional and aesthetic rehabilitation some problems are still unsolved.

The function of the tongue is a much more basic and biological one than speech for also the factors of chewing, sucking, and swallowing are impaired as a result of glossectomy. For this reason

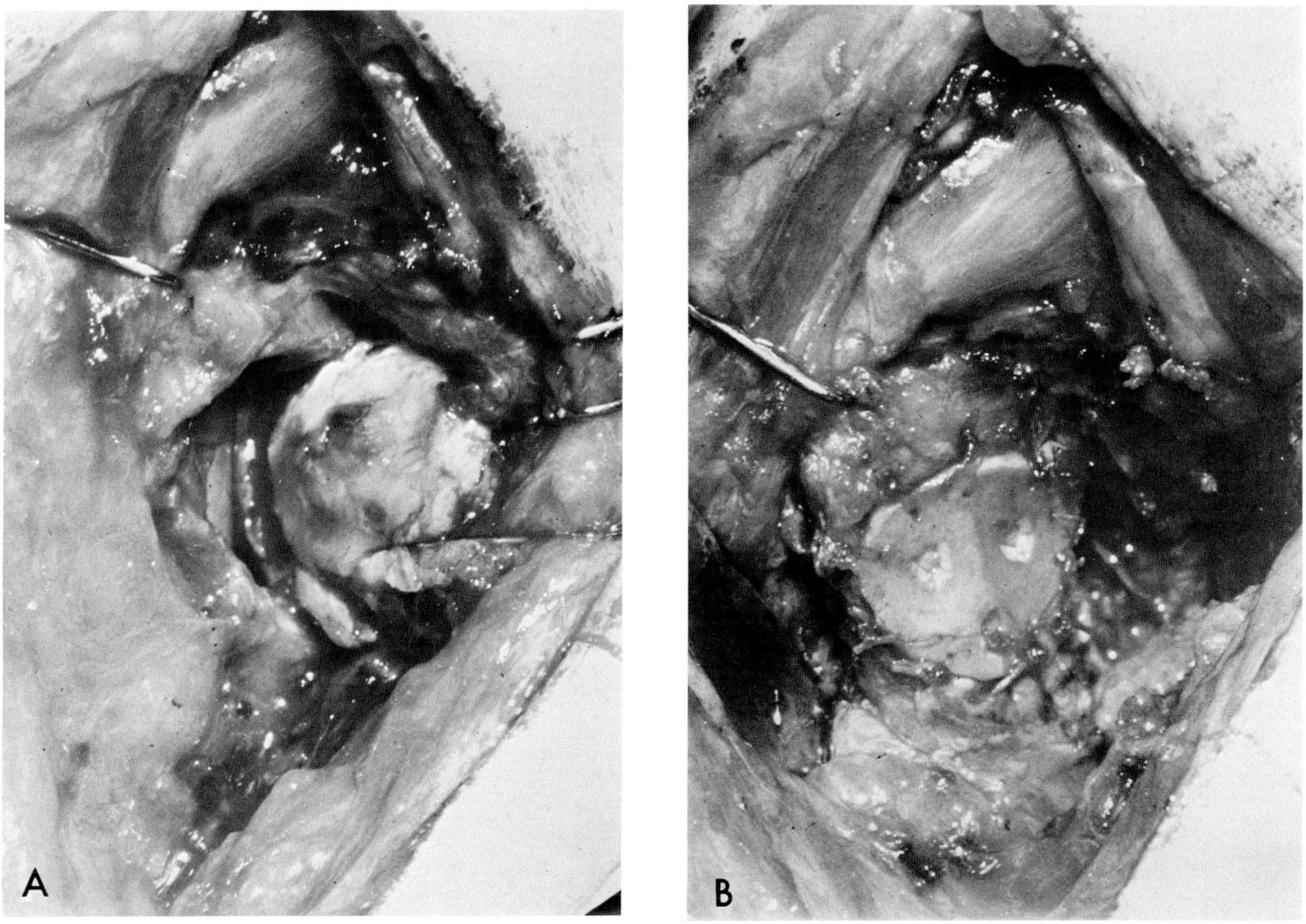

Fig. 5. (A) The tumor about to be resected with the lateral posterior wall. (B) The defect covered with a composite graft from the nasal septum.

we think that an immediate primary provisional repair is important not only for the life of the patient but—just as important—for the quality of survival.

Usually we distinguish between tumors of the movable part of the tongue and tumors of the base of the tongue. Resections of the former present no technical difficulties and in general only lead to difficulties in articulating and chewing. Radical resections of tumors situated at the base of the tongue include all the adjacent tissues and the epiglottis with additional impairment of deglutition and sometimes even breathing. Such operations require therefore always tracheotomy and often pharyngostomy. Some time after the operation substitute mechanisms take over the role of the sacrified epiglottis and also phonation becomes possible after closure of the tracheostoma. But the chief complaints of the patient remain continuous and uncontrolled salivation, inability to swallow solid food, regurgitation of liquids through the nose and unintelligible speech.

A classic procedure was to wait for the secondary definitive reconstruction until all danger of recurrence had passed. This concept has changed somewhat in the last ten years and it has been contested by oncologic and plastic surgeons such as Conley,[7] Edgerton,[8] and others. In our opinion, a patient should be given the chance to lead an acceptable life by replacing the amputated tongue with a substitute that will at least improve mastication and deglutition, sometimes even speech.

For the reconstruction of the anterior part of the tongue, we use either a forehead visor flap (Dufourmentel)[9–11] or a Champion[12] flap. These two procedures are well-known techniques. Although only static operations, the gain of substance is for the patient a considerable help to perform the above-mentioned functions.

If a radical operation en bloc has been performed including partial glossectomy, hemimandibulectomy and neck dissection the resulting defect can be covered primarily with a pectoral flap (Fig. 6A). In order to cover a persisting perforating defect in the former submandibular region (Fig. 6B) and the pharyngobuccostoma we raised a controlateral deltopectoral flap with its distal end duplicated (Fig. 6C). This flap did not only serve as coverage for the above mentioned defects (Fig. 6D) but could also be used to reconstruct the missing soft tissues of the cheek, the partially amputated tongue and the sinus piriformis (Fig. 6E,F).

In cases of more extensive tumour growth where the entire tongue has to be sacrified, accompanied as well by subtotal or total mandibulectomy and neck dissection, we have the opportunity to reconstruct the tongue.

Figure 7 (A,B) show how in such a case the incisions are planned and how the en bloc resection is carried out. A privisional pectoral flap provides the primary coverage of the defect (Fig. 7C). Some 12 months later an abdominobrachial flap plus iliac bone grafts are used in a first step to reconstruct the missing lower third of the face (Fig. 7D). A forehead visor flap (Fig. 7E) is now carried down and it furnishes tissue for lip reconstruction and tongue reconstruction (Table 1), the latter being made out of the two united pedicles of the visor flap after having been severed very near their base. The last two parts of the figure (Fig. 7F,G) show the visor flap sutured to the future lower lip and the final result with the clearly visible tongue which—although practically not actively movable—is appreciated by the patient as a help in deglutition.

If only the base of the tongue has to be reconstructed, we prefer the skin-muscle flap described by Bakamjian.[13]

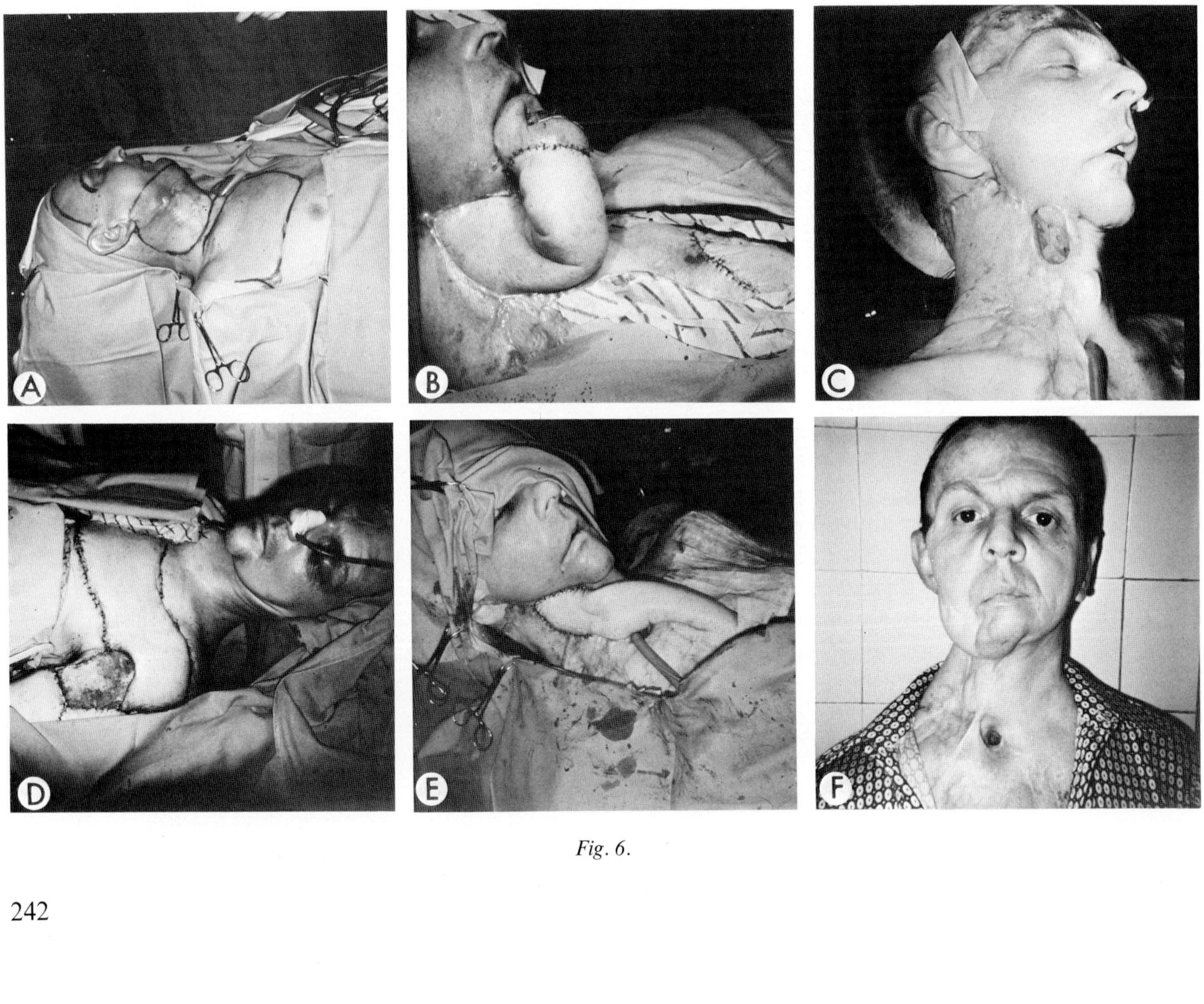

Fig. 6.

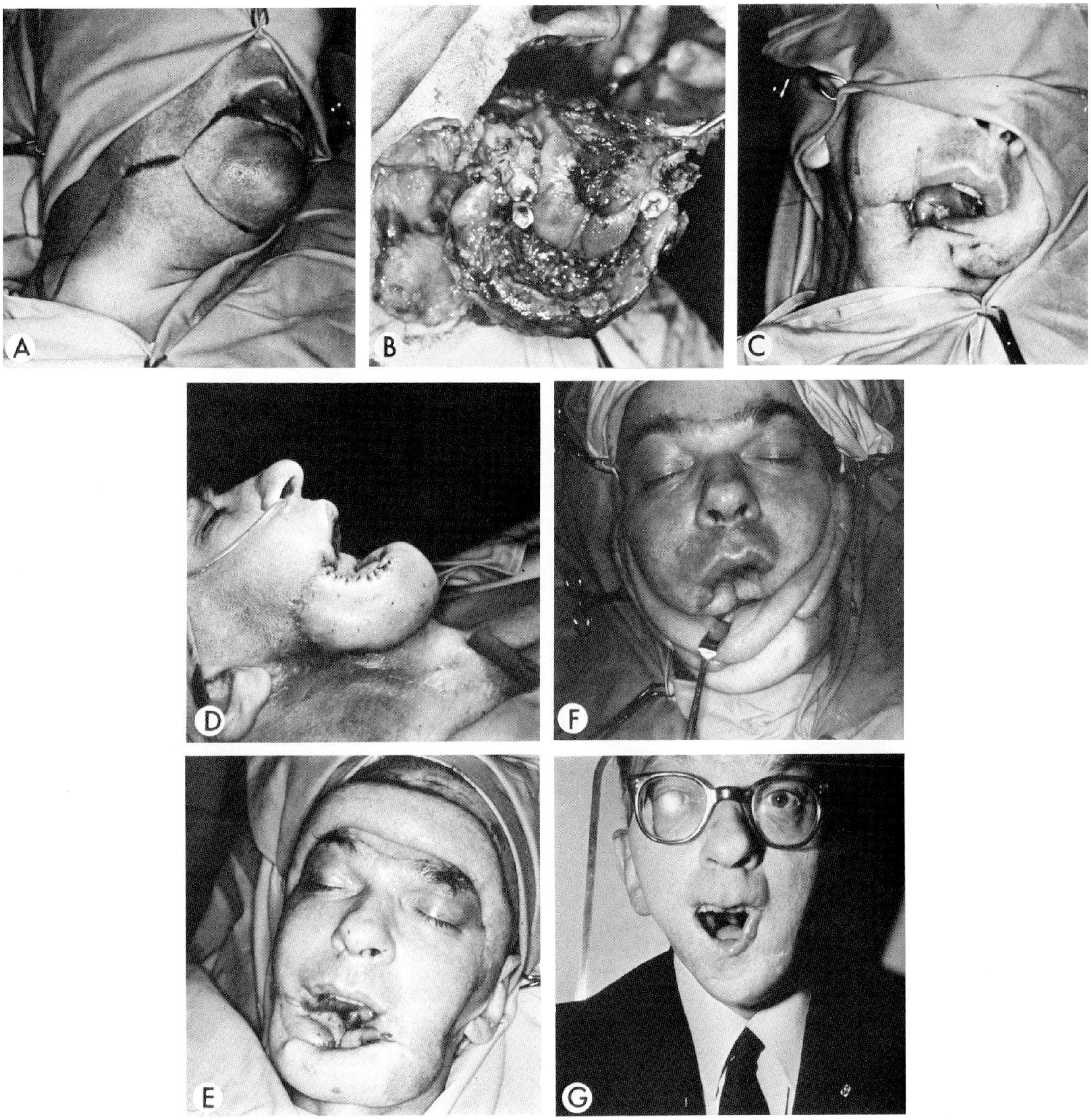

Fig. 7.

Total Reconstruction of the Larynx and the Upper Trachea

The technique was developed from other reconstructive methods for surgical treatment of laryngotracheal and tracheal stenosis and for repair of tracheal wall after tumor resection, as described above, and from reparative procedures after ablative head and neck tumor surgery.

We hope to succeed in adopting the same or similar procedures for the reconstruction of the larynx also in laryngectomized patients and to develop valuable operative techniques for more extensive surgery in the middle tract of the airways where resections and anastomoses are not possible.

Table 1

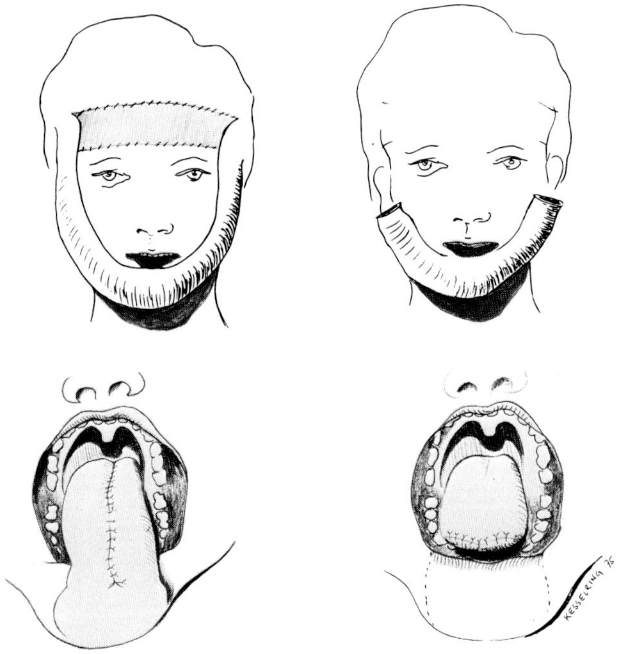

In a case of total destruction of all the cartilaginous structures of the larynx and the cricoid by overirradiation of a struma maligna Langhans with secondary total necrosis of the larynx where only a strip of mucosa without contour of vocal cords was present, we succeeded in reconstructing the whole larynx and the upper part of the trachea.

Similar to the above-mentioned procedures we prepared a composite flap with mucosa and cartilage on the right side of the neck. In a second operation two oval cartilage struts from the 7th and 8th rib were placed on either side of the defect beneath the skin forming two vertical dams with a groove inbetween. At the same time the prepared flap was turned onto the upper end of the hollow in order to form part of the future anterior wall. Into the gutter-like groove we placed a Portex tube No. 9 to connect the pharynx at the level of the base of the tongue where only a rudimentary epiglottis was left with the low tracheostoma.

In a third session a deltopectoral flap and a submental flap were brought onto the persisting defect.

In the fourth operation a further composite flap was prepared with a coffin-lid-shaped cartilage implant just beyond the tracheostoma. This armed flap was then used in the fifth session to construct the anterior vault of the neo-larynx. Due to a still quite high, cavinalike bifurcation of trachea and pharynx swallowing is completely functional. The width of the reconstructed segment of the respiratory tract gives an ample respiratory capacity and yet allows a distinctive speech.

References

1. Meyer R: Rekonstruktion des Trachealllumens durch Haut- und Knorpeltransplantation. Pract oto-rhino-laryng 22:161, 1960
2. Meyer R: Behandlung der Trachealstenosen. Arch klin exp Ohr-Nas- u Kehlk Heilk 199:292, 1971
3. Meyer R: La chirurgie de la trachée. Rev méd de la Suisse rom 90:87, 1970
4. Meyer R: New concepts in laryngotracheal reconstruction. Trans Amer Acad Ophthalmol Otolaryngol 76:758, 1972
5. Meyer R: Traitement chirurgical des sténoses trachéales et laryngotrachéales au moyen de greffes et de lambeaux. JFORL 23:409, 1974
6. Wilflingseder P: Tracheal stenosis reconstruction by means of nasal septum graft. Transactions of the 5th International Congress of Plastic and Reconstructive Surgery, p 1219, Butterworths Australia, 1971
7. Conley JJ: Rehabilitation in radical head and neck surgery. New York St J Med 15:224, 1962
8. Edgerton MT, Zovickian A: Reconstruction of the trachea and in infraglottic larynx. Plast Reconstr Surg 13:167, 1964
9. Dufourmentel C, Preaux J: Le bénéfice apporté au traitement des cancers par les greffes et autoplasties. Méd et Hyg 26:549, 1968
10. Meyer R: Plastische Chirurgie bei Verstümmelungen an Kopf und Hals. Helv Chir Acta 37:296, 1970
11. Meyer R: Reconstruction plastique après intervention chirurgicale mutilante de la face et du cou. In: Oncologie chirurgicale. F Saegesser & J Pettavel, Hans Huber Berne, 1971
12. Champion R: Reconstruction of cervical trachea. Brit J Plast Surg 12:259, 1959
13. Bakamjian VY: The reconstructive use of flaps in cancer surgery of the head and neck. In: Reviews in plastic surgery: General plastic and reconstructive surgery. Saad MN, Lichtveld P Excerpta Medica Amsterdam, American Elsevier Publishing Co Inc, New York, 1974

Reconstruction of the Subglottis and Upper Trachea in Pediatric Patients

Robin Cotton, Cincinnati, Ohio and Blair Fearon, Toronto, Canada

The Clinical Problem

The problem of both acquired and congenital subglottic stenosis in infants has been recognized for a long time. Logan Turner[1] writing in 1916 discussed stenosis of the larynx in children following intubation and tracheotomy.

In 1964 Holinger reported that congenital subglottic stenosis formed "the largest single group of congenital laryngeal anomalies requiring tracheotomy under one year of age."[2] The following year McDonald and Stocks[3] advocated the practice of long term intubation for the management of airway problems. Since then the number of cases of subglottic stenosis of the acquired type secondary to long term intubation has increased: these acquired cases of subglottic stenosis form the largest proportion of cases presently seen in clinical practice.

In the past decade, there has been much published data on the surgical correction of such lesions in adults. Judging from the literature, there has been a reluctance to operate on the pediatric patient with similar problems. Lapidot et al[4] have stated that "we have been unable to find a report in the literature which describes a method of reconstruction and subsequent decannulation in the infant or child in his first decade of life with a subglottic stenosis." Grahne,[5] in 1971 seems to be the first in the literature on this subject.

The accepted method of treating laryngotracheal stenosis in this young age group is by a long-term tracheotomy, with or without periodic laryngeal dilation depending on the surgeon's preference. This prevailing attitude is based on two assumptions that the present authors believe to be untrue.

First is the belief that the laryngotracheal complex increases in size as the infant grows with eventual outgrowth of the problem. This disregards the fact that the life of an infant with a severe laryngeal stenosis requiring tracheotomy is indeed tenuous. Despite the best of care, small tracheotomy tubes readily become blocked. Oliver et al[6] have reported a fearful 25 percent mortality with patients handled this way, and this is supported by our own study.[7] It is devastating to witness a child, otherwise recovered from an illness requiring prolonged endotracheal intubation, die from complications of long term tracheotomy necessitated by an iatrogenic subglottic stenosis.

The second assumption is that extensive surgery on the larynx of the growing child will interfere with normal growth producing a "minilarynx." Careful experimental data collected by us in the past four years strongly suggests that this is not the case.[8] These studies support that of Calcaterra et al[9] who report that midline vertical thyrotomy in dogs does not interfere with subsequent laryngeal development and vocal function.

The authors have developed a surgical procedure for infants with severe subglottic stenosis; it has the promise of excellent success and illustrates certain new principles concerning laryngotracheal surgery in this age group. The procedure was developed over a four year period of careful experimental surgery on the African Green monkey.

Principles

Certain principles for surgery on the pediatric laryngotracheal complex have emerged from our experimental and clinical work.

1. Thyrotomy and cricotomy in the growing larynx does not interfere with the growth potential of the larynx.

2. The cartilage of the infant larynx and trachea is extremely plastic; thus anterior transection of the cricoid in primates produces a "U"-like structure. The elasticity of infant growing cartilage allows the incised ends to spring apart, the gap anteriorly filling in with soft tissue, with resultant considerable enlargement of the cricoid lumen. This plasticity of the infant cricoid cartilage is quite unlike the rigidity of the calcified or ossified cricoid of adults. Anterior section of the cricoid in patients with subglottic stenosis does not produce this ideal situation, since the intraluminal fibrous tissue tends to hold the incised ends together. However, placement of an autogenous cartilage graft holds the incised ends apart most satisfactorily.

3. We are strongly opposed to the use of intraluminal stenting in the pediatric patient. If a satisfactory lining is provided for the laryngotracheal lumen, then granulation tissue does not form and intraluminal stenting is not required. Avoidance of such stenting decreases ulceration, infection and granulation tissue formation, with much improved healing. Thomas and Stevens[10] have recently reported on the satisfactory management of acute laryngotracheal injury in dogs without intraluminal stenting.

Indications

Many cases of subglottic stenosis are mild enough to be handled without tracheotomy; those cases should clearly not be subjected to the laryngotracheoplasty to be described. Selected for the procedure should be those patients who have a subglottic lumen that cannot be dilated above 12 French gauge after three examinations at monthly intervals. These are the patients who are at such a risk should the tracheotomy become occluded or misplaced, because they have no "reserve" airway above the tracheotomy.

There are no specific contraindications. However, we are only prepared to operate on those patients who do not have other medical problems that would preclude a successful rehabilitation at home. We do not believe that there is a lower age limit.

Preoperative assessment includes an accurate estimate of the stenotic segment by endoscopy, supplemented by high kV radiographs of the tracheal air shadow. We have found that xerography is a useful confirmatory study.

Operative Technique

The larynx is exposed by a horizontal skin incision centered on the cricoid and an incision made in the midline through the thyroid cartilage below the anterior commissure, the cricoid and upper 2 to 4 tracheal rings, depending on the extent of the stenosis. The intraluminal scar and mucosa is incised along the length of the stenotic segment. No attempt is made to remove the scar; attempts to do so will produce a raw intraluminal surface that will become infected and form further granulation tissue with subsequent scar formation. We advocate leaving the well-healed mucosally covered mature scar in place.

An autogenous cartilage graft is used to hold the incised cartilaginous ends apart. Having initially used thyroid cartilage for this, we now prefer costal cartilage. This is removed so as to preserve the lining perichondrium on one surface. An elliptically shaped piece of cartilage is now fashioned according to the following principles.

1. The largest piece of cartilage that may comfortably be placed between the cut end of the thyroid, cricoid and tracheal cartilages should be used.

2. The perichondrial lining is placed towards the lumen.

3. The edges of the graft are bevelled to prevent "settling" of the graft into the lumen.

Prolene sutures are used to sew in the graft, which can be well immobilized by carefully placed sutures. It is important to position the sutures extramucosally. The wound is closed in layers and a small drain left in place.

We have no hesitation in bronchoscoping the patient immediately after the procedure and observing the increase in the size of the subglottic and upper tracheal lumen.

Reports of Cases

At the present time we have performed the operation on six patients. These patients have been followed carefully postoperatively and have had bi-

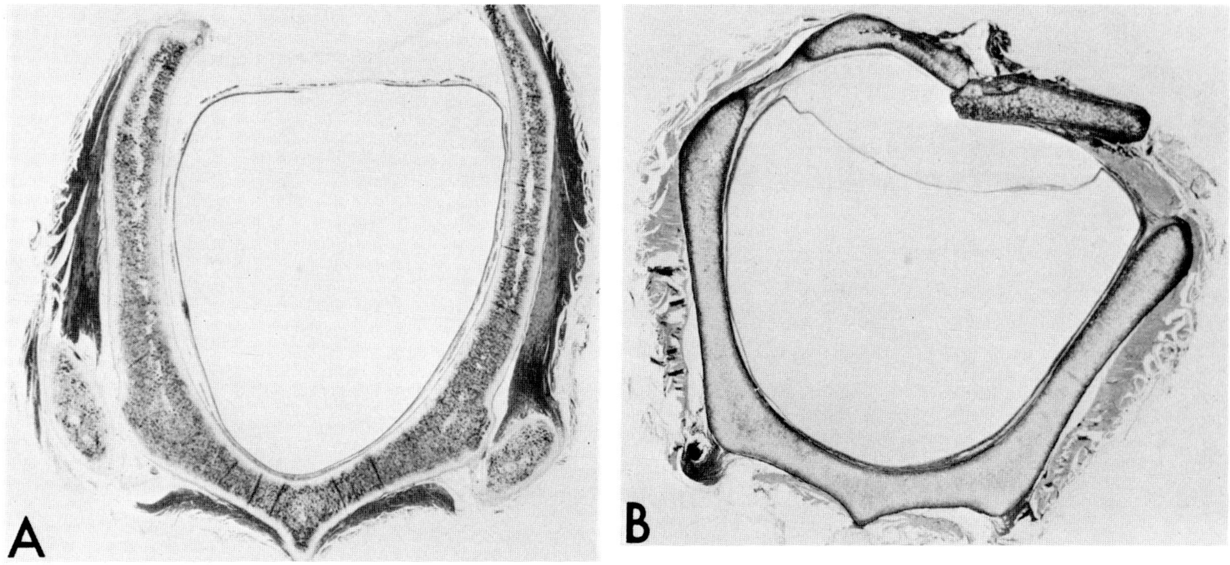

Fig. 1. (A) Cross section of the cricoid which had been incised anteriorly at the midline, twelve months prior to sacrifice in a growing primate. (B) Cross section of cricoid which had been incised anteriorly in the midline with the placement autogenous cartilage graft, twelve months prior to sacrifice in a growing primate.

weekly endoscopic examinations for the first six weeks. At the time of these examinations there has been a notable lack of granulation tissue and the initial enlargement of the lumen has been maintained. There have been no cases in which the graft has "settled" into the lumen. So far as it is possible to tell from endoscopic examination all the cartilage grafts have survived intact.

There have been no postoperative complications and no mortality. The youngest patient was seven months and the oldest five years old. The longest follow-up is $2\frac{1}{2}$ years. Five of the six patients have been successfully extubated. The first two patients were able to plug their tracheotomies within a month of surgery. They wore a small plugged tracheotomy for the next four months without incident and then were extubated. The next three patients were extubated at 6 weeks, 8 weeks, 2 weeks postreconstruction. One patient operated on in the last month should be extubated in the near future. The voice of each patient is satisfactory; there are no cases of hoarseness since the anterior commissure has not been violated.

Comments

After many years of teaching that extensive surgery should not be performed on the infant laryngotracheal area, we conclude from our experimental and clinical studies that the assumptions on which this opinion was based are false. Our endeavors are supported by the observations of others.[5,9,11]

We have encountered fewer problems with our pediatric patients than our adult patients. The plasticity of the pediatric cartilage led us to develop this technique of reconstruction: careful mucosal apposition and provision of a perichondrial lining on the graft dispenses with the need for conventional intraluminal stenting. We are pleased to note the absence of reparative granulation tissue formation, and this has been a most important fact in our success. The development of techniques of subglottic reconstruction in adults without intraluminal stenting would be a fruitful area of further investigation.

References

1. Turner AL: Stenosis of the larynx in children following intubation and tracheotomy. J Laryngol 31:313–324, 1916
2. Holinger PH: Congenital subglottic stenosis. J Laryngol 75:1–25, 1964
3. McDonald IH, Stocks J: Prolonged nasotracheal intubation. Brit J Anaesth 37:161–167, 1965
4. Lapidot A et al: Experimental repair of subglottic stenosis in piglets. Arch Otolaryn 88:529–533, 1968
5. Grahne B: Operative treatment of severe chronic traumatic laryngeal stenosis in infants up to three years old. Acta Otolaryngol 72:134–137, 1971

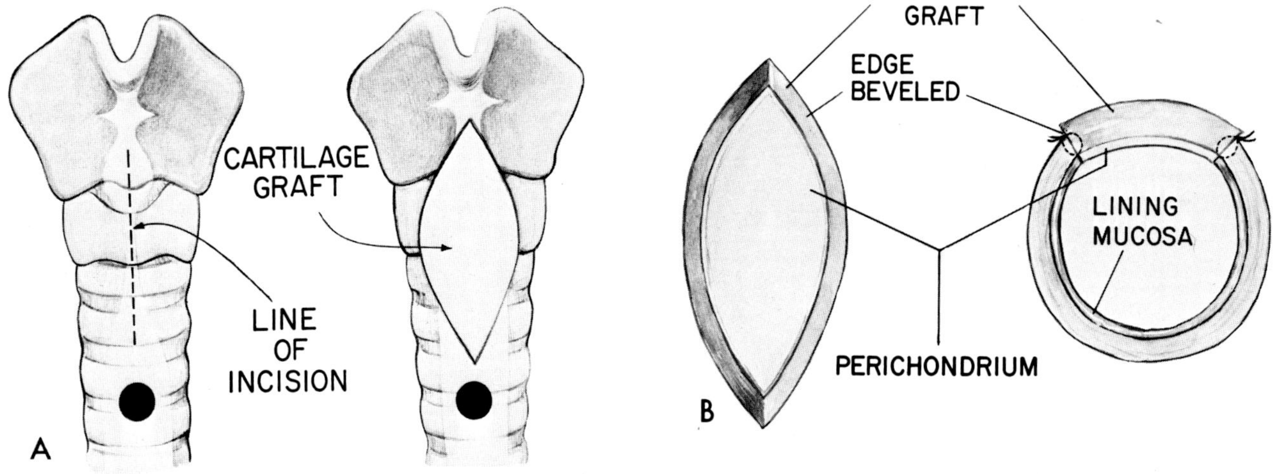

Fig. 2. (A) A schematic of laryngotracheal incision and placement of cartilage graft. (B) Details of fashioning of cartilage graft.

6. Oliver P, Richardson JR, Clubb RW, et al: Tracheostomy in children. N Engl J Med 267:631–639, 1962
7. Fearon B, Cotton RT: Subglottic stenosis in infants and children: the clinical problem and experimental surgical correction. Can J Otolaryngol 1:281–289, 1972
8. Cotton RT, Fearon B: unreported data, 1975
9. Calcaterra TC, McClure R. Ward PH: Effect of laryngofissure on the developing canine larynx. Ann Otol Rhinol Laryngol 83:810–813, 1974
10. Thomas GK, Stevens MH: Stenting in experimental laryngeal injuries. Arch Otolaryngol 101:217–221, 1975
11. Robin PE, Dalton GE: Subglottic stenosis in infants. Eight cases and their surgical conservative management. J Laryngol Otol 88:233–247, 1974

Tracheo—Innominate Artery Fistula—Problem and Prevention*

Norman W. Thoms, and Agustin Arbulu, Detroit, Mich.

Tracheo-innominate artery fistula was a lethal complication in one patient out of a series of 16 patients who have required tracheal resection and end to end anastomosis for symptomatic tracheal stenosis secondary to prolonged endotracheal cuff inflation. In ten of these patients, the innominate artery was entrapped in the peritracheal fibrous tissue in the area where the innominate artery crossed the stenotic tracheal segment. The first patient in whom we encountered fibrous entrapment of the innominate artery had only loose areolar tissue placed between the innominate artery and the tracheal anastomosis at the time of tracheal repair. Ten days postoperatively he developed a fatal tracheo-innominate artery fistula.

In the next nine cases in whom the innominate artery was bound down to the tracheal scar, we have protected the thinned-out innominate artery from the tracheal repair site with a double thickness pericardial flap. All these patients recovered and none developed a tracheo-innominate artery fistula.

Tracheo-innominate artery fistula was a fatal postoperative complication in one of our patients

* Supported by the Research Corporation, Detroit General Hospital, Detroit Michigan.

who had a segmental tracheal resection for stenosis of the trachea. When we operated upon this patient, we found that the stenotic segment of the trachea and the innominate artery were firmly fused by scar tissue. Dissection of the innominate artery away from the trachea left a thinwalled innominate artery. The postmortem examination showed that suppuration at the tracheal anastomosis had eroded through the thinned and fibrotic innominate artery resulting in a tracheo-innominate artery fistula. Subsequently, we have interposed a double-thickness pedicled pericardial flap between the tracheal repair and the innominate artery in order to prevent the formation of a fistula. In this paper, we will describe our clinical experience with the fibrous entrapment of the innominate artery and the technique for preventing a tracheo-innominate artery fistula following tracheal repair: interposed double thickness pericardial flap.

Methods

In the past five years, we have treated twenty-three patients who have developed tracheal stenosis secondary to tracheostomy or prolonged endotracheal cuff inflation. One patient died in an extended care facility due to an unrecognized tracheal stenosis. One patient had local excision of exuberant granulation tissue in the region of a tracheostomy stoma. One patient had a Montgomery stent placed through a stenosis at the cricoid level. One patient has a permanent tracheostomy. Three patients who have normal pulmonary functions are being followed. Table 1 shows our patients that had segmental tracheal resection for tracheal stenosis. In ten of these patients, the innominate artery was entrapped in the peritracheal fibrous tissue at a level where the artery crossed the stenosed tracheal segment. In the first patient in whom we encountered

Table 1. Tracheal Resection and End to End Anastomosis—A Consecutive Series.

Case No.	Age and Sex	Tracheal stenosis and innominate-artery adherent	Pericardial flap	Results
1	20 M	No	No	Excellent
2	46 M	No	No	Excellent
3	27 M	Yes	No	Died Bleeding T-I Fistula
4	21 F	Yes	Yes	Saphenous Vein Graft Excellent
5	24 M	Yes	Yes	Excellent
6	52 M	Yes	Yes	Excellent
7	58 M	Yes	Yes	Excellent
8	21 F	Yes	Yes	Excellent
9	19 M	No	No	Excellent
10	60 F	Yes	Yes	Excellent
11	33 W	No	No	Excellent
12	21 M	Yes	Yes	Excellent
13	65 M	Yes	Yes	Excellent
14	68 F	Yes	Yes	Granulation Tissue at Anastomosis Good
15	27 M	No	No	Excellent
16	80 F	No	No	Excellent

this problem (Case No. 3), we interposed only loose areolar fibroadipose mediastinal tissue between the innominate artery and the tracheal anastomosis at the time of the tracheal repair. On the seventh postoperative day, the tracheogram showed an intact anastomosis with no evidence of leak or stenosis. Three days later, he developed a fatal tracheo-innominate artery fistula. At autopsy, the following pathologic changes that predisposed to the development of a tracheo-innominate artery fistula were found: (1) a small "stitch abscess" at the anterior aspect of the tracheal anastomosis; (2) suppuration necrosis of the thinned-out posterior wall of the innominate artery; and (3) replacement of the arterial elastic media by fibrous tissue.

In the next nine patients in which the innominate artery was bound down to the tracheal scar, the innominate artery was dissected from the trachea very carefully because fibrous tissue formed a common wall between the innominate artery and the trachea. This fibrous tissue represented scar replacement of the tracheal wall and the media and adventitia of the innominate artery. In these nine cases, an anterior pericardial flap was interposed between the tracheal repair and the innominate artery. The technical details of the operation are as follows: A median sternotomy incision is made. The left innominate vein is divided. The stenosed tracheal segment is resected and an end to end tracheal repair is performed using interrupted non-absorbable sutures.[4,5] The anterior surface of the pericardium is fashioned into a flap which has its base cephalad and its free end caudad. The base is made wider than the distal end so that the pericardial flap will remain viable. The flap is passed under the innominate artery and placed between the tracheal repair and the innominate artery. The pericardial flap is sutured to the fibroadipose tissue adjacent to the trachea and is doubled back so that two layers of pericardium protect the innominate artery from the tracheal anastomosis. The pericardial flap should not be wrapped completely around the tracheal anastomosis because if this were done, contraction of the flap would constrict the trachea.

The pericardial flap technique has been used to complement tracheal repair in nine patients in whom the innominate artery was involved in peritracheal fibrosis at the level of the tracheal stenosis (Table 1).

Results

A tracheo-innominate artery fistula occurred in one patient, the patient described in Table 1 as Case No. 3. The postmortem examination suggested that the formation of the tracheo-innominate artery fistula was initiated by a stitch abscess at the tracheal anastomosis that led to perforation of the diseased posterior wall of the innominate artery by a process of suppuration necrosis. This perforation of the innominate entry in the vicinity of a small peritracheal abscess at the tracheal anastomosis resulted in a tracheo-innominate artery fistula and fatal hemorrhage ensued. No tracheo-innominate artery fistula has occurred in any of the patients who have had the pericardial flap procedure.

Comment

Tracheal stenosis is a complication of prolonged ventilatory support resulting from pressure necrosis of the tracheal wall.[1,2] This lesion has been reproduced experimentally[3] and observed clinically many times. Repair of this lesion by resection of the stenotic segment and end to end reconstruction of the trachea has been described and is widely used in surgical practice.[4]

The problem of tracheo-innominate artery fistula complicating tracheal repair has been previously described.[5,6] Grillo describes a patient that "suffered a hemorrhage from the innominate artery three days postoperatively and required resection of the artery . . .".[7] The bleeding of a tracheo-innominate artery fistula may be temporarily tamponaded by an endotracheal tube cuff and gauze packing as reported by Myers and Pilch.[8] However, in the best of circumstances, the bleeding often happens so suddenly that the patient suffocates and exsanguinates before help arrives. The logical solution to this problem is, therefore, its prevention. The pathological findings at the autopsy of one of our patients who died of a tracheo-innominate artery fistula suggested to us that placing a tough pericardial buttress between the weakened innominate artery and the tracheal repair would prevent the dreaded fistula.

The findings at operation and at autopsy suggest that the following situations and events led to the tracheo-innominate artery fistula in our patient

No. 3. The innominate artery became involved in the peritracheal inflammation and fibrosis that followed tracheal injury because of its proximity to the trachea as it passes through the anterior mediastinum. The gross and microscopic examination of the innominate artery in two of our patients (Case No. 3 at autopsy and Case No. 4 at operation) showed that fibrosis extends into the wall of the innominate artery. During resection of the tracheal stenotic segment, the arterial wall is detached from the tracheal scar leaving a thinned-out fibrotic innominate artery. If such a damaged artery is placed unprotected against the tracheal repair, a tracheo-innominate artery fistula may occur at the tracheal suture line.[5,6] The placement of a pericardial flap between the tracheal repair and the thinned-out innominate artery will prevent the development of this serious complication. The desirable features of this operation are as follows: (1) the pericardial flap is easy to construct; (2) the flap offers a strong, autogenous structure that obviates the problems encountered when one uses foreign material; (3) the flap acts as a seal to the tracheal anastomosis and a shield to the damaged innominate artery; (4) the pericardial flap allows lateral drainage of any purulent collection that develops after tracheal repair because it is a double thickness sheet of fibrous tissue that is placed in a frontal plane; and (5) the pericardial flap will not constrict the trachea because it is not wrapped circumferentially around the tracheal repair.

We have presented our experience with one tracheal innominate artery fistula which followed the resection of a segment of stenotic trachea and end-to-end anastomosis. We have suggested a technique for preventing a tracheo-innominate artery fistula in patients who had similar findings at operation: an innominate artery bound down to the stenotic segment by dense peritracheal adhesions, resulting in a fibrotic union of the trachea and innominate artery. In nine subsequent patients, who had the above findings at operation, a pericardial flap was interposed between the tracheal repair and the thinned-out innominate artery wall preventing the formation of a tracheo-innominate artery fistula. The technique and rationale for constructing a pericardial flap between the tracheal repair and innominate artery is presented in detail.

References

1. Cooper JD, Grillo HC: Evaluation of tracheal injury due to ventilatory assistance through cuffed tubes—a pathologic study. Ann Surg 169:334, 1969
2. Pearson FG, Golberg M, da Silva AJ: Tracheal stenosis complicating tracheostomy with cuffed tubes—clinical experience and observations from a prospective study. Arch Surg 97:380, 1968
3. Cooper JD, Grillo HC: Experimental production and prevention of injury due to cuffed tracheal tubes. Surg Gynec Obst 129:1235, 1969
4. Arbulu A, Thoms NW: Post-tracheostomy tracheal stenosis. J Am Nurse Anesthetists, pp 119–126, 1973
5. Arbulu A, Thoms NW: Tracheo-innominate artery fistula following tracheal stenosis repair—problem and prevention. J Thoracic Cardiovasc Surg 67:936, 1974
6. Deslauriers J, Ginsberg RJ, Pearson FG: Innominate artery rupture: a major complication of tracheal surgery. Soc Thoracic Surgeons. p 54, Jan 1975
7. Grillo HC: Surgery of the trachea. Current Probl Surg p 22, July, 1970, Year Book Medical Publishers, Inc, Chicago
8. Myers RS, Pilch YH: Temporary control of tracheal innominate artery fistula. Ann Surg 170:149, 1969

Clinical Experience with Thyroplasty for Dysphonia

Nobuhike Isshiki, Kyoto, Japan

An attempt was made to change the position and tension of the vocal cord through reformation of the thyroid cartilage. The experimental studies on 14 dogs indicated the usefulness of various types of reformation of the thyroid cartilage for dysphonias artificially produced in dog. Four types of thyroplasty were proposed for functional purposes.[1] Their effects on the vocal cord are: (1) lateral compression; (2) lateral expansion; (3) relaxation (shortening); and (4) stretching (lengthening) (Fig. 1). This paper describes our clinical experiences with thyroplasty in 12 cases of dysphonia.

Thyroplasty Type I

Various types of thyroplasty type I were performed on nine patients with dysphonia, seven with recurrent laryngeal nerve paralysis and two with vocal cord atrophy. Prior to surgery, manual compression tests of the larynx and cricothyroid approximation should be performed on each patient in order to decide the indication of thyroplasty. These tests not only indicate the prognosis after surgery rather well but also help relieve the patient's anxiety as to what the voice would be like after surgery.

The surgery can be performed on either in- or out patients, but always under local anesthesia. The types of incisions in the thyroid ala were varied with the cases, but the most typical is a kind of rectangular one 10 × 3 mm, the upper margin of which should be at the level of the vocal cord (Fig. 2). Anatomical study of the human cadaver larynx indicated that the anterior commissure of the vocal cord (upper surface) is positioned almost at the level of the midpoint between the thyroid notch and lower margin of the thyroid cartilage or slightly higher than that level. Prior to incisions, we draw a rectangular window with pyocutanine so that the upper horizontal line should lie at the midpoint between the thyroid notch and lower margin of the thyroid cartilage and go further back in parallel to the lower margin of the thyroid ala. After gentle and careful marginal separation of the rectangular

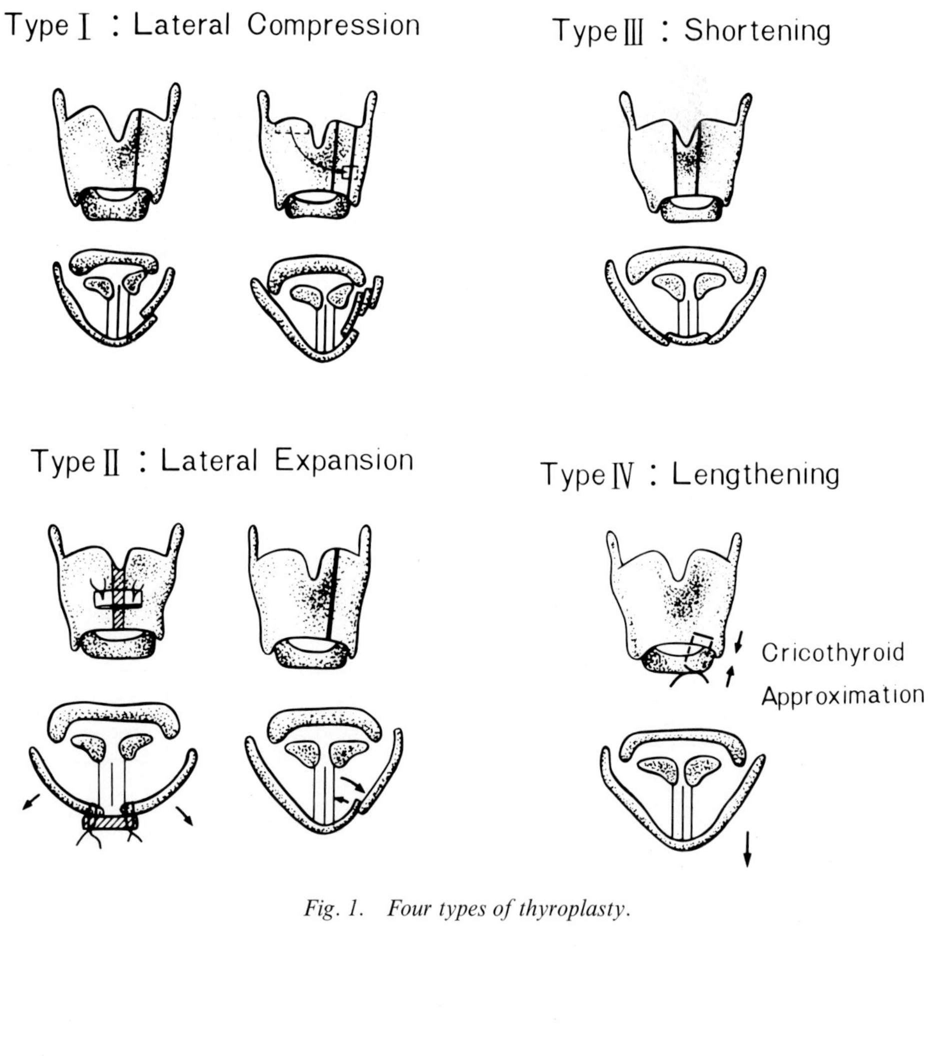

Fig. 1. Four types of thyroplasty.

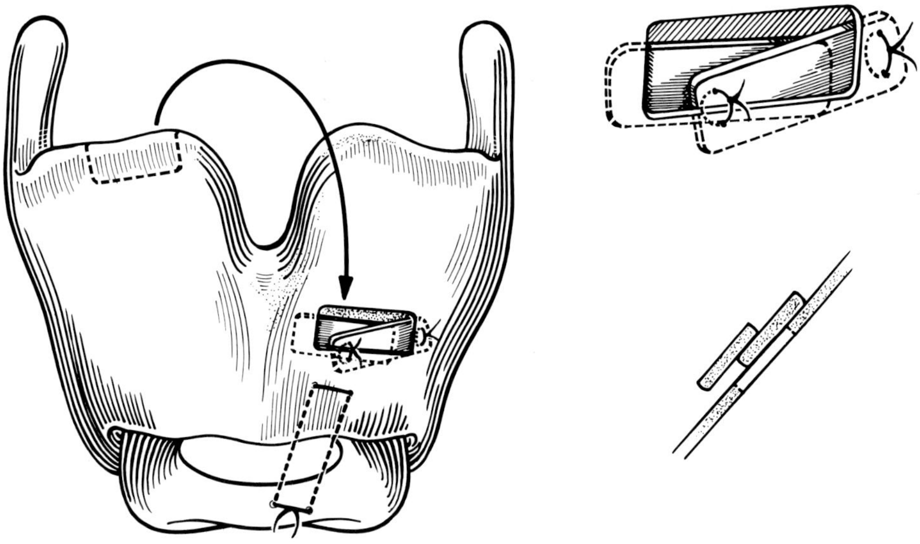

Fig. 2. Typical thyroplasty type I.

fragment with rather fine raspatrium, it is depressed inward to varied depth to know the optimal depression for voice. If slight depression is sufficient for optimal voice, the fragment is displaced 1 mm downward (caudal direction) behind the remaining frame of the thyroid ala (Fig. 3). If further depression is required for maximal voice improvement, a wedge taken from the opposite side of thyroid ala is inserted and fixed with nylon sutures between the rectangular fragment and the remaining thyroid ala (Fig. 2). Usually a wedge pared off to a half thickness is sufficient for adequate compression of the vocal cord.

In aged patients, an oscillating saw was required for cutting the calcified cartilage. In cases where the paralyzed vocal cord is positioned higher than the intact one, cricothyroid approximation on the involved side is tested routinely to determine whether the procedure further improves the voice or not. If voice improvement is obtained by the tentative approximation, the thyroid and cricoid cartilages should be fixed in approximation with one or two 3–0 nylon mattress sutures. In 3 cases, thyroplasty type 4, cricothyroid approximation was added to thyroplasty type 1.

Voice was much improved after surgery in all the cases except in one case of vocal cord paralysis due to traffic trauma on the neck. The poor result in this case was attributed to scarring and granulation of the vocal cord. Generally speaking, the compression effect of thyroplasty type I was not so marked in vocal cord atrophy as in vocal cord paralysis. Functional aspect in vocal cord atrophy should be taken into consideration in deciding the indication for the surgery. No complications such as strider or dyspnea occurred.

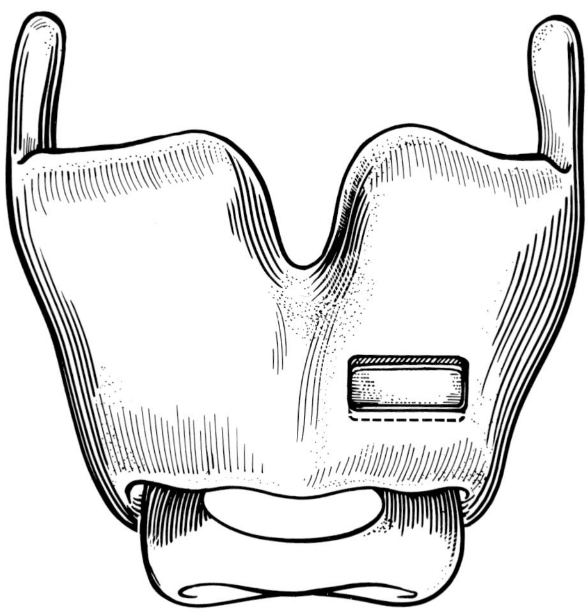

Fig. 3. Thyroplasty type I without a wedge.

Thyroplasty Type II

So far we have no experiences with thyroplasty type II. Hyperfunctional dysphonia such as dysphonia plica ventricularis may be an indication for this type of thyroplasty. However, the expansion of the thyroid ala seems rather difficult to perform and more experimental trials are needed before clinical application. Simulation of hyperfunctional voice disorder per se is difficult to make in the dog.

Thyroplasty Type III

Combination of types III and I was utilized for one case of mutational voice disorder. Two parallel vertical incision in the thyroid cartilage as in Figure 1 resulted in much lowered but slightly hoarse voice. Then the median vertical fragment was depressed inward inside the right lateral ala (thyroplasty type III) and on the left side the lateral ala was slipped in the medial fragment (thyroplasty type I), as shown in Figure 4. The effect of lowering the vocal pitch was reduced but the voice was not hoarse.

Thyroplasty Type IV

Thyroplasty type IV or cricothyroid approximation was performed on two cases of androphonia due to administration of anabolic hormone. Cricothyroid distance was shortened by two 3–0 nylon mattress sutures on each side. Cartilage fragment taken from the upper margin of the thyroid ala was used as a mattress in order to prevent the thyroid cartilage from being cut by the nylon sutures. Elevation of the vocal pitch after surgery was substantial from 119 to 176 Hz, and from 142 to 180 Hz. One year after surgery, the vocal pitch in one case was found further raised.

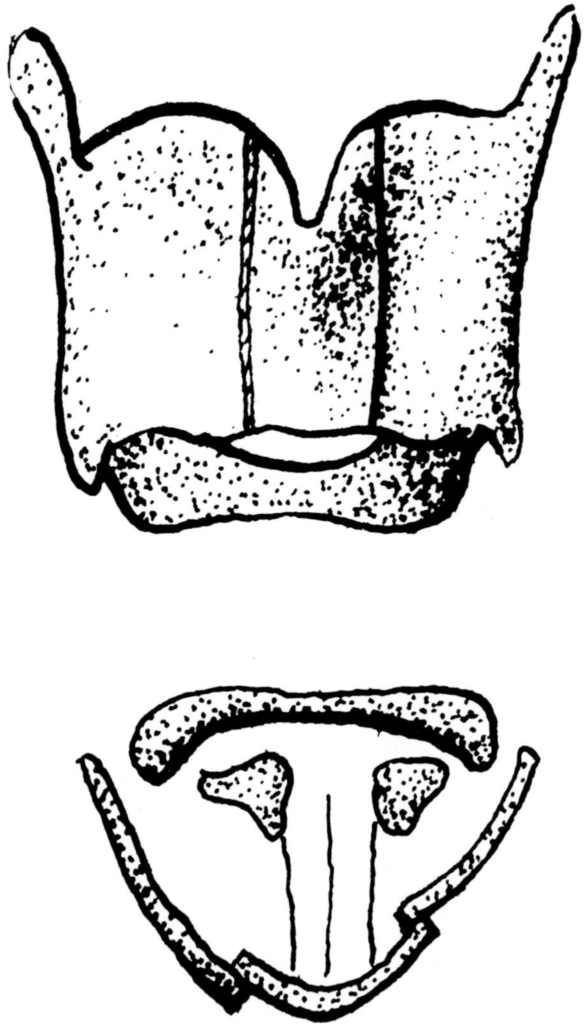

Fig. 4. Combination of types I and III for mutational voice disorder.

Thyroplasties as we proposed are rather simple and easy to perform and can be modified during surgery so that the best voice is obtainable.

References

1. Isshiki N, Morita H, Okamura H, Hiramoto M: Thyroplasty as a new phonosurgical technique. Acta Otolaryngol 78:451–457, 1974

Lips, Oral Cavity, and Pharynx

Pharyngo-Esophagcal Reconstruction (Panel)

D. F. N. Harrison:

The closure of the pharyngo-eosophageal defect resulting from radical extirpation of malignant tumors in this region, must in no way influence the choice of the initial oncological operation. Consequently, in those neoplasms which extend into the cervical esophagus, the resulting operative deficiency may require the surgeon to venture deep into the superior mediastinum. Although primary repair may be technically possible using skin—this may not be possible nor desirable. In addition, clinico-pathological studies may advise complete oesophagectomy. On such occasions repair with the whole stomach brought up through the posterior mediastinum and anastomosed to the cut pharynx, is the treatment of choice. Personal experience of 50 such procedures will be briefly described together with relevant statistics.

Where radical resection leaves a more accessible and smaller deficit between pharynx and divided esophagus—intervention of a revascularized segment of small or large bowel should be considered. However, such a procedure (performed only five times by the author) has inherent disadvantages and should be reserved for those patients where simple techniques are inappropriate.

John M. Loré, Jr.:

When the entire circumferential portion of the hypopharynx is resected combined with total laryngectomy and radical neck dissection, reconstruction of this portion of the digestive tract can be achieved in a one-stage operation utilizing a posterior tongue flap and dermal graft.

Sisson[1] and Hiranandani[2] independently have described posterior tongue flaps to reconstruct the anterior wall of the hypopharynx following laryngectomy and partial hypopharyngectomy.

The technique consists of a horizontal incision in the base of the tongue, thus developing a sliding advanced posterior tongue flap which when tubed 270° forms the anterior and lateral walls of the food conduit. The posterior wall is formed by a dermal graft sutured to remnant of the prevertebral fascia and the anterior spinal ligament.

Outline of Technique[3]

1. Defect reconstructed can be up to 8 cm in total length including 1.0 cm to 2.0 cm of the cervical esophagus.
2. Liberal mobilization of oropharynx and esophagus. Flexion of head and neck aids in reducing tension on the anterior suture lines and reduces the length of the defect.
3. Suture all mobilized oropharyngeal and esophageal mucosa and underlying muscle to prevertebral fascia and the anterior spinal ligament. This avoids tension on mucosal suture lines.
4. Suture dermal graft to prevertebral fascia and the anterior longitudinal ligament. This forms posterior wall of the new gullet.
5. Tongue flap is a sliding advanced flap with the base anteriorly and forms the anterior and lateral walls of the new gullet. The flap can extend anterior to the circumvalate papillae and is 10 mm to 12 mm in thickness.
6. Vertical incision in esophagus to widen lumen at the anastomotic suture line.
7. Radical neck dissection is easily combined with resection in the standard method.
8. The skin incisions for the radical neck dissection should be planned to facilitate the use of a deltopectoral flap in the event the tongue flap is too short and has to be abandoned.

The main limitations of the use of this type of reconstruction is involvement of the base of the tongue and/or extension of disease into esophagus. Regardless of the type of reconstruction planned, or finally used, the ablative phase of the operation must never be limited to accommodate the reconstructive phase. It also must be emphasized that squamous cell carcinoma of the hypopharynx, like the esophagus, spreads submucosally and also may be multicentric. Free use of frozen sections and wide margins are important. In any event, nothing is lost if the tongue flap and dermal graft method is planned and then must be discarded for another method. If it is adequate, a great savings is afforded the patient in this one-stage method of reconstruction. Radiation treatment can be combined with the operation, either preoperatively or postoperatively.

John Conley:

My assignment on this panel, in a discussion of pharyngo-esophageal reconstruction, places me in the role of coming to this meeting to qualify Caesar's death, if not to bury him. Regional neck flaps were at one time popular in rehabilitating ablative wounds of the pharynx. Their appeal was based primarily on the advantages one encounters with the immediate availability of regional tissue and their ability to accommodate a small resection in the hypopharynx and postcricoid, usually associated with a midline incision and without incorporating a radical neck dissection. This concept eventually proved to have the disadvantages of limited square surface availability for transfer, design often restricted, the resultant gullet may be narrowed and tight, the concept of repair may not comply with the demands of the resection, and frequently these regions of the neck have been previously damaged by irradiation.

With this list of deterrants, and with the increase in the dimensions of the ablative procedures, more accommodating rehabilitative techniques were developed. Before departing from these neck flaps, however, one must recognize the original and splendid contribution of Dr. Wookey, who in his time developed the use of neck flaps in reconstructions of the gullet into a standard procedure. Prior to that there was nihilism and chaos. The flaps were usually designed horizontally on the neck, formed into a trough at the site of the deformed pharynx, and then this stoma was closed at a second stage. The donor areas on the neck were dressed with split skin grafts. There is no question about the rationale and beauty of this concept and that it unconsciously pointed the direction for new developments.

Free skin grafts had been used extensively to resurface all types of wounds, and a wave of energy and enthusiasm carried us in this direction, as far as rehabilitation was concerned. The technique was direct, simplistic, and merely required the connecting of a free skin tube to the upper segment of the pharynx and the lower segment of the esophagus. At one time it was felt that this could be combined with unilateral or bilateral radical neck dissection. Things have a way of proving themselves, however, and these evangelical hopes succumbed to loss of the graft, stenosis of the passageway, wound infection, carotid artery hemorrhage, and unpredictability. Stenosis of the food passageway was partially controlled by stenting, but this often proved impractical, and occasionally dangerous. Only an exceptionally unique and highly imaginative aspect of free skin grafting remains. The surviving aspect of the concept avoided the use of split skin and employed only full-thickness skin grafts. The donor area was the penis, and the operation originated, understandably, in Israel. Dr. Kaplan created a penile skin tube from the shaft of the penis and connected this full-thickness skin graft to the deficient gullet. The skin did not unduly contract, stenting was not necessary, and the limitations imposed by size and the anxiety of surgically touching this organ were well received by this romantic race. This operation has not become extremely popular in the United States, however.

These semi-artifactual medical epitaphs are counterbalanced at the other end of the spectrum by the philosophy of a comprehensive combination of radical ablation, irradiation, and reconstruction of the gullet by the transposition of the large bowel with a segment of ileum. This series of surgical stages in management is applied to the advanced cancer of the cervical esophagus which is presumably amenable to resection through the cervical route but where immediate reconstruction is contraindicated. The cervical esophagus is cut at the lowest level, transfixed, and then dropped into the mediastinum. The larynx, hypopharynx, and cervical esophagus are removed, with or without the thyroid gland, and the hypopharynx is sutured closed and a gastrostomy is performed. There is therefore no connection between the pharynx and the esophagus. A complete course of irradiation is delivered to the low neck and mediastinum and, within an interval of six to eight weeks, the bowel is transposed through the mediastinum and left inferior neck to be anastomosed to a new opening in the hypopharynx.

Preparation for such an undertaking should consist of an accurate documentation of the lower limits of the primary cancer, the status of the mediastinum, and the local resectability of the lesion. Tribulations often supersede these sincere efforts, with unexpected extensions and biological compromises. These may be accommodated by retreat from the wound when this is feasible, subtotal resection of the area, and postoperative irradiation.

I have, therefore, taken you on a short surgical journey of earlier attempts to reconstruct these treacherous deficiencies and to extend some of the qualified expertise in the direction of those with the gravest aspects of the disease. It is done with the full knowledge of more rewarding and more efficient techniques that will be presented by the other speakers.

V. Y. Bakamjian:

The deltopectoral flap, carrying deltoid skin on the end of a parasternally based pedicle of pectoral skin, is relatively nonhairy usually. With a rich vascularity in axial pattern from the perforating intercostal branches of the internal mammary artery, it is usually safe when used undelayed. And, obtained pararegionally rather than regionally from the head and neck, it is usually not affected adversely by any prior surgery or irradiation for head and neck lesions. Consequently, it is almost ideally suited for use in a relatively simple and safe reconstruction technique to restore pharyngoesophageal continuity after a total laryngopharyngectomy and radical neck dissection for cancer. Essentially, the technique comprises introducing the flap subcutaneously into the neck, tubing it skin-surface-inward, thus creating a hollow replacement for the missing gullet, and anastomosing it end-to-end with the oropharynx above, and side-to-end with the stump of the cervical esophagus below. The resultant fistulous outlet that remains at the base of the neck is closed in a second stage when the pedicle is divided and the anastomosis between the skin tube and esophagus is revised.

Siegfried Zehm:

In extirpative surgery of the head and neck one tries to preserve the vagus nerve because loss of its function causes dysphagia.

This is seen in radical surgery in the posterior cranial fossa such as exploration for extensive acoustic neuroma or removal of a solitary extracranial neuroma from the main trunk of the vagus nerve. It is possible to completely remove the tumor by sharp dissection leaving some anatomical continuity of the nerve; however, the nerve fails to regain normal function.

This is also seen in extensive ablative surgery of the temporal bone which includes structures to the level of the internal carotid artery, the internal jugular vein, the sigmoid sinus, the mandible, and the neck. When the pharyngeal muscles are denuded, small pharyngeal nerve fibers cannot be identified nor preserved; therefore the vagus nerve may lose its function and a paralyzed hemipharynx with dysphagia results.

To restore deglutition, a major portion of the paralyzed pharynx is removed.

In 1961 Rethi[4] a Hungarian otolaryngologist, after studying patients with motor neurone diseases, presented the idea of invaginating those parts of the parapharyngeal wall in which the muscles had been become atrophic and the pharynx dilated on the paralyzed side. Denecke[5] suggested at the same time the excision of parts of the atrophic muscles, excluding the mucosa, and then narrowing the pharynx by suture. Prior to operation he studied the exposed paralyzed pharyngeal wall under local anesthesia several months after primary tumor removal in order to be able to recognize the atrophic muscle parts during the act of swallowing.

Instead of waiting several months for the muscle fibers to become atrophic I excise all structures of the pharyngeal wall, either at the time of primary surgery or 6 to 8 weeks later at a second stage.[6] The excision includes approximately one third of the circumference of the denervated pharynx, so that the remainder of the newly formed and narrowed gullet is 80–90 percent innervated by the contralateral vagus nerve (Fig. 1). The excision extends

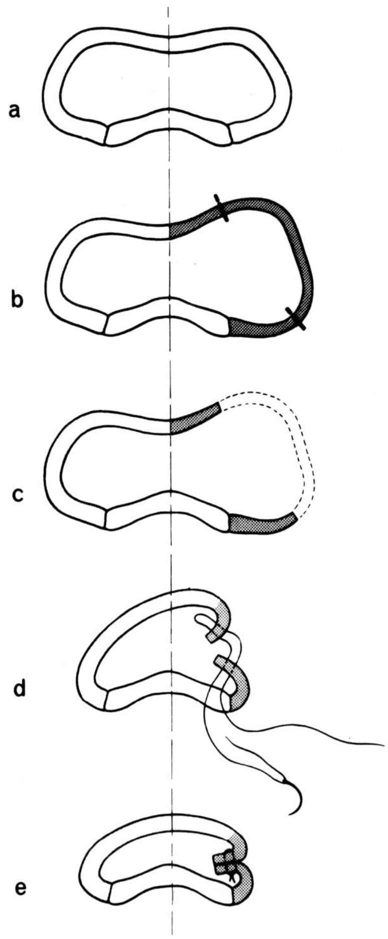

Fig. 1. Diameter of the gullet: (a) normal; (b) paralyzed site outlined; (c) resected area outlined; (d,e) pharynx narrowed on the paralyzed site.

from the inferior tonsillar pole to the level of the cricopharyngeal muscle and is usually 10–12 cm in length and 2–3 cm wide (Fig. 2). Because it is important to ensure that no food is trapped into the postericoid space during swallowing an extramucosal myotomy must be performed before this excision. X-Ray studies should not be obtained before the end of the 3rd postoperative week. A barium swallow will show the narrowed gullet and movie x-ray studies demonstrate the increase of food intake during the following weeks (Fig. 3).

My personal experience with this procedure is based on 5 patients since 1967. Subsequently postoperative examinations have demonstrated normal function, and all patients have been able to lead a normal family life.

In some cases of pharyngeal paralysis, nasopharyngeal regurgitation may present a problem because of the insufficient closure of the velopharyngeal muscles. This occurs in extensive ablative tumor surgery of the lateral nasopharyngeal wall, the soft palate, the pterygoid fossa including parts of the tongue, the mandible and the neck. In certain circumstances surgery can be extended to the midportion of the external part of the base of the skull and may include resection of the cartilagineous part of the Eustachian tube; to prevent stenosis of the remainder of the tube, a small silicone–rubber tube is passed through the nose into

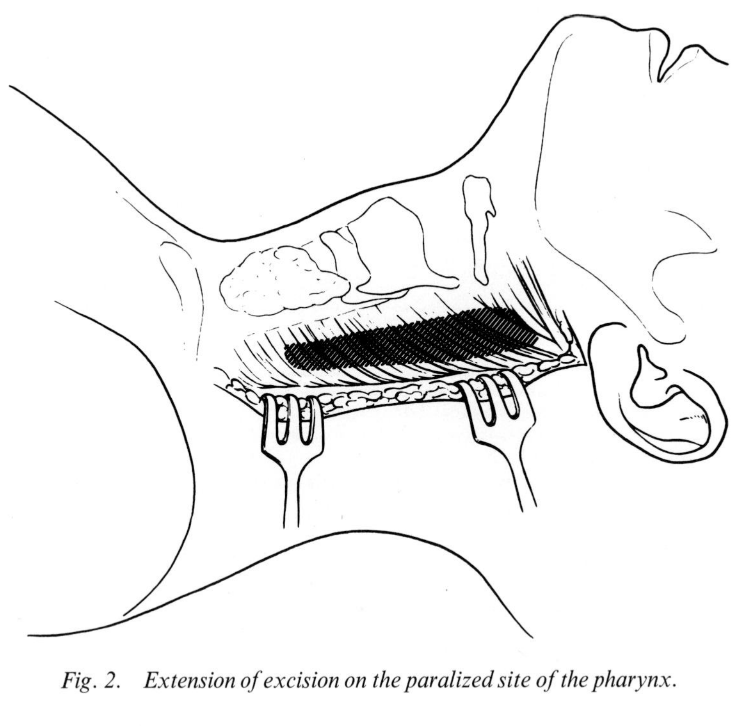

Fig. 2. Extension of excision on the paralized site of the pharynx.

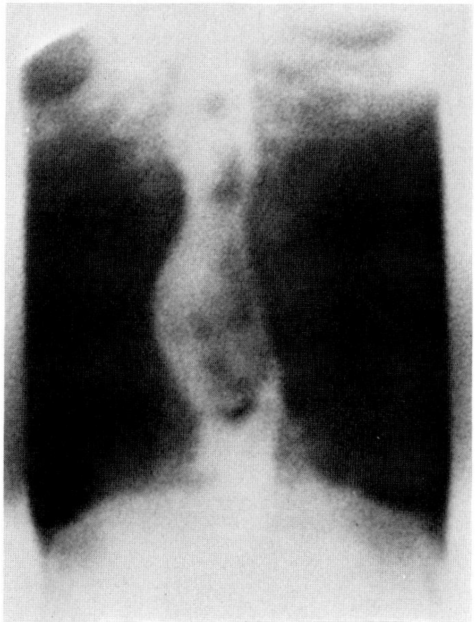

Fig. 3. X-ray movie study demonstrates the functioning and narrowed gullet, right side.

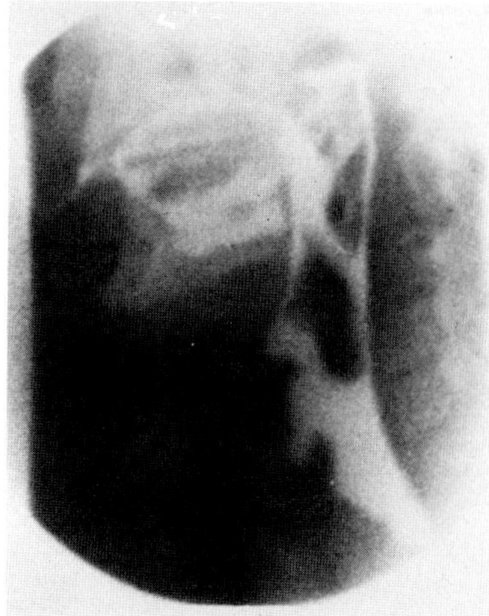

Fig. 4. Regurgitation of liquids into the nasopharynx (→), X-ray movie.

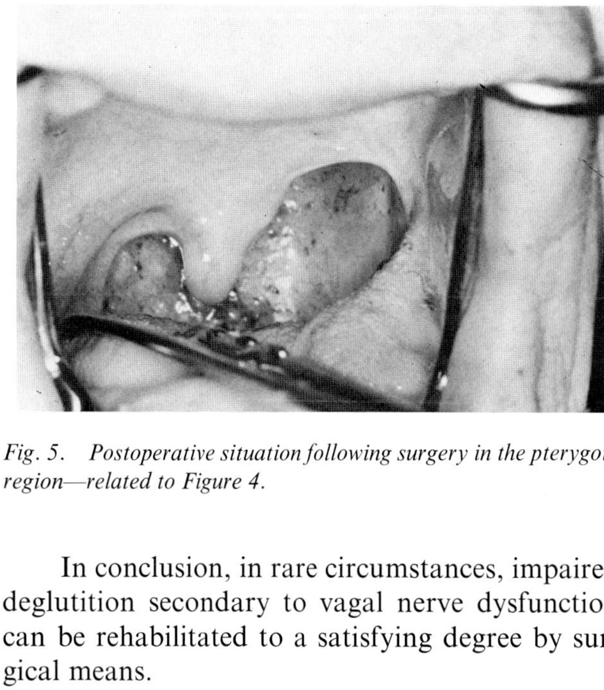

Fig. 5. Postoperative situation following surgery in the pterygoid region—related to Figure 4.

the middle ear. The area to be rehabilitated is covered with split skin grafts, while the remainder of the pharyngeal wall, the soft palate, and the tongue are brought together with suture to establish useful velopharyngeal function.

Insufficient closure of the nasopharynx may occur permitting liquids to be trapped into the nasopharynx and to enter the nasal cavity (Figs. 4 and 5). Therefore, it may become necessary several weeks after the first operation to narrow the entrance into the nasopharynx by the use of two local flaps—one from the soft palate, based superiorly, and the second from the posterior pharyngeal wall, based inferiorly (Figs. 6 and 7). Both flaps are created on the side of the primary operation and extend almost to the midline of the velum. When healing is complete nasal regurgitation is eliminated.

The latter procedure was used in the case of a 39-year-old Caucasian male, who had a primary anaplastic carcinoma at the pharyngeal end of the Eustachian tube. There was no evidence of malignancy at the base of the skull, but there was in the regional lymphatics which were along the entire length of the internal carotid artery up to the base of the skull—an extension which could not be made in an ordinary neck dissection. This patient is demonstrated on slides 10 years following surgery and is free of recurrence.

In conclusion, in rare circumstances, impaired deglutition secondary to vagal nerve dysfunction can be rehabilitated to a satisfying degree by surgical means.

Summary

Pharyngeal dysfunction resulting from radical tumor surgery is caused by loss of the function of the vagus nerve. Impaired deglutition can be satisfactorily rehabilitated by excision of parts of the denervated musculature and mucosa of the paralyzed pharynx. Before this, an extramucosal myotomy is performed. This allows 80–90 percent of the remainder of the narrowed and newly formed

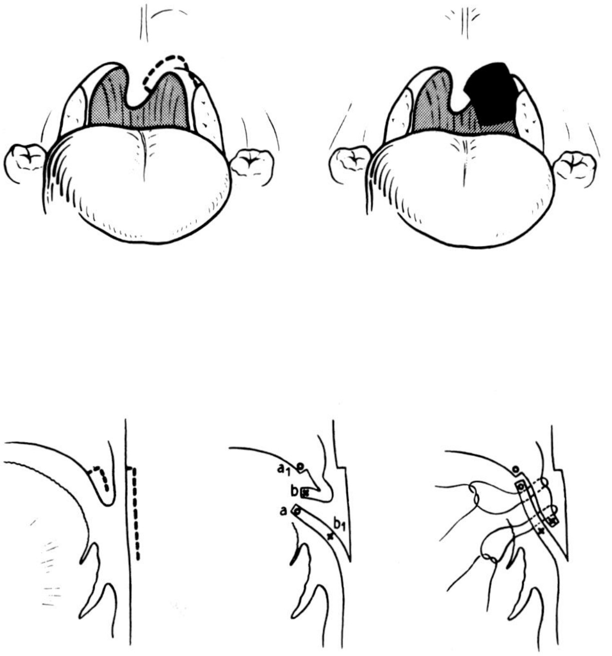

Fig. 6. Narrowing of the nasopharyngeal entrance by creating two flaps in the paralyzed pharyngeal site.

gullet to be innervated from the contralateral vagus nerve; swallowing is facilitated by division of the cricopharyngeal muscle.

Nasal regurgitation as the consequence of the insufficient closure of the nasopharynx on the operated side can be corrected by the use of local flaps which approximate the posterior pharyngeal wall to the soft palate on the paralyzed side.

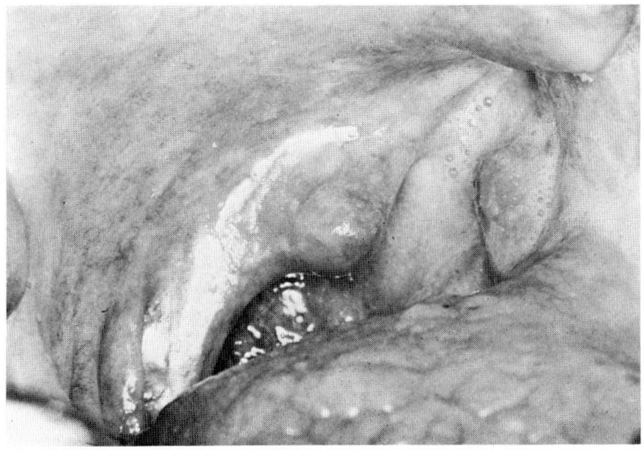

Fig. 7. Flaps in position—10 years following primary surgery (compare Figure 5).

References

1. Sisson GA: Reconstruction of the hypopharynx and cervical esophagus after radical excisional surgery. Laryngoscope 66:1268–1290, 1956
2. Hiranandani LH: Tongue and pedicle flap for reconstruction of pharynx in one-stage laryngopharyngectomy. Rev Laryngol Otol Rhinol (Bord) 1–2: January–February, 1967
3. Loré JM, Jr: Atlas of Head and Neck Surgery, ed 2, Philadelphia, WB Saunders Company, 1973
4. Rethi A: Retablissement de le déglutitions dans le cas de paralysie bulbaire et hémibulbaire Ann Otolaryngol (Paris) 78:372–377, 1961
5. Denecke HJ: Korrektur des Schluckaktes bei einseitiger Pharynx-Larynxlähmung. HNO 14:351, 1961
6. Zehm S: Functional Restitution of the Denervated Gullet Arch Otolaryngol 99:279–280, 1974

The Reconstruction of the Oral Cavity and the Pharynx Using a Muscle-Skin Island Flap of the Sternocleidomastoid Muscle Pediculated at the Caudal End

H. L. Wullstein, R. Baumann, and W. Richter, Wurzburg, Germany

In the case of large defects of the floor of the mouth in cancer surgery, Bakamjian and Littlewood[1] left the sternocleidomastoid muscle attached to the mastoid process turning it together with a cervical skin island on the caudal end into the defect, thus repairing the floor of the mouth.

Concerned about the deep supraauricular defect in neck dissection occasionally filled with seroma or chylus and ugly in the cosmetic effect, I had started since the same year (1964) to fill the defect with the help of the lower third of the muscle, in every case suturing it with the cut end into the deep triangle between the ligated jugular vein and the subclavicular vein (Fig. 1). Not in one case did any late metastasis happen in any deep lymph nodes left behind.

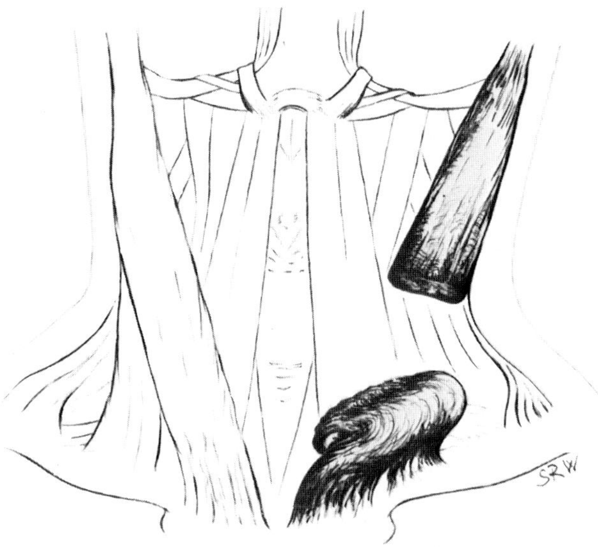

Fig. 1.

In the meantime in all carcinomata superior to the glottis I made it a rule in my Department to cut away the mastoid process with the purpose of reaching the uppermost lymph nodes underneath the external auditory meatus and the squama occipitalis behind the mandibular joint. This is especially important when we preserve the mandible as we wish to do.

I—therefore—have discarded the method of Bakamjian. Instead of that I form a composite flap out of the sternocleidomastoid muscle pediculated with the caudal end of the sternum and at the clavicle and covered with a long skin-island at the cranial end of this muscle including the retroauricular skin together with the periosteum up to the border of the scalp. The flap offers ample material to fill the whole floor of the mouth down to the vallecula and to cover the tonsillar area with vital tissue and skin. This method of reconstruction of the oral cavity and the wall of the pharynx can be performed with or without splitting the mandible. It depends upon the topography and the extension of the malignoma, whichever method is preferred (Fig. 2).

In case of extensive and deeply infiltrating carcinomata or metastases perforating the capsule of the lymph nodes there may be objections against the use of the sternocleidomastoid muscle of the tumor side. In such a case—honestly spoken—more and more often we shy away from using this side to do a typical neck dissection. Instead of that we form the composite flap out of this muscle together with the skin of the healthy side. The flap of the healthy side can be fitted in as well in the oral-pharyngeal defect (Fig. 3). If possible this muscle flap is pulled through medially to the anterior venter of the digastric and the mylohyoid muscle, it—therefore—adapts better to the profile of the floor of the mouth. This composite muscle skin flap of the healthy side is always combined with the bilateral suprahyoidal excision of the lymph nodes including the bilateral resection of the mastoid process (Fig. 4). The pneumatisation of the mastoid is then covered with a piece of fascia or periosteum to avoid effusion into the middle ear

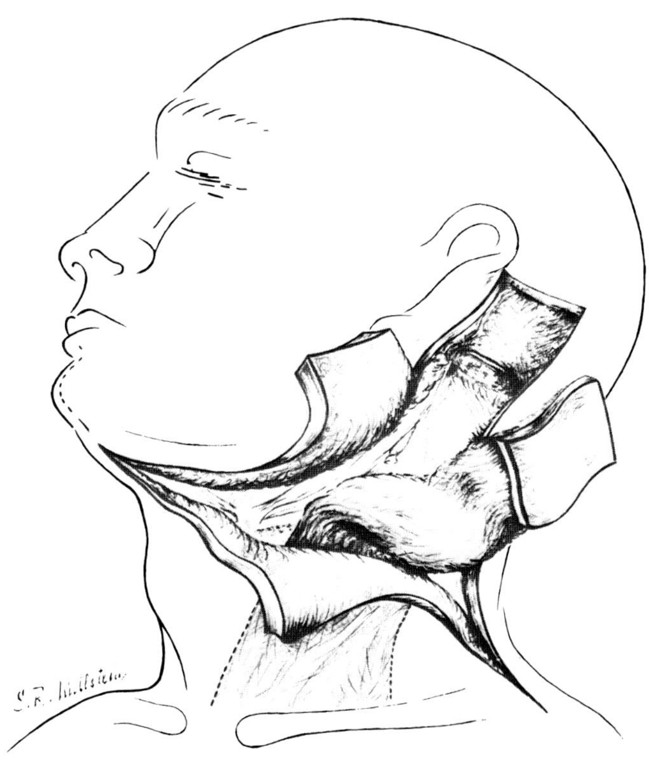

Fig. 2.

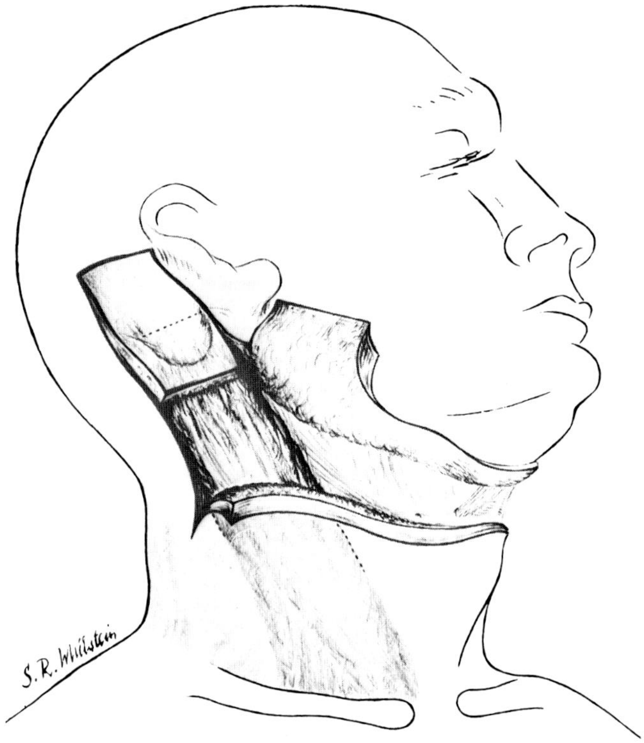

Fig. 3

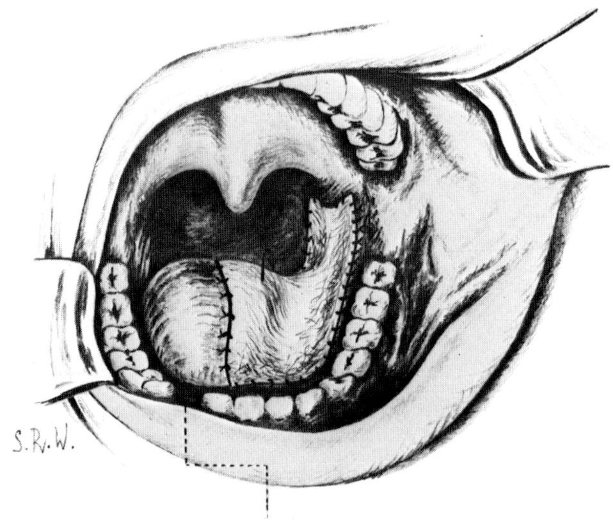

Fig. 4.

spaces. The tip of the mastoid process can be left incorporated in this flap as Conley does.[2]

For these purposes the skin incision shows slight variations on each side compared to those already known (Conley Y-L, Ducuing).[3] It is essential that the vertical incision runs along the posterior margin of the sternocleidomastoidal muscle starting on the retroauricular bone. On the side of the carcinoma it reaches down into the trigonum omoclaviculare for neck dissection, on the healthy side we need only the upper half. The horizontal incision branches off at the upper margin of the thyroid cartilage thus preserving the innervation of the sternocleidomastoid muscle.

This muscle flap always heals quickly and without disturbances, the full skin as an island, too, especially if it is not too large. The full thickness of the skin on top of the muscle flap offers a solid protection of the internal lining in the oral cavity or the pharynx against deterioration of the flap by contamination through saliva. In case the skin shows partial necrosis we should wait a while and only then cut it away superficially; out of the deep layers it can regrow safely. When complete local defects of the dermis result, the surrounding mucosa quickly overgrows this area. Under adequate treatment the mucosa proves to be the great friend of the surgeon in oto-rhino-laryngology as I have repeatedly demonstrated also in ear surgery.

This composite flap was also useful in case of excision of cancer in the base of the tongue together with horizontal partial extirpation of the larynx.

The sternocleidomastoid muscle transferred into the pharynx and the oral cavity forms the best protection possible for the arteries of the neck.

There is no objection to performing this operation on the side of the carcinoma and the healthy side in one and the same stage, if there is any indication as to the extension of the tumor, the development of the metastasis or the size of the defect. Together with my two collaborators in this subject, Dr. Baumann and Dr. Richter, we have made use of this method in plastic reconstruction more and more often with great satisfaction, even when half of the irradiation with cobalt on the primary tumor and the metastasis had already been administered.

References

1. Bakamjian V, Littlewood M: Cervical skin flaps for intraoral and pharyngeal repair following cancer surgery, Brit J Plast Surg 17:191–210, 1964
2. Conley J: Concepts in head and neck surgery, Stuttgart: Thieme 1970.

3. Conley J: Regional composite pedicle flaps in surgery of the head and neck In: Arslan M, Ricci V (Edit.): Otorhinolaryngology Proc. X World Congr., Venice May 21–25, 1973 Amsterdam: Excerpta Medica 1974
4. Ducuing J, Ducuing L: Les tumeurs malignes des voies aéro-digestives supérieures. Paris: Masson, 1949
5. Wullstein HL, Zehm S: Der Verschluß des Ductus thoracicus bei der Exstirpation carcinomatöser Lymphknotenmeta stasen, insbesondere nach vorausgegangener Bestrahlung. Arch Ohr-, Nas-u Kehlk-Heilk. 182:392–399 (Kongreßber 1963)

Lip Reconstruction: Emphasis on Electrical Burns

Stephen D. Proffitt and Robert H. Sorosky, Pomona, California

Introduction

Morphologic and histeopathologic defects caused by the passage of electrical current through tissue are in general indistinguishable from those produced by hyperthermia. Much of the damage caused by electrical injury is due to direct production of heat. Current tends to flow omnidirectionally, passing in a broad front through the tissue. The burn is characterized by destruction of epidermal, dermal, and deep fascial structures[1]; histologic changes are essentially the same as those described in the third degree burn with increased inflammatory and vascular response.

Electrical injury thus causes extended thermal damage in both depth and plane. Voltage/duration/contact are obvious principle factors in the extent of burn.[2] An important point is that extreme temperature of high voltage transmission may coagulate blood in vessels some distance from the contact points; with principle veins and arteries thus damaged, a vascular gangrene may develop. The subsequent gangrene necrosis is somewhat different than that caused by crush injuries or other vascular trauma or insufficiency and its possible extent has been coined "4th degree burn".[3] Controversial areas of opinion have been proposed regarding allowing the burn lesion to demarcate and slough, i.e., the concept of "progressive necrosis." Many surgeons[4–6] advocate immediate excision of burned tissue to prevent bacterial invasion of adjacent tissues with "depressed vitality." In these regions, however, histologic examination reveals spotty areas of coagulation necrosis and vascular damage. Use of sulfa mylon, silver nitrate or Sulfadiazine is not recommended in local injury, as these substances may depress the formation of healthy granulation tissue and obscure the landmarks of future excision and repair.[3]

Wounds caused by mechanical violence can be contrasted primarily in the self-limited extent of their damage; devitalization is usually readily apparent. In these cases debridement of nonviable tissue can be approached directly. Blood, lymphatic, and neural supporting structures adjacent to the wound are not generally subject to toxic effects and the subsequent devitalization and necrosis which occurs so often in thermal injury. Areas of marginal viability in a mechanical wound can be thus appraised directly with less fear of hidden underlying damage. Without the effects of extensive coagulation, devascularization and necrosis, immediate inflammatory changes and their subsequent wound healing events commence.[7] With minimal tissue damage and loss, the healing cellular exudate rapidly becomes mononuclear in preparation for the ingrowth of granulation and fibrous tissue elements.

Thus we contrast mechanical wounds with their minimal, nonviable debris, and subsequent rapid responding sequence of healing elements with electrical-thermal injury, its radiating degrees of superficial and deep appendage injury, and delayed, intensely fibrotic reactivity.

Outline of Repair Methods

The preceding discussion forms the basis for our varying approaches in wound repair. Mechanical trauma of the lip requires the same considerations of management as any soft tissue injury of the face. Distorted flaps and fragments of lip are splinted and protected from further vascular compromise, until definitive repair can be undertaken. Repair is optimally performed within 24 hr of injury, when the patient's general situation permits. Tetanus prophylaxis is routine. Anesthesia varies with the patient's age and extent of injuries.

Antibiotic coverage is indicated; several studies[8,9] suggest high concentration of Tetracycline compounds in dermal and epidermal appendages, with possible reduction in cutaneous bacterial flora of surgical concern in wound in-

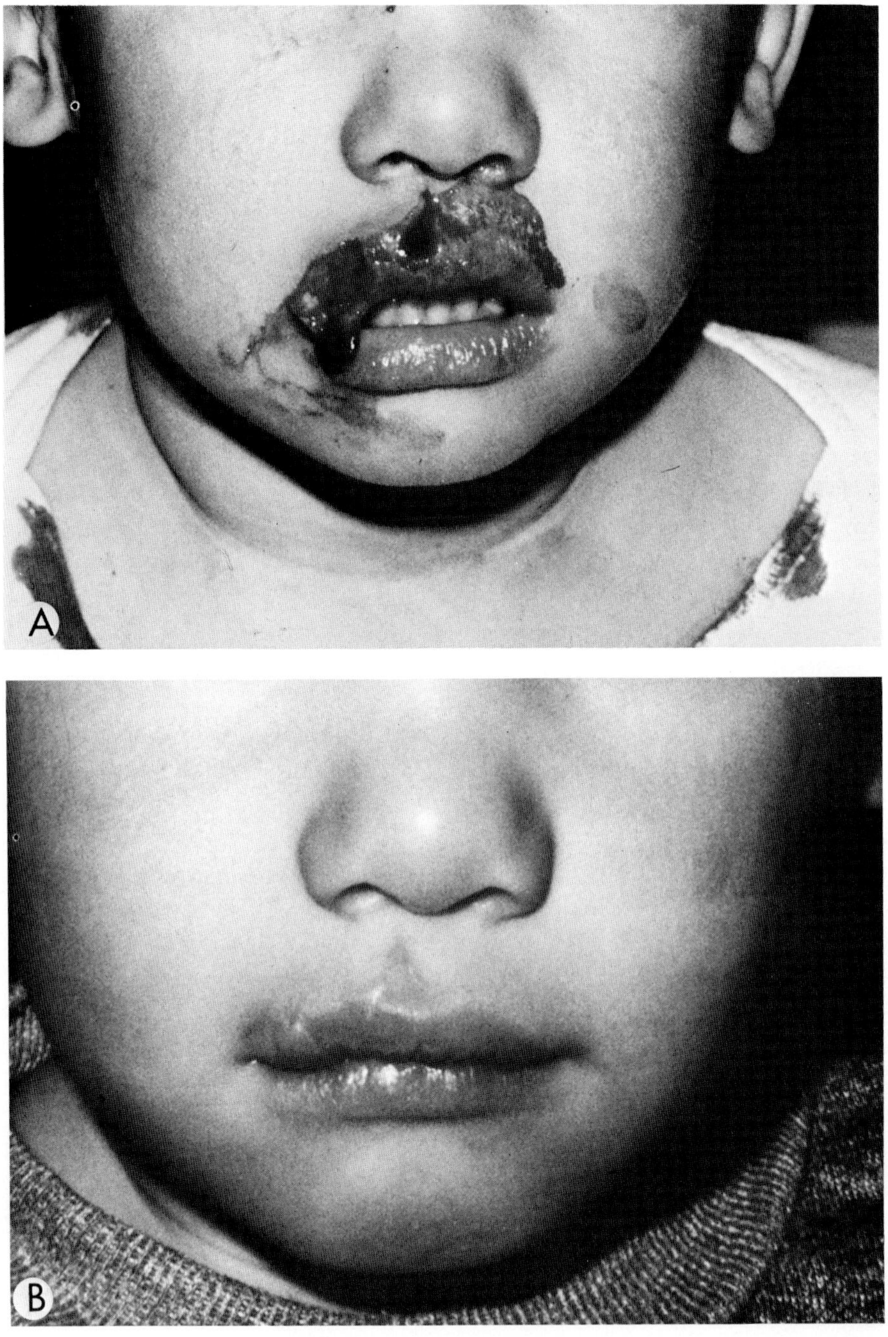

Fig. 1. (A) Avulsion laceration. (B) Post repair.

fection; other products elaborated by the wound's edges are also favorably suppressed, aiding a problem-free healing process.

Wound preparation should be atraumatic and only mildly antiseptic; toxic wound preparations and mechanical debridement compromise the wounds and reduce the marginally viable surrounding tissues. Zepharin or normal saline solution in generous quantity usually suffice. Intelligent wound exploration and conservative debridement need only be mentioned in passing, and are strictly adhered to. Mechanical wounds involving superficial structures without tissue loss respond to a variety of different suture techniques, materials and closures of compromised tissue (Figs. 1,2). Full thickness tissue loss is approached immediately and directly with functional restoration in mind.

The oral muscles of expression are unique in

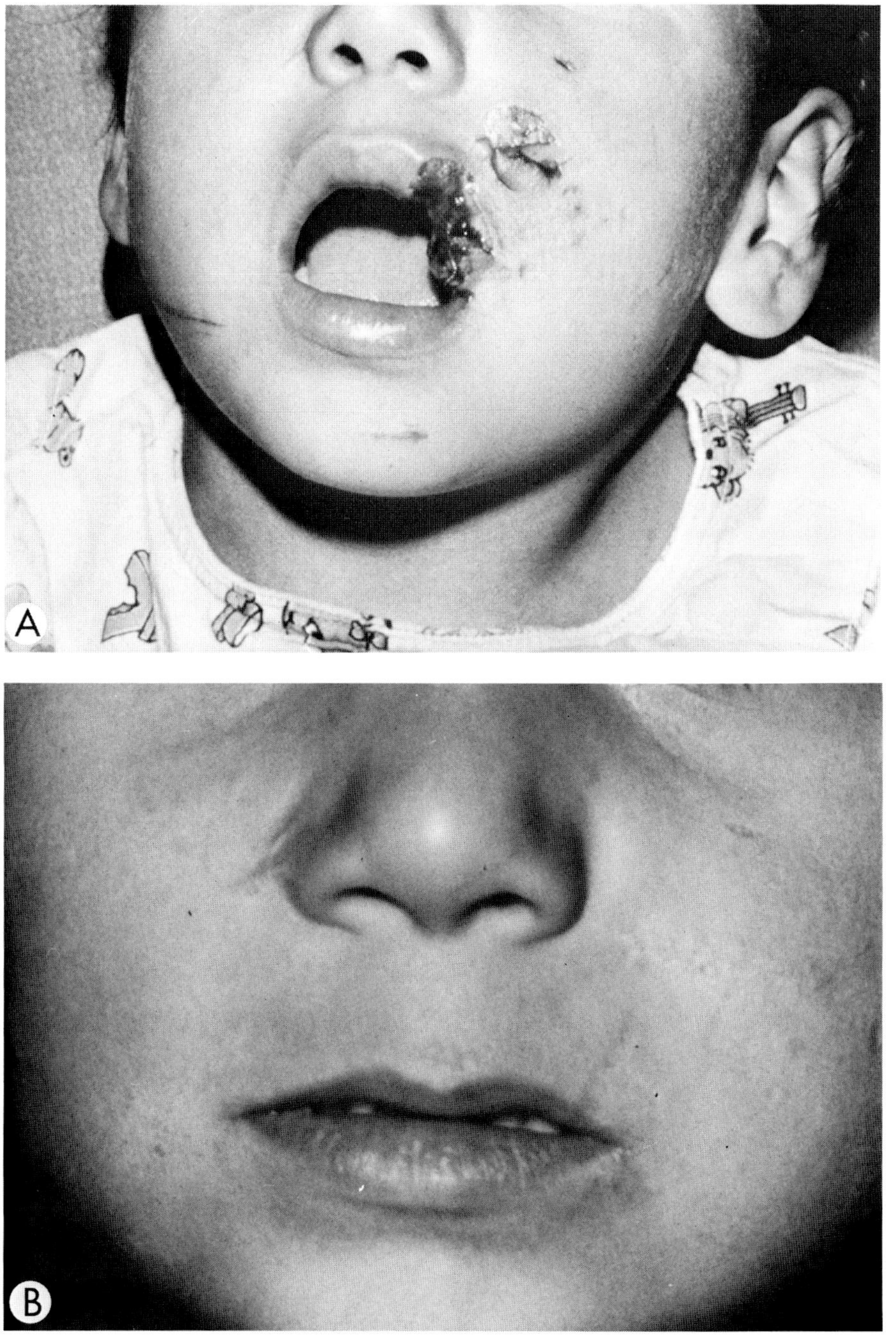

Fig. 2. (A) Avulsion injury with loss of tissue. (B) Post repair.

that they move soft tissue structures of the face rather than acting to move underlying bony structures. They may be characterized into a superficial and deep group (Fig. 3). It is our experience that attention to these muscles primarily is crucial. The superficial secondary skin flaps and the total results hinge on these primary techniques. Most descriptions of such surgery emphasize full thickness, composite flaps and their subsequent rotation.[10,11]

By considering the variety of forces that the individual muscles of expression exert on the mouth, concepts for approaching these repairs have been formulated for presentation. It becomes apparent, that if possible, the muscle groups should be more individually considered.

Selective muscle flaps can be designed where applicable in traumatic wounds. Severed muscle groups can be isolated with ease and the extent of loss directly evaluated at the time of primary repair. Creation and dissection of isolated "sliding muscle pedical flaps" can proceed if necessary, and each advanced to recreate the normal functional anatomy; by attending to deep muscle flaps, followed by superficial structures, anatomic reconstruction develops.

The following examples will illustrate the concepts. Figure 4—A full thickness avulsion defect of the upper lip involving obicularis oris and quadratus labii muscles; repair proceeds with these muscles in mind and permanent buried suture material is used (monofilament nylon or tycron). Figure 5—Loss of lateral commissure with buccinator and zygomaticus primarily involved. Buccinator is closed primarily and zygomaticus muscle flap can be developed to attach to reconstructed lateral commissure. Figure 6—Full thickness avulsion loss of the right upper lip involving the quadratus labii, attached to a primarily sutured

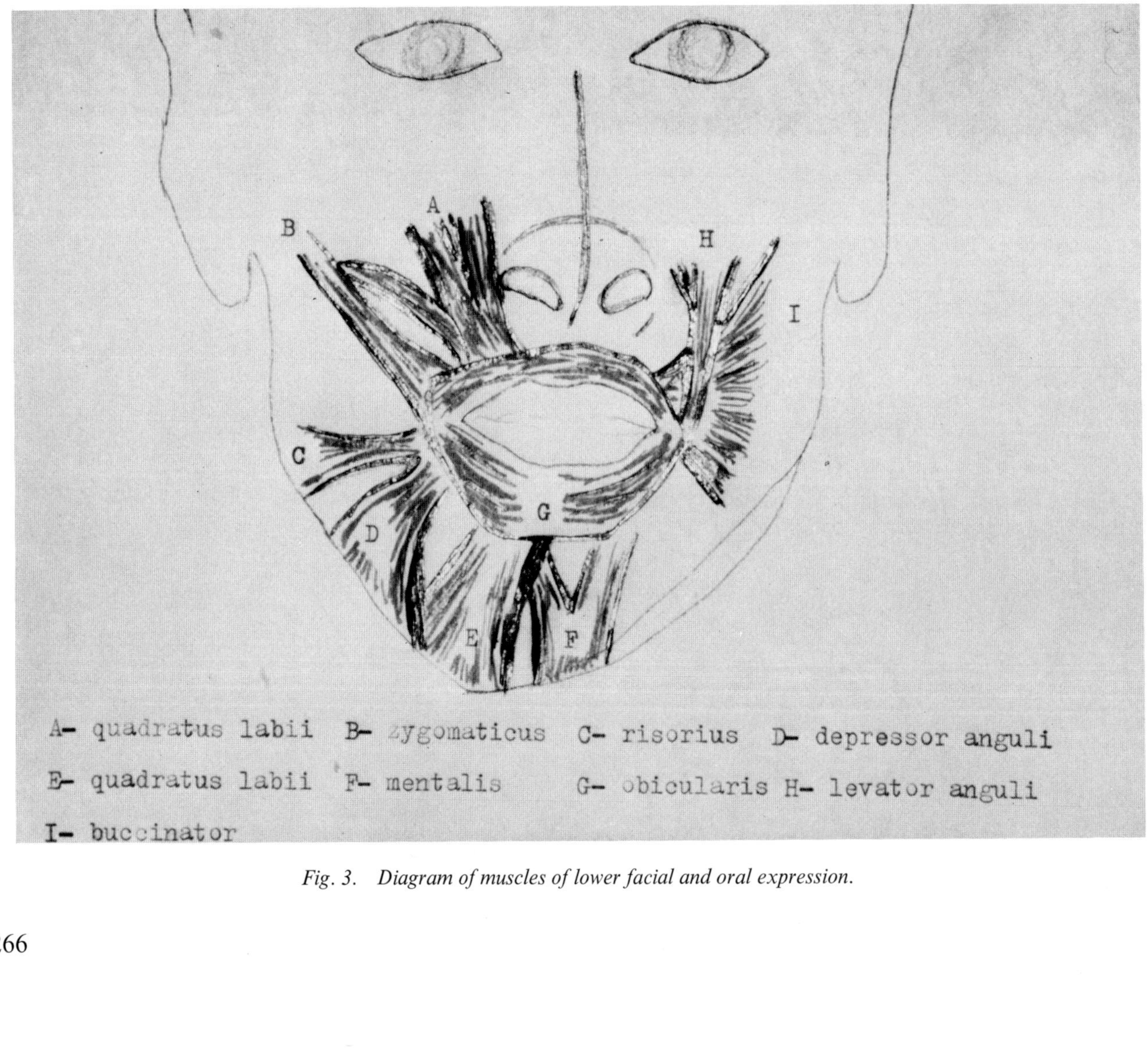

Fig. 3. Diagram of muscles of lower facial and oral expression.

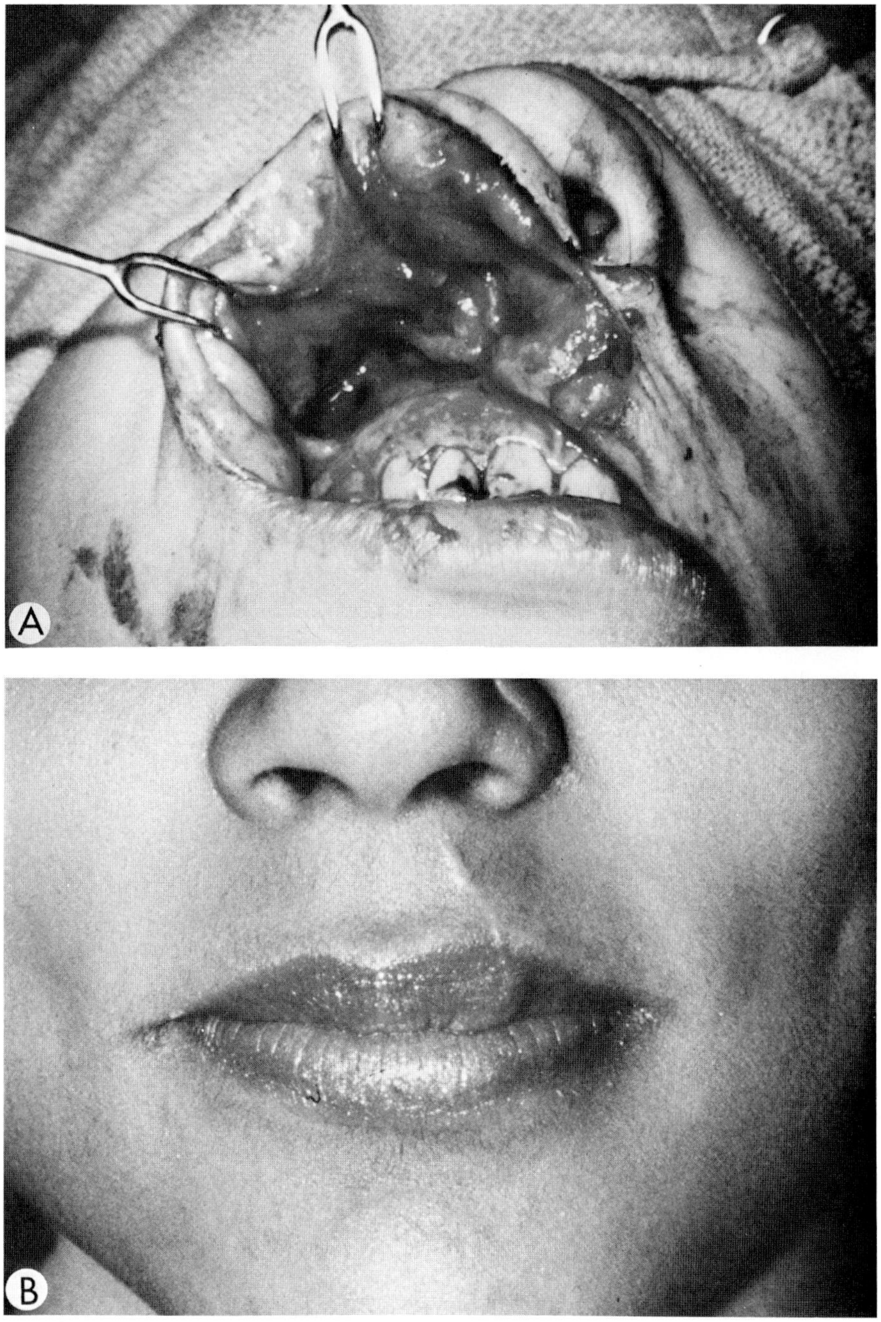

Fig. 4. (A) Avulsion laceration, extensive. (B) Early postop result.

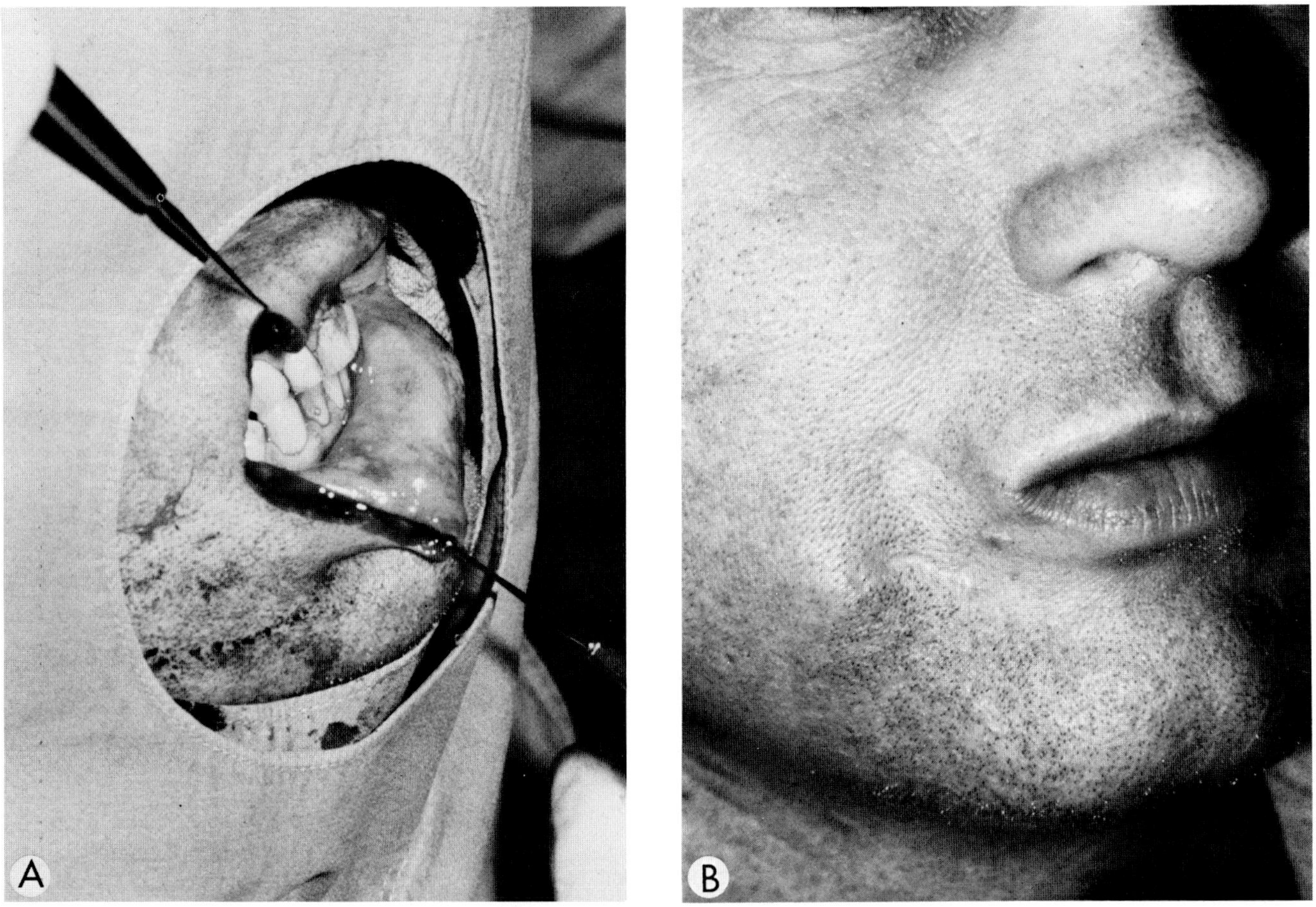

Fig. 5. *(A) Lateral lip and commissure defect. (B) Post reconstruction.*

obicularis oris closure. Figure 7—Total loss of upper lip with demarcation of nasal labial flaps. These skin flaps, however, are at right angles to the underlying pull of the superficial muscle groups and thus primary consideration should be given to muscle pedicle flaps for upper lip function.

Isolated electrical burns of the lip respond most favorably to a contrasting sequence of procedures and care. Because of the charring "4th degree" aspect of the injury,[3] hemorrhage is virtually nonexistant. Initial evaluation of the wound is cautious; the very pathologic processes that are generated by the burn strongly influence the course, and thus the timing of repair. Though the pathogenesis of the burn's thermal damage is well known and repeatedly documented, many surgeons[4–6] still advocate immediate debridement and repair. Our admonition is that superior results will be obtained when the tissues are observed expectantly prior to surgical intervention.

The local lip wound is handled gently with nontoxic moist dressings, appropriate anti-bacterial ointments, and generous systemic prophylactic antibiotics. Thus the viable tissues are supported, and the peripheral partial coagulation necrosis that is occurring in the burn wound can proceed without the invasion of bacteria. Expectant treatment can preserve marginally viable tissues which may play an important role in reconstruction. Early debridement can only destroy marginally viable tissues which, if appropriately supported, could survive.

Timing of staged debridement and reconstruction varies, of course, with the extent of burn. Signs of surrounding edema and distortion must be

(*Text continues on page 279.*)

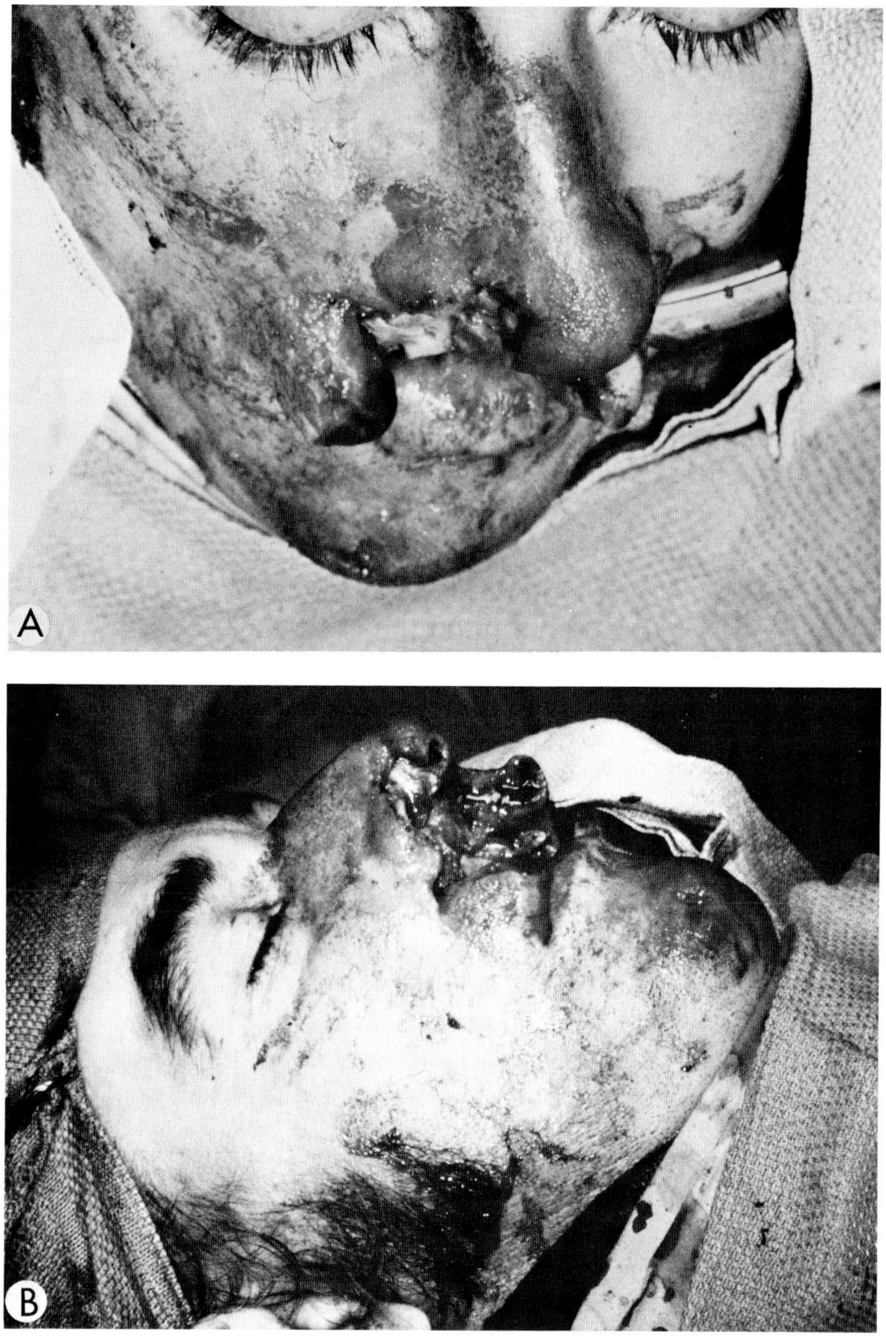

Fig. 6. (A) Avulsion loss of upper lip and right lateral ala. (B) Same.

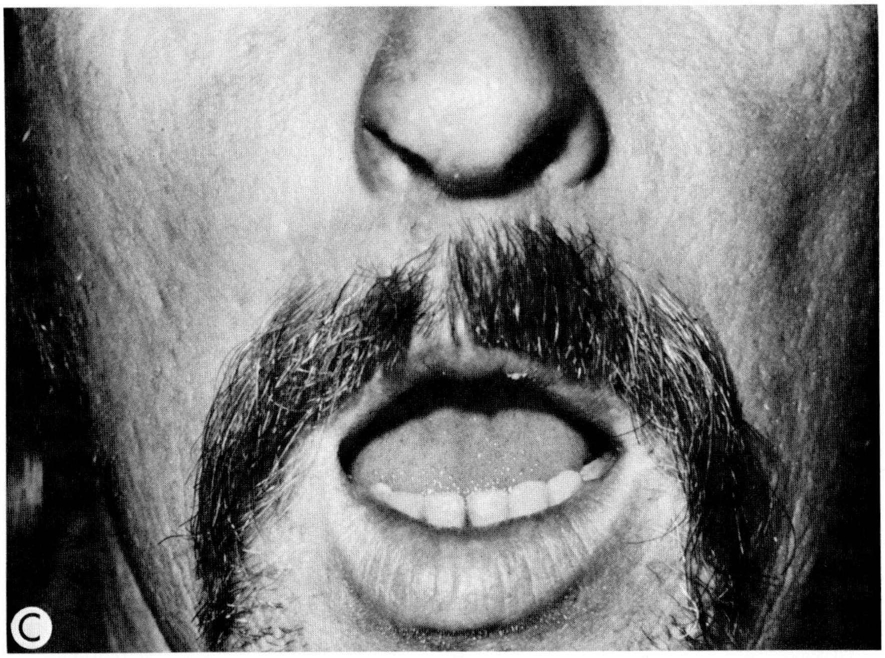

Fig. 6. (C) Post reconstruction.

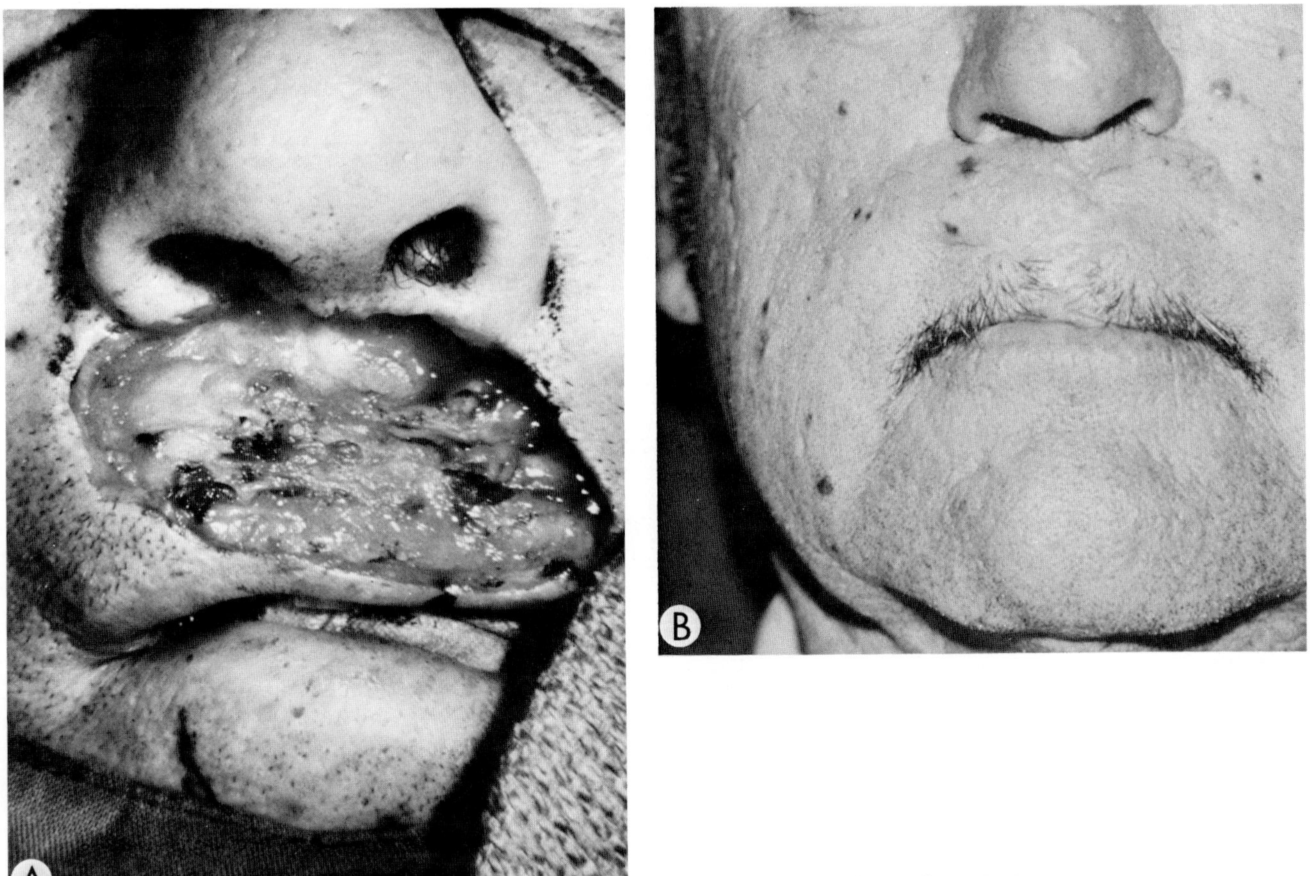

Fig. 7. (A) Loss of upper lip. (B) Postop reconstruction.

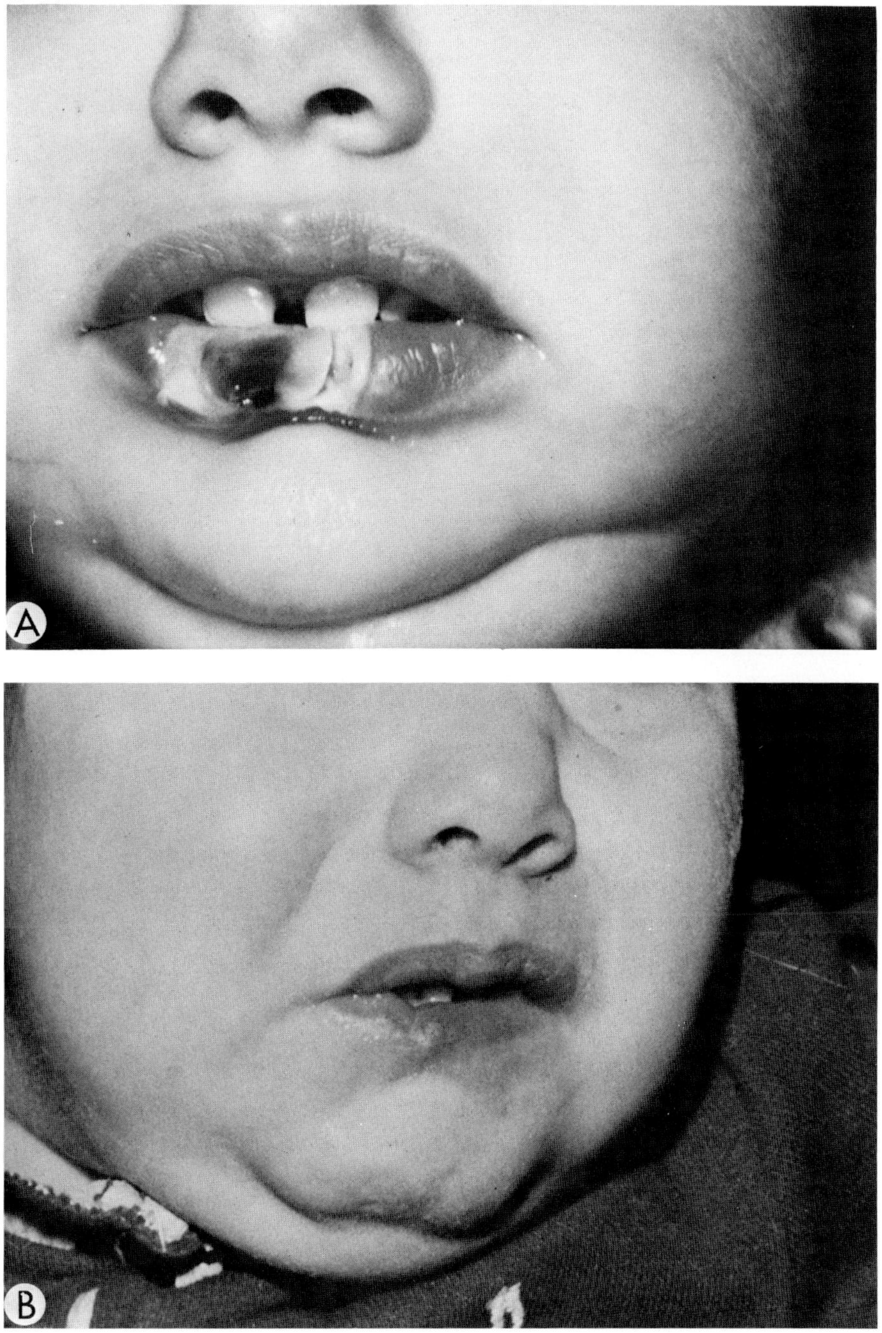

Fig. 8. (A) 2 days post electrical burn, lower lip. (B) Early postop.

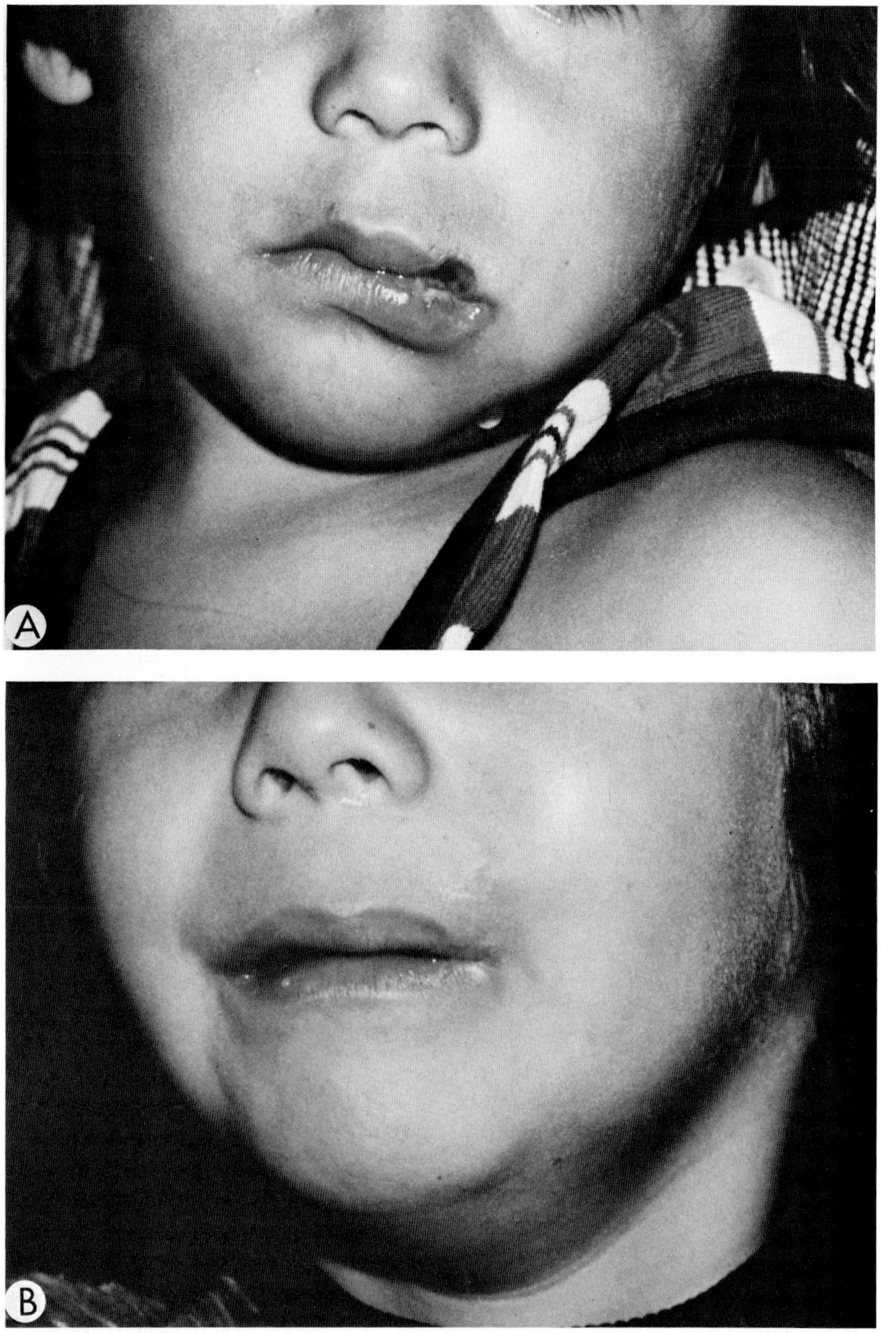

Fig. 9. (A) 48 hours post electrical burn of upper lip and lateral commissure. (B) Postop reconstruction.

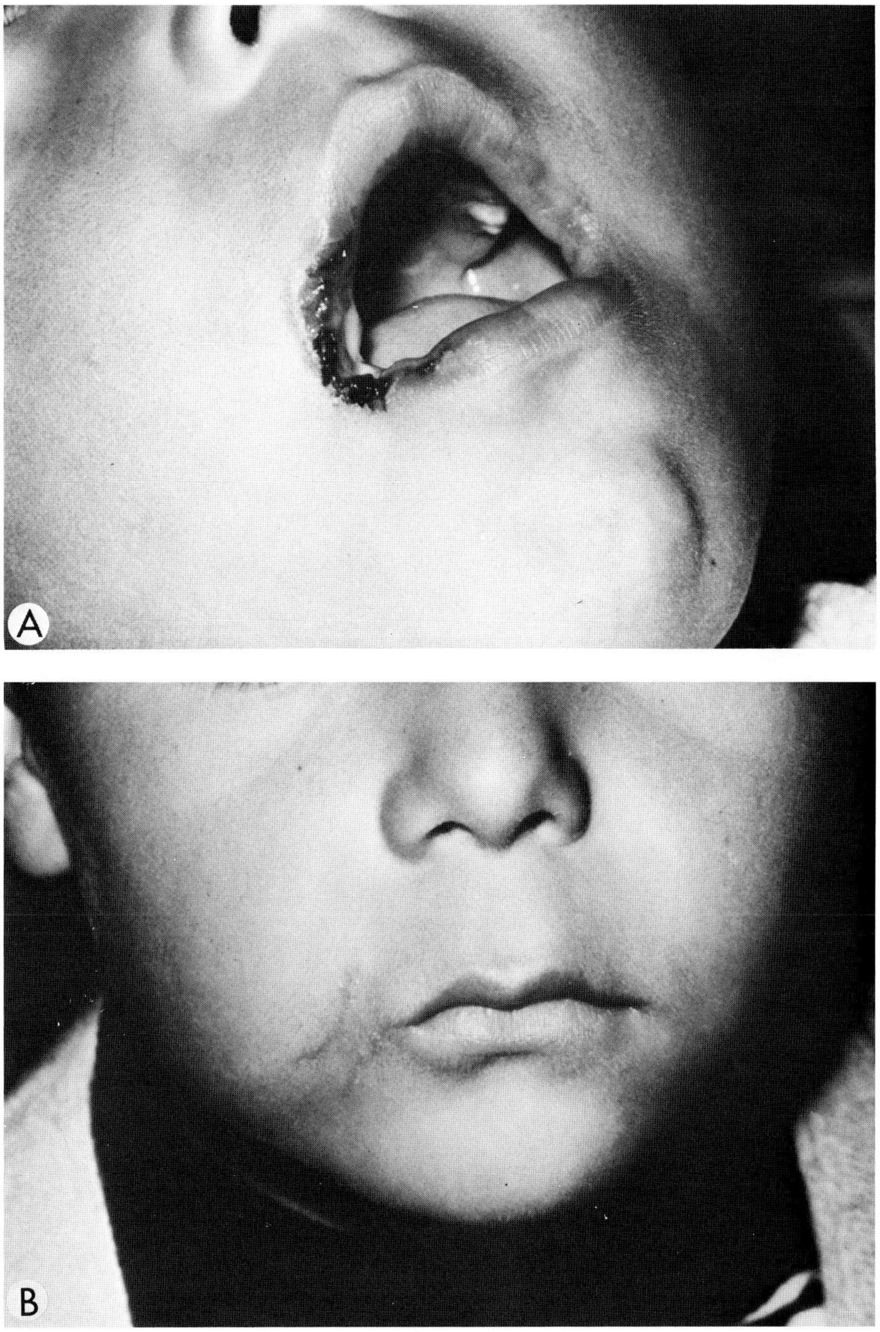

Fig. 10. (A) 48 hours post lateral commissure burn. (B) Postoperative appearance of reconstruction.

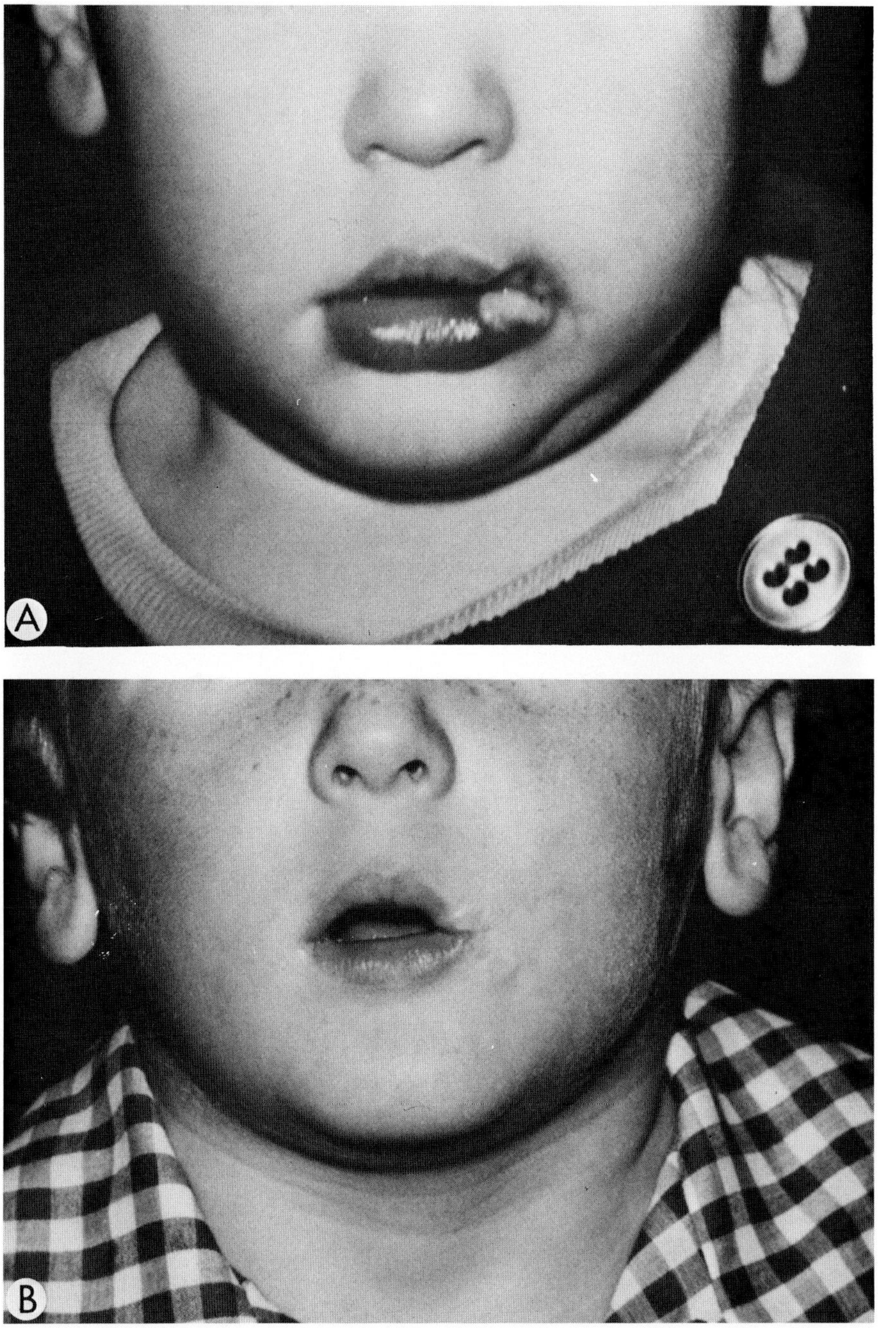

Fig. 11. (A) Lateral commissure and upper lip burn, 48 hours. (B) Postop reconstruction.

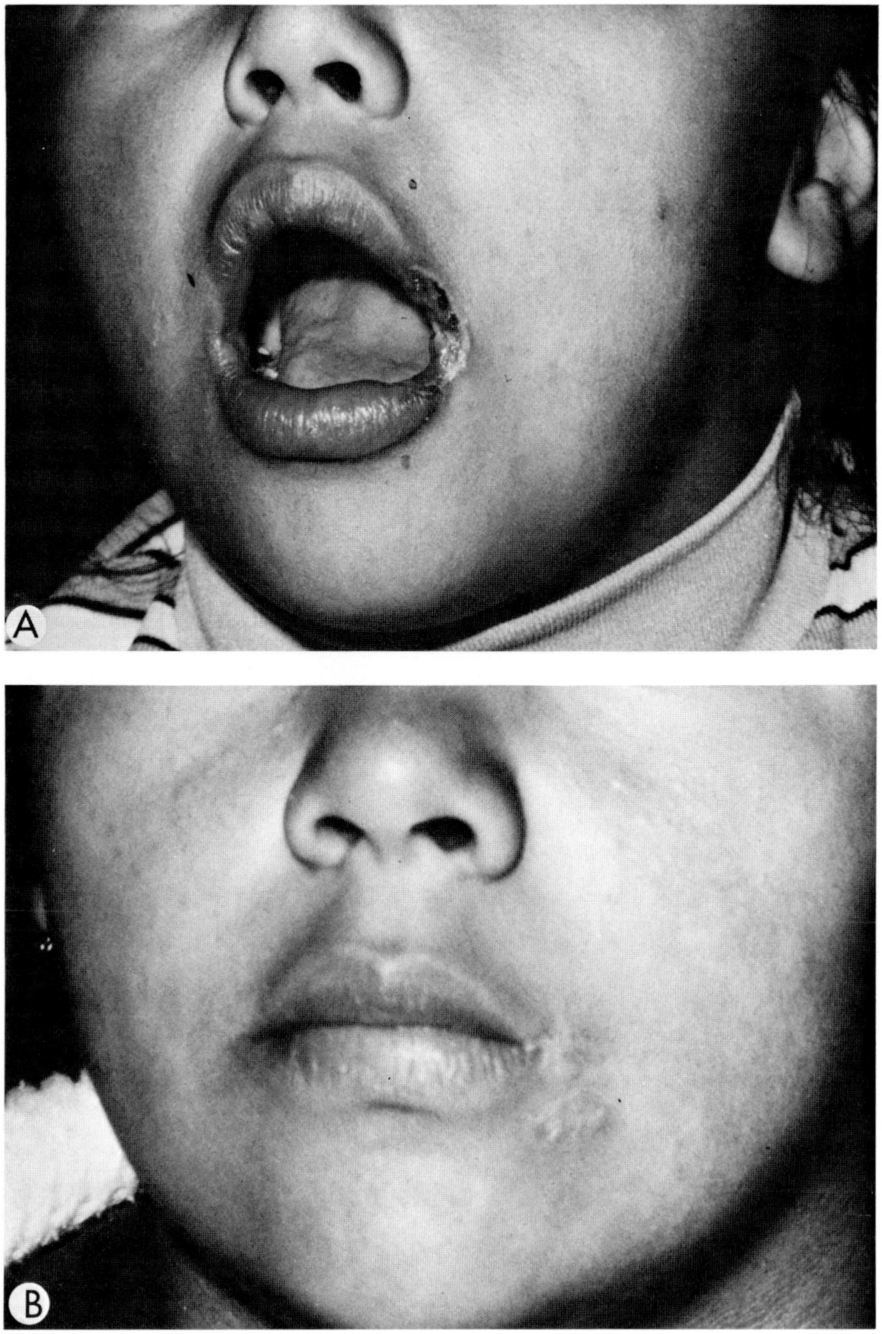

Fig. 12. (A) Lateral commissure and upper lip burn, 48 hours. (B) 2 years postop reconstruction.

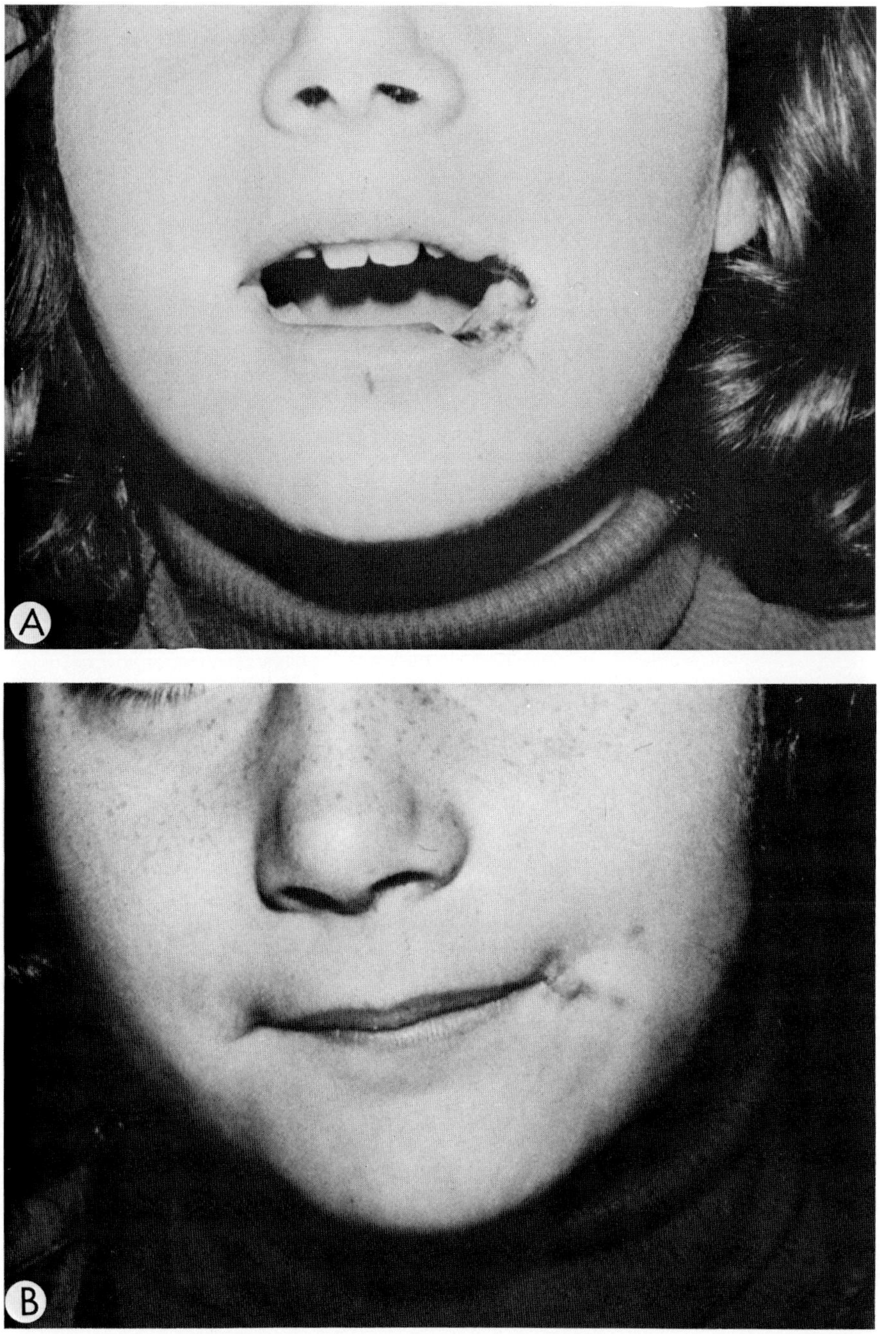

Fig. 13. (A) Extensive lateral commissure and upper and lower lip electrical burn. (B) Postop reconstruction.

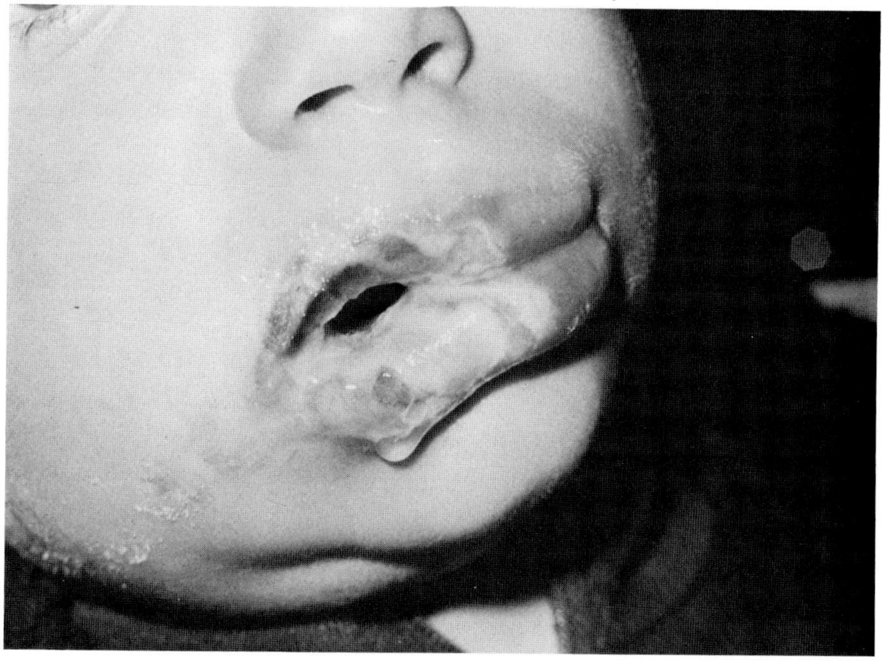

Fig. 14. Severe burn with total loss of right upper lip, lateral commissure, and right lower lip (50% of mouth).

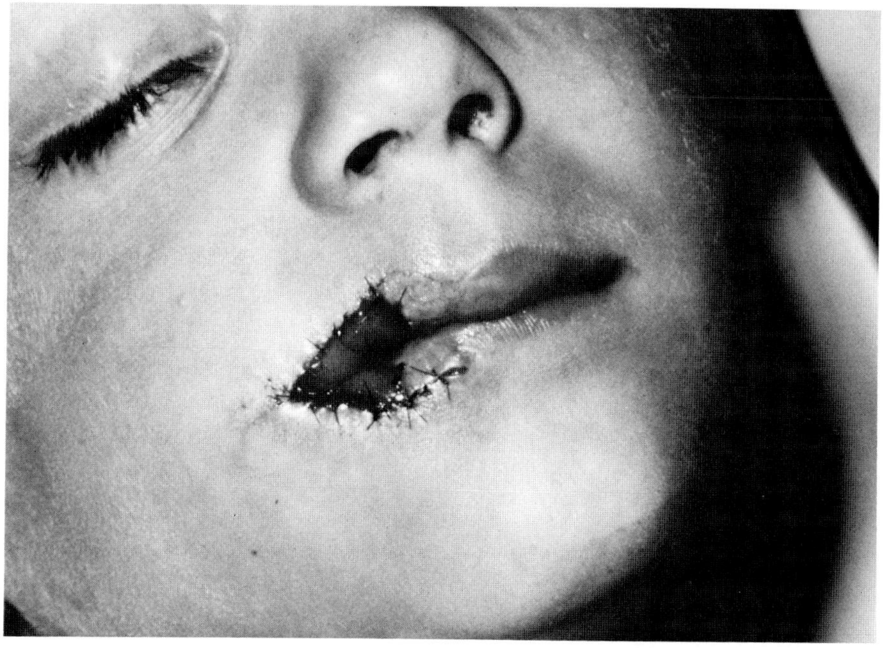

Fig. 15. Early appearance of second stage reconstruction utilizing muscle and vermillion border flaps for reconstruction.

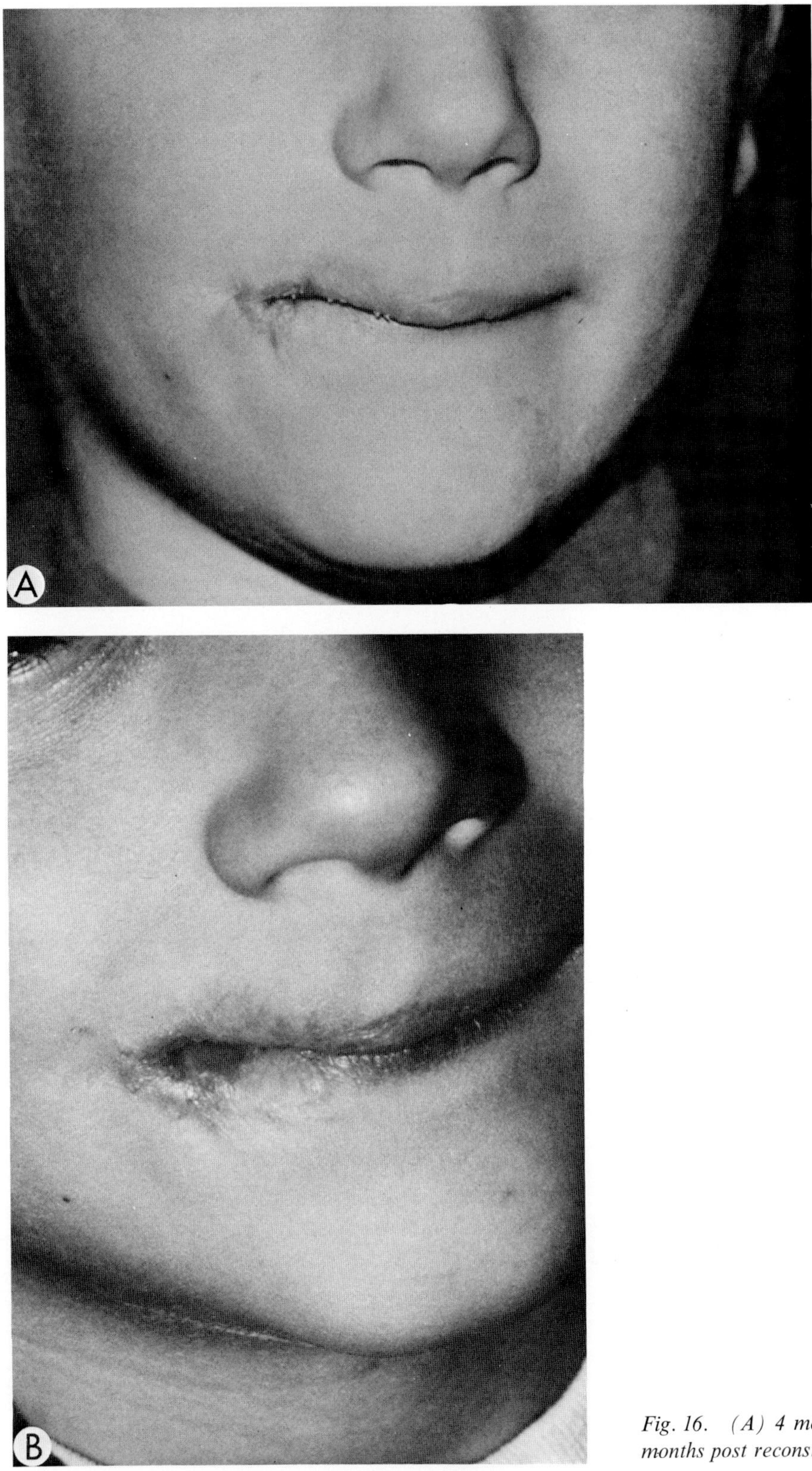

Fig. 16. *(A) 4 months post reconstruction of lower lip. (B) 5 months post reconstruction of lip.*

evaluated closely in order that appropriate surgery time can be instituted; several days of periodic observation is suggested. The devitalized tissues demarcate and slough very slowly with a moderate surrounding tissue reaction, and spontaneous repair, in our hands, has been very slow to occur. We have avoided the use of silver nitrate, sulfamylon and other standard forms of burn therapy, because of their local tissue toxicity, as well as their tendency to depress important formation of granulation tissue. Topical and systemic steroids have been used with satisfactory results, delaying a premature fibrocytic response.

In isolated, well-circumscribed lesions, a one-stage reconstruction is the treatment of choice. Wound margin excisions with approximation (Figs. 8–10) may also lend themselves to "sliding muscle pedicle flaps" of both buccinator and zygomaticus fibers (Figs. 11–13). The more extensive burn (Fig. 14) is staged, with primary concern being preservation of marginal tissue and closure of the defect. No attempt is made to reconstruct muscle or function initially. The definitive repair being best achieved after healing of the burn wound, and after allowing a significant period of time to elapse while the scars soften. Thus the tendency toward hypertrophic scarring is anticipated and does not include the muscle groups in its fibrosis. Second stage reconstruction (Fig. 15), including techniques of muscle flaps, are considered at an appropriate time when definitive margins can be ascertained, and the muscles can be dissected free of the binding fibrosis (Fig. 16).

The suture materials we utilize in all burn wounds are permanent monofiliment products and we avoid reactive materials such as braided synthetics and animal fiber.

References

1. Harkins HN: Research in the pathology of burns, Arch Path 38:147–154, 1944
2. McLaughlin CW et al: Management of electrical burns. Arch Surg 68:531, 1954
3. Robbins SL: Textbook of pathology. Philadelphia: Saunders, 1962
4. Bowe JJ: Primary excision of third degree burns. Plast Reconstr Surg 24:240–247, 1960
5. Hyslop VB et al: Treatment of electrical burns of the lips, Plast Reconstr Surg 20:315, 1957
6. Peterson RA: Electrical burns (in) plastic surgery, Boston: Little Brown, 1973
7. Schultz RC: Facial injuries, Chicago: Yearbook Medical Publishers, 1970
8. Scheimann LG et al: Role of bacteria in formation of free fatty acids in human skin surface, J Invest Derm 34:171–194, 1960
9. Freinkel RK: Pathogenesis of acne vulgaris, NEJM 280:1161, 1969
10. Converse et al: Reconstructive plastic surgery. Philadelphia: Saunders, 1964
11. Kazanjian/Converse: Surgical treatment of facial injuries. Baltimore, Williams & Wilkins, 1974

Oral Reconstruction after Cancer Surgery: The Lingual Flap

Lawrence W. DeSanto, Rochester, Minn.

The choice of reconstruction technique after excision for cancer of the oral cavity and pharynx often determines whether a patient will heal quickly and leave the hospital or suffer wound disruption, infection, fistulization with prolonged hospitalization, or even die from infection or hemorrhage after wound breakdown. The reconstruction decision likewise determines the functional end result in terms of voice, swallowing, and appearance.

Many factors are considered in deciding on a reconstruction technique. One of these is the type of surgery, particularly whether a portion of the lower jaw is to be sacrificed or spared. This decision is significant because sacrifice of a portion of the mandible makes primary closure safer in that local tissues fall together more directly. Also of importance is the size of the surgical defect, the use and amount of preoperative radiation, and the length of time from radiation to surgery. Other factors considered are the patient's age, occupation, general health, and sex.

Primary closure after resection of cancers of the oral cavity and upper pharynx pulls the remaining tongue mucosa to cheek, palate, and pharynx. This draws the anterior portion of the tongue backward and laterally, with restriction and shortening of the mobile tongue.

Free skin grafts have been advocated for oral and pharyngeal reconstruction. The frequent use of external or interstitial radiation before surgery, however, makes this method hazardous. Also, free grafts tend to shrink, lessening functional mobility.

Regional flaps such as those from the forehead and chest wall are popular reconstruction methods after ablation of oropharyngeal cancers. Both areas provide safe and predictable flaps. The major difficulty with regional techniques is the need for staging and cosmetic consideration. In both types of flaps, the greatest percentage of tissue that is moved is used as the carrier portion, and only the distal few centimeters of either flap are used for the final reconstruction.

The pharyngostome separates ablation from reconstruction and is useful in the patient who has been heavily radiated as well as in the debilitated or elderly patient in whom surgery is best terminated as quickly as feasible. The length of time required to complete reconstruction can be demoralizing to patient and physician, particularly if the flaps fail during closure or recurrence is recognized during reconstruction. Nevertheless, a few patients are best managed with the pharyngostome.

The tongue flap is useful for intraoral and upper pharyngeal reconstruction. This flap includes a portion (usually half) of the adjacent remaining tongue and is used as a rotation flap rather than in primary closure. This portion of the tongue can provide nearly 100 cm^2 of a thick, well-vascularized mucosal surface that is native to the oral cavity. The entire pedicle is used for reconstruction, and none is needed as the carrier portion. Reconstruction is completed in one stage. In our practice, tongue flaps have been successful after radiation, after ligation of the ipsilateral lingual artery, and in conjunction with mandibular reconstruction.[1] Tongue flaps have been used after resection of the soft palate,[2] tonsillar area, floor of the mouth,[3] tongue base, lateral pharynx,[1] and buccal mucosa.[4] These flaps are desirable options to the larger regional flaps such as the forehead and various chest flaps.

Mayo Clinic Series

In a series of 38 consecutive patients in whom the tongue flap was used for reconstruction, 20 of the tumors were situated at the base of the tongue, 12 in the tonsillar region, 2 in the buccal mucosa, 3 in the floor of the mouth, and 1 in the lateral pharynx.

In another series of 82 consecutive patients treated surgically for squamous cancer of the tonsillar area and tongue base, lingual flaps were used for 32 patients, and primary closure was accomplished in 42 patients. In the total experience with 38 tongue flap reconstructions, there was one surgical death from myocardial infarction and four patients had salivary fistulas that closed spontaneously. One flap that was used to reconstruct buccal mucosa was revised. Speech and swallowing were not major problems. Some flaps are used with the hypoglossal nerve intact, which in time becomes integrated as dynamic functioning tissue in swallowing and phonation.

The tongue flap is ideal for covering the site of mandibular reconstruction after osteotomy has been performed to gain access to the site of the primary tumor. This combination has been utilized in 20 patients in whom the jaw was divided, cancer excised, and jaw rewired. In 15 of the 20 patients, radiation preceded resection either in a planned sequence or with intent to cure by use of surgery at recurrence.

Technique

After neck dissection and resection of the primary site, the appropriate tongue flap is developed.

The Posterior-Based Tongue Flap

This flap is used when the tongue base and lingual artery are intact. It is best suited for reconstruction of the floor of the mouth and the buccal area but can be used in reconstruction of defects of the palatal and tonsillar area or of combinations of these defects. The flap is developed by dividing the tongue down the midline, as is done in hemiglossectomy. The lateral border is then "unrolled" by sculpturing the flap open, as in spreading a tubed pedicle. A flap of full-thickness tongue mucosa and 1 or 2 mm of muscle are available for rotation. Bleeding is managed with surgical diathermy. After being rotated, the flap is attached in the submucosa and mucosal edges by the use of interrupted absorbable sutures. The degree of rotation depends on the recipient site. Only a few degrees of rotation are needed to reconstruct the floor of the mouth, about 45° of lateral rotation are needed for the buccal area, and a full 90° of rotation are needed to repair the tonsillar area and palate. The degree of twisting does not seem to be critical for flap survival. The flap usually retains its hypoglossal nerve innervation, and such innervation is preferable, although a noninnervated flap does not present any difficulty.

The Lateral Tongue Flap

This type of tongue flap is based on the anterior and lateral floor of the mouth. It is designed for use after a portion (or even half) of the tongue base has been resected and the lingual artery has been divided. The flap uses the remaining mobile portion of the tongue; this portion is rotated into the base defect and, if needed, into the adjacent tonsillar area in order to retain a more nearly normal movement of the tongue. Unlike that in primary closure, the tongue is narrowed rather than shortened. The remaining portion of the tongue is sutured on itself, as in closure after hemiglossectomy.

The viability of this type of flap depends on anastomotic ipsilateral and contralateral circulation. Because of this dependence, if the ipsilateral external carotid artery is ligated, the viability of the flap is not as predictable and the flap should not be used. The hypoglossal nerve is usually divided. To develop the lateral tongue flap, the tongue is divided down the middle so that the base defect can be joined in the midline. The lateral free edge of the tongue is unrolled in the same manner as was done in the posterior flap technique, the entire mucosal flap is rotated into the defect and sutured in place in layers, and the donor tongue is closed primarily on itself. Stay sutures or an immobilizing sponge bolus is not necessary.

Comments

Continued experience with the surgical treatment of malignant disease in the oral cavity and upper pharynx of radiated and nonradiated patients provides the opportunity to reconsider and refine reconstruction techniques. There are five options for this reconstruction: (1) primary closure, (2) regional pedicle flap closure, (3) primary skin grafting, (4) the pharyngostome, and (5) the use of a pedicle flap from an adjacent portion of the tongue.

The excellent blood supply of the tongue and the position of the tongue adjacent to the defect permit the use of these flaps as an important option for immediate reconstruction. Nondelayed repair without alteration of appearance is likewise an important advantage.

These flaps are useful if carefully developed in the radiated patient, after ligation of the ipsilateral lingual artery (but not lingual and external carotid arteries). The flaps are useful to cover the site of mandibular reconstruction either after composite resection or after mandibular osteotomy has been used to gain access to the primary neoplasm.

References

1. DeSanto LW: Lingual flap reconstruction after resection for cancer. Trans Am Acad Ophthalmol Otolaryngol 78:135–139, 1971
2. Klopp CT, Schurter M: The surgical treatment of cancer of the soft palate and tonsil. Cancer 9:1239–1243, 1956
3. Papaioannou AN, Farr HW: Reconstruction of the floor of the mouth by a pedicle tongue flap. Surg Gynecol Obstet 122:807–810, 1966
4. Ganguli A: Use of tongue flap to line cheek defects in surgery for cancer. Plast Reconstr Surg 41:390–392, 1968

Total Reconstruction of the Lower Lip

Alvin J. Novack, Seattle, Washington

Total reconstruction of the lower lip for malignancy is indicated in extensive carcinoma of the lower lip (Fig. 1). Reconstruction is entirely adequate with bilateral cheek flaps, and when planned correctly, reconstruction should allow full restoration of lip function and contour.

The total resection of the lower lip is first done with or without preservation of the oral commissure of either side. Two lateral nasolabial flaps are outlined, each with the base corresponding to the newly planned muco-cutaneous junction, and the medial border in the nasolabial fold (Fig. 2).

The skin and muscles of each triangle are next excised to the cheek mucosa, and the skin-muscle triangle is discarded. The mucosa is preserved, and retained as a triangular flap, to be used for the new lower-lip vermillion (Figs. 3, 4).

The cheek flaps are then mobilized and shifted medially (Fig. 5). As this is done, final corrections are completed to the mucosal margin to create a precise vermillion border. The final closure (Figs. 6, 7) should present a pleasing nasolabial fold, and a soft vermillion border.

The complete reconstruction after healing forms a functioning lower lip with adequate sphincter action and good cosmetic contour and projection (Figs. 8, 9).

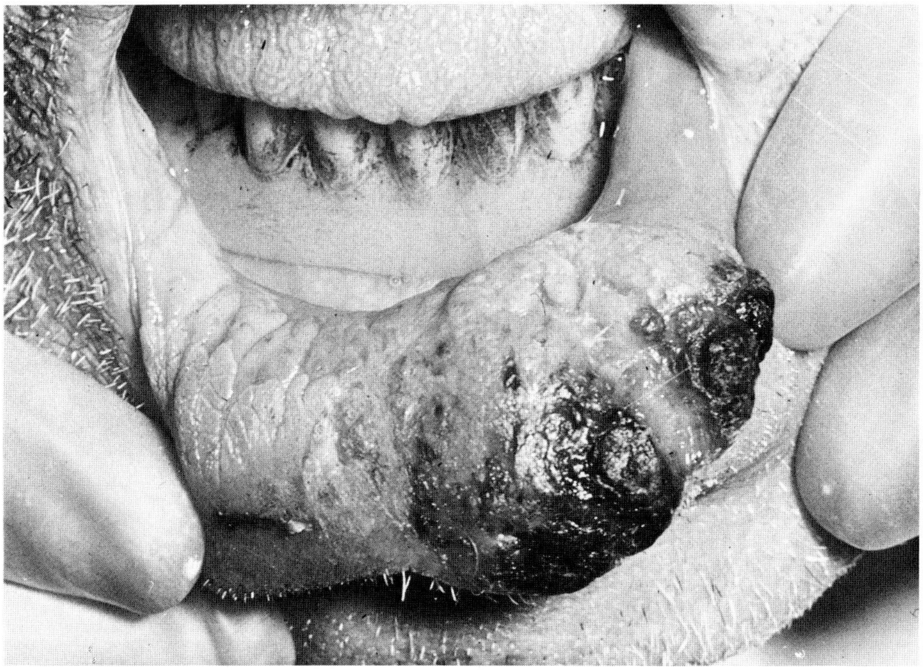

Fig. 1. Infiltrating carcinoma of the lower lip. Note extent near the commissure on each side. Total lower lip resection is indicated. Primary resection and reconstruction may be done on irradiated tissue. If neck dissection is done, conserve the external maxillary artery on each side or complete as a secondary stage.

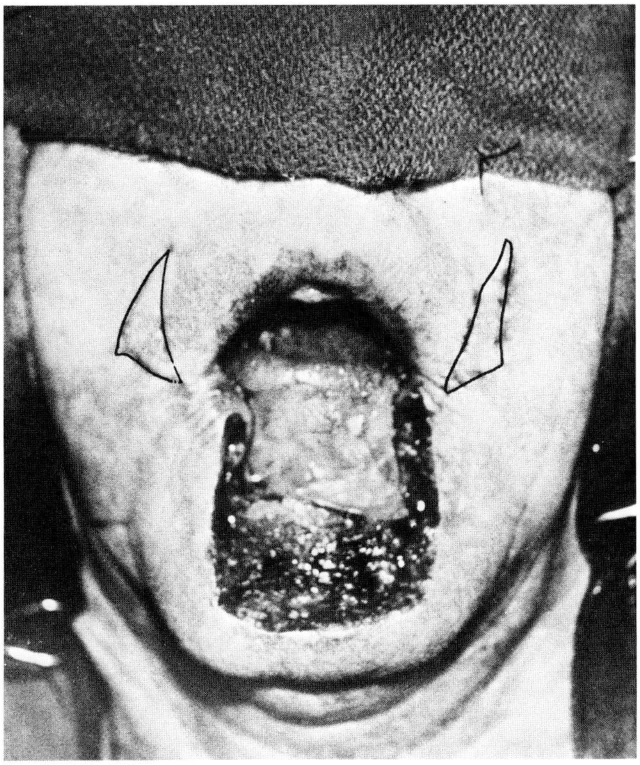

Fig. 2 Resection of the lower lip carcinoma has been completed, and two nasolabial flaps have been outlined in preparation for the primary reconstruction. The base of each triangle corresponds to the newly planned vermillion border.

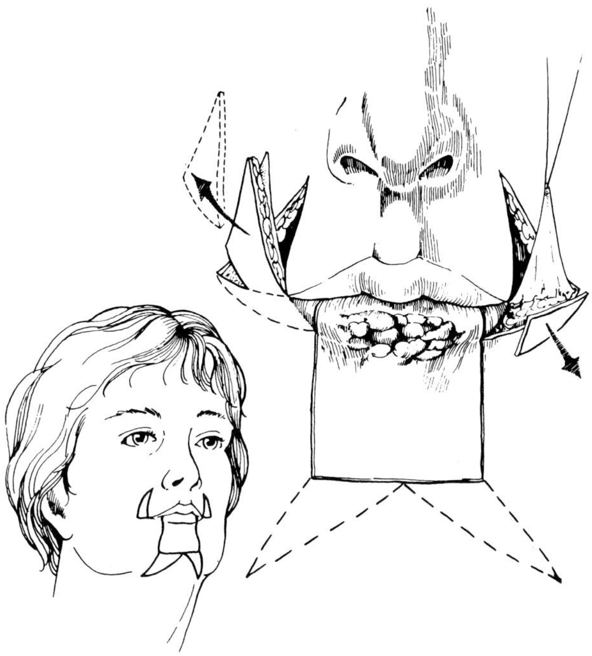

Fig. 3. The outline of the cancer operation in shown. The triangular nasolabial flaps have been outlined, and the skin-muscle portion discarded. The mucosal flaps are retained, and a small portion of skin is removed next to each base for final placement of the vermillion border.

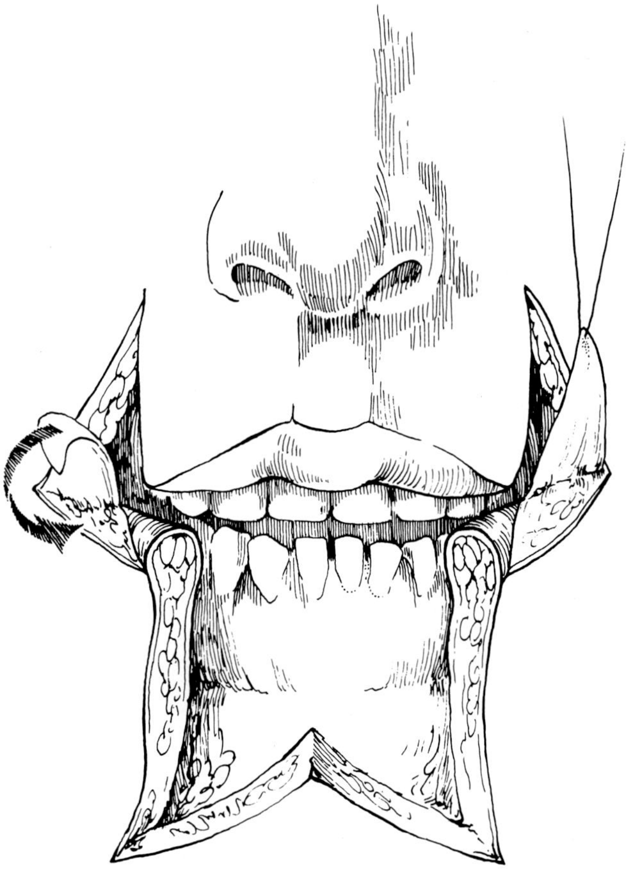

Fig. 4. The mucosal flap is shown on each side in preparation for formation of the new vermillion.

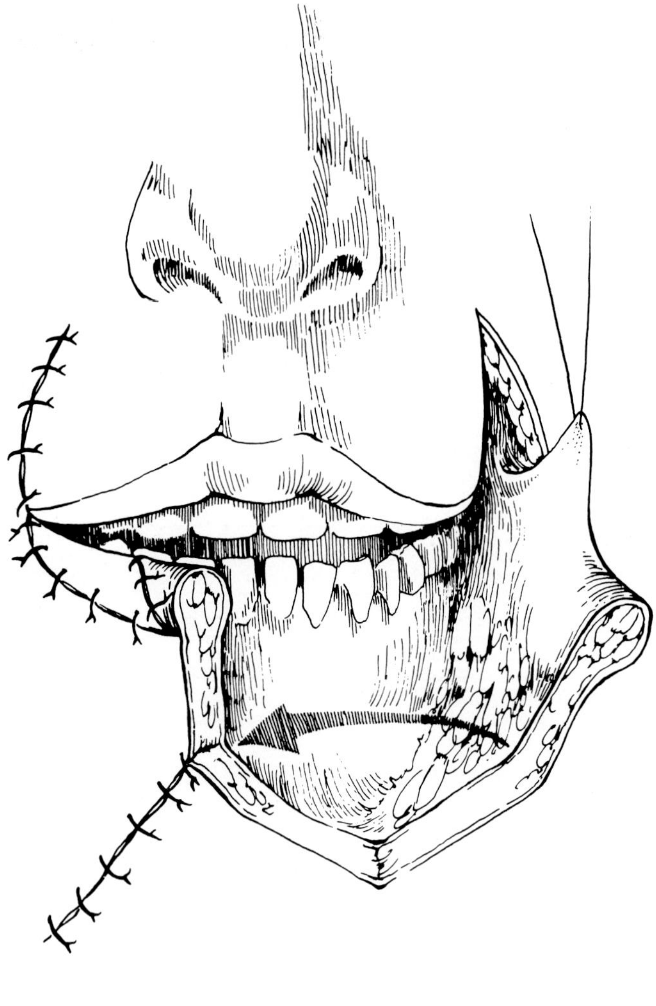

Fig. 5. The mucosal flap has been sutured in position, and the cheek flaps are mobilized for a medial rotation and closure.

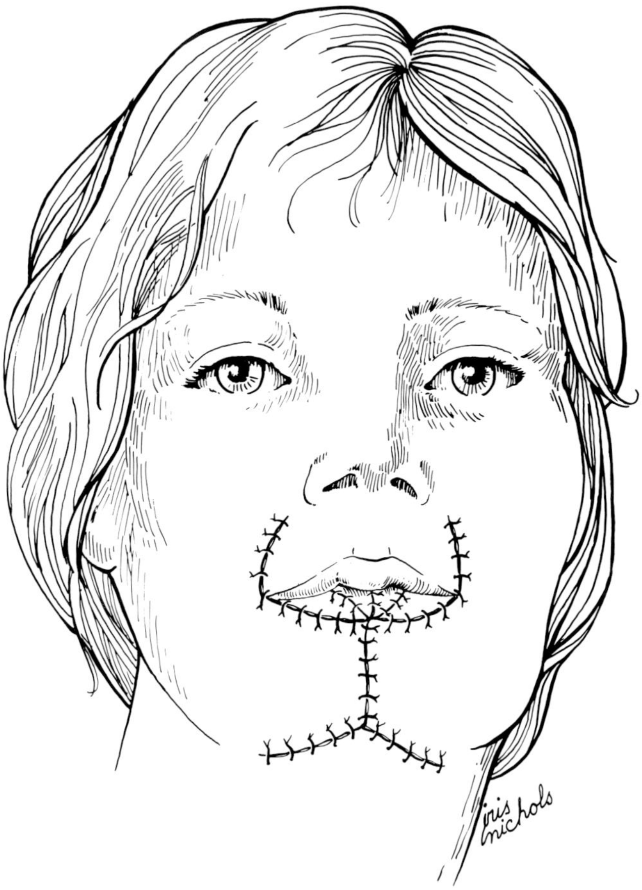

Fig. 6. The final closure should effectively reconstruct the oral commissure, the lower lip and the chin, without distortion to the nose, upper lip, or cheek.

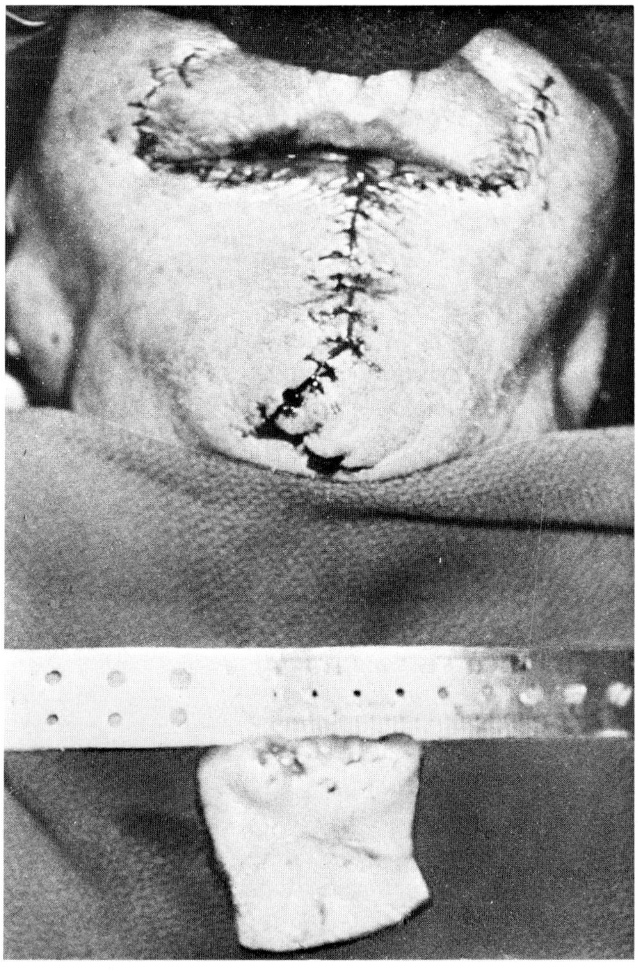

Fig. 7. Final closure after complete lower lip resection.

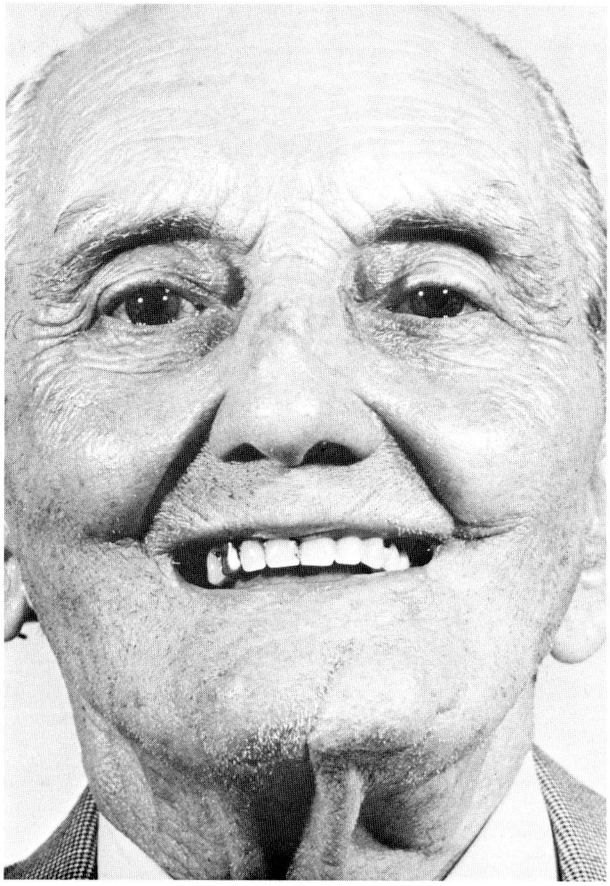

Fig. 8. Final healing and function three months after total lower lip resection.

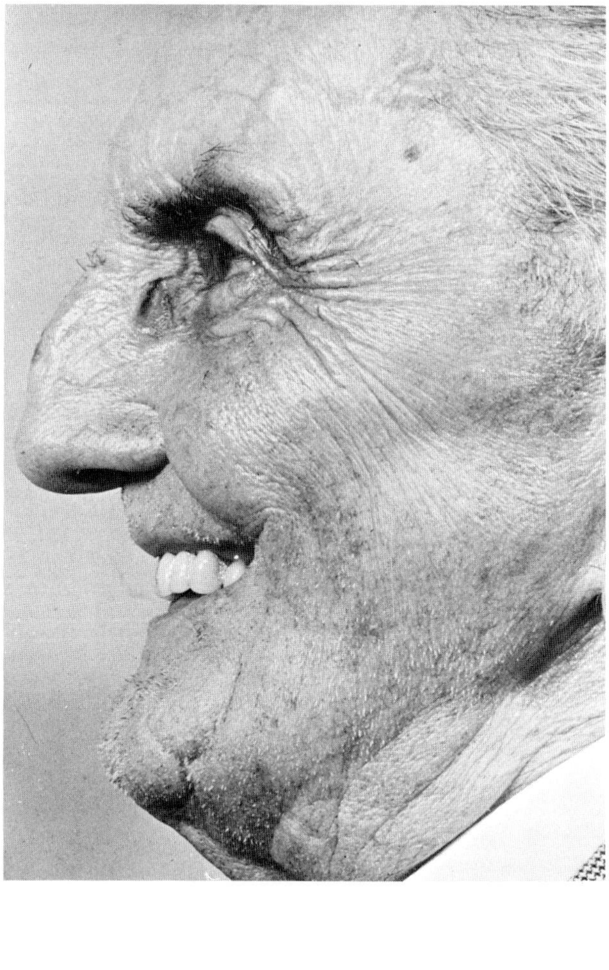

Fig. 9. Lateral view, three months after total lower lip resection.

Factors Affecting Lingual Blood Flow

James M. Toomey and
G. Gordon Snyder, III, Newington, Conn.

In recent years lingual flaps have been increasingly used for the reconstruction and resurfacing of surgical defects in the oral cavity and oropharynx.[1,2] In addition, lingual remnants have long been employed to reconstitute oral mucosal continuity after major resections involving portions of the tongue, floor of mouth or alveolus. It has been assumed clinically that the tongue has an abundant blood supply which generally assures the viability of narrow lingual remnants and permits rotation of tongue flaps with minimal fear of necrosis. On the other hand, some surgeons have the impression that wide ablative procedures in the region of the base of the tongue may present a threat to tongue survival, particularly if both lingual arteries are sacrificed.

The present study was designed to measure blood flow in the canine tongue and to determine the relative contribution of several larger vessels to lingual circulation. It is hoped that this information will provide the surgeon with a more rational basis for his operative manipulations of lingual tissue.

Method

Thirty-six mongrel dogs of medium size and weight were used. After each animal had been anesthetized with intravenous thiopentol (15 mg/lb) an endotracheal tube was inserted and connected to a Harvard respiratory pump with an intermittent hyperinflation valve. A membrane mass spectrometric probe as described by Roberts and Owens[3] was inserted into the central portion of the ipsilateral half of the oral tongue and a second probe was placed in the abdominal aorta through a femoral cutdown. The spectrometers were connected to a Model 7 Grass polygraph so that the partial pressures of argon (pA), oxygen (pO_2) and carbon dioxide (pCO_2) in both sites could be monitored continuously, directly and simultaneously by the spectrometer digital display and recorded by the polygraph. The argon washout method of blood flow determination[4] was used, with both absolute and relative flows being obtained. All washouts were done only after alterations in local circulation due to probe insertion, vessel ligation or soft tissue disruption had stabilized. The data were analyzed with the 9810A Hewlett-Packard programmable calculator.

Baseline blood flow was measured in each animal initially. The upper carotid and lingual vasculature was then surgically exposed and small umbilical tapes placed about each. The appropriate vessels were then ligated and divided, with subsequent repeat determination of flow. Each animal was examined one week later in order to assess the status of the tongue.

In four dogs, regarded as a pilot group, the contralateral lingual artery was ligated and divided and a washout done, followed by sequential division of the ipsilateral artery with repeat blood flow determination.

In a second group of fourteen dogs, the contralateral and ipsilateral lingual arteries were ligated and divided at the same time and the washout repeated.

Another twelve dogs had all accessible named vessels supplying the tongue (lingual, facial, external carotid and maxillary arteries plus the external maxillary, lingual, pharyngeal, facial, and submental veins[5]) ligated and divided in rapid succession and blood flow measured after pO_2 and pCO_2 had stabilized.

A final six animals were subjected to division of all soft tissues of the base of the tongue except mucosa and with the major vessels and nerves being left intact.

Results

The mean absolute lingual blood flow in twenty-seven animals was 14.19 ± 0.67 ml/100 m tissue/min.

In the pilot group of four dogs, division of the contralateral lingual artery produced a mean reduction of local blood flow of 10.1 percent. Subsequent interruption of the ipsilateral artery resulted in a total 45.1 percent flow reduction.

Simultaneous ligation and division of both lingual arteries produced a mean reduction of 59.4 percent in blood flow to the tongue.

A mean decrease in lingual blood flow of 56.9 percent occurred in the twelve animals in which all named, accessible vessels were divided.

Surgical division of the soft tissues of the base of the tongue, with neurovascular bundles and most of the mucosa intact, in six animals resulted in a mean 37.9 percent reduction of flow.

In no case did necrosis of the tongue result. Three of the seventeen dogs in the first two groups had moderately cyanotic, but clearly viable, tongues seven days postoperatively. By contrast, seven of the twelve animals in the third experimental group showed similar lingual cyanosis.

Comment

The mean absolute lingual blood flow of 14.19 ± 0.67 ml/100 m/min determined in this investigation demonstrates that the tongue does indeed have a generous blood supply which, for example, approximates that of brain.[6] These results generally agree with the less direct measurements of blood flow to the tongue made by Meyer[7] in which he reported a flow rate of 16 to 19 ml/min/100 gm tissue in dogs using ^{42}K or ^{86}Rb as ionic tracers and a flow of about 22 ml/min/100 gm employing ^{196}Yb labelled carbonized microspheres as a particle tracer. Whang et al[8] recorded a mean total lingual blood flow of 16.5 ml/min in 20 dogs as determined with an electromagnetic flow probe. Although no figures were published, Davis and Baker[9] stated that blood volume changes in the tongue were closely comparable whether ^{51}Cr or ^{32}P or a photoelectric plethysmographic technique was used.

The results of vessel ligation and soft tissue disruption in this study suggest that the vessel contribution to lingual blood flow is nearly 60 percent of the total, with the soft tissues adding almost 40 percent and, by implication, the mucosa accounting for the remaining 5 percent or less. The minimal effect of contralateral lingual artery division is in agreement with anatomic studies in which lingual artery distribution was largely confined to one half of the organ. The Acid Blue and Renografin 60 studies of Maloney et al[10] and the intravital staining results reported by Hellekant[11] lead to this conclusion. Maloney et al did note, however, that, in the majority of dogs in their investigation, the contralateral lingual artery played the dominant role in providing collateral circulation following ligation of the ipsilateral artery. Shepherd et al[12] provided additional evidence in their experimental study of control of lingual artery hemorrhage in which they reported that ipsilateral lingual artery ligation was ineffective in fourteen of sixteen dogs, while additional ligation of the ipsilateral external carotid produced a control rate of 50 percent and bilateral common and external carotid plus lingual artery ligation controlled bleeding in all sixteen dogs studied.

Specific studies of physiologic mechanisms controlling lingual blood flow have been sparse. In 1952, Erici and Uvmas[13] reported that the chorda tympani contained efferent vasodilator fibers. Subsequently Bishop and Dorman[14] confirmed this observation and noted that this atropine-resistant effect was first reported by Heidenhain in 1883. Hellekant[11,15] found that the taste response of the anterior two-thirds of the tongue was related to blood flow rather than to the oxygen content of the blood perfusing the organ.

There has been a number of clinical reports documenting lingual necrosis or gangrene attributed to a variety of etiologic agents. Howard and Cremin[16] had a patient with massive lingual necrosis secondary to bacterial infection of the tongue with acute thrombosis. In 1961, Missen[17] described the microscopic findings at autopsy in ten lingual arteries of five patients with giant cell arteritis. Nine vessels were inflammed, one was occluded, five severely stenosed and one moderately stenosed. All five tongues appeared normal. A number of cases of lingual gangrene secondary to giant cell of temporal arteritis have appeared in the literature since.[18,22] Gangrene may be preceded by attacks of pain or paroxysmal blanching.[19]

Other reported causes of gangrene of the tongue have included athero-sclerotic arterial occlusion or arterial embolism secondary to auricular fibrillation,[20] progressive systemic sclerosis presenting with Raynaud's phenomenon of the tongue,[21] the use of ergotamine in temporal arteritis,[22] and occasionally following the use of lingual flaps for reconstruction.[1,23] Consequently it would appear that lingual viability may be threatened in a variety of clinical circumstances in which there is either diffuse involvement of intrinsic vasculature or widespread occlusion of the carotid system with or without major soft tissue disruption.

It would appear that there is a rational basis for the use of lingual flaps and remnants as well vascularized, dependable and readily available tissue in the oral and oropharyngeal region. The surgeon should, nonetheless, be aware of the possibility of occasional necrosis in the situations mentioned which can produce a reduction in blood flow to levels incompatible with viability.

References

1. Chambers RG, Jaques DA, Mahoney WD: Tongue flaps for intraoral reconstruction. AmJ Surg 118:783–786, 1969
2. DeSanto LW: Lingual flap reconstruction after resection for cancer. Trans Am Acad Ophth Otol 78:135–139, 1974
3. Roberts M, Owens G: Direct mass spectrographic measurement of regional intracerebral oxygen, carbon dioxide, and argon. J Neurosurg 37:706–710, 1972
4. Roberts M, Vilinskas J, Owens G: Mass spectrographic quantitation of regional cerebral blood flow. Med Res Eng 11:25–28, 1972
5. Davis ME: Anatomy of the dog. W. B. Saunders Co., Philadelphia and London, 1964, pp 294 and 395.
6. Silver DJ, Roberts M, Owens G, Rembish R: Measurement of regional cerebral blood flow. Neurology 24:322–324, 1974
7. Meyer MW: Distribution of cardiac output to oral tissues in dogs. J Dent Res 49:787–794, 1970
8. Whang CJ, Mozingo JR, Rhoton AL: Comparison of flow in arterial and vein grafts to basilar artery. Surg Forum 25:449–451, 1974
9. Davis DL, Baker CH: Comparison of changes in blood volume and opacity in dog digital pad and tongue. J Appl Physiol 27:613–618, 1969
10. Maloney PL, Doku HC, Shepherd NJ: Collateral circulation after ligation of the lingual artery in dogs. J Oral Surg 27:395–397, 1969
11. Hellekant G: The effect of changes in the blood flow to the tongue on the chorda tympani response in the rat. Acta Physiol Scand 82:145–153, 1971
12. Shepherd NJ, Maloney PL, Doku HC: Control of lingual artery hemorrhage in dogs. Oral Med, Oral Surg, Oral Path 31:298–301, 1971
13. Erici F, Uvmas B: Efferent and antidromic vasodilator impulses to the tongue in the chorda lingual nerve of the cat. Acta Physiol Scand 25:10–14, 1952
14. Bishop JG, Dorman HL: Control of blood circulation in oral tissues. Adv Oral Biol 3:1–44, 1968
15. Hellekant G: On the relation between the chorda tympani nerve response, arterial oxygen tension and blood flow in the tongue of the rat. Acta Physiol Scand 82:453–459, 1971
16. Howard S, Cremin MD: Acute parenchymatous glossitis with gangrene of the tongue. Lancet 2:410–411, 1959
17. Missen GAK: Gangrene of the tongue. Brit Med J 1:1393–1394, 1961
18. Henderson AH: Tongue pain with giant cell arteritis. Brit Med J 4:337, 1967
19. Grahme R, Bluestone R, Holt PJL: Recurrent blanching of the tongue due to giant cell arteritis. Ann Int Med 69:781–782, 1968
20. Reed C Inglis MJ: Acute massive gangrene of the tongue. Brit Med J 2:575–576, 1965
21. Casey EB, Lawton NF: Progressive systemic sclerosis presenting with Raynaud's phenomenon in the tongue and sensory trigeminal neuropathy. Rheum Phys Med 11:131–133, 1971
22. Wolpaw JR, Brottem JL, Martin HL: Tongue necrosis attributed to ergotamine in temporal arteritis. JAMA 225:514–515, 1973
23. Sessions DG, Dedo DD, Ogura, JH: Tongue flap reconstrution of the oral cavity. Arch Otolaryngol 101:166–169, 1975

The Accelerated Surgical Treatment of Electrical Burns of the Mouth in Children

Allen Small, Washington, D.C.

Introduction

The most common cause of microstomia in the pediatric age group is electrical burns of the mouth.[1] The difficulty in early determining the depth of the injury has led to a controversy in the surgical management.[2–4] The advocates of early debridement and repair suggest that early repair leads to decreased hospitalization, decreased morbidity and better cosmetic results.[5–9] They also report decreased secondary infection and therefore less scarring.[6,8]

Hyslop advocated debridement within the first 12 hr.[5] Within this time there is a demarcation line that is dissectable. This line locates the deepest penetration of injury.

The majority of authors advocate late debridement and suggest that the true level of necrosis becomes evident only after three to four weeks.[11–15] At that time repair could be facilitated. Earlier debridement will remove some normal tissue which could be used in the repair.[11,14,16]

There are others who recommend debridement and repair at four to seven days.[6,9]

Thomsen et al, has reviewed forty-three cases of electrical burns of the mouth in children. He noted no difference in the results if surgery was done within the first four weeks of injury or far later.[17] Pitts et al, recommended deferring repair anywhere from six months to several years after injury.[18] They reported early repair results in a tight lower lip which may lead to orthodontic disturbances.

The controversies and arguments presented suggest that a critical review of the topic is required.

Electrical burns are classified into two types; contact or flash burns, and arc burns. The contact burn is usually a superficial or second degree burn while the arc burn is a full-thickness type with destruction down to and often including bone.[19] The severity of the burn is determined by the following factors.[10,21,22]

1. AC or DC current. Alternating current is more destructive.
2. High tension or low tension. High tension is more destructive and implies a current of greater than 1000 V.
3. Cycles per second. Normal domestic current is 60 cycles per second. The lower the cycles, the greater the chance for arrhythmias.
4. Conduction of the patient. A poorly grounded child will incur less damage than a well-grounded child.
5. Size of the contact site. The larger the site, the greater the injury.

The initial burn in the mouth presents as a grey–yellow depressed area with loss of skin, vermillion and surrounded by hyperemia. The lesion is bloodless, cold, and painless (Fig. 1). Anesthesia of the local area is caused by damage to the sensory nerve fibers. The local muscle necroses and atrophies leaving a depressed scar. The permanent teeth usually are unaffected. However, the alveolar ridge, floor of the mouth and buccal sulcus may be involved. The main complications of electrical burns of the mouth in children are:

1. Microstomia[1,21,23]
2. Cosmetic deformity
3. Malocclusion[18]
4. Incontinence of saliva[23]
5. Loss of deciduous teeth
6. Psychological sequelae

Other reported complications have been death,[22] gas gangrene,[24] and traumatic cataracts.[10] The latter complications are most often noted following high tension injuries.

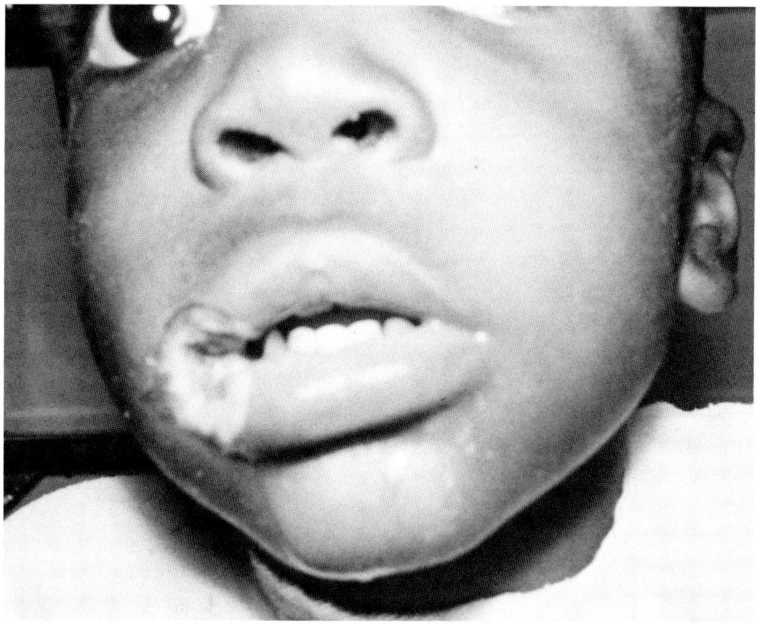

Fig. 1. A typical commissure lesion.

Study Group

Thirty-six patients were treated from 1969 through 1974 for electrical burns at the Children's Hospital National Medical Center. All patients were admitted. Five additional patients were seen and treated by the author. The study group consists of forty-one patients.

The age range was seven months to nine years and the sex ratio was sixteen females to twenty-seven males. Thirty-three cases occurred between seven months and four years of age. Three of the burned children were mentally retarded.

The burns occurred most often by biting on live electrical cords or plugs (Fig. 2). Several occurred by sucking on electrical sockets. The appliances most often involved were lamps, air conditioners, toasters and uncapped electrical outlets.

Epidemiology (Fig. 2)

Muir reported an incidence of two to three cases a year in a British population of five million.[8] Thomsen reported on forty-three cases in Toronto in an eighteen year experience.[17]

Forty-five percent occurred in the summer months and twenty percent in the winter months.

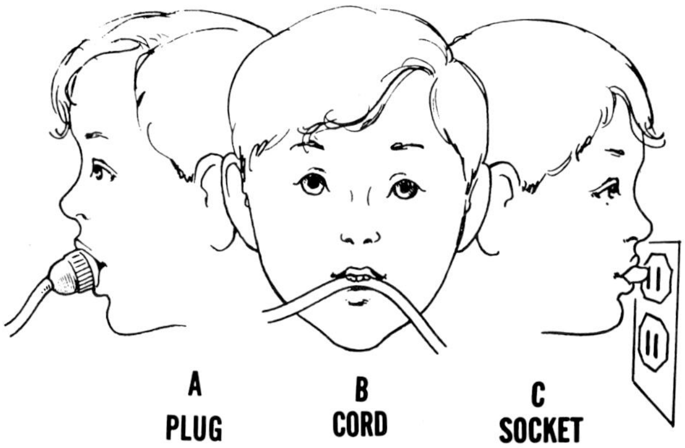

Fig. 2. Etiology of burns.

It is speculated that thirst and dryness may be factors causing children to chew or suck on electrical cords.

Twenty-seven of the thirty-six children treated at Children's Hospital were available for examination. All surgically treated patients were available for follow-up.

Results

Forty-one cases of low tension injuries were evaluated. No deaths were noted. Thirty children incurred injury of the commissure while eleven had mid-lip injuries only. The conservatively treated patients were all admitted and had an overall average hospital stay of nine days. They were treated by tetanus immunization, oral mouth care and antibiotic ointment application. The eschar was allowed to fall off spontaneously. Follow-up surgical therapy occurred from four weeks to adolescence. Nineteen of the twenty-seven children available for follow-up required surgery. Four superficial mid-lip and two very small commissure lesions required no repair at all. They may be considered partial-thickness burns. The best results of the group of conservatively treated patients were the mid-lip small lesions. The poorest results were the commissure and large lesions.

Twenty-two percent of the total group (9/41) had labial artery bleeding. In several patients, this was the only reason the parent brought the child in for examination. Two bleeding episodes occurred after the child was discharged following eschar separation. The bleeding usually occurred on the fifth to ninth day following injury. Only one patient required transfusion. No patient who underwent surgical repair during the first week had bleeding.

In the surgical group, mid-lip lesions had very satisfactory cosmetic results. The success decreased with the larger lesion. All surgery was carried out at the fifth to sixth day post-injury. A sickle buccal mucosal flap was the method of repair with two small full-thickness injuries. One child with a mid-lip burn required wedge excision with muscle and mucosal flap advancement (Fig. 3). Two children with commissure lesions were treated in the first week.

A small commissure lesion treated at four days by vermillion advancement had satisfactory results. One patient with a larger commissure lesion underwent eschar removal and buccal mucosal advancement (Fig. 4). This case required two revisions. The commissure edge was thin. Drooling and webbing occurred in this patient. Labial artery bleeding was absent in this group. No patient developed further necrosis and no flap failed. The average period of hospitalization was less than three days for the group. No microstomia occurred in this group.

The impression was that the residual scarring in the lesion site was considerably less in the surgical group.

Discussion

Progressive Necrosis

The advocates of conservative therapy stress that one must wait for demarcation of the eschar to occur before repair.[9–12] Early debridement, they contend, will not prevent progressive necrosis of

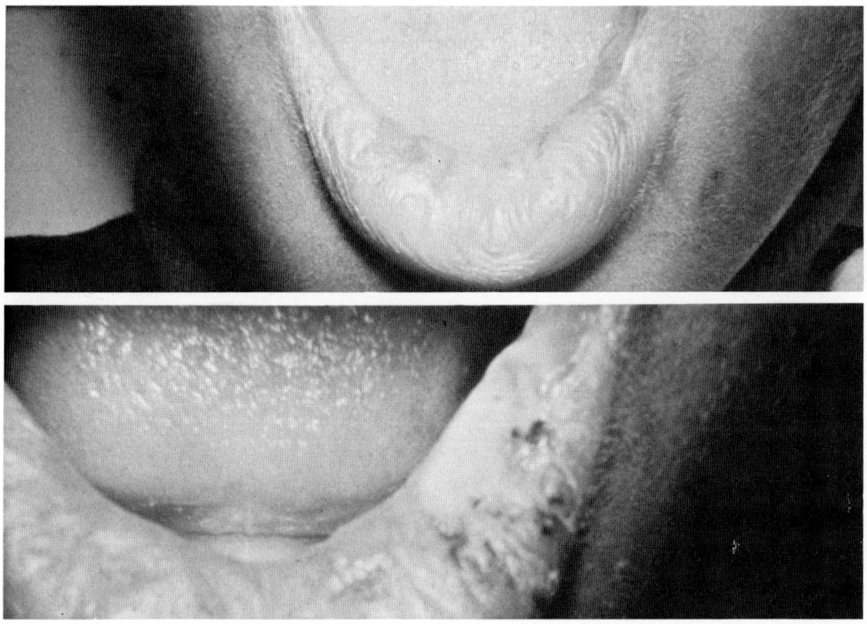

Fig. 3. Before (bottom) and after (top) of mid-lip buccal advancement repair.

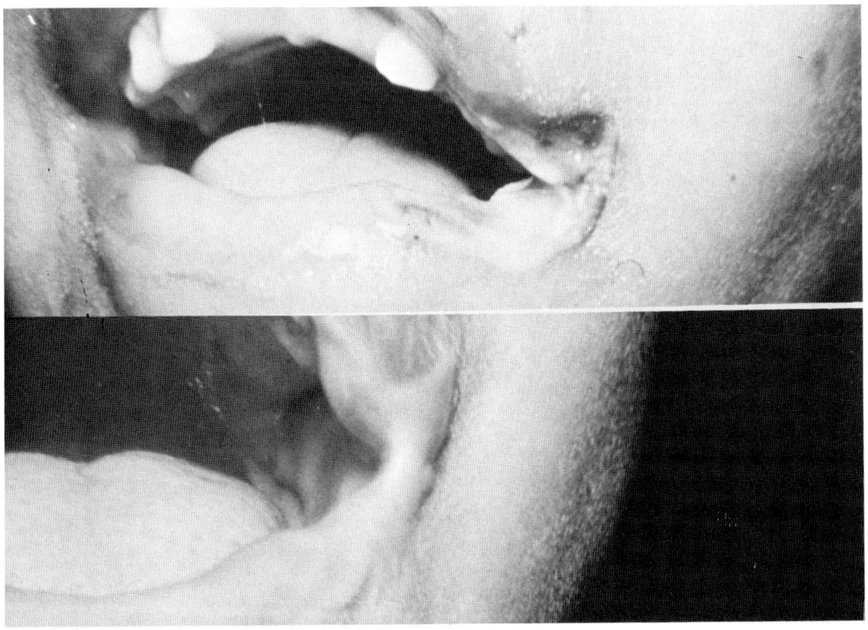

Fig. 4. Commissure repair using buccal mucosal flap. Note thin lower lip (bottom).

this surrounding normal appearing tissue which could be used in repair. The concept or myth of progressive necrosis should be analyzed.

High tension injuries will involve thermal injury to the arteries leading to coagulation necrosis.[8,10] This may occur over a long distance from the original electrical injury. The vascular injury will affect the graft viability and lead to a poor result. Household injuries, however, are low tension injuries with 110 to 120 V involved. Progressive arterial thrombosis is usually not a factor in these injuries.[8,10] Venous thrombosis and local edema does occur.[10]

Studies in patients with electrical burns of the extremity demonstrate that primary repair utilizing flaps is a safe procedure.[9,10,12,24] Transposition flaps had a reduced success rate due to the early local edema which occurs.[10]

The evidence for progressive necrosis is thus lacking. No evidence of progressive necrosis was evident in the series of patients presented.

Surgical Timing

The controversy over treatment approach also requires an understanding of just what time limits "early surgical repair" implies. George Frank offers a useful classification to describe the timing of surgical repair of electrical burns.[9]

1. Primary repair-either immediate of delayed (within twelve or before forty-eight hours).
2. Accelerated early-between three and fourteen days post-injury.
3. Late-plasty-early-late-plasty or late-late-plasty.

This terminology will surely clarify the distinctions and reports of results. Thomsen et al[17] noted no difference in cosmetic results between those patients having surgical repair within the first four weeks and those having repair after four weeks. They noted that early repair implied that surgery was performed before the eschar had demarcated. Other reports indicate that early repair is feasible and have been successful anywhere from twelve hours to one week following the initial injury.[5–8,10,14] Hyslop[5,10] reports that a line of demarcation forms within the first twelve hours and repair is best facilitated then. This could be classified as immediate repair.[5,10]

Fleury[6] advocates repair at four to five days post-injury in order to prevent the consequences of infection which leads to increased scarring. This timing may be classified in the accelerated-early group according to Frank.[6] Pitts et al advised waiting until the scar has matured and softened before attempting any repair.[18] This might be considered advocating late-late-plasty.

Classification

A program for management of the injury based on an admittedly simplified classification is offered (Fig. 5). This classification is based on the clinician's ability to distinguish between partial and full-thickness injuries and the capability of determining the deepest extent of necrosis. The latter capability is limited. Numerous articles allude to this problem.[2–4] Its solution is the key to success in an early surgical treatment program. Techniques utilizing intravenous flourescein, radioisotopes, dyes, thermography, and sensation analysis have all been offered as methods to determine the deepest level of injury. In the final analysis, the clinician at the operating table makes the decision. With this limitation noted, this classification is offered as a useful overall approach to the treatment of electrical burns of the mouth in children.

A. PARTIAL THICKNESS

B. FULL THICKNESS

CLASS I - 15% OF UPPER AND/OR LOWER LIP

CLASS II - 15%–50% OF UPPER AND/OR LOWER LIP

CLASS III - GREATER THAN 50% AND/OR FLOOR OF MOUTH

Fig. 5. Classification of electrical burns.

There is no controversy with regard to the treatment of the partial-thickness burns. All are treated by conservative therapy. Epithelialization takes place from the surrounding uninvolved epidermal elements. The subcutaneous tissue is uninvolved so scarring and contracture are not problems. Healing takes place leaving no deformity.

The treatment of full-thickness burns according to this classification is variable depending on the size and extent of injury.

Class III burns are best treated by surgical delay. Life support is primary; airway control, Levine tube feedings[23,24] and fluid control may be necessary before definitive management of the burn site. The floor of the mouth is repaired first. Definitive repair of the lips occurs only later.

Factors operating against primary immediate repair are the following:

1. The patient often presents after the first twelve hours.
2. The burned child may require other considerations prior to surgical repair-tracheostomy, treatment of shock, fluid maintenance etc.
3. Technical considerations such as pedicle flap rotations, very extensive burns, bone exposed, or floor of mouth involved, favor delay.

Surgical delay is definitely indicated in those children with airway compromise, shock, nutritional feeding problems, floor of mouth involvement, cardiac or similar systemic abnormalities. In this group of injured children life support is the primary consideration.

It is also evident that primary or accelerated repair is feasible and desirable. The hospitalization stay is shortened. Labial artery hemorrhage may be prevented. Note that 23 percent of the cases in some series have this complication which occurs from the fourth to tenth day post-injury.[17] No case in the surgical group presented had this complication and to the author's knowledge, no case has been reported in the literature. There is the distinct impression that the amount of scarring is less in the primary and accelerated surgical group. This is supported by others.[5,6,8–10] It is also important to consider that the principle of delay implies healing by contracture. This violates one of the principles of wound repair. In no other area do surgeons advocate healing by contracture. Recall that the treatment of thermal burns were treated by delay for many years with scars resulting in very extensive contractures and severe cosmetic and functional problems. Today the treatment has changed to early grafting techniques which avoid the stage of contracture.

If the mandible or alveolar ridge is involved, a sequestrum is allowed to develop and this may delay reconstruction for four to six weeks at the very minimum. Definitive repair may require a cheek flap, pedicle flap or other rotational flaps (Fig. 6).

The author prefers to repair the Class I burn during the first week post-injury. Conservative methods which allow the eschar to demarcate and then repairing the resulting deformity will also achieve acceptable cosmetic and functional results, eventually.

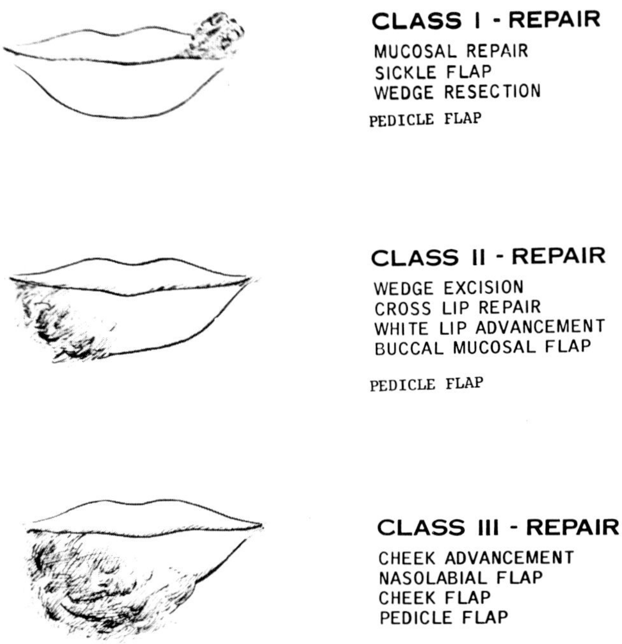

Fig. 6. Various techniques of repair.

It is with the Class II burns that repair, primary or accelerated-early repair offers the maximum benefit over late-plasty techniques. The small Class I burn will leave a small defect. With lip growth this will become less noticeable with time. The larger Class III burn requires delay. The mid-size lesion offers the maximum benefit for utilizing primary or accelerated early repair. Decreased scarring and distortion, a decreased incidence of microstomia and improved cosmesis are likely dividends for utilizing this early approach.

The repair of Class II type burns during the first week post-injury is supported by several authors.[5–10,14] The techniques utilized may be by wedge resection, cross-lip flaps, pedicle flaps, cheek advancements and buccal mucosal advancement techniques or any combination thereof.

The Class II commissure lesions in the author's surgical group, though satisfactory, required revisions. No result was excellent. The conservatively treated commissure group required corrections as well. Several articles in the literature note that the results of commissure procedures are often unsatisfactory.[11,23] Recall the words of Brown and Fryer, "plastic surgery cannot build normal sphincters which is what the lips are . . .".[13] Anderson et al noted, "that commissure procedures have only fair results as to cosmesis and function." "The vermillion cannot be duplicated by mucosal flap, pedicle or skin graft. Mucous membrane repairs are often incontinent of saliva . . .".[23] Class II type mid-lip repairs reviewed in the literature similarly required revisions.[5,6,8,14] For this reason, the parents may be told that several procedures may be necessary.

The routine management of the child requires a complete history and physical exam including opthalmologic exam on presentation post-injury. The size, shape, and location of the burn should be noted. A drawing is often helpful. A notation as to the cause should be written, i.e., by socket, plug or cord. All Class III burns and many Class II type burns should be admitted. All superficial and Class I type burns may be treated at home. The child may have tetanus toxoid, topical antibiotic ointment, cleansing mouth care and a liquid diet with avoidance of acid containing and spicy foods. Systemic antibiotics may be used depending on the philosophy of the physician. If the child is sent home, the parents should be instructed to stop the labial artery bleeding by compression of the bleeding lip between two fingers.

Summary

It is clear that the best treatment is prevention in the first place. In this regard, the following preventative steps have been advocated[14]:

1. Heavy rubber cords utilized for electrical appliances.
2. Sockets located at three-foot level from the floor.
3. Master switch to control wall sockets.
4. Outlet covers made available.

Many of these preventive measures are now available and can be utilized.

A classification is submitted in order to delineate treatment groups according to the size and extent of the lesion.

A method of discussing surgical timing is presented.

Commissure burns cause more cosmetic and functional disabilities than mid-lip burns.

Labial artery bleeding may be eliminated by the initiation of early surgical debridement and resurfacing of the burns.

The further developement of better techniques to judge early post-injury the deepest depth of tissue damage will facilitate the general acceptance of the early surgical approach for the treatment of electrical burns of the mouth in children.

Acknowledgments

Gratitude and appreciation is expressed to G. Gaunoux, Medical Records Children's Hospital National Medical Center who assisted in the research for this study. Illustrations were ably provided by M. Wilhoite, Department of Medical Illustrations, National Naval Medical Center, Bethesda, Maryland.

References

1. Evans AJ: The treatment of burns in infancy and childhood Mustarde JC, 1st ed., Plastic surgery in infancy and childhood, Phila. Saunders WB 1971 pp 558–559
2. Dingman RO, Bennett J: Evaluation of burn depth by the use of radioactive isotopes: Plast Reconstr Surg 20:261–272, 1957
3. Jackson DM: The diagnosis of the depth of burning, Brit J Surg 40:588–596, 1953
4. Cope O, Langohr JL, Moore FD, Webster RC: Expeditious care of full-thickness burn wounds by surgical excision and grafting, Ann Surg 125:1–22, 1947
5. Hyslop VB: Treatment of electric burns of the lips, Plast Reconstr Surg 20:315–317, 1957
6. Fleury AF: Electrical burns of the lips: a modified pland of treatment Am Surgeon 25:328–331, 1959
7. Wells DE: Treatment of electrical burns by immediate resection and skin graft, Ann Surg 90:1069–1078, 1929
8. Muir IFK: The treatment of electrical burns, Brit J Plast Surg 10:292–299, 1958
9. Frank G: primary and accelerated early plastic surgery for burns, Plast Reconstr Surg 23:313–329, 1959
10. Hyslop VB, Miller EW: The treatment of electrical burns, J Int Coll Surg 23:481–486, 1955
11. Kazanjian VH, Roopenian A: The treatment of lip deformities resulting from electrical burns Am J Surg 88:884–890, 1954
12. Dale RH: Electrical accidents: a discussion with illustrated cases Brit J Plast Surg 7:44–66, 1954
13. Brown JB, Fryer MP: Reconstruction of electric injuries including cranial losses with preliminary report of cathode ray burns, Ann Surg 146:342–351, 1957
14. Schultze LW, Vazironi SJ: Electrical burns of the mouth, Am J Surg 98:921–922, 1959
15. Skoog T: The surgical treatment of burns, Acta Chir Scand Supplementum 305, 1963
16. Ackerman B, Goldfaden G: Electrical burns of the mouth in childhood Arch Dermatol 104:308–311, 1971
17. Thomsen HG, Juckes AW, Farmer AW: Electric burns to the mouth in children, Plast Reconstr Surg 35:466–477, 1965
18. Pitts W, Pickrell K, Quinn G, Massengill R: Electrical burns of the lips and mouth in infants and children, Plast Reconstr Surg 44:471–479, 1969
19. Baldridge RR, Fryer MP: Electrical burns, New Engl J Med 250:46–48, 1954
20. Sturmer FC Jr: Electrical burns, Ann Surg 154:120–124, 1954
21. Sturim HS: The treatment of electrical burns, Surg Gynec Obstet 128:129–133, 1969
22. Oeconomopoulos CT: Electrical burns in infancy and early childhood: a review of the current literature, Amer J Dis Child 103:35–38, 1962
23. Anderson R, Kurtay M: Reconstruction of the corner of the mouth, Plast Reconstr Surg 47:463–464, 1971
24. Poate WJ, MacAfee AL: Gas gangrene following electrical burns, Brit J Plast Surg 15:17–19, 1962
25. Davies MR: Burns caused by electricity: a review of 70 cases, Brit J Plast Surg 11:288–300, 1959

Reconstruction of the Floor of the Mouth and Tongue Mobilization by Skin Grafting

Stanley E. Thawley, Gershon J. Spector, and Joseph H. Ogura, St. Louis, Mo.

Impaired speech and swallowing difficulties are debilitating results in some cases of oral cancer resections. Several factors contribute to these problems. Resection of the lateral tongue and mandible often obliterates the sulcus between the tongue and alveolar ridge. This space serves as a collecting area for saliva and provides for tongue mobility. If the sulcus between the tongue and alveolar ridge is or becomes obliterated the saliva has a tendency to pool in the center of the mouth. Once there it either drools out or is swallowed with difficulty. If the gutter is absent the edentulous patient has difficulty retaining his dentures, preventing mastication of a solid diet.

In most tongue-mandible resections the defect is repaired by suturing the buccal flap to the cut edge of the tongue, thus creating a scar and obliterating the natural sulcus. The tongue may then be unable to perform the movements necessary for good speech (Fig. 1). This limitation is particularly evident for the fricative sounds such as "this" and "that" which require that the tongue be able to slightly protrude through the anterior teeth.[1] The tongue should also be able to touch the palate in order to propel a bolus of food toward the pharynx. A relatively simple skin grafting technique can remedy these problems by recreating the floor of the mouth and the sulcus.

The clinical use of intraoral skin grafting has had a long history. In 1894, Schnitzler and Ewald[2] successfully skin grafted a granulating area in the mouth. Following this the use of intraoral skin grafting was not reported until 1915 when Moszkowicz[3] used the technique of epithelial inlay for reconstruction of the alveolar sulcus. During World War I, Esser[4,5] popularized the inlay method. He recreated the lower labial sulcus in patients in whom it had been obliterated by scarring. Through an incision in the submental region he created a pocket on the outer aspect of the mandible, which extended up to the scarred mucous membrane. Into this pocket he inserted a mold of dental compound covered with a split thickness skin graft with the inner surface out. The wound was closed and seven to ten days later an incision opened up the scar area overlying the stent. After the stent was removed the skin graft remained, creating a new skin-lined labial sulcus. The approach was external rather than intraoral because at that time, asepsis was considered the most important principle in successful application of skin grafts. Waldron, working with Gilles[6] in England, modified Esser's procedure by inserting the graft-covered stent through the mouth and closing the mucous membrane over it. The success of this modification increased the application of intraoral skin grafting. The realization that immobilization and not asepsis was the most important factor in the success rate of intraoral skin grafting, extended graft applications immensely.

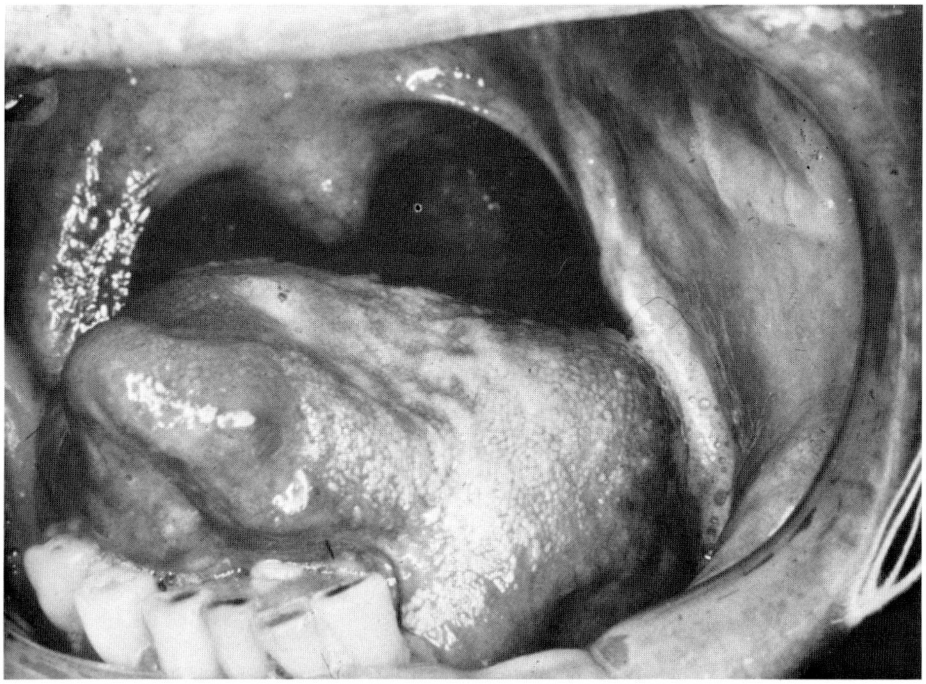

Fig. 1. A postoperative oral resection closure showing limitation of tongue mobility.

Intraoral skin grafting continued to find new uses during the next several decades. They were utilized to recreate the labial sulcus in a cleft lip repair[7] and for correction of nasopharyngeal stenosis.[8] After World War II the use of intraoral skin grafting spread widely. Conley used skin grafts in maxillectomies,[9] and tongue resections[10] and Edgerton used them for oral reconstruction after cancer resections.[11] Skin grafting was also used for immediate reconstruction of one stage radical laryngo-pharyngo-esophagectomies by Negus[12] and Conley,[13] and surgeons frequently used skin grafting to recreate a lingual sulcus after dental extractions.[14,15]

There are four methods by which scarred areas of the mouth may be epithelized. The least efficient method is the establishment of an epithelized tract in the normal tissue adjacent to the fibrosis. The scar is opened into this tract and the epithelium prevents the edges from growing together.

The second method involves using a pedicle or sliding mucous membrane flap from the immediate area. In tongue mobilization this would leave a considerable raw area to be closed by wide undermining or skin grafting.

The third technique involves a pedicle skin flap from outside the mouth. This involves at least two stages and offers no advantage except extra bulk of tissue.

The fourth technique is utilization of split thickness skin (Fig. 2). In some of our postoperative tongue-mandible resections with significant drooling or speech problems we use a modification of the previously described Esser inlay method (Fig. 3). A 3 × 4 in. split thickness skin graft approximately 18 to 20 thousandths of an inch thick is taken. The graft, raw surface outward, is wrapped around a 2-1/2 in. red rubber tube which has a circumference of about 3 cm. The two edges of skin are sutured together along the long axis of the tube with no. 3–0 chromic sutures (Fig. 3C). The skin is not stretched on the tube as this diminishes the width and thickness of the graft which will line the recreated sulcus. A one cm. stab wound is made in the anterior border of the scarred area, and by using a long blunt clamp a tunnel is created in an anterior-posterior direction into the scarred area (Fig. 3b). The tunnel is not connected to the surface, and the superficial layer of scar remains intact. The graft-covered stent is then inserted into the tunnel and secured using no. 2–0 silk sutures applied through the stent and anchored to both sides of the tongue. After seven days the scar area overlying the buried stent is incised down through the

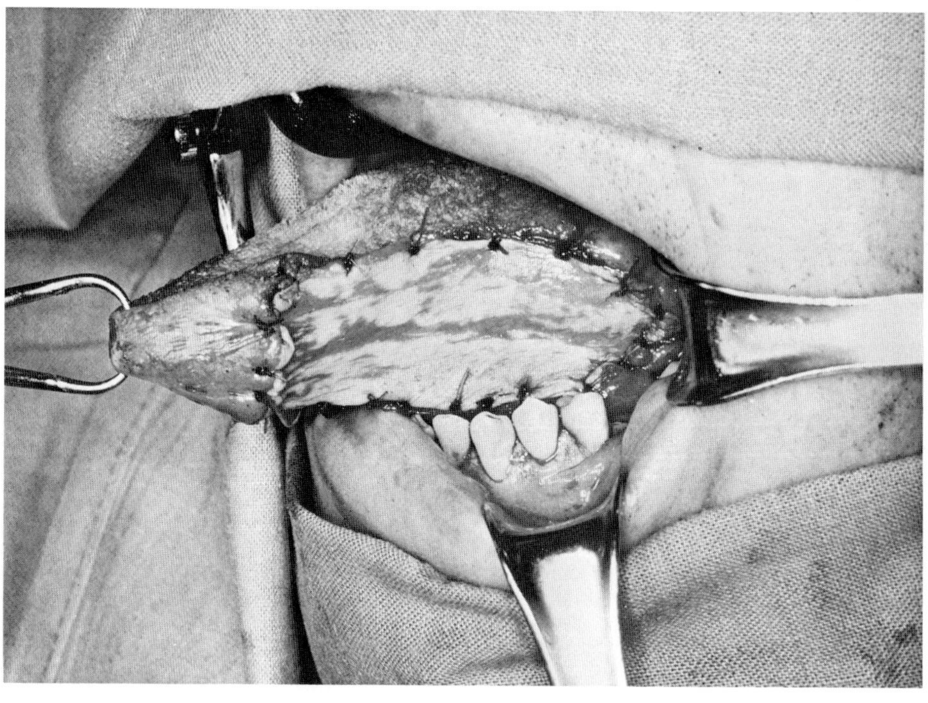

Fig. 2. Hemiglossectomy with applied skin graft to lateral tongue surface.

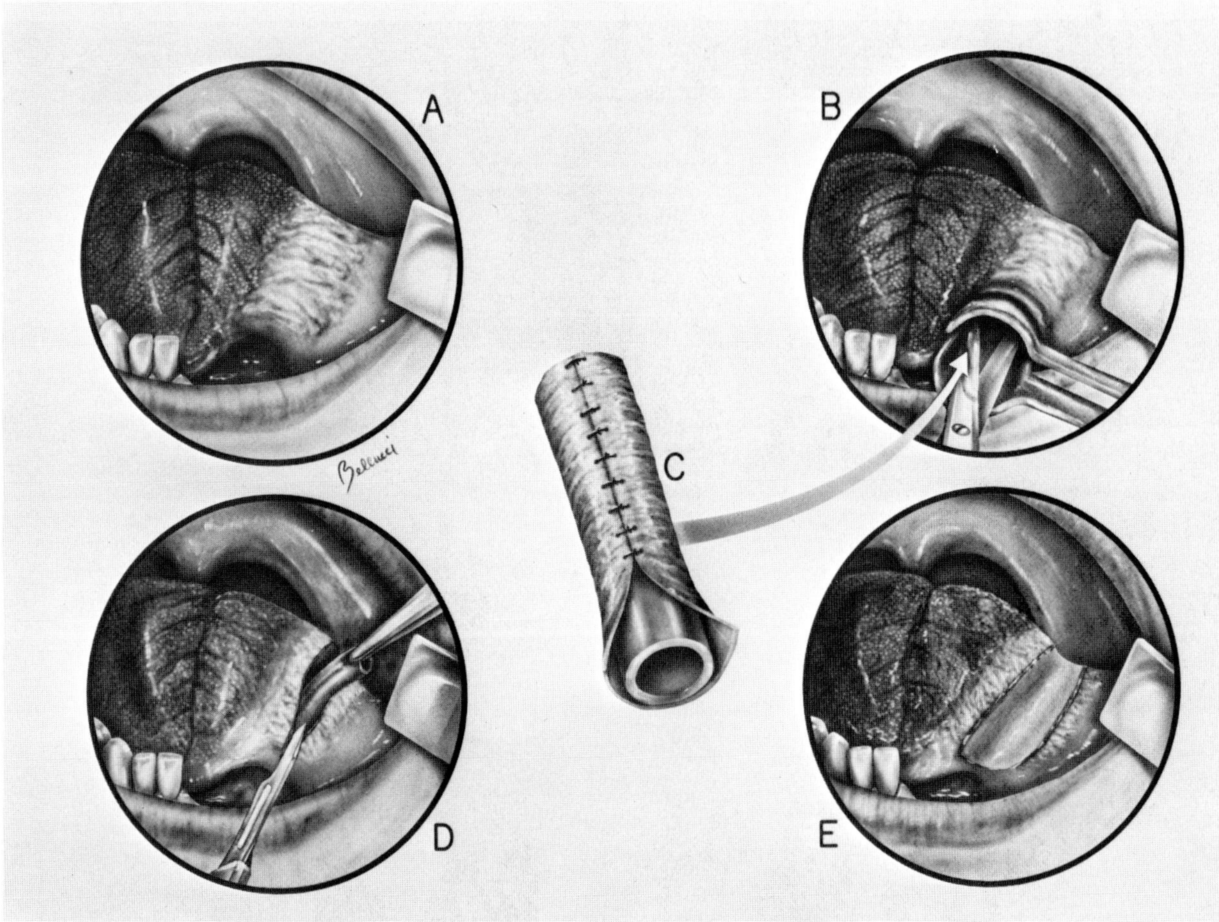

Fig. 3. Technique of skin grafting and tongue release. (A) lateral oral scarring limiting mobility with obliteration of salivary sulcus. (B) creating tunnel. (C) skin graft applied to stent. (D) removal of stent. (E) skin graft in place.

top portion of the graft covered tube, which is then removed and the skin graft remains in the recreated sulcus (Fig. 3D, E).

We use this technique primarily after jaw-neck dissection for carcinoma of the mouth or oral pharynx. In our cases a segment of the mandible is normally removed; however, this technique may also be used in marginal resections of the mandible. We feel that this method is simpler and quicker than cutting through the scar initially to place the graft as this would involve more sutures, involve potential hemostasis problems and would not create as tight a tunnel immobilizing the graft-covered stent.

We do not routinely use this technique at the time of primary surgery as many of these patients will not have significant problems to warrant the additional time in an already long surgical procedure. Six to twelve months after surgery, if the patient continues to have significant speech or swallowing difficulty attributable to tongue immobilization, the tongue release and grafting is performed as a secondary procedure (Figs. 4 and 5).

A technique of secondary reconstruction by applying the stent through an external incision has been described,[1] but we have not used it because it offers no significant advantage except asepsis, and we feel that immobilization is by far the most important factor in the graft take. Also, it would involve an extra incision through irradiated skin.

Some technical points are important to remember in the technique. The tunnel should be created along the axis of the mandible and should be as close to the overlying scar as possible. Occasionally, if the patient's main problem is poor speech because of inadequate anterior tongue projection, the tunnel may be angled slightly toward the middle

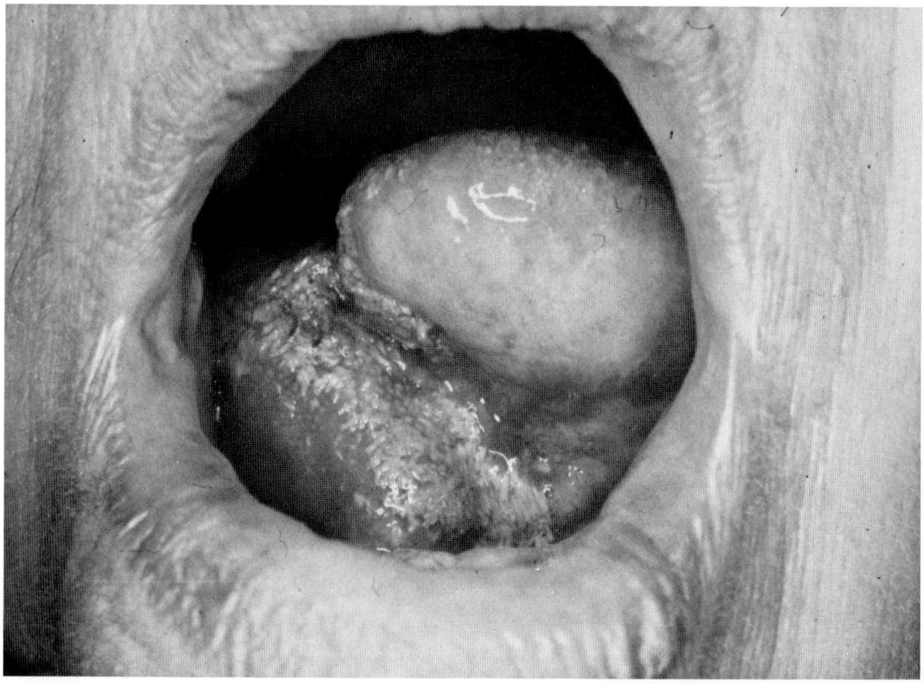

Fig. 4. Postoperative skin grafting and tongue release with tongue in resting position.

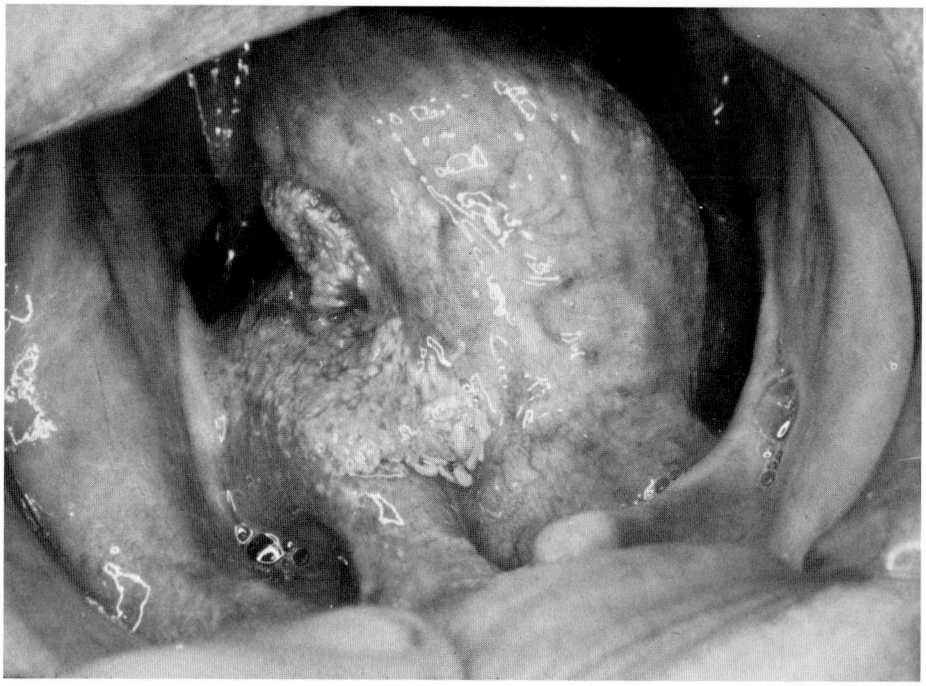

Fig. 5. Postoperative skin grafting and tongue release showing mobility of tongue.

of the tongue posteriorly. The tongue would then be released in a more anterior direction. However, this is somewhat risky as one may inadvertently denervate the ipsilateral side of the tongue secondary to cutting the lingual nerve. We have not had this complication but are alert to its possibility.

The split thickness skin graft should be thick to decrease postoperative contracture. Hemostasis should be good as a hematoma will prevent the graft take. And finally, the graft must be checked prior to insertion to prevent inadvertent reverse skin application.

When grafting skin into the mouth it is wise to avoid skin from hair-bearing donor sites. Postoperatively it is helpful to remember that skin grafts rarely attain the high sensory qualities of normal skin but the ability to appreciate pain, touch, and temperature change return to some extent, usually in that order.[16] All grafts are devoid of sensation immediately following transplantation, but begin to recover sensation as early as one to two months after the operation. Skin grafts are rarely able to sweat, but the sebaceous glands remain functional.[17]

Summary

A relatively simple technique has been described for secondary reconstruction of the floor of the mouth and for tongue mobilization. This is helpful in those patients who have speech and swallowing problems secondary to obliteration of the salivary sulcus. The resultant loss of an adequate floor of mouth, and tongue immobilization secondary to the scar formation can thus be relieved.

References

1. Corso PF, Gerold FP: Immediate and secondary reconstruction of the floor of the mouth and mobilization of the tongue by a new technique. Amer J Surg 104:727–731, 1962
2. Schnitzler J, Ewald K: Zur technik der haut transplantation nack thiersch. Centrif Chir 21:148–149, 1894
3. Moszkowicz L: Uber verpflanzung thiersch'scher epidermoislappschen in die mundhohle. Arch Klin Chir 108:216–220, 1915
4. Esser JFS: Neue wege fur chirurgische plastiken durch heranziehung der eahnarztlichen technik. Beitr Klin Chir 103:547–560, 1916
5. Esser JFS: Studies in plastic surgery of the face. III. The epidermic inlay. Ann Surg 65:297–315, 1917
6. Gillies HD: Plastic Surgery of the Face. London, Oxford University Press, 1920
7. Figi FA: Skin grafting in the mouth: report of two cases. Proc Staff Meet Mayo Clin 9:740–742, 1934
8. O'Connor GD: Pharyngeal reconstruction for nasopharyngeal stenosis. Ann Otol 46:376–382, 1937
9. Conley JJ: Free skin grafting in the sinus, oral and pharyngeal areas in radical surgery of the head and neck. Cancer 7:444–450, 1954
10. Conley JJ: A technique of skin grafting to the tongue and case report. Plast Reconstr Surg 5:450–453, 1950
11. Edgerton MT, Desprez JD: Reconstruction of the oral cavity in the treatment of cancer. Plast Reconstr Surg 19:89–113, 1957
12. Negus VE: Reconstruction of pharynx after pharyngo-esophago-laryngectomy. Brit J Plast Surg 6:99–106, 1953
13. Conley JJ: A one stage operation for the immediate reconstruction of the pharynx and cervical esophagus following radical resection. West J Surg 63:355–360, 1950
14. Gorney HS, Forney AJ, Famon S: Creation of mandibular ridge by deepening labial sulcus and lining with skin graft. J Amer Dent Ass 29:751–754, 1942
15. Colley DO: A method for deepening the mandibular and maxillary sulci to connect deficient endentulous ridges. J Oral Surg 10:279–283, 1952
16. Davis L: The return of sensation to transplanted skin. Surg Gynec Obstet 59:533–540, 1934
17. Ponten B: Grafted skin: observations on innervation and other qualities. Acta Chir Scand (Suppl) 257:1–78, 1960

Surgical Management of Carcinoma of the Lip

James R. Leonard, Altanta, Ga.

Introduction

The primary purpose of this presentation is to review some of the many surgical techniques involved in reconstruction of the lip after excision of carcinoma. This will be accomplished by a progressive review of a series of cases, with a small amount of pathophysiology discussed when necessary. We will attempt to mention most of the major surgical techniques involved but will concentrate on those that the author finds most useful. By necessity, some of the tumor biology, radiobiology, and natural disease history must be mentioned as well.

General Considerations

Carcinoma of the lip is primarily a disease of the lower lip and is related to exposure to the actinic rays of the sun, exposure to the heat of pipe smoking and similar chronic irritant situations. Fortunately, this disease is unique in several respects. First, it shows little tendency to metastasize in the early stages. This is indeed very fortunate because to include the nodal drainage system (Fig. 1) in any surgical extrapative maneuver could result in significant debilitating cosmetic deformity. The disease generally shows little tendency to recur regardless of whether treated by surgical or radiotherapeutic means. Obviously, there are exceptions to this last statement. Near the conclusion, further mention of this particular topic will be made. Also, fortunately, the lip is particularly well supplied in vascularity and, therefore, many liberties can be taken with surgical extirpation and reconstruction. Additionally, numerous mucosal surfaces in close proximity of the lip can be used to reline the surface of the lip.

Illustrative Cases

Figure 2 shows a 56-year-old white male farmer (Patient A) with a 1.5 cm ulcer on the left lateral portion lower lip that on biopsy proved to be squamous cell carcinoma. The author prefers an incisional biopsy to punch types as the pathology is frequently more clear in this fashion. In fact, we do not hesitate to excise the lesion in toto for biopsy purpose. Figure 3 represents a V-shaped excision with simultaneous lip shave with advancement of the buccal mucosa with straight line closure. Superimposed on the photograph is the excised portion of the lip as well as the V-shaped wedge enclosing the entire carcinoma with adequate margins. It should be noted at this point, that a little more than one-half of the lower lip can be excised in this fashion, depending somewhat on the age and the tissue flaccidity of the patient. One should not compromise the stoma by making the orifice too small in using this technique but this can be judged at the time of surgery cand a flap swung if necessary. Figure 4 represents the healed state of the patient approximately three months postoperatively. With the passage of additional time, this scar becomes even more unnoticeable. The patient is alive and well with no evidence of recurrence five years postoperatively.

Figure 5 represents a patient, 62-year-old white male (Patient B), with a recurrent carcinoma on the lateral portion of the left side of the lower lip outlined lightly with the inside marking. This had

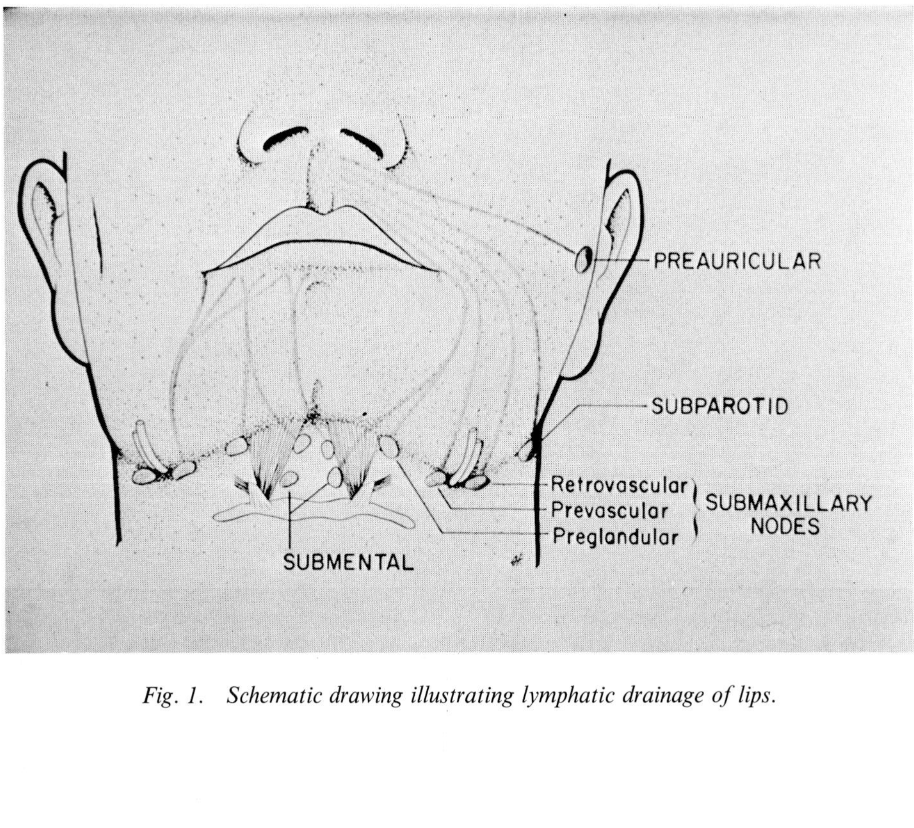

Fig. 1. Schematic drawing illustrating lymphatic drainage of lips.

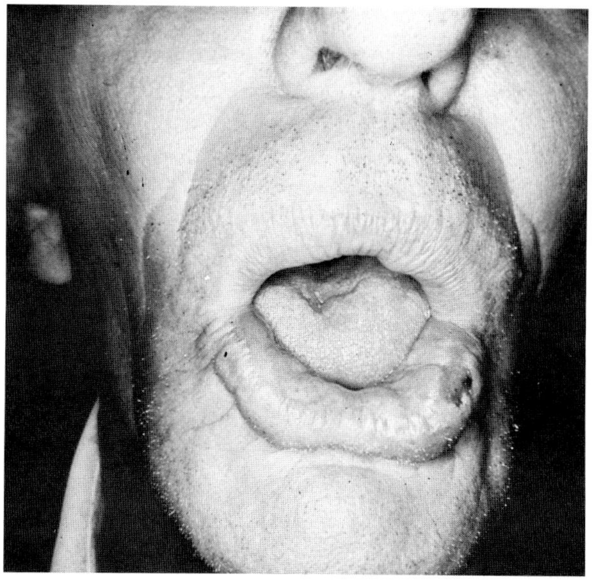

Fig. 2. Patient A. Small carcinoma of lower lip, left.

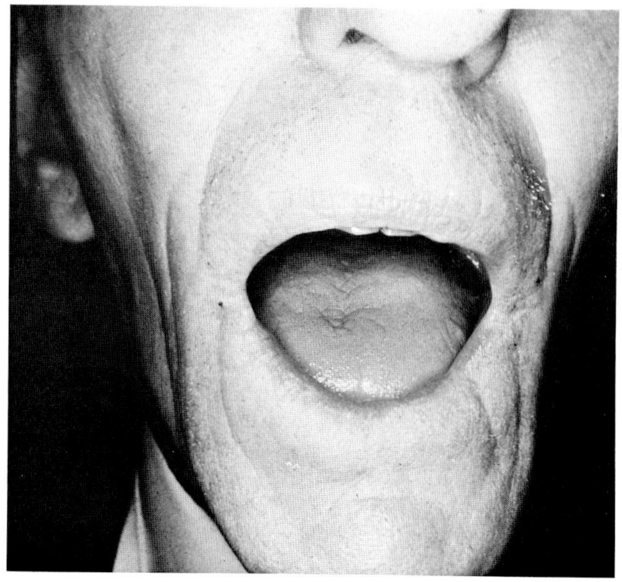

Fig. 4. Patient A. Three months postoperatively.

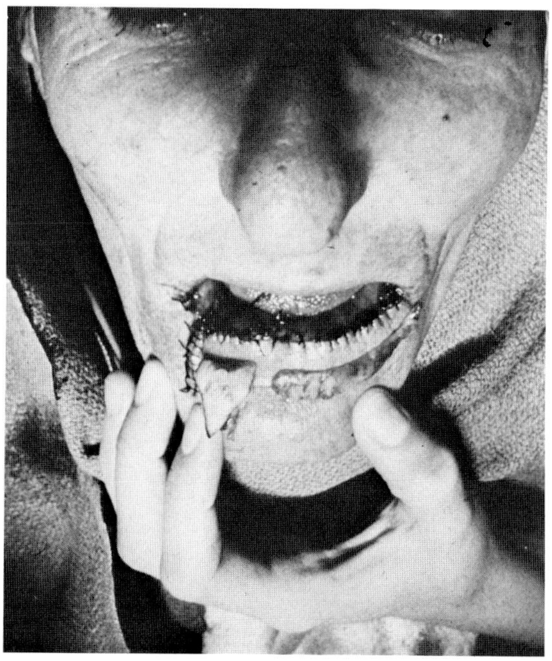

Fig. 3. Patient A. Immediately postoperatively, showing lesion and repair.

recurred three years postradiation therapy and proved to be squamous cell carcinoma on biopsy. The outer drawing represents the excisional portion of the lip, extending across the midline and going completely to the left lateral commissure. Outlined above is an Estlander's flap.

At this point, it should be noted that a triangular shaped flap in the midline lower lip swung to the midline upper lip was described by Abbe in 1856. Abbe was a New York otolaryngologist. Estlander described the swinging of a triangular flap from the lateral upper to the lateral lower lip. This was described sometime after Abbe's flap. Any modification of these two operations should properly be called a modified Abbe-Estlander flap.

Figure 6 represents the immediate conclusion of the operation with the carcinoma excised and the Estlander flap swung and sutured into position. This results in a slight rounding of the commissure but this is easily corrected by a secondary procedure should the patient so desire. In the author's own experience, patients very seldom desire to have this minor correction made.

This patient is now three and one-half years postop with no evidence of recurrence. As one can imagine, this is one of the most useful techniques in reconstructing of the lip whether it be the upper or lower.

The next patient (Patient C) is a 93-year-old white female (Fig. 7) with a recurrent verrucous carcinoma of the squamous cell variety of the midline lower lip. This patient had had previous surgical excision and simple repair for carcinoma and

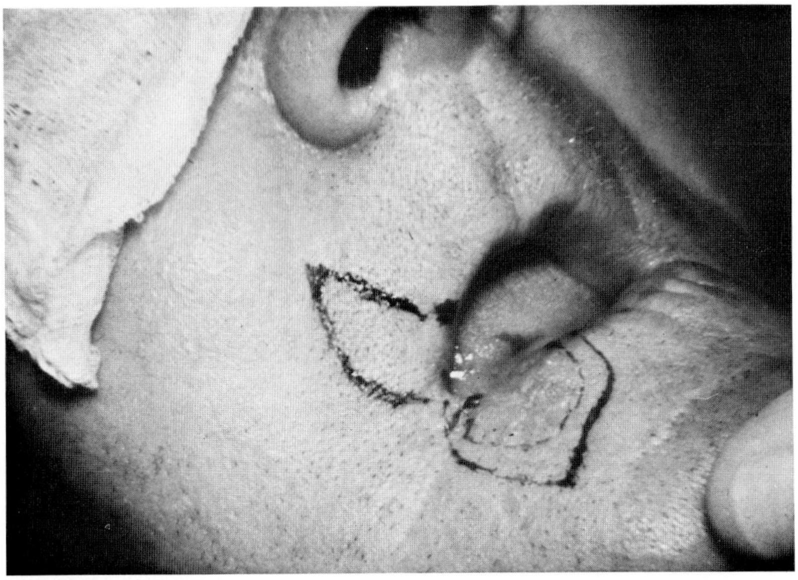

Fig. 5. Patient B. Recurrent squamous carcinoma of the left lower lip.

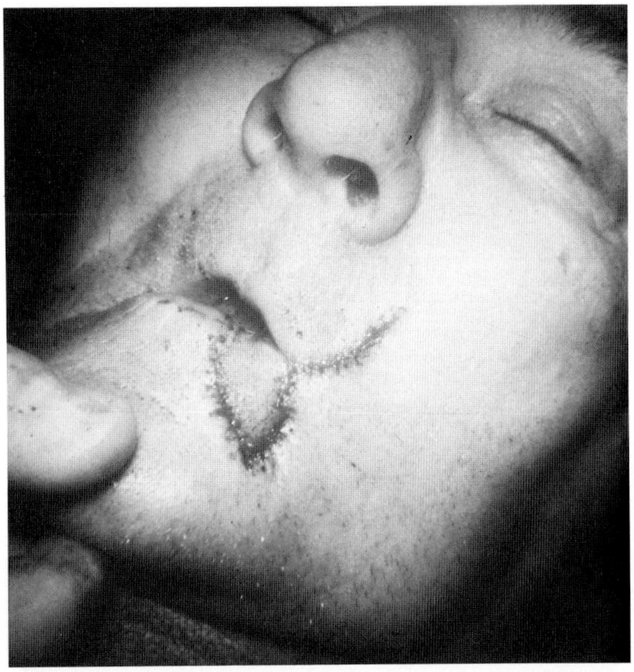

Fig. 6. Patient B. Immediately postop, with the Estlander flap in position.

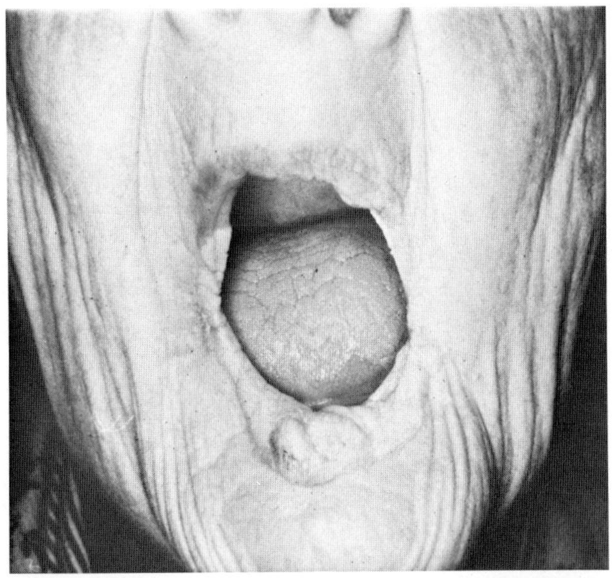

Fig. 7. Patient C. Large verrucous carcinoma of the lower lip.

also previous radiation therapy. She additionally had profuse leucoplakia on the remaining lower lip as well as throughout the oral cavity. Figure 8 reveals the extensive resection of the entire lower lip with extensive loss of chin-lip substance at this point.

The technique used to reconstruct this lip is shown in Figure 9. A large filleted tongue flap with considerable muscle tissue included was made to reline and reconstitute the lower lip. One has considerable flexibility in this flap in the amount of thickness desired whether it be only the mucous membrane or to include some muscular bulk as well. The author typically detaches this type flap three weeks later. Patients are able to communicate

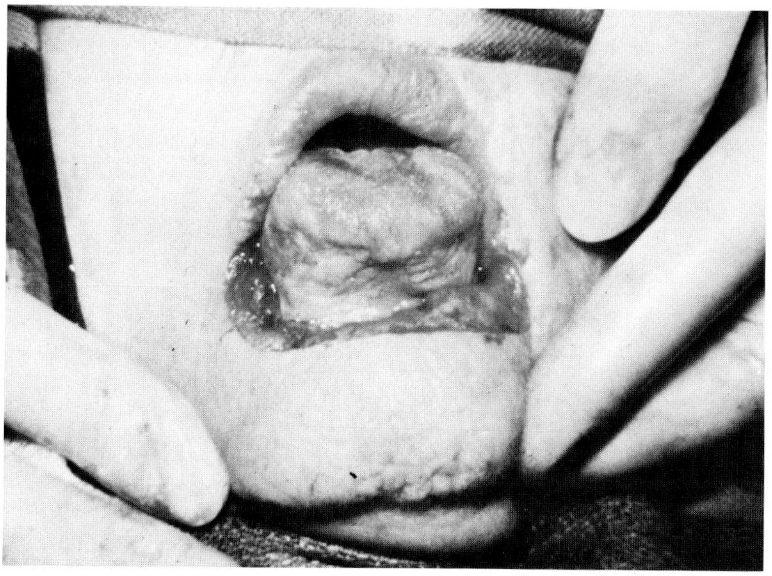

Fig. 8. Patient C. Operative defect.

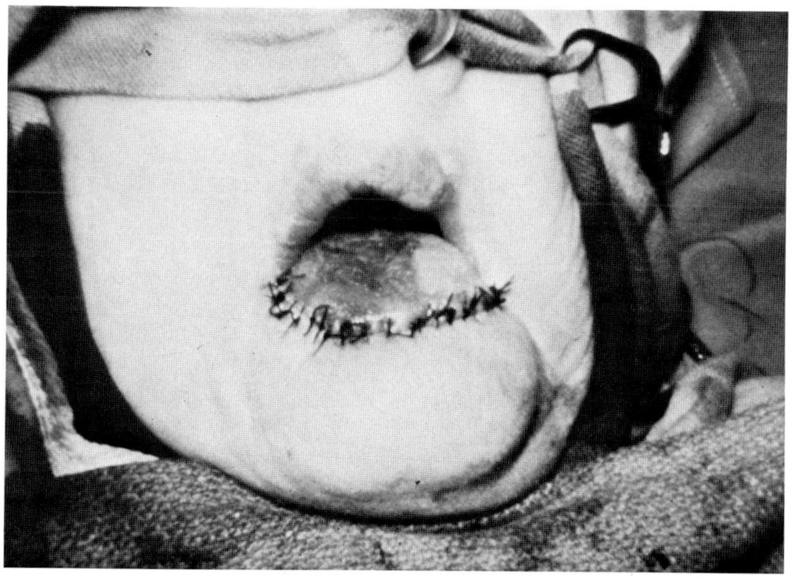

Fig. 9. Patient C. Immediately postop, with tongue flap in position.

and feed surprisingly well during this three week period.

This patient is alive and well with minor recurrences and resections in the oral cavity three years postoperatively.

The tongue flap is also one of the most useful techniques in reconstructing the lip, particularly the lower.

The next patient is a 63-year-old white male (Patient D), outdoorsman, with a recurrence in the middle third of the lower lip. Figure 10 represents the preoperative outline of the excisional phase of the lower lip which will consist of almost the entire surface of the lip except for two small lateral segments. Also shown in the drawing is the outline of the Burow's triangle in the nasolabial groove to allow advancement of the lower lip flaps. One has the option of using the mucosal surface of the Burow's triangle to reline the lip or as in this case as shown in Figure 11, a tongue flap was used. In

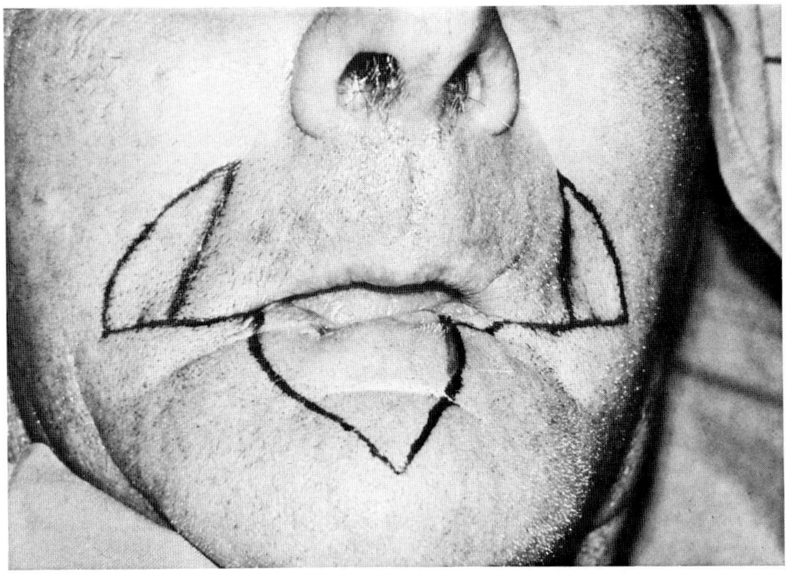

Fig. 10. Patient D. Recurrent squamous carcinoma (after radiation therapy), large, approximately 3.5 cm.

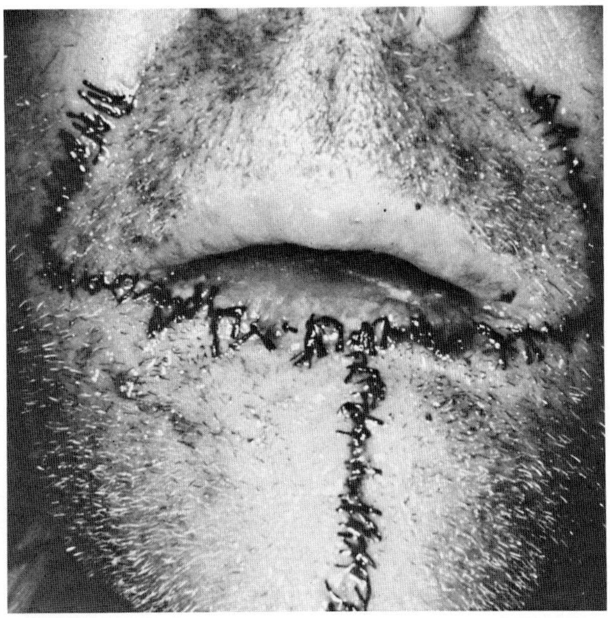

Fig. 11. Patient D. Immediately postop, with Burow's triangles excised and tongue flap in place.

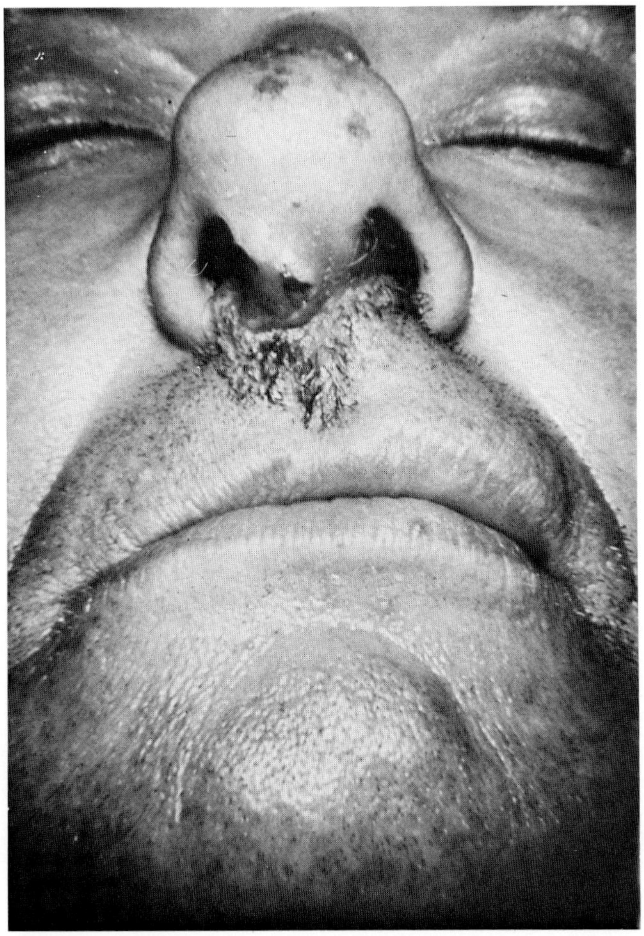

Fig. 12. Patient E. Carcinoma of the columella with extension into the upper lip.

referring back to Figure 10, if one possibly can avoid the resection past the mental crease, a much more acceptable cosmetic result occurs.

This patient is alive and well six years postoperatively with no evidence of recurrence.

This next patient does not represent carcinom of the lip per se (Patient E) but does illustrate some of the reconstructive problems and techniques. Figure 12 shows a 53-year-old white male with carcinoma of the columella with extension into the left upper lip. Close examination of the lip revealed the peau d'orange effect with carcinoma in the dermal lymphatics. Figure 13 represents the very extensive surgical excision of approximately two-thirds of the upper lip, part of the anterior maxilla and complete rhinectomy. This presented a tremendous reconstructive challenge. We elected (one must plan completely in advance) to reconstruct the upper lip by swinging bilateral Gilles' fan flaps as illustrated in Figure 14. This, of course, represented acceptable reconstruction of the lip but does not suffice for the nose. Figure 15 shows him approximately two months postoperatively with acceptable scars and with the initial nasal prosthesis in place. Not shown in this photograph is his upper denture which further accentuates the normality of the situation. Despite the extensiveness of this patient's problems, and there were correlary ones as well, he is free of carcinoma three years postoperatively.

A number of techniques exists for reconstituting the upper lip, including direct flap advancement, modifications of the Abbe and Esthlander as well as a number of forehead, visor, and scalp flaps.

The final patient represents an exception to the general considerations presented earlier. He serves primarily to illustrate some of the exceptions.

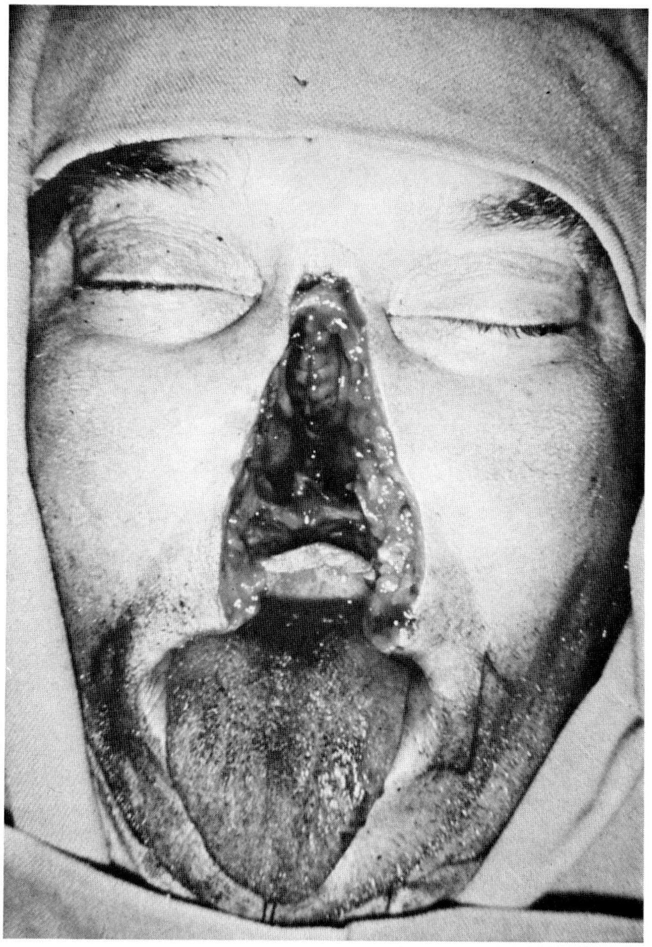

Fig. 13. Patient E. Operative defect.

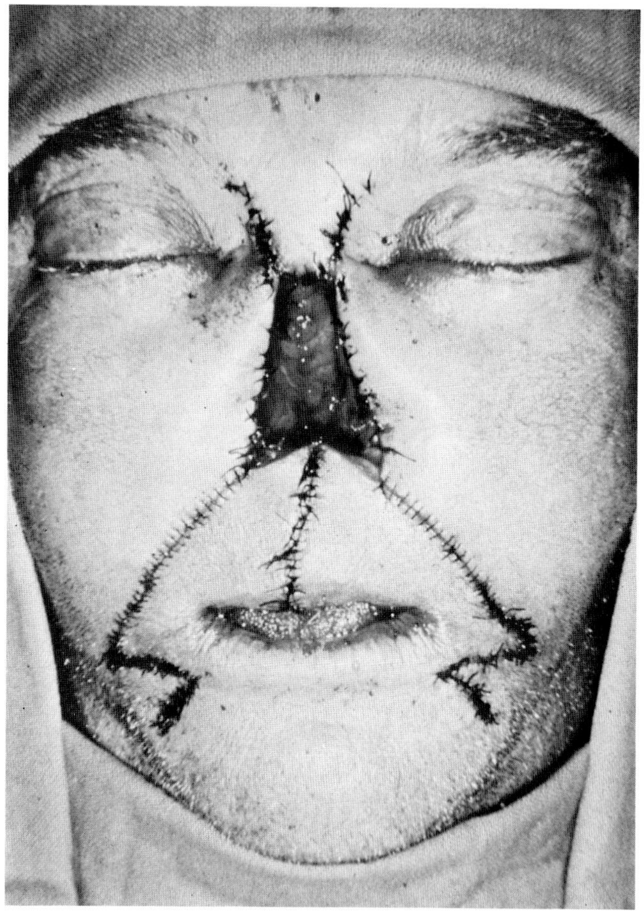

Fig. 14. Patient E. Immediately postop, with Gilles' fan flaps

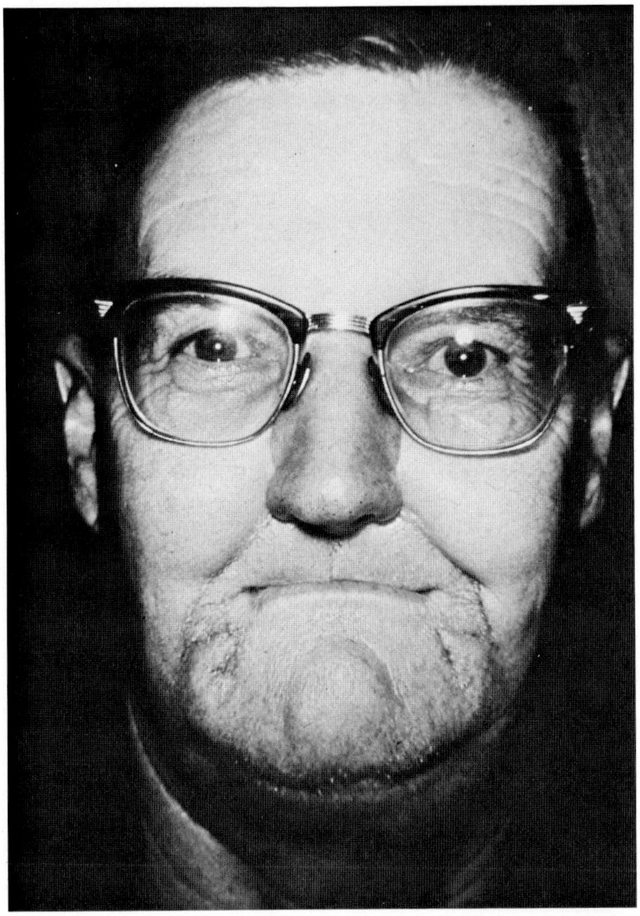

Fig. 15. Patient E. Two months postop, with nasal prosthesis, but without dental prosthesis.

Figure 16 (Patient F) shows a very extensive carcinoma of the lip in a patient that has just completed 8500 rads of cobalt radiation therapy. The lesion not only did not respond to radiation therapy as they usually do quite well, but continued to grow throughout the course of therapy. Rather than discontinue the treatment, it was carried on beyond the normal dosage. At the time we first saw him, the tumor had extended into the dermis as shown in the photograph as well as into the lymph nodes of the submandibular triangle on the right. Additionally, it had invaded the mandibular alveolus and the labial sulcus. Because of the gravity of the situation, the patient's unusual cosmetic and social plight, and in view of other cases preceding this one, we elected to do a total resection of the lower lip, anterior mandible, and chin. The surgical defect is shown in Figure 17. Reconstruction of the mucosal lining of the lip and the lip per se was done with buccal mucosa and an anterior tongue flap and reconstruction of the chin and lower lip was through bilateral undelayed deltopectoral flaps, Figure 18.

The patient has required three minor revisions in the chin after detachment of the deltopectoral flaps and eventually, one and a half years following the original surgery, developed positive modes in the right cervical chain necessitating a right radical

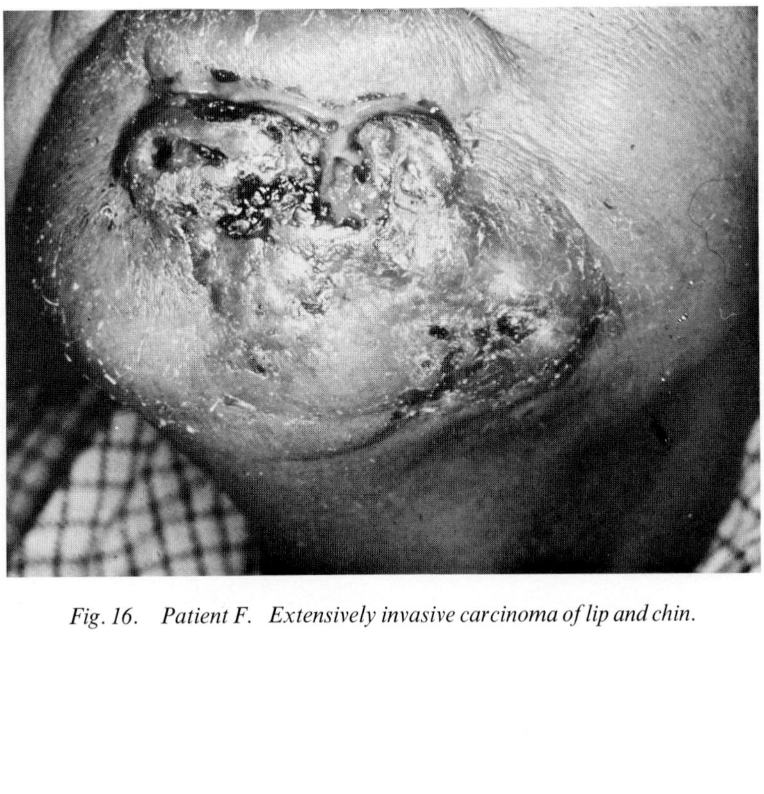

Fig. 16. Patient F. Extensively invasive carcinoma of lip and chin.

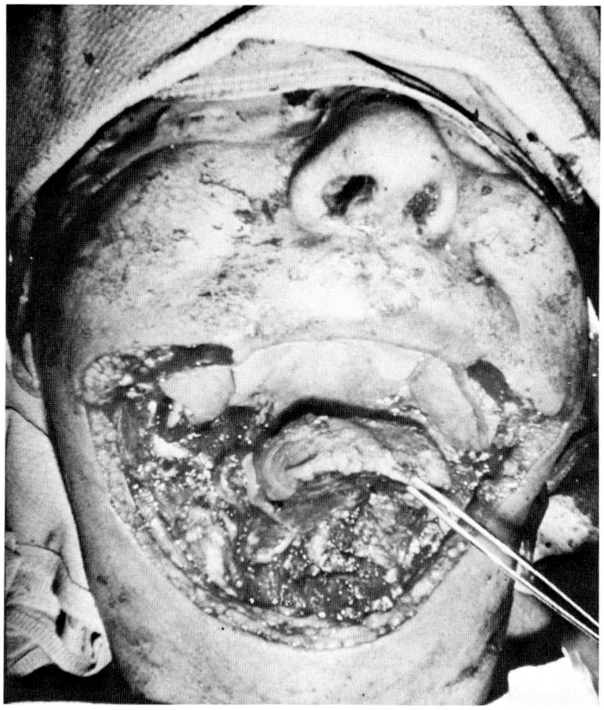

Fig. 17. Patient F. Surgical defect.

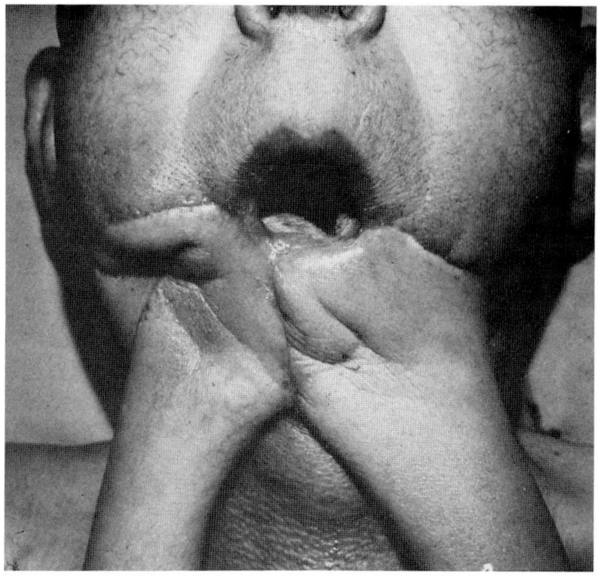

Fig. 18. Patient F. Reconstruction by use of bilateral deltopectoral flaps, buccal mucosal flaps and anterior tongue flaps.

neck dissection. In spite of these matters, the patient is alive and free of carcinoma more than three years after the original operation.

Conclusion

The author has presented a small series of patients primarily with carcinoma of the lower lip that serve to illustrate some of the natural history of this disease and primarily to demonstrate some of the surgical techniques that may be employed reconstructing the lip following surgical excision.

Esophagoplasty Following Resection of Postcricoid Carcinoma

Henry J. Heimlich,* Cincinnati, Ohio

If cancer of the cervical esophagus is to be cured, the surgeon must be able to resect as much of the esophagus as he deems necessary, since cancer cells have been detected in the esophageal submucosa as far as 8 cm distal to the palpable lesion.[1]

* This work supported by the Dysphagia Foundation, Inc., Cincinnati, Ohio.

He will, however, be restricted from doing this if he plans to incorporate the distal portion of the esophagus in the reconstructive process. Such limitations are often the reason for inadequate resection of carcinoma of the cervical esophagus.

Various kinds of skin tubes, plastics, or interposition of the small or large intestine have been used to span the gap between the pharynx and the thoracic esophagus. To accommodate these forms of reconstruction, the distal margin of resection is often inadequate since the distal cervical or upper thoracic esophagus must be kept intact. Skin tubes are united to the distal esophagus at the thoracic inlet, and intestinal grafts are anastomosed to the upper thoracic esophagus. The latter is an especially difficult maneuver in view of the confines of the mediastinum. In addition, should leakage occur at the intrathoracic anastomosis the resulting mediastinitis is often fatal.

The effectiveness of preoperative radiation therapy is compromised by having to limit dosage to preserve the viability of tissue when the surgeon plans to create a skin tube. If an appropriate full course of radiation is administered, the patient is then in the unfortunate situation of having to undergo multiple-stage plastic repair to bring nonirradiated skin to the site of reconstruction.

Laryngectomy is often necessary for adequate resection of cancer of the cervical esophagus. This results in a permanent tracheostoma which obliterates the retrosternal route, precluding the use of a colon transplant, which does not function well in the subcutaneous plane.

Ideally, esophageal replacement after resection of carcinoma of the cervical esophagus must allow for the following: (1) No limitation should be put on the length of esophagus to be excised. (2) The most satisfactory route for esophageal replacement, whether retrosternal, intrapleural, or subcutaneous, should be available for the needs of any particular patient. (3) The blood supply to the substitute esophagus must be good. (4) The patient should be able to eat a regular diet postoperatively.

Reversed gastric tube (RGT) esophagoplasty meets these criteria. It also restores a normal physiologic status in that no foreign material or intestinal organ is interposed between the esophagus and the stomach. In addition, the patient is not subjected to the complication of peptic esophagitis because the antrum of the stomach (which secretes a minimal amount of acid) is the portion that is brought upward and anastomosed to the esophagus.[2,3] Furthermore, 80 per cent of the stomach remains in the abdomen and maintains its normal storage function. Another significant advantage is that the new "esophagus" grows at a normal rate in children. In addition, "esophageal speech" is possible by means of swallowing and expelling air through the RGT.

Reversed Gastric Tube Operation

Experience indicates that the RGT operation is most effectively performed when done two to four weeks after resection of the neoplasm. The abdomen is entered through a left subcostal incision. The tail of the pancreas is freed from its bed and the splenic vessels are ligated in the hilum preserving the origin of the left gastroepiploic vessels. Splenectomy is then performed. Blood passing through the splenic vessels is now directed into the left gastroepiploic vessels which nourish the greater curvature of the stomach.[4]

A pedicle tube, 1 ft long and approximately 1 in. in diameter, is constructed in the following manner: An incision is made into the greater gastric curvature 2 in. proximal to the pylorus. Using a stapling instrument, a double row of metal staples, 6 in. in length running parallel to the greater curvature of the stomach and 1 in. from it, is inserted. An incision is made between the staples, then a second double row of staples, 6 in. long and proximal to the first row, is inserted (Fig. 1).

Since the staples unite the anterior and posterior walls of the stomach, an incision between them forms a tube from the greater curvature and, simultaneously, the remainder of the stomach is already sealed by the staples. The staples are then inverted into the gastric tube and into the residual stomach by a continuous seromuscular silk suture (Fig. 2).

The RGT is reversed in direction, its antral portion brought upward to the neck. The tube can be directed to the neck subcutaneously, retrosternally, or intrathoracically. In general, the subcutaneous route is preferred for older and debilitated patients because it does not enter the chest or mediastinum. The retrosternal or intrathoracic planes offer a cosmetic advantage, a point to be taken into consideration for children and young women. When a permanent tracheostoma is present following laryngectomy, a subcutaneous tunnel is the only available route. The open antral end of the RGT is anastomosed end-to-end to the proximal cervical esophagus or the pharynx (Fig. 3).

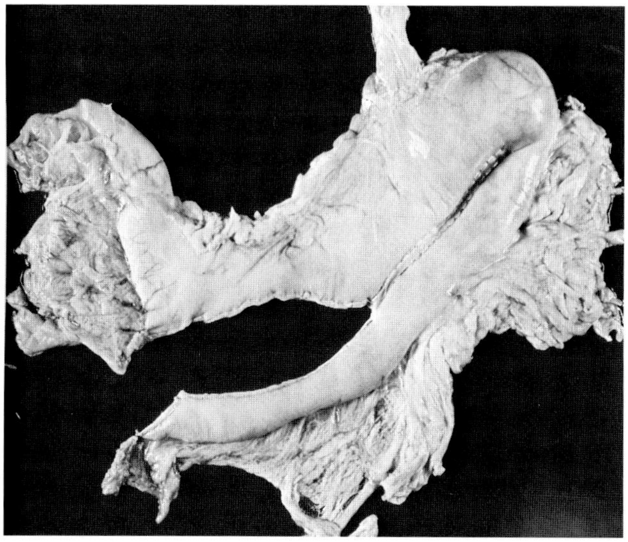

Fig. 1. Specimen of stomach shows double row of staples 1 foot long, parallel to and 1 inch from the greater gastric curvature. Staples were inserted with two applications. An incision has been made between the staples and will be continued for their full length, approximating the anterior and posterior walls of the stomach, thereby forming the gastric tube from the greater curvature.

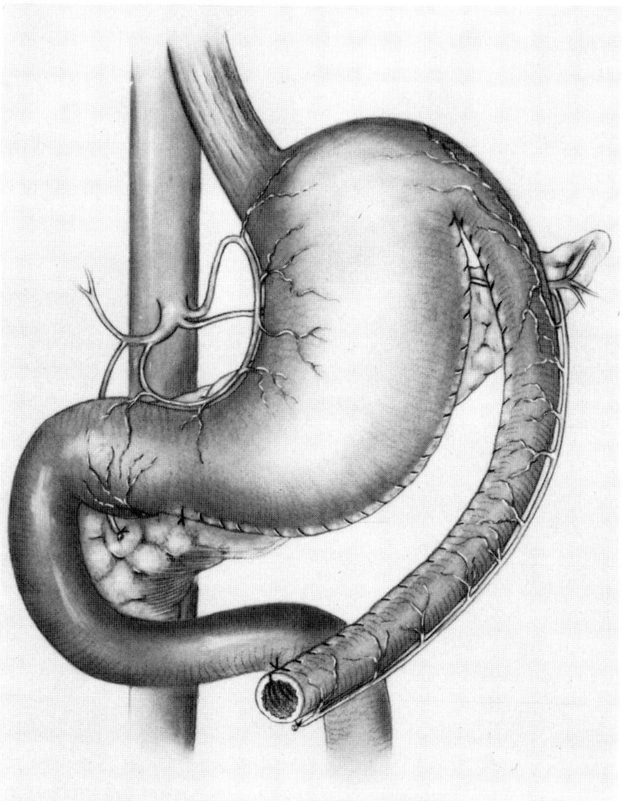

Fig. 2. Diagram of the completed gastric tube after staples have been inverted into the stomach with continous seromuscular silk suture. Figures 2 and 3 are from the motion picture "Reversed Gastric Tube Esophagoplasty Using Stapling Technique" (American College of Surgeons Film Library).

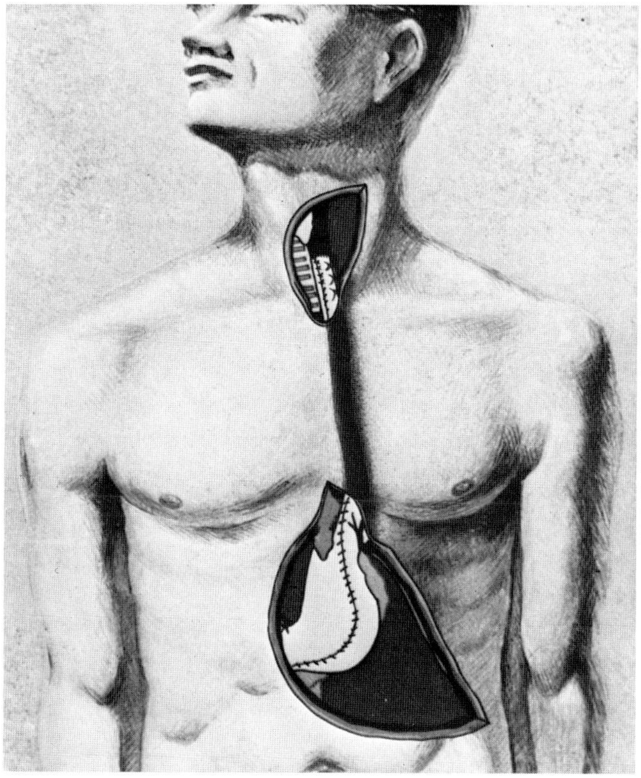

Fig. 3. Completed operation. Reversed gastric tube has been anastomosed to the cervical esophagus or the pharynx. (See Fig. 2.)

Case Reports

Case 1

This 62-year-old woman had the following surgical procedures prior to admission to Montefiore Hospital. August 1958, excision of cervical esophagus for postcricoid carcinoma. A Teflon graft prosthesis was unsuccessful as a replacement for the cervical esophagus. Laryngectomy was performed to prevent aspiration. A permanent tracheostoma was formed, and a Levin tube was inserted through a distal cervical esophagostomy for feeding.

On June 5, 1959, she was admitted to Montefiore where barium swallow studies showed pharyngeal obstruction (Fig. 4a). On July 1, 1959, a RGT was anastomosed to the hypopharynx. Later, reanastomosis was required since the original one was made too narrow (Fig. 4b). The patient was able to eat a normal diet until she died of recurrence of her disease, May 30, 1960.

Case 2

A 57-year-old man was admitted to Montefiore Hospital in July 1960, because of increasing dysphagia and a loss of 20 pounds. Barium swallow study, esophagoscopy and biopsy provided a diagnosis of squamous cell carcinoma of the cervical esophagus. The lesion involved the esophagus from the hypopharynx to the aortic arch.

On August 9, 1960, in a one stage procedure, head and neck service (H&N) resected the cervical and thoracic esophagus to well below the aortic arch using a sternal splitting incision. The distal end of the esophagus was closed. The author then performed RGT esophagoplasty with anastomosis of the gastric tube to the pharynx.

A small fistula developed postoperatively at the site of the anastomosis but healed spontaneously. The patient was able to eat a regular diet when discharged. Six months later, carcinoma recurred which partially occluded the pharynx. The patient died from metastasis on February 5, 1961.

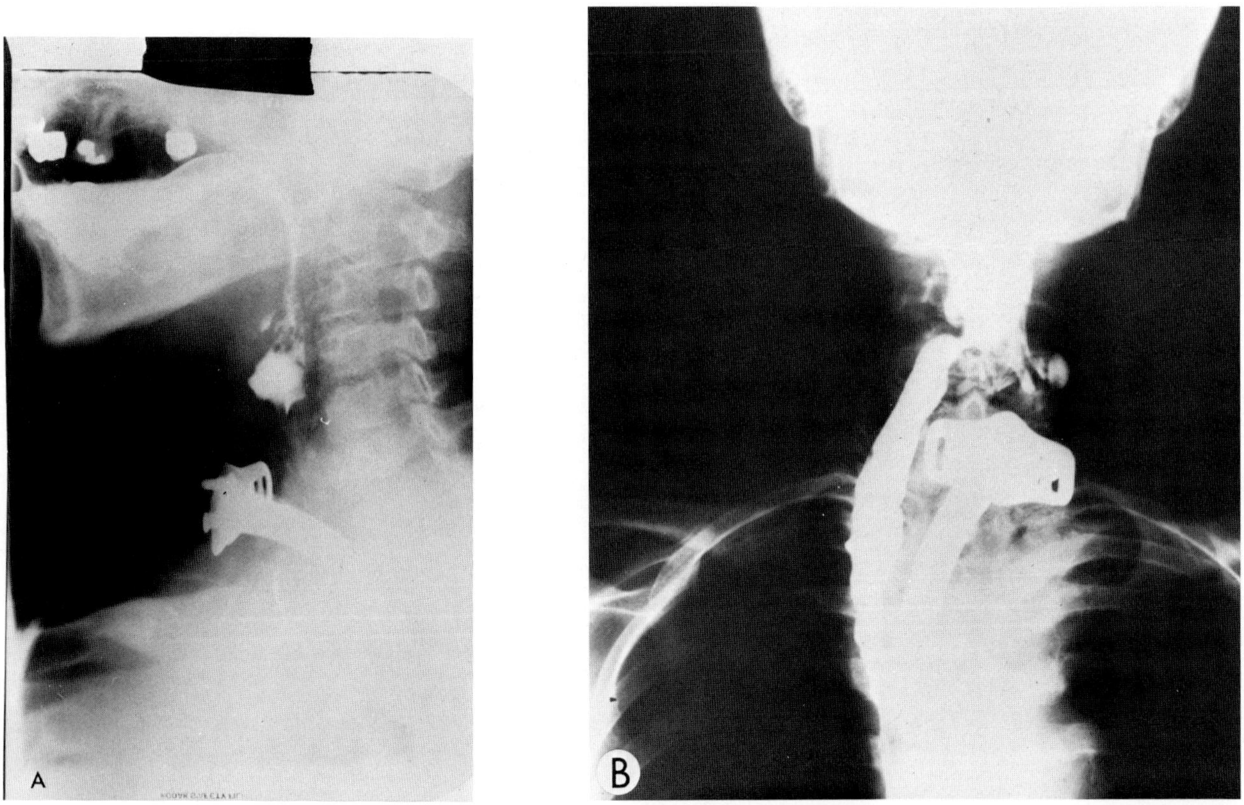

Fig. 4. Case 1. (A) Preoperative barium swallow demonstrates total obstruction of the hypopharynx. Note permanent tracheostoma. (B) RGT is anastomosed to hypopharynx at the level of the pyriform fossa.

Case 3

On June 17, a 61-year-old woman was admitted because of dysphagia and loss of 20 pounds. Barium swallow roentgenography revealed a filling defect from the pharyngoesophageal junction to the thoracic inlet. Squamous cell carcinoma was diagnosed on biopsy.

Pharyngo-esophago-laryngectomy was performed and a tracheostoma created, June 29, 1967 (H&N). A free jejunal transplant was not successful, consequently the distal thoracic esophagus was closed and a pharyngostoma was constructed and gastrostomy tube inserted. On August 1, 1967, RGT esophagoplasty with end-to-end anastomosis to the pharyngostoma was performed (HJH) (Fig. 5). The patient was able to eat a regular diet and learned esophageal speech. Three and one-half years postoperatively she died at home when tracheostomy tube was accidentally removed.

Case 4

A mass that involved the thyroid was resected from a 49-year-old man on August 22, 1967 (H&N). Pathology reported adenocarcinoma, primary in the trachea. A tracheoesophageal fistula developed postoperatively. A month later, a pharyngo-esophago-laryngectomy and mediastinal lymph node dissection was performed (H&N) and, simultaneously, an RGT was constructed (HJH).

During the neck dissection, the innominate artery tore at its origin with the aorta. The defect was closed and a Teflon graft was inserted between the innominate artery and a new site on the aorta. It was decided that the surgical procedure should be prolonged; therefore, tracheostoma and pharyngostoma were created. The RGT was brought subcutaneously to the neck and its open end was exteriorized under the mandible, thus isolating it from the area of the neck dissection. Anastomosis

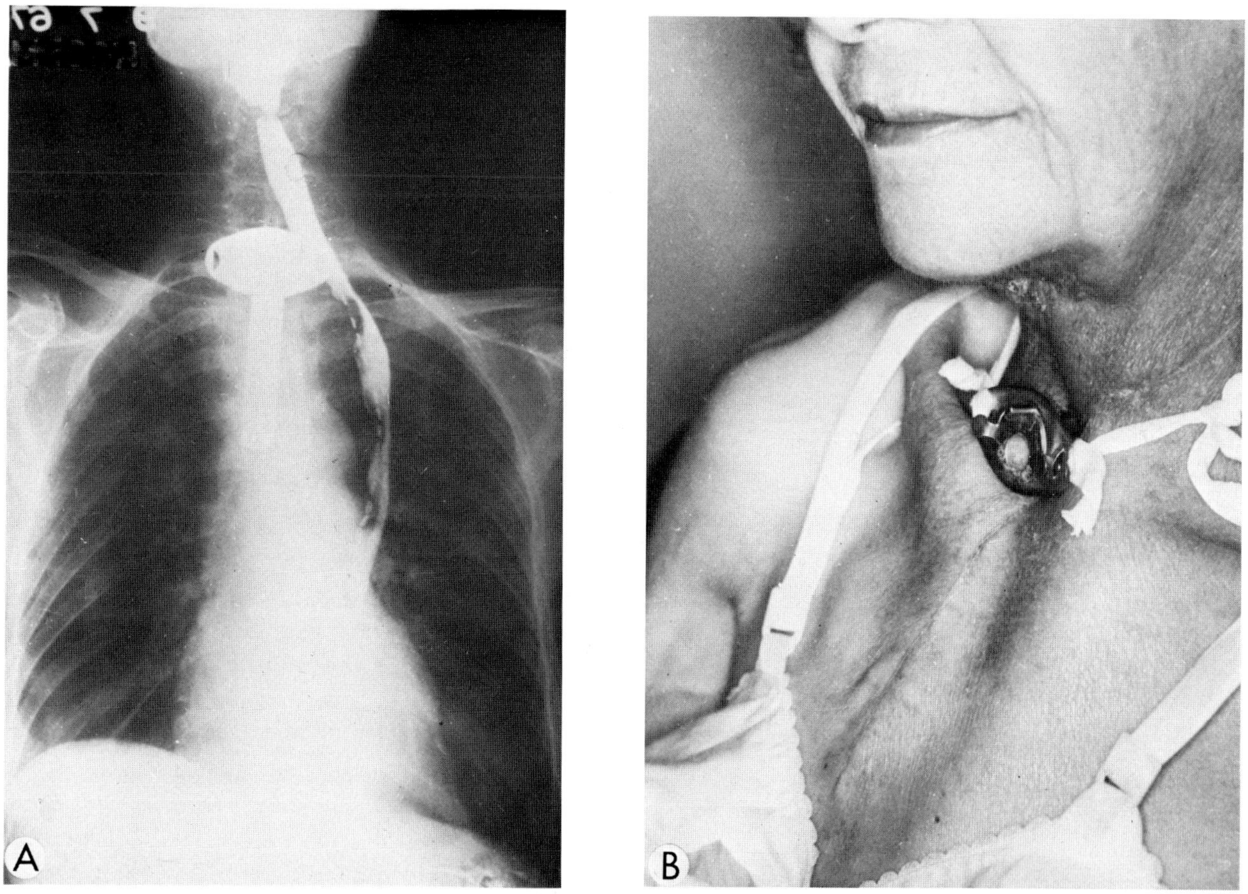

Fig. 5. Case 3. Postoperative barium swallow. (A) RGT is anastomosed to pharyngostoma at base of the tongue. (B) The RGT is seen beneath the skin to the left of the tracheostoma. Sternal splitting incision and extensive scarring are evident. These factors did not interfere with passage of RGT subcutaneously nor with its anastomosis to the pharynx.

of the RGT to the pharyngostoma was postponed, a procedure that has been used in other patients. The patient hemorrhaged several times, secondary to laceration of the innominate artery. He died on October 28, 1967. Autopsy showed that the RGT had remained healthy and viable and had not interferred with the care of the patient.

Case 5

A 65-year-old woman had radiotherapy for squamous cell carcinoma of the cervical esophagus 6 months before admission to Montefiore Hospital on July 16, 1968. Severe dysphagia brought about a 30 pound weight loss. Also, she had not eaten for several weeks because of constant aspiration owing to a high tracheoesophageal fistula. Right middle and lower lobe aspiration pneumonia was present, also stridor and fever that had not responded to intensive therapy for one week.

It was emergent to overcome the aspiration, so on July 23, 1968, a pharyngo-esophago-laryngectomy with formation of tracheostoma, pharyngostoma, and gastrostomy was performed (H&N). Tissue specimen showed carcinoma at the tracheoesophageal fistula well within the margins of resection.

The patient's nutritional status improved and pneumonia resolved gradually. On September 5, 1968, RGT esophagoplasty was performed (HJH) with anastomosis of the tube to the pharynx at the level of base of the tongue. She was able to eat a regular diet, although complaining of some regurgitation when discharged on November 9, 1968. Eight months after her operation, recurrence was detected at the tracheostoma. It regressed after radiotherapy, but she died of metastatic carcinoma on May 30, 1969.

Case 6

A 62-year-old woman had pharyngo-esophago-laryngectomy on January 3, 1967, and esophageal reconstruction with a vascularized free jejunal transplant (H&N). Dilatation was performed every several weeks resulting in perforation into the right chest in January 1969. Thoracotomy for empyema and neck exploration revealed that the transplant had fibrosed immediately after the first surgical procedure, and that food had been passing through a fistulous tract into the distal esophagus.

RGT esophagoplasty (HJH), February 19, 1969, required anastomosis of the gastric tube to a rim of skin attached to the pharyngostoma, since the mucosa was higher than the base of the tongue and could not be freed. A fistula occurred at this site but healed spontaneously in three weeks. She died of cardiac disease July 8, 1971.

Discussion

The ideal surgical therapy for carcinoma of the esophagus is resection of the entire esophagus. Segmental resection too often leads to incomplete removal of the tumor. In our experience and from reports of others, a more adequate resection of a carcinomatous cervical esophagus can be performed when RGT esophagoplasty is used for esophageal replacement. Since the distal esophagus need not be preserved for reconstruction, resection can be carried as far distally as is considered necessary. The RGT reaches to the base of the tongue without difficulty, and when a retrosternal tunnel is not feasible (such as after laryngectomy), normal swallowing can be restored by bringing the gastric tube to the neck in the subcutaneous plane.

We prefer that the head and neck surgeon do the esophageal resection and neck dissection. The distal esophagus is closed at least 8 cm beyond the tumor. This can be accomplished through a sternal-splitting incision. A thoracic incision, however, can be made should one wish to excise the entire esophagus. The pharynx is closed or a pharyngostomy is constructed, and if laryngectomy is necessary a tracheostoma is also created. A Stamm gastrostomy is performed through a small midline abdominal incision. The gastrostomy tube is inserted high on the lesser curvature of the stomach so as not to interfere with the subsequent RGT procedure. It is then brought out through a stab wound in the right side of the abdomen.

If the patient is in otherwise good health, and laryngectomy is not necessary, reconstruction can be performed by a second surgical team at the same time the resection is being done. In such instances, it is sometimes desirable to bring the RGT up to the neck through a retrosternal tunnel.

Reversed gastric tube esophagoplasty has been performed by the author in 68 patients since 1957 for benign or malignant esophageal disease. Three patients died in the early postoperative period, a mortality of 4.4 percent.

Patients 1, 3, and 6 had pharyngo-esophago-laryngectomy for management of carcinoma of the cervical esophagus. Attempts to replace the resected esophagus with a Teflon graft in one[5] and a free jejunal graft in the other two had failed. In patient 5, a tracheoesophageal fistula developed secondary to irradiation of pharyngoesophageal carcinoma. Pharyngo-esophago-laryngectomy was performed to relieve intractable aspiration pneumonia. In each of these patients, however, it was possible to restore swallowing at a second stage operation by RGT esophagoplasty, the gastric tube being anastomosed near the base of the tongue.

Case 2 had resection of the cervical and upper two-thirds of the thoracic esophagus for esophageal carcinoma without laryngectomy. The RGT was anastomosed to the pharynx at the same operation.

The innominate artery was lacerated in one patient (Case 4). The RGT was brought to the neck subcutaneously, its open end forming a stoma beneath the mandible, totally isolating the gastric tube from the area of neck dissection, yet maintaining it for subsequent anastomosis to the pharyngostoma. Unfortunately, the patient died from complications of vascular laceration five weeks postoperatively.

The most frequent complications are salivary fistula at the cervical esophagogastric anastomosis, which usually heals spontaneously, and too narrowly constructed esophagogastric cervical anastomosis. These complications have occurred in patients with extensive scarring due to irradiation or multiple surgical procedures prior to RGT esophagoplasty. The stenoses respond satisfactorily either to dilatation or to revision of the anastomosis.

Our experience[5] and reports by others,[6,7] substantiate that reversed gastric tube esophagoplasty offers the following advantages over other surgical procedures for esophageal reconstruction after resection of carcinoma of the cervical esophagus:

1. A more adequate cancer operation can be performed with the RGT procedure because the distal esophagus can be resected, since it will not be needed for reconstruction.
2. The vascular supply to the RGT is excellent.
3. The RGT can be brought to the neck subcutaneously, retrosternally, or intrapleurally.
4. The RGT easily reaches the base of the tongue.
5. Patients who require concomitant laryngectomy can be taught "esophageal" voice by expelling air through the mouth via the reversed gastric tube.

References

1. Watson WL, Goodner JT, Miller TP, Pack GT: Torek esophagectomy: the case against segmental resection for esophageal cancer. J Thoracic Surg 32:347–359, 1956
2. Heimlich HJ: Peptic esophagitis with stricture treated by reconstruction of the esophagus with a reversed gastric tube. Surg Gynecol Obstet 114:763–767, 1962
3. Heimlich HJ: Elective replacement of the oesophagus. Brit J Surg 53:913–916, 1966
4. Heimlich HJ: Esophageal replacement with a reversed gastric tube. Dis Chest 36:478–493, 1959
5. Heimlich HJ: Esophagoplasty with reversed gastric tube. Am J Surg 123:80–92, 1972
6. Alvarez, AF, Colbert JG: Lye stricture of the esophagus complicated by carcinoma. Can J Surg 6:470–476, 1963.
7. Hawk JC Jr: Total laryngectomy and cervical esophagectomy and reconstruction employing a greater curvature gastric tube, Am J Surg 102:789, 1961

The Diagnosis of Orocutaneous Fistulas and Their Management Prior to Surgical Reconstruction

Douglas D. Dedo, William A. Alonso, and Joseph H. Ogura, St. Louis, Mo.

Various surgical approaches for the rehabilitation of orocutaneous and pharyngocutaneous fistulas complicating head and neck surgery have been discussed in the literature.[1–9] However, there is a paucity of information regarding the early diagnosis and management of this complication prior to closure. This healing interval between wound demarcation and spontaneous or surgical repair requires daily management of a draining wound. Adherence to sound principles of wound management will enhance and thereby shorten this dynamic period of healing.

An approach for the early diagnosis and subsequent management of pharyngocutaneous fistulas will be described. It is based upon experience with 36 oro- and pharyngocutaneous fistulas, following 369 major head and neck cases, treated over a two-and-one-half year period.

Clinical Material

The daily progress notes, temperature and postoperative course were reviewed for the 36 patients complicated by a cutaneous fistula. It was possible to identify and tabulate the early wound changes which occurred prior to the diagnosis of a fistula. Warning signs, although often subtle, suggested an interruption in normal healing and heralded an impending catastrophic dehiscence.

The number of days between primary resection and the diagnosis of the cutaneous fistula was recorded. Commonly, there was a delay of several days between the warning signs of a wound irregularity and the diagnosis of a fistula. The daily management and final closure of the oro- or pharyngocutaneous fistula were also reviewed.

Results

The 369 major head and neck procedures and the corresponding fistulas are summarized in Table 1. Thirty-six fistulas represented a 9.6 percent complication rate. The highest incidence (20.8 percent) of postoperative fistulas was associated with partial laryngopharyngectomy and radical neck dissection. The lowest incidence (5.9 percent) was seen after a total laryngectomy. The predisposing factors and features influencing the incidence of postoperative fistulas among the various surgical procedures were presented previously.[10]

Daily management of a major postoperative head and neck patient involves inspection and palpation of the cervical flaps for edema, discoloration, tenderness, hemovac function and fluid accumulation. In the majority of the 36 patients, one or more signs of abnormal healing developed several days before the diagnosis of a fistula. Fluid accumulation was identified in 17 cases (Table 2). Fever elevations of 0.5°C to 2°C with occasional

Table 1. Incidence of Fistulas With Respect to Surgical Treatment of Primary Tumor

	No. Cases	No. Fistulas
Composite jaw-neck resection	120	9 (7.5%)
Partial laryngopharyngectomy with radical neck dissection	72	15 (20.8%)
Supraglottic subtotal laryngectomy with radical neck dissection	60	5 (8.3%)
Total laryngectomy	117	7 (5.9%)
Total	369	36 (9.6%)

Table 2. Early Wound Changes and Signs of Altered Healing Prior to the Diagnosis of a Fistula

	Jaw-neck dissection	Partial laryngopharyngectomy	Subtotal supraglottic laryngectomy	Total laryngectomy	Total
Fluid accumulation	6	7	2	2	17
Fever	1	6	2	3	12
Persistent flap edema and discoloration	6	5	3	3	17
Pus at incision	2	6	3	2	13
Persistent edema of arytenoids preventing decannulation	0	4	2	0	6
Air leak	0	2	0	0	2

spiking temperatures were recorded in 12 patients. Persistent flap edema and discoloration were observed in 17 cases. Purulent discharge at the incision was recorded in 13 patients. Air leaks from the trachea or the perichondrial suture line, characterized by billowing of the flaps on coughing, were seen in two instances.

Healing of the endolarynx following conservation surgery may be adequately followed postoperatively by indirect laryngoscopy. Edema of the mucosa and arytenoids usually subsides within two weeks permiting tracheal decannulation. However, six patients had persistent arytenoid and laryngeal edema during five weeks of follow-up. In each case the edema resolved after exteriorization and treatment of a pharyngocutaneous fistula.

Despite these early signs, an average of 18 days elapsed from the day of surgery to the diagnosis of fistula in these 36 cases. Table 3 summarizes the range, distribution, and average number of days required to diagnose a fistula after each procedure. For comparison, the time of appearance of the various wound irregularities is recorded in the same table. Study of the distribution of the early wound changes suggests that any deviation from normal healing during the first nine days postoperatively may herald eventual dehiscence over the next 12 days. To avoid an unnecessary delay in diagnosing a fistula, we encourage removal of a few sutures and gentle exploration of the wound if the local changes do not resolve after 48–72 hr of local and systemic antibiotic therapy.

Seventy-two percent of the fistulas were identified within three weeks of surgery. Those wounds that drained within six days postoperatively either had massive areas of flap necrosis with slough, or necrosis of the pharyngeal suture line secondary to excessive tension. The maximum time for diagnosing a fistula was 37 and 40 days postoperatively. Both patients had established peroral feeding and tracheal decannulation. In each a small wound abscess traced to the neopharyngeal suture line was discovered. Pharyngeal dehiscence developing six weeks or more after primary resection is not considered a surgical complication.

Impending difficulty should first be suspected before surgery. Identification of the high risk patient likely to develop a cutaneous fistula is frequently possible with careful preoperative screening. This information and a postoperative course characterized by unexplained fever, flap edema, tenderness along the neopharyngeal suture line, persistent arytenoid edema or fluid accumulation can lead one to suspect a fistula. When wound disruptions do not resolve within 48–72 hr after high dose intravenous antibiotics, local drainage, warm compresses, and Barton dressings, a diagnosis of a fistula is almost certain. Pharyngeal leak is confirmed by having the patient swallow a small amount of methylene blue and identifying the dye under the flaps. The test is repeated after three to four days if the local wound changes persist. After a positive test, the fistula is immediately exteriorized. A counterincision is placed through the cervical flaps over the area of pharyngeal dehiscence. The carotid artery is avoided by placing the incision anterior. A penrose drain or gauze wick is inserted through the counter incision into

Table 3. Number of Days Following Primary Resection for Early Warning Signs and Fistula Diagnosis

Number of Days	JND	PLP	SSL	TOTAL LARYNG.
›29	°40	°39 °34	°30	°31
28				
27				
26			X °	
25	°	°		
24	°	°		
23				
22		°		
21		X	X ϕ 21	
20				
19	ϕ 19	°	°	
18 (avg.)	°	X °		°
17		X		
16		X ϕ 16.8	X	
15	X ° ° °	° ° °		ϕ 15
14		X °		X °
13				
12	°	X ° °	X °	°
11		X		X
10	X °	X °	X	
9	XX	° °		X
8	X	XX		
7		X		X °
6	XXXXX	XXXX °	XX	
5	XXX	XXX	X	X °
4	XX			
3	X	XXX		
2	X	XXXX	XX	XX
1	XXX	XXXXX		X
0				
PROCEDURE	JND	PLP	SSL	TOTAL LARYNG.

° Day postop diagnosed
X Day postop for warning signs
ϕ Average for each procedure

the pharynx to divert the fistula. The combination of the drain and light gauze packing saturated with povidone–iodine ointment under the cervical flap, prevents the accumulation of secretions inferiorly.

A bulky dressing is changed two or three times daily. During each dressing change the packing is replaced after hydrogen peroxide irrigations. Necrotic tissue is periodically debrided from the edges and base of the wound. Debridement in the operating room is necessary if the wound does not respond to conservative therapy, or when large areas of flap necrosis and pharyngeal slough are present.

Systemic treatment includes high dose intravenous antibiotics. A regimen of 2.0 g of cephalothin every six hours is continued until the acute inflammatory changes subside. The oral route (1.0 g every 6 hr) is then substituted until fistula closure. Supplemental parenteral and oral vitamins are used. Blood is transfused to maintain the hematocrit above 35 percent. High caloric intake with any of the commercially available preparations is started as soon as the patient tolerates nasogastric feedings.

The outcome in these 36 cases is summarized in Table 4. Fifteen fistulas (41.6 percent) closed spontaneously with eight requiring some form of surgical manipulation in the operating room. Thirteen fistulas (36 percent) required surgical closure and reconstruction. Eight fistulas (22.4 percent) failed to close.

Table 4. Outcome of 36 Fistulas

Closed spontaneously		15 (41.6%)
Required surgical manipulation before closing	8 (22.2%)	
Closed spontaneously	7 (19.4%)	
Required surgical closure		13 (30%)
Failed to close		8 (22.4%)

Discussion

The importance of an early diagnosis of impending pharyngeal dehiscence cannot be overemphasized. By recognizing subtle wound irregularities and instituting vigorous local and systemic therapy, the subsequent disaster of a pharyngeal breakdown may be avoided. Failure to recognize early wound irregularities and failure to diagnose a fistula for several days will prolong the normal healing process and increase patient morbidity and hospitalization.

Meticulous wound management postoperatively is the best approach to ensure the early diagnosis of a cutaneous fistula. Erythema of the cervical flaps with edema and tenderness over the neopharyngeal suture line represents an early cellulitis. Failure to treat these signs with high dose intravenous antibiotics can lead to an abscess and attendant pharyngeal slough. Fluid accumulation under the cervical flaps may represent hemovac malfunction, chyle leak, hematoma, or a small pharyngeal leak. Opening the incision will allow identification and drainage of the fluid.

Purulence at the incision may represent local wound infections or a pharyngeal leak. Frequently, a localized wound infection not responding to conservative therapy is being fed by a pharyngeal fistula. This is readily confirmed by having the patient swallow methylene blue.

The source of even minor fever elevations must be identified. Ten of these patients became afebrile after drainage and exteriorization of the cutaneous fistula.

Persistent arytenoid and laryngeal edema within the first six weeks of surgery preventing tracheal decannulation may be due to a subacute infection or chondritis. After exteriorizing the fistula, the edema usually subsides. However, Ward et al[11] reported that prolonged laryngeal and arytenoid edema beyond six months may represent an occult persistence of the tumor which must be investigated with direct laryngoscopy and deep biopsy.

The physiology of a healing wound may be conveniently divided into three phases.[12] The lag or substrate phase primarily involves the inflammatory response, with the removal of blood clots, necrotic tissue, and bacteria. The fibroblastic phase begins with fibroblast migration, differentiation, and collagen synthesis. It ends with wound contraction as the fibroblast syncytium adheres to the wound base and prepares for collagen maturation. The last phase of healing, maturation, continues indefinitely. For the first few weeks the wound gains tensile strength reaching a maximum at six weeks[13] as the collagen fibrils form intermolecular bonds. Thereafter, a dynamic equilibrium exists between collagen synthesis and degradation. Each phase overlaps the next, but progression of the healing process if dependent upon success of the preceding phase. For example, the presence of fluid or necrotic debris in a wound prolongs the lag phase and inhibits fibroblastic proliferation and maturation.

The management of postoperative oro- and pharyngocutaneous fistulas may be divided into two periods. The first period involves handling the acute changes as the fistula demarcates. The basic approach during the acute phase is to: (1) provide drainage and allow demarcation of the fistula; (2) facilitate contraction and adherence of the flaps; (3) protect the carotid artery; and (4) encourage wound granulation and epithelialization. The exteriorization of the fistula through the cervical flap directly over the area of pharyngeal dehiscence provides a more direct route for drainage of secretions. By directing the drainage latero-inferiorly, away from the cervical flap, contraction and adherence of the flap to the wound base are enhanced. The carotid artery is protected by exteriorizing the fistula. Without diversion, the secretions would drain across the carotid artery and pool in the inferior aspect of the wound. A penrose drain or iodoform wick placed through the counter-incision prevents its closure. A light packing of iodoform gauze saturated with a topical antimicrobial agent is placed under the flap. Frequent dressing changes with gradual reduction in the volume of packing allows the wound to close. Failure to pack the wound lightly and frequently will result in the accumulation of bacteria, necrotic tissue, and wound exudate in a warm environment. The subsequent proliferation of bacteria and wound exudation increases the area of flap elevation.

The gauze packing accomplishes several purposes. First, its frequent removal followed by hydrogen peroxide irrigation serves to debride the wound. Second, two raw surfaces that continually rub against each other form a fibrin layer that prevents adherence of the flaps.[12] The insertion of gauze between the two surfaces discourages this fibrin formation. Third, the gauze acts as a carrier for the topical antimicrobial agent.

The use of a topical antimicrobial agent in the management of a cutaneous fistula is based upon the physiology of a draining wound. When a fistula develops, tissue loss with necrosis, bacterial overgrowth, and acute inflammation occurs. A cycle of altered tissue pH, cell lysis, enzymatic digestion and subsequent bacterial proliferation ensues. If bacterial overgrowth is impeded by systemic and topical antibiotics, the cycle is interrupted with resultant potentiation of the healing process. Povidone–iodine ointment[14] possesses several qualities which make it particularly suitable for use in head and neck surgery. It has a built-in color indicator of its effectiveness, and will not stain since it is water soluble. It also has the broad antimicrobial spectrum of iodine without its side effects.

After the acute phase of fistula demarcation, the chronic prolonged management of these wounds begins. This second period involves maintaining the wound for spontaneous or surgical closure. If the fistula is to close spontaneously, it must do so by secondary intention. The prime consideration is to promote flap contraction and epithelial migration. Occasionally, relaxing incisions in the cervical flaps are necessary to allow the flap to seat properly on the wound base. Epithelialization will not begin until the wound has contracted with adherence of the flaps to the wound base. Fine mesh gauze impregnated with an antimicrobial ointment is placed at the edges of the fistula. A bulky dressing holds the gauze in place and absorbs secretions. The ointment prevents drying and crusting in addition to reducing the bacterial concentration and odor. The fine mesh gauze acts as a scaffold for the granulation tissue and protects the flap edges.

Debridement of the wound in the operating room is selected when large amounts of the wound sloughs or after a poor response to local management. Recently nine patients have been debrided under general anesthesia. From this and a prior study[10] it was found that the time required for spontaneous closure was reduced after patients were debrided in the operating room rather than treated at the bedside. The size of the fistula was greater in those patients debrided in the operating room after a Bakajamian chest flap was staged but not used. This accelerated wound response may be explained by the second wound phenomenon.[12,15,16] Simply stated, it is the observation that rewounding results in an acceleration of the healing of the first wound. This phenomenon was observed in eight patients.

Summary

Meticulous wound management postoperatively provides the safest ambient approach for diagnosis of a cutaneous fistula. The majority of the 36 patients complicated by a pharyngocutaneous fistula, had subtle wound changes noted 7 to 12 days before the fistula was actually diagnosed. Vigorous local and systemic therapy for any wound irregularity is recommended to limit and possibly prevent the ultimate pharyngeal dehiscence. Failure of abnormal wound changes to resolve after 48–72 hr of treatment should be followed by gentle exploration of the wound. Confirmation of a pharyngeal leak is made by having the patient swallow methylene blue and identifying it in the wound. A positive test is managed by immediately exteriorizing the fistula through the cervical flap.

Management of a pharyngocutaneous fistula is divided into an acute phase (as the fistula demarcates) and a chronic phase (awaiting spontaneous closure or surgical reconstruction). The basis for the daily maintenance of these wounds is discussed.

Forty-one percent of the oro- and pharyngocutaneous fistulas closed spontaneously. Thirty-six percent required surgical closure and 22 percent failed to close.

References

1. Barretto PM: New techniques of plastic surgery to repair the pharyngo-esophageal segments using cervico-acromial flaps. Acta Otolaryng 65:236–243, 1968
2. Bellinger CG: Classification of pharyngostomes: a guideline for closure. Plast Reconstr Surg 47:54–60, 1971
3. May AR, Lavelle RJ: The management of postoperative pharyngocutaneous pharyngeal fistulae. J Laryng 86:795–805, 1972
4. Monihan RM, Lipshutz H: Method for closure of pharyngocutaneous fistula. Plast Reconstr Surg 47:384–385, 1971
5. Myers EN: The management of pharyngocutaneous fistula. Arch Otolaryng 95:10–17, 1972
6. Ogura JH, Dedo HH: Repair of large pharyngostoma utilizing bilateral non-delayed regional pedicle flaps. Laryngoscope 75:588–600, 1965
7. Siirala U, Lauerma S: Stubborn postoperative pharyngeal fistula. Arch Otolaryng 95:274–276, 1972
8. Vieta LJ, Quintana RA, Obregon MA: Plastic repair of pharyngeal fistulas. Arch Otolaryng 87:78–81, 1968
9. Zovickian A: Pharyngeal fistulas: repair and prevention using mastoid occiput band shoulder flaps. Plast Reconstr Surg 19:355–372, 1957
10. Dedo DD, Alonso WA, Ogura JH: The incidence, predisposing factors, and outcome of pharyngocutaneous fistulas complicating head and neck cancer surgery. Accepted for publication, Ann Otol
11. Ward PH, Calcaterra TC, Kagan AR: The enigma of post-irradiation edema and recurrent or residual carcinoma of the larynx. Laryngoscope 85:522–529, 1975
12. Peacocke EE, VanWinkle W Jr: Surgery and Biology, Philadelphia, WB Saunders Co, 1970
13. Levenson SM, Geever EF, Crowley LV, et al: The healing of rat skin wounds. Ann Surg 161:293–308, 1965
14. Shelanski HA, Shelanski MV: PVA-iodine: history, toxicity and therapeutic uses. J Inter Col Surgeons 25:727–734, 1956
15. Dunphy JE, Jackson DS: The practical applications of experimental studies in the case of the primary closed wound. Amer J Surg 104:273–282, 1962
16. Dingman RO: Factors of clinical significance affecting wound healing. Laryngoscope 83:1540–1554, 1973

Simplification of Superiorly Based Pharyngeal Flaps

Stephen C. Ferguson, Evansville, Ind.

The most widely utilized method of repair of velopharyngeal insufficiency is a superiorly based pharyngeal flap.[1] The major disadvantage to this type of reconstruction is the difficulty in preparing an adequate palate flap or bed.[2] Historically the palate surface has been denuded or a "flap" created in a retrograde manner from the posterior aspect of the palate, although other methods have been suggested.[3] In my hands no flap was created and a great deal of time was involved in attempting to prepare the nasal aspect of the palate.

Therefore, somewhat over a year ago, it was decided to split the palate in the midline for obtaining the palate flap. The operating time has been cut in half and healing improved. This technique has now been used for two patients with insufficiency secondary to tonsillectomy and adenoidectomy, one patient with palate paralysis secondary to cerebral vascular accident and two patients with residual defect following cleft palate repair. Success, as judged by the patient, family, and surgeon, was based on normal sounding speech, absence of nasal leak during swallowing, adequate nasal airway, and absence of ear problems. One patient with tonsillectomy and adenoidectomy scored 100 percent in all regards. One still has ear problems but less than preop and is otherwise excellent. The patient with palate paralysis still has slight to moderate hypernasality but is now understandable to a casual observer and otherwise excellent. One 40-year-old

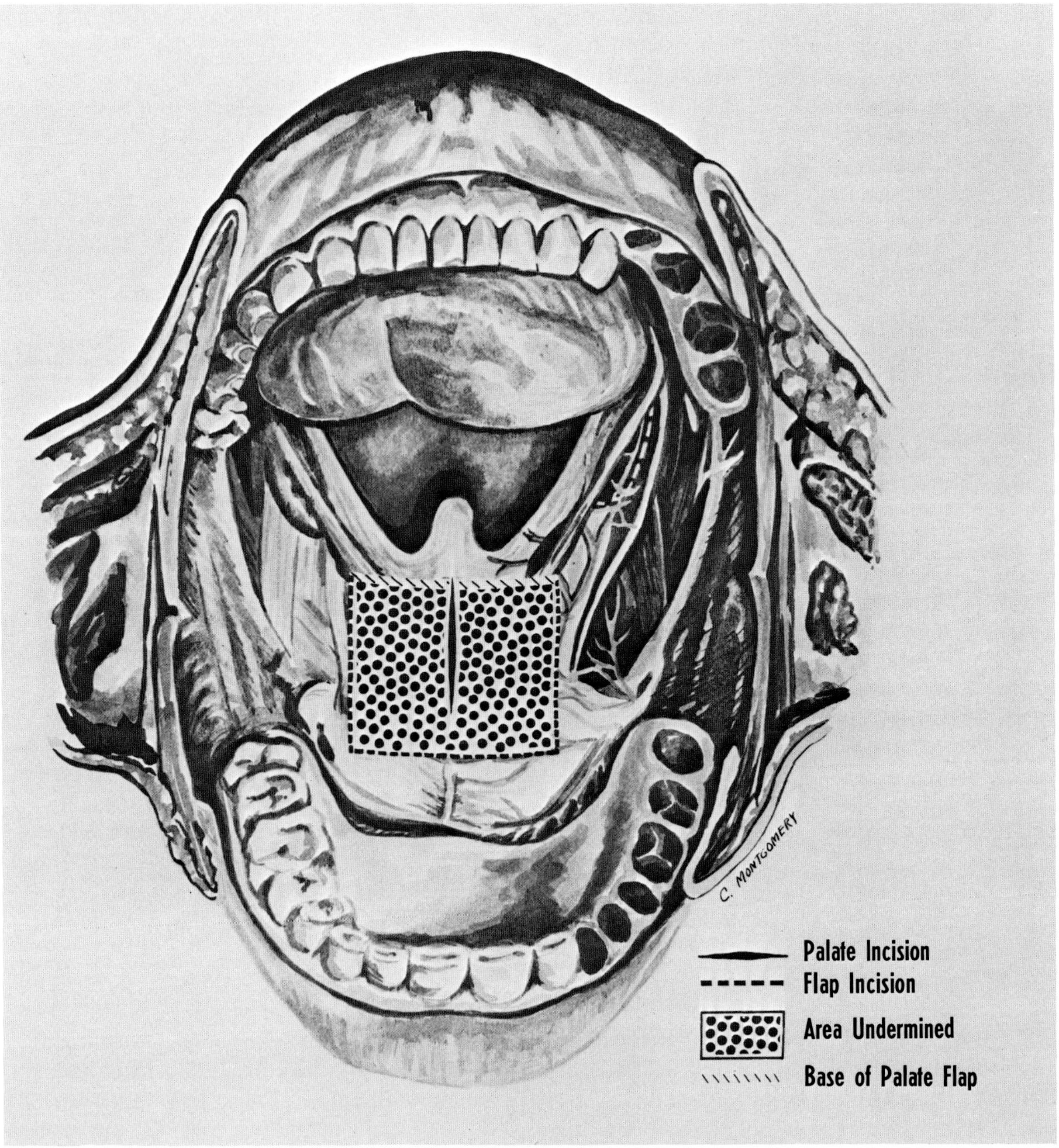

Fig. 1. Palate as visualized in the Rose position.

patient with cleft palate still has hypernasality but is able to close off the nasopharynx and has been sent to a speech therapist. The other 14-year-old patient with cleft palate has essentially a 100 percent result.

Operative Procedure

The palate is approached in the Rose position under general endotracheal anesthesia using a McGivor mouthgag. One percent Xylocaine with 1 to 100,000 epinephrine is locally infiltrated into the palate and posterior pharyngeal wall. A 1.5–2 cm incision is made in the midline of the palate approximately 0.5 to 1 cm anterior to the uvula or posterior edge of the palate (Fig. 1). Using Foman, Metzenbaum, and Knapp scissors, a palate flap is elevated in a natural plane superior to the palatoglossus muscle. The flap is composed of palatopharyngeus muscle and portion of levator and tensor veli patatini muscles. The dissection is carried laterally to approximately the width of the anticipated pharyngeal flap, and anteriorly to the hard palate. The flap is then cut free with a knife and the anterolateral edges tagged with 3–0 chromic sutures.

The superiorly based pharyngeal flap is then created in the usual manner as wide, as long, and as high as can reasonably be obtained. The pharyngeal flap is then tagged with 3–0 chromic and the two flaps are interdigitated through the midline palate incision (Fig. 2). The pharyngeal flap is then secured to the palate as far anteriorly as possible with 3–0 chromic mattress sutures. The palate flap

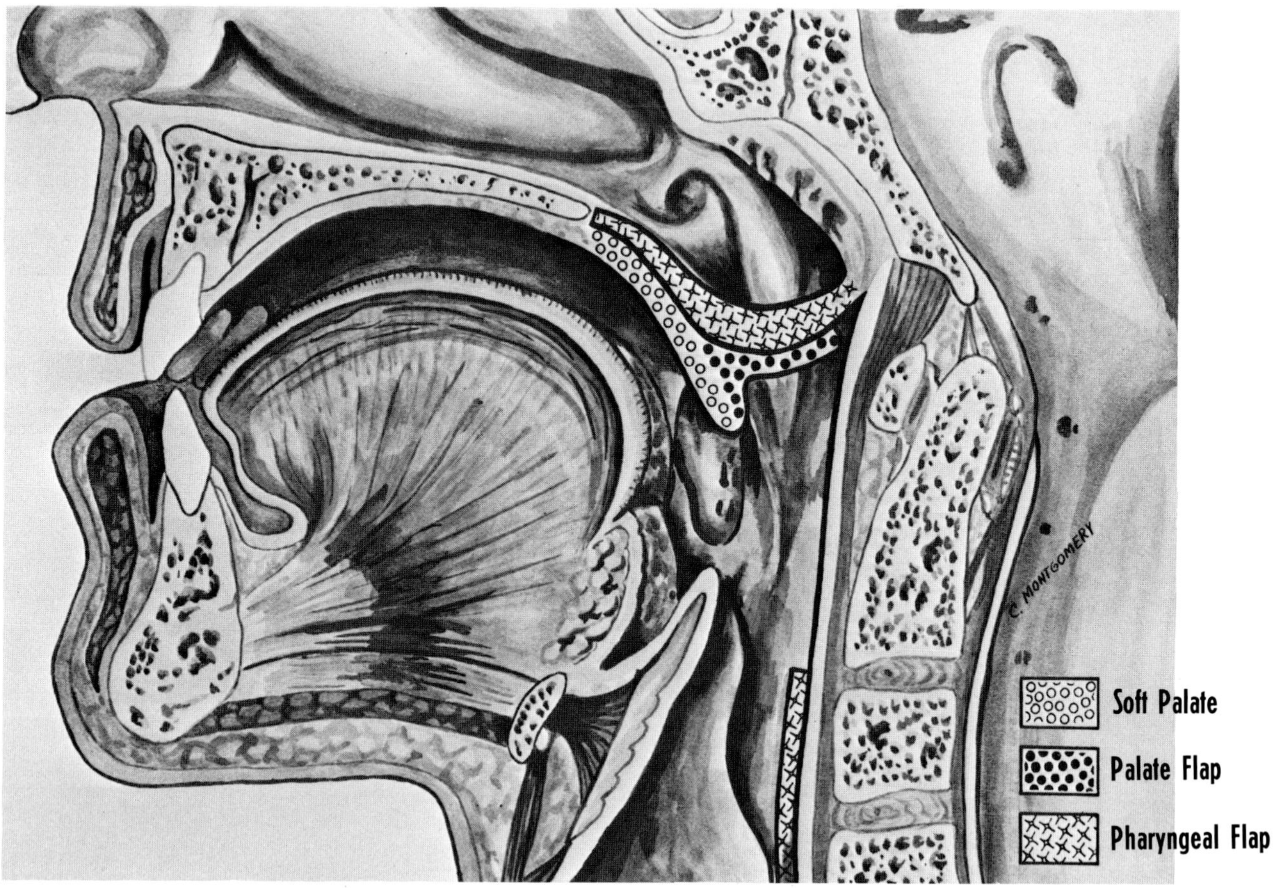

Fig. 2. Lateral cross section of interdigitated palate and superiorly based pharyngeal flap.

is then secured to the pharyngeal flap, again using the already placed 3–0 chromic sutures. Additional sutures are placed as required. The midline palate incision is then closed with horizontal everting mattress sutures and a running simple suture. The posterior pharyngeal wall is then closed with a running 2–0 chromic. The nasopharynx is then thoroughly irrigated with saline and the patient extubated.

Comment

This procedure may or may not improve the overall results, in that a stiff board-like or nonfunctioning palate will still not totally close off the nasopharynx during phonation and swallowing if a nasal airway is maintained. The major advantage to the procedure appears to be the ease with which it can be done and decreased operating time to approximately 30–45 min. There does not appear to be a problem with fistulization of the palate and, in fact, preexisting fistulae have been closed with this technique.

Summary

A technique is described for a closure of velopharyngeal insufficiency utilizing a superiorly based pharyngeal flap and posteriorly based palate flap that is elevated through a midline partial palate split incision.

References

1. Yules RB, Chase RA: Pharyngeal flap surgery: a review of the literature, Cleft Palate J 6:303–8, 1969
2. Yules RB, Chase RA: Secondary techniques for correction of palatopharyngeal incompetence, in Grabb WC, Rosenstein SW, Bzoch KR (eds), Cleft Lip and Palate, Boston: Little, Brown, 1971, Chap 32
3. Bernstein L: Treatment of velopharyngeal incompetence, Arch Otolaryngol 85:67–74, 1967

Congenital Defects

Choanal Atresia—An Approach to Unilateral Atresia in the Adult

A. L. Roper, Norfolk, Va.

Choanal atresia occurs with sufficient frequency for the busy Otolaryngologist to encounter this condition several times per year. Surprisingly, many of these cases are of the unilateral type, which account for about ten percent of the total. Most will present with the complaint of a persistent "cold," or be referred with the diagnosis of "foreign body in the nose." The teenager comes because the symptoms represent an increasing social handicap.

Surgical procedures on the choanae can be accomplished through the nose, thereby obviating the need for extensive palatal incisions, prolonged anesthesia, and increased blood loss. With experience, this method has been found to be practical for the surgical correction of the bilateral condition in the infant as well.

Method

Anesthetization is accomplished by topical cocaine crystals on nearly dry epinephrine pledgets. Two percent lidocaine with epinephrine 1:100,000 is used for local infiltration and a transpalatine sphenopalatine block.

Using a large ear speculum, and obtaining binocular vision through the operating microscope, incisions can be made, and flaps created, as if one were operating in the auditory canal and tympanum. A septoplasty may be required when found to be deviated.

The anterior mucosa of the atretic area is incised superiorly, inferiorly, and *laterally*. The medial side (toward the septum) is left attached to the septal mucosa while this flap is elevated from the bony or fibrous atresia. Tynpanoplasty instruments and fine otologic suctions are employed with ease. The underlying bone or fibre-cartilage is then removed using mastoid curettes and fine chisels, along with the posterior bony septum. Care is exercised to avoid injury to the mucosa lying posterior to the atresia. This posterior mucosa is then incised superiorly, inferiorly, and *medially*, forming a flap based on the lateral nasal wall.

The anterior flap is now reflected posteriorly, while the posterior flap is drawn anteriorly. The result of this maneuver is to prevent the circumferential opposition of raw surfaces which tend to form stenosis. This is the major advantage of this technique over simple "punch-through" or "cut-out" procedures.

Direct visualization of the operative area should make it more difficult to inadvertantly injure the spheno-palatine canal, or to enter the sphenoid sinus.

A soft stent is placed through the choana and left in place for four to five weeks. I originally used a portion of Foley catheter, however Silastic or Teflon seems to be less reactive. This is secured to the septum with a single suture, and is allowed to protrude through the nostril. A light packing of Vaseline gauze is inserted for two days, then removed. At this time the stent is trimmed to lie entirely within the nose. Ointment is applied to the nostril daily as long as the stent is in place, to decrease irritation and to loosen crusts which tend to form.

Antibiotics and decongestants are administered until the stent is removed.

I have found this method to be simple and effective. No further procedures nor dilitations have been necessary to maintain an adequate airway. The patients for whom I have performed this procedure have been among the most grateful for the elimination of a severe social handicap.

Scalp

Scalp Reconstruction

William R. Simpson and John W. Miles, Los Angeles, Calif

The Department of Otolaryngology at the Los Angeles County-University of Southern California Medical Center has dealt with a variety of major scalp injuries over the years. Our patients have been the victims of animal attacks, machete assaults, bicycle and motorcycle accidents, as well as auto and pedestrian accidents. The principles of scalp reconstruction rest on a basic knowledge of scalp anatomy, which shall be the first topic of our discussion.

Scalp Anatomy

The thinner frontal, temporal, and mastoid areas of scalp skin are attached to the origin areas of the frontalis, occipitalis, and galea aponeurotica by connective tissue bridges. This combination of thin skin and restraining connective tissue bridges creates the predictable and actual sites of many of the initial points of scalp tearing and avulsions. The inelasticity of the galea prevents many of the ruptured scalp vessels from retracting and stemming severe scalp hemorrhage.

There are three surgical layers of the scalp. The outer layer is composed of skin, subcutaneous fat, and galea. An intermediate loose areolar connective tissue layer is followed by an inner division of pericranium or periosteum. The vascularity of the periosteum nourishes the outer table of the skull, as does the vascularity of the dura mater nourish the inner table of the skull. The traumatic plane of separation in scalp avulsions usually passes through the loose areolar connective tissue. Surgical separation and rotation of reconstructive scalp is also carried out through this loose areolar connective tissue.

The network of vessels external to the galea is made up of a companion arterial and venous system that is supplied by branches of the internal and external carotid arteries. This network of vessels must not be needlessly injured in the surgical separation and rotation of scalp flaps or when multiple parallel galea incisions are used to provide stretch to the scalp.

The variety, width, and length of scalp flaps is made possible by the richness of the vascular supply to the scalp. The vessels supplying this network pass from a superficial to a deeper anatomical plane in the base of the temporal, mastoid, and occipital scalp flaps, and must not be injured in a scalp flap construction.

Scalp flaps of the frontal, temporal and occipital areas are supplied by specific arteries (Fig. 1) The base of the frontal area scalp flap contains the supratrochlear and supraorbital branches of the internal carotid artery. An anterior branch of the superficial temporal artery that originates from the external carotid also supplies this flap. A temporal area based scalp flap is supplied by the superficial temporal artery and the posterior auricular branch of the external carotid artery. Occipital area scalp flaps contain the posterior auricular and posterior occipital branches of the external carotid artery, as well as paramidline and midline emissary vessels of the skull.

The rupturing of cervical and scalp veins and the opening of diploic spaces of the skull in a patient with markedly lowered venous pressure exposes that individual to the possibility of fatal air embolism.

The use of bone wax to seal the diploic spaces or dressings to seal torn vessels will help avoid the danger of air embolism and infection. Uncontrolled infection in these cases of scalp avulsion and skull destruction may lead to venous sinus infection, thrombosis, meningitis, and/or brain abscess.

Initial Evaluation and Treatment

Life-threatening scalp hemorrhage, is controlled in most cases, at the accident scene with the

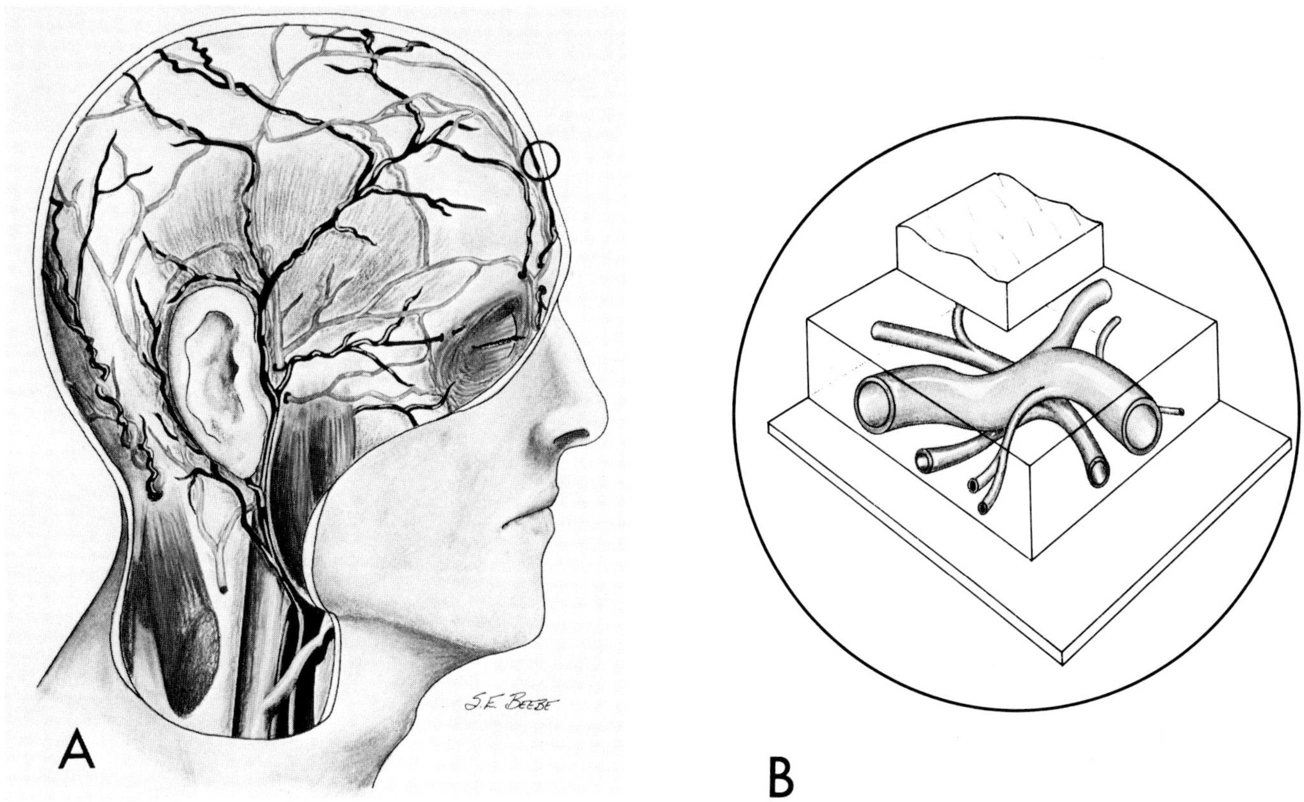

Fig. 1. (A) SCALP ARTERIES Anterior scalp is supplied by the supraorbital and supratrochlear arteries; Lateral scalp is supplied: by the superficial temporal and posterior auricular arteries; Posterior scalp is supplied by the occipital and emissary vessels. (B) The vascular compartment of the scalp lies just above the galea aponeurotica and must not be injured in elevation or rotation of the scalp flap.

aid of pressure dressings. There are a number of ways to control scalp hemorrhage in the emergency room or in surgery prior to initial repair of the scalp. Specific bleeding arteries are clamped and stick tied. General scalp bleeding may be controlled by grasping the galea with an instrument and everting the cut scalp edge and then folding the loose scalp back on itself. A running lock suture may be placed about two centimeters from the bleeding edge. Excellent scalp hemostasis is achieved by the application of Raney clips to the cut edge of the scalp. Whatever the method of hemostasis, it must never reach the extremes of causing avascular necrosis of viable scalp.

Attainment of airway and hemorrhage control is accompanied by a simultaneous effort to restore the hemodynamics of the patient. Care must be taken not to overload the circulatory system or jeopardize the patient with possible cerebral edema. Intravenous catheters provide a rapid route of infusion for the appropriate crystalloid, blood fraction, or whole blood.

Motorcycle and pedestrian accidents frequently result in a number of serious injuries that must be placed in the proper priority of evaluation and treatment (Fig. 2). These patients frequently sustain a triad of scalp injuries including lacerations, avulsions, and friction burns of the scalp. These scalp burns contain borderline viable tissue that may take ten to twelve days for the thrombosed vessels in the area to recover or cause necrosis of the tissue.

Infection has not been a serious problem in most of the cases where there has been an opportunity to carefully clean and debride the foreign material and necrotic tissues. The wound debridement has either been carried out under local or general anesthesia, depending upon the patient's total condition. A few of our cases that involved a delay in referral to our service or exhibited severe and extensive burns did have a resistant infection of *Staphylococcus aureus* and *Pseudomonas*. The Staphylococcus infections responded to the appropriate antibiotics indicated by the culture and

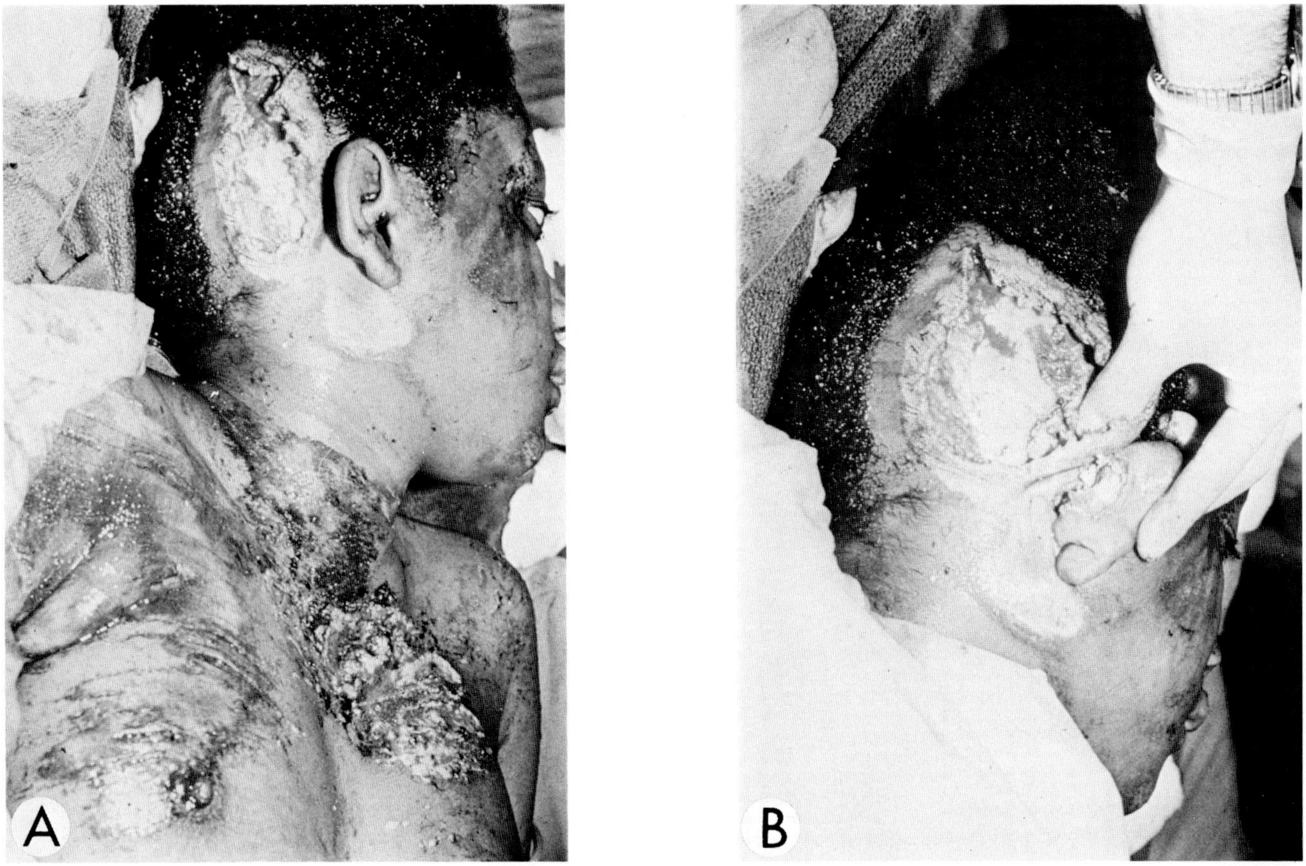

Fig. 2. (A) This 19-year-old patient was thrown from a car to the street and received abrasions, lacerations and avulsions of soft-tissue of the head, neck, and chest. (B) illustrates an occipital temporal bone skull fracture.

sensitivity studies. The presence of Pseudomonas deeply imbedded in the scalp tissue required extensive local wound care, involving the use of Sulfamylon cream and Gentamycin sulfate systemically. The patient's general metabolic condition, including renal function, was closely monitored in these cases.

The intensive local wound care by the entire medical team is an absolute necessity. Wet to dry dressings utilizing saline, quarter percent acetic acid, or diluted half strength Dakin's solution are combined with meticulous debridement of necrotic and infected tissues.

Exposed pericranium or skull is covered with autografts or scalp flaps (Fig. 3). When a patient sustains injuries to the scalp that do not permit immediate autografts or scalp flap coverage, various dressings are employed. Moist, sterile saline dressings, homografts, and porcine skin are used in combination with the appropriate systemic antibiotic. When there is a reasonable chance of success with autografts or scalp flaps, surgery is carried out as soon as possible. We have maintained patients with exposed pericranium and skull for eight to twelve days without serious problems or complications.

Choice of Scalp Reconstruction

Depending on the patient's age, general condition, and type of trauma causing a specific scalp defect, avulsion measuring three or four centimeters in diameter can be repaired by wide scalp undermining and scalp flap advancement and rotation (Fig. 4).

Large areas of scalp avulsion that do not involve the pericranium and are not grossly contaminated are covered with thick split autografts. The disadvantage to applying permanent skin grafts

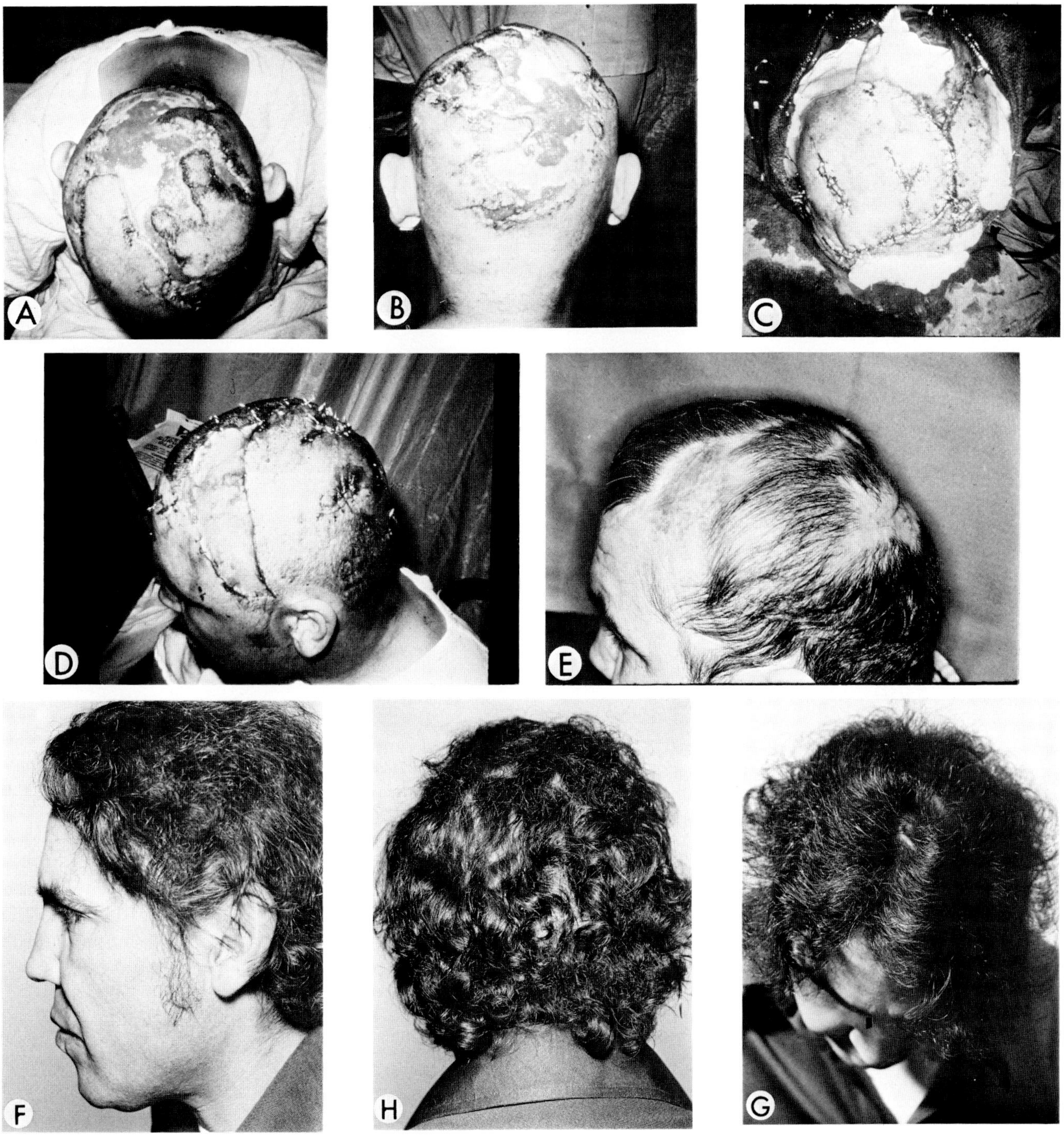

Fig. 3. (A–H) Illustrations of severe scalp lacerations and loss of scalp due to machete assault on the patient. The reconstruction period extended over a 12 month period and required the use of rotation scalp flaps, outer skull table decortication and split thickness skin grafts.

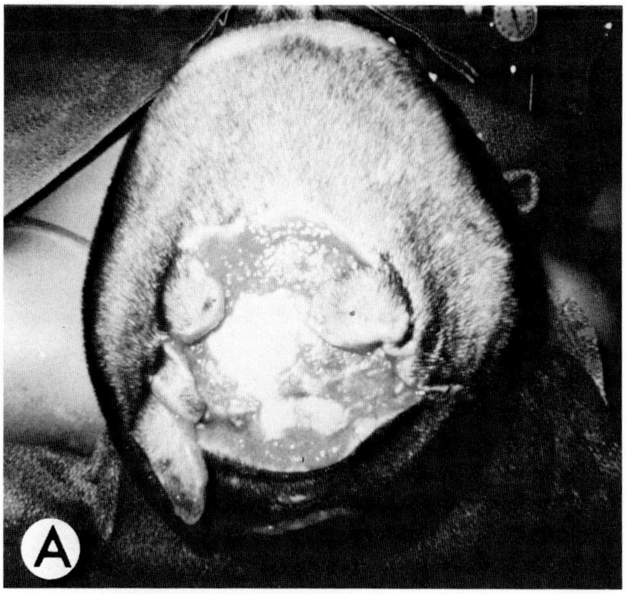

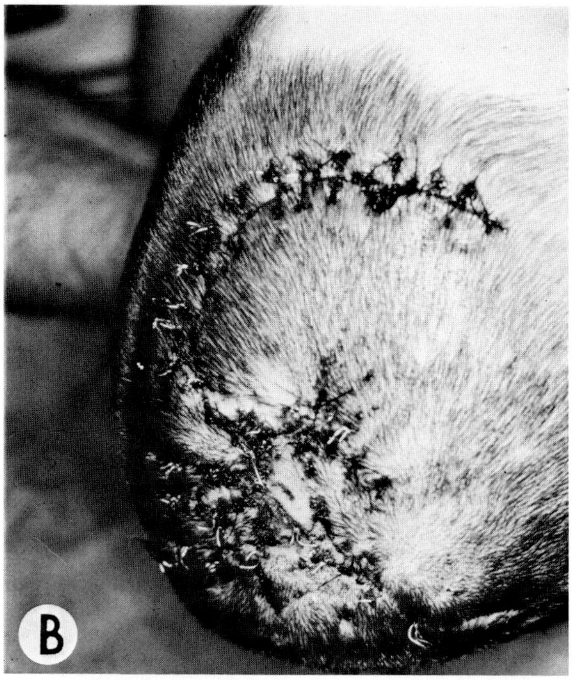

Fig. 4. *(A,B) Illustrates a combined laceration and avulsion injury of the scalp closed by a single anterior based-scalp rotation flap, combined with extensive undermining of the scalp.*

directly over the pericranium is that they are subject to recurrent trauma, ulceration and infection. Carcinoma has reportedly developed in these long standing, repeatedly traumatized autografts after many years.

When the avulsion injury has removed the pericranium and the surrounding remaining scalp is not suitable for scalp flap development, the outer table of the skull is burred off with a large cutting ear burr (Fig. 5). Sterile wet saline dressing and/or porcine skin is used to encourage the development of granulation tissues from the exposed diploic spaces. This granulation changes from its initial pale color to a rich red vascular granulation tissue in sixteen or seventeen days. This vascular granulation easily nourishes autografts and gives a satisfactory contour if the granulation is allowed to reproduce to a height of the surrounding subcutaneous tissue.

The feeder arteries of the prospective flap area are palpated and marked on the scalp skin prior to designing, infiltration of epinephrine containing local anesthetic, or incision of any part of the flap. This marking of scalp arteries allows the designing of scalp flaps with the least amount of vascular supply destruction.

The Site of Defect and Flap Design

Midline occipital and parietal-vertex scalp defects may be closed in a number of ways (Fig. 6). (1) The smaller defects may be closed with undermining and a single rotation flap. (2) A moderate-sized defect is closed with double rotation flaps that are rotated in clockwise or counterclockwise direction (Fig. 7). (3) The bipedicle laterally based temporal flap provides a double vascular supply to the midline area of the flap. This double blood supply is extremely valuable in large or long flaps and when other scalp lacerations have injured the blood supply on either side of the scalp. Large flaps result in exposure of pericranium in the donor bed and require temporary or permanent split thickness autografts (Fig. 8).

The most distal corner opposite the proximal pivot corner is the area most likely to suffer avascular necrosis in a rotation flap. Only an essential number of sutures should be placed in this distal corner. A dog ear of scalp tissue routinely develops at the proximal pivot corner of a rotational flap. This dog ear will flatten out and provide extra scalp if only the skin layer of the scalp is sutured in this area. The 3-0 and full-thickness monofilament

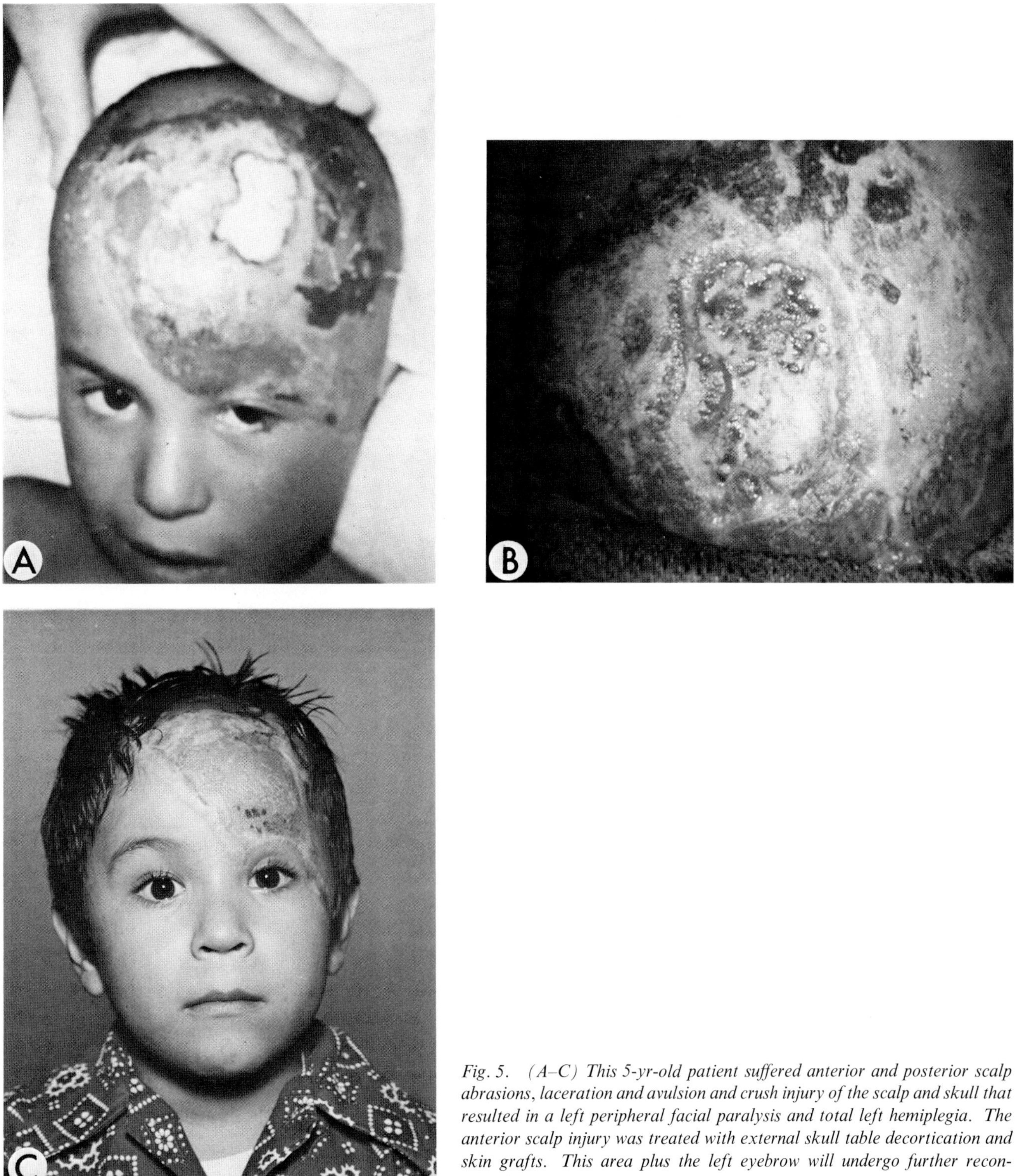

Fig. 5. (A–C) This 5-yr-old patient suffered anterior and posterior scalp abrasions, laceration and avulsion and crush injury of the scalp and skull that resulted in a left peripheral facial paralysis and total left hemiplegia. The anterior scalp injury was treated with external skull table decortication and skin grafts. This area plus the left eyebrow will undergo further reconstruction.

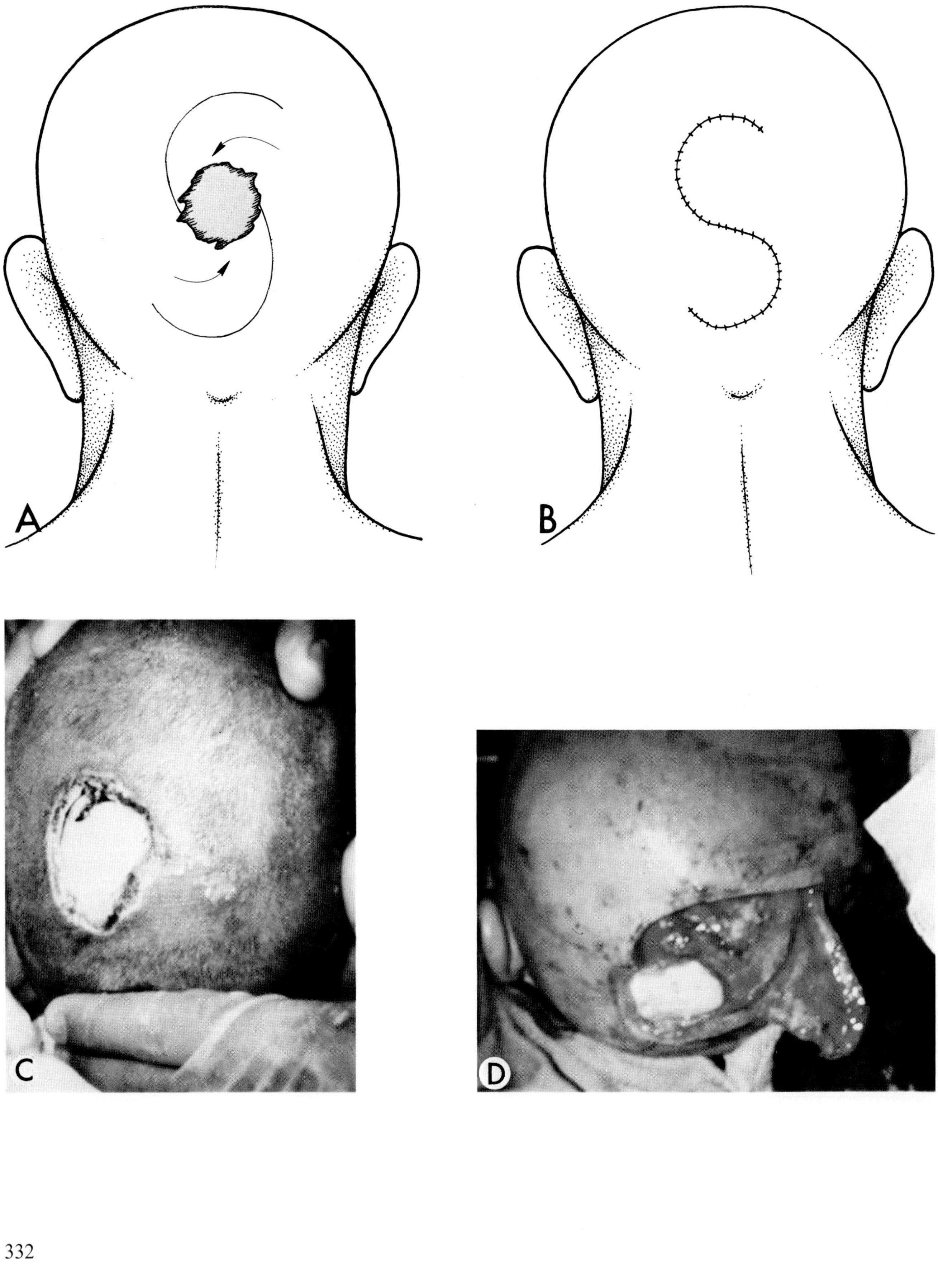

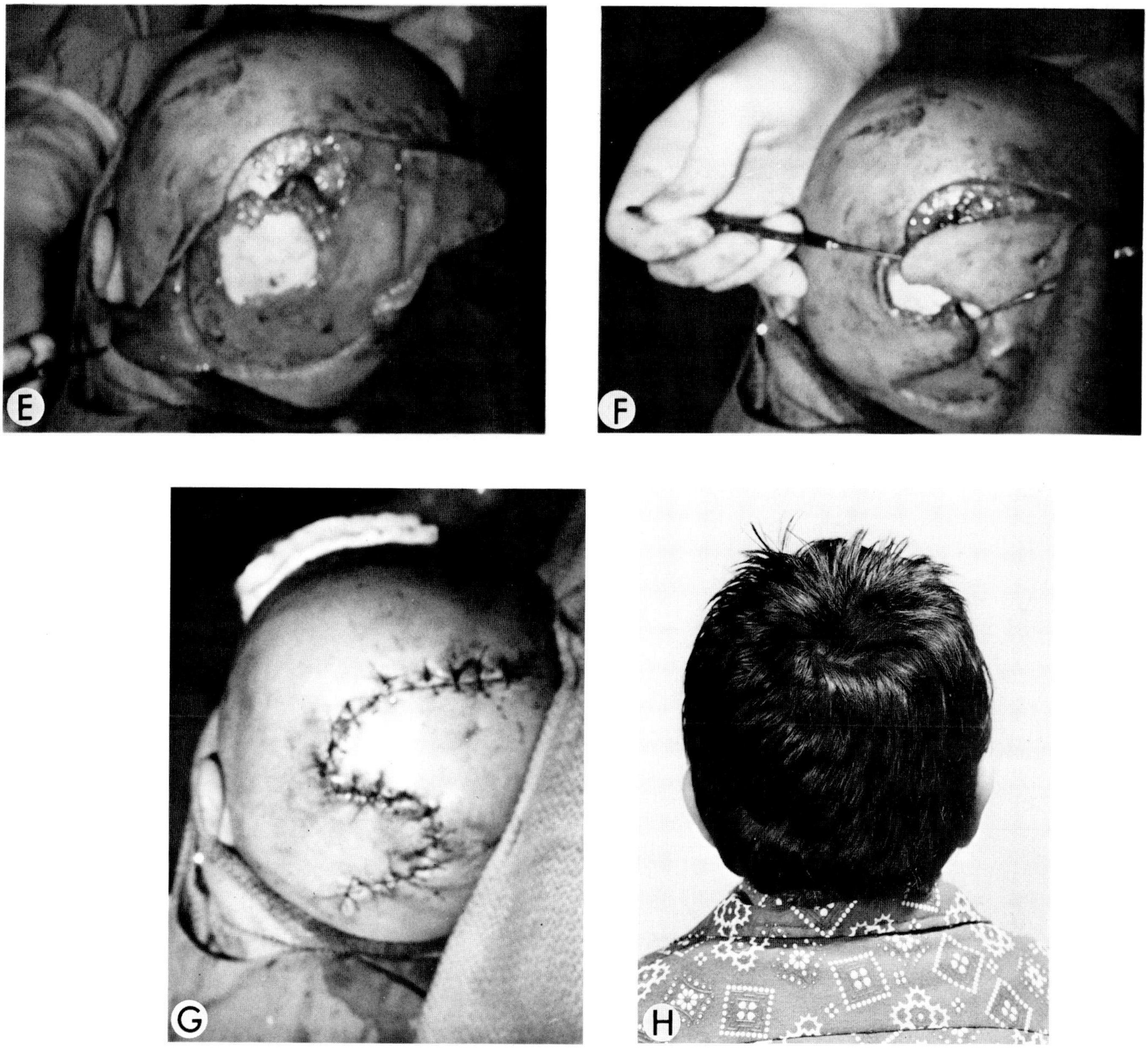

Fig. 6. (A–H) Same patient as in Figure 5, in which the posterior scalp defect was closed by double rotation scalp flaps.

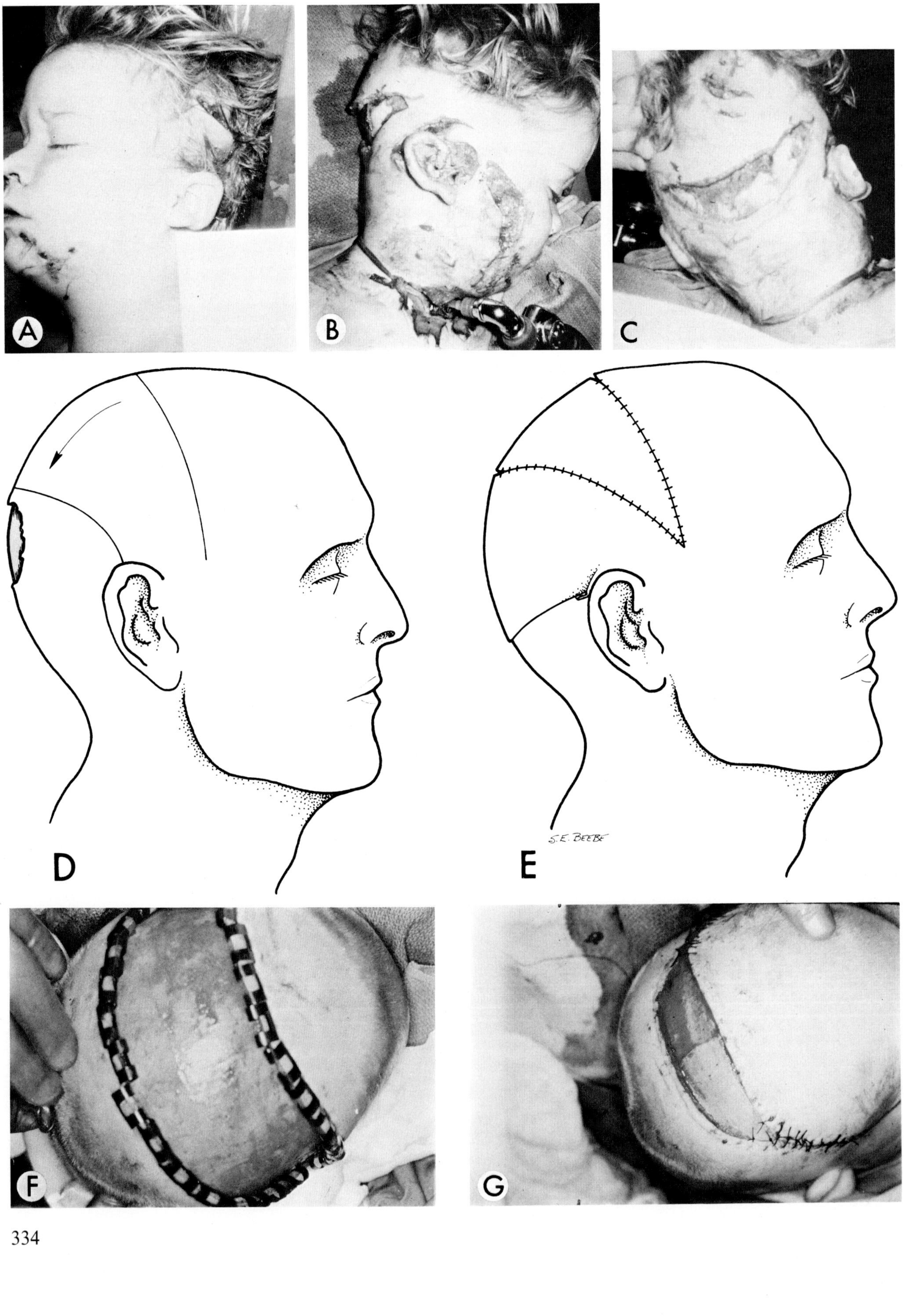
A
B
C
D
S.E. BEEBE
E
F
G

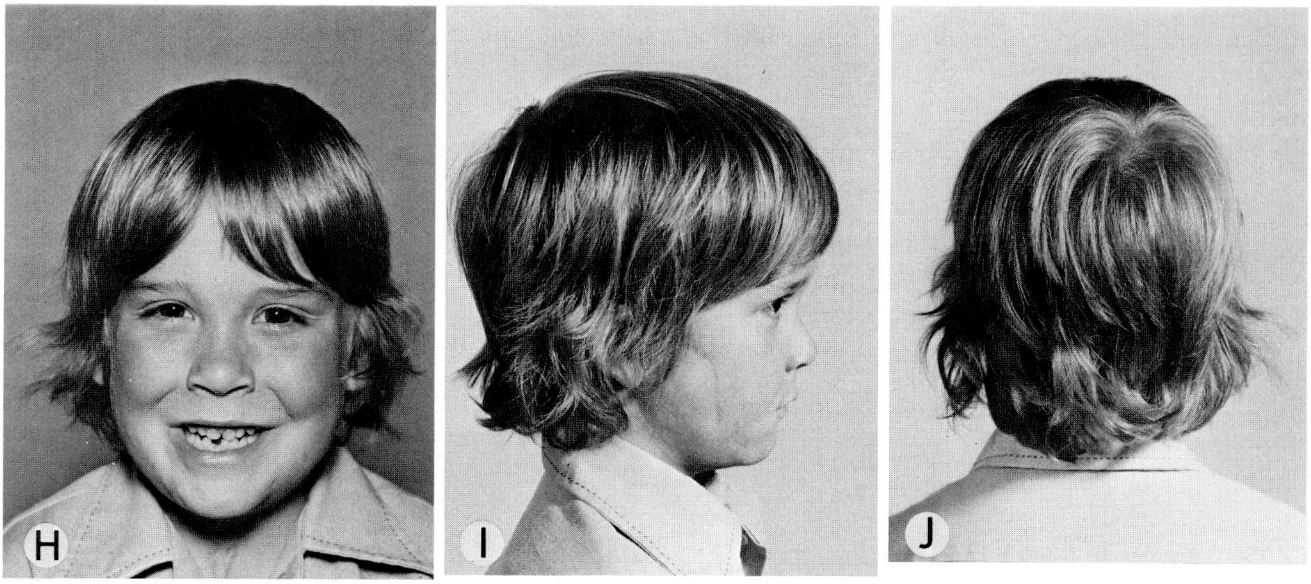

Fig. 7. (A–J) This 5-yr-old was attacked by a pack of dogs. The left postauricular, the right superficial temporal and posterior auricular arteries were destroyed in the attack. A bipedicle flap was chosen because of injury to major Temporal Area Arteries.

nylon sutures remain in critical places along the flap for twelve to fourteen days to insure a satisfactory connective tissue scar bridge.

Often the midline occipital-parietal area defects and mastoidtemporal area defects may be closed by rotational flaps based on either the homolateral or contralateral occipital, parietal, and temporal areas (Fig. 9). A bipedicle anterior and posterior based flap is useful in closing large defects in the lateral parietal and temporal areas. The anterior base of this bipedicle flap does not result in as nice a cosmetic result as the posterior based flaps. The destruction of the superficial temporal artery may force the use of a widely based single anterior scalp flap that again has the same cosmetic drawbacks as the previously mentioned bipedicle flap.

The timing of the single or serial excision of the temporary split thickness autografts and their staged replacement with advancement and rotation scalp flaps required experience and good clinical judgment (Fig. 10). The looseness of remaining scalp decreases after each serial excision and scalp stretch until a final limit of available scalp is reached. The time interval between the serial graft excision runs between four to ten months in most of the major scalp loss cases. When gentle squeezing pressure moves the scalp edges bordering the graft toward each other and a general looseness of scalp is apparent, the surgeon can expect to achieve a significant or complete reduction in the scalp defect.

Anterior scalp hairline defects, and hair and forehead defects in general present a challenging problem in reconstruction and cosmetic rehabilitation. The hairline, when possible, is reconstructed with the aid of more posteriorly based flaps. Moderate sized forehead defects are repaired with the use of forehead advancement flaps. Attempts at horizontal closing of large forehead defects may lead to upper eyelid ectropion or the anterior hairline being just superior to the eyebrow.

Areas of scalp that lack hair may receive small free grafts or hair plugs in the final stages of a patient's cosmetic rehabilitation. We have found that these hair plugs can be placed in scalp scar tissue after a reasonable blood supply has been allowed to develop in the scar area. Eyebrows may be constructed from a temporal area pedicle or from hairline free grafts from the postauricular area. Best results are obtained with hair scalp grafts that do not exceed 4 or 5 mm in width.

Postoperatively, scalp incisions are bandaged with Kerlix bandages for gentle pressure and absorption of discharge from the incision or drain sites. Soiled dressing must not be allowed to remain in contact with the scalp for any extended period

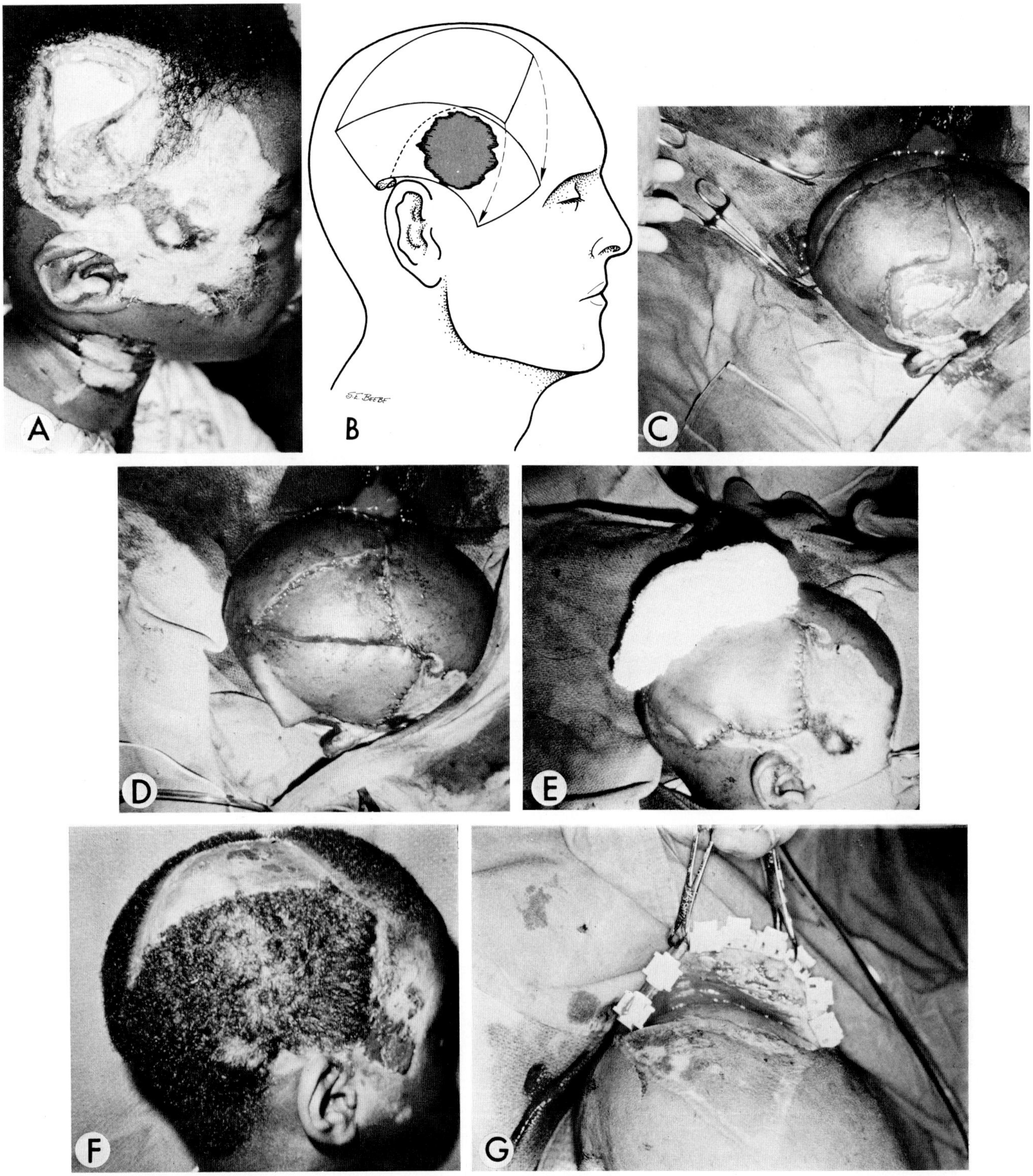
A
B
C
D
E
F
G

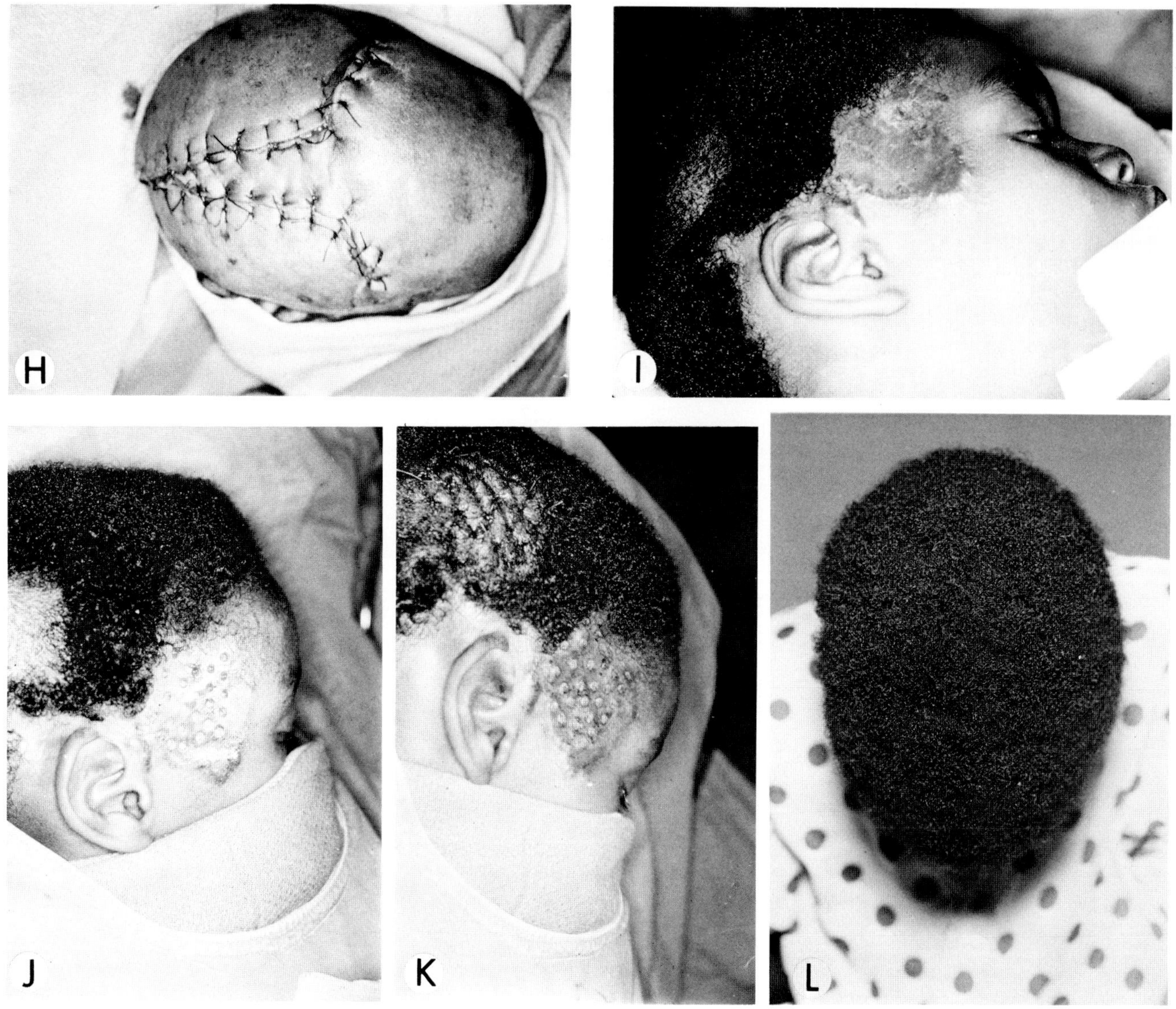

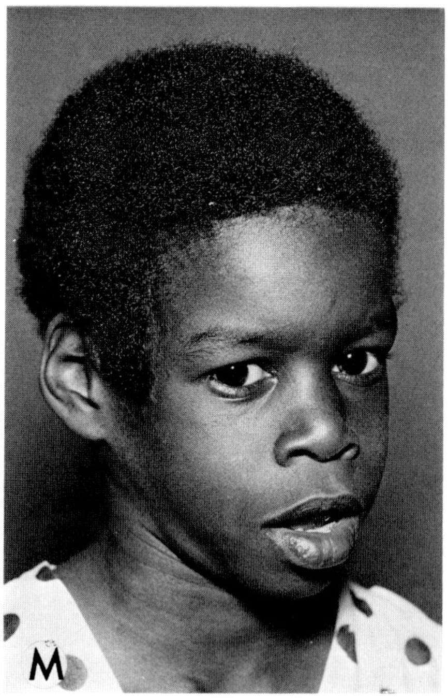

Fig. 8. (A–M) This 6-yr-old child was involved in an auto versus pedestrian accident and was thrown to the ground sustaining abrasions. lacerations and avulsion of the right lateral scalp area. There was a wide area of third degree friction burns. He has undergone reconstruction of the scalp with the aid of a large scalp rotation flap and progressive excision of intermediate stage skin grafts. Hair transplants were used to reconstruct the right temporal area.

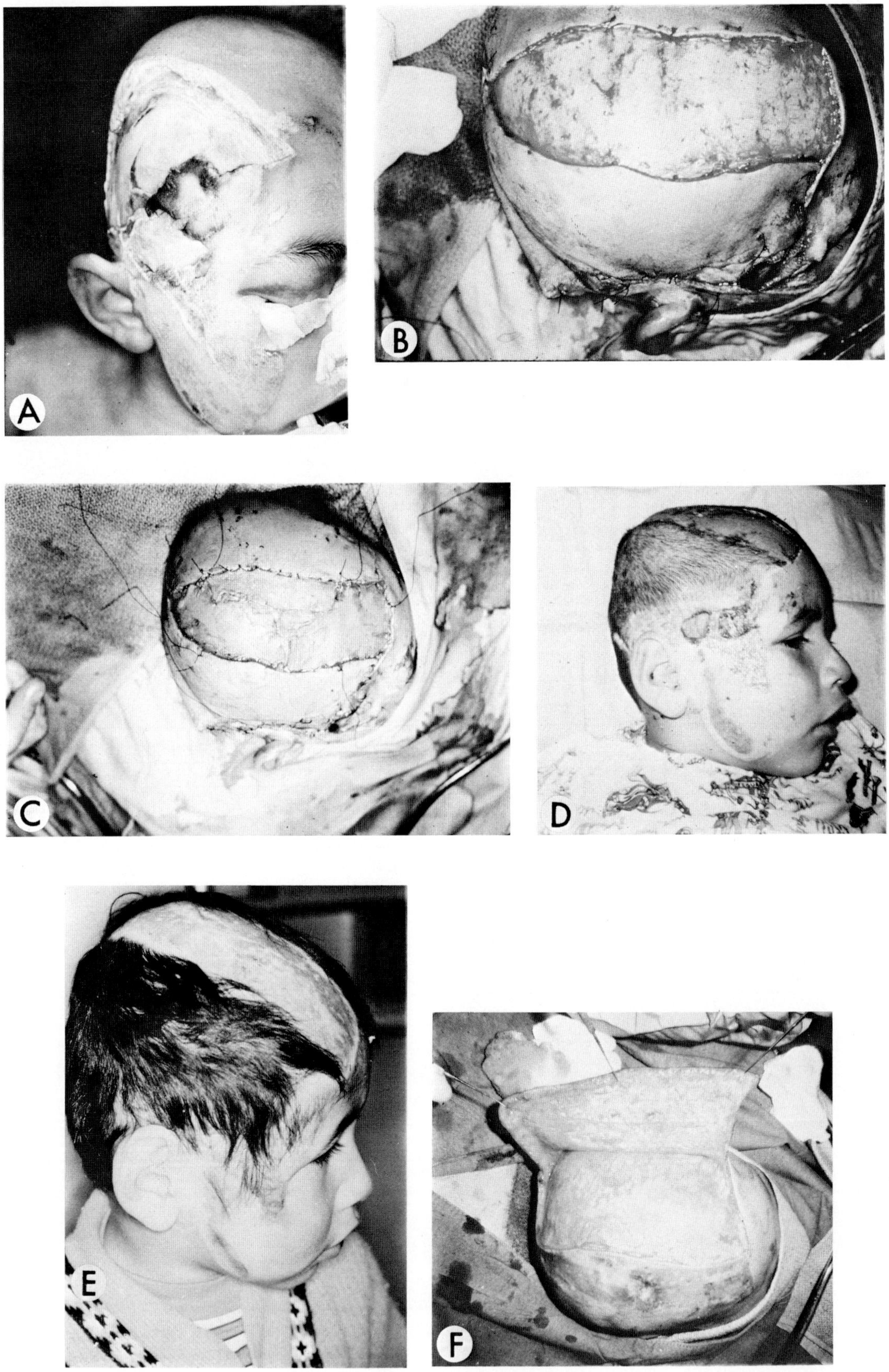

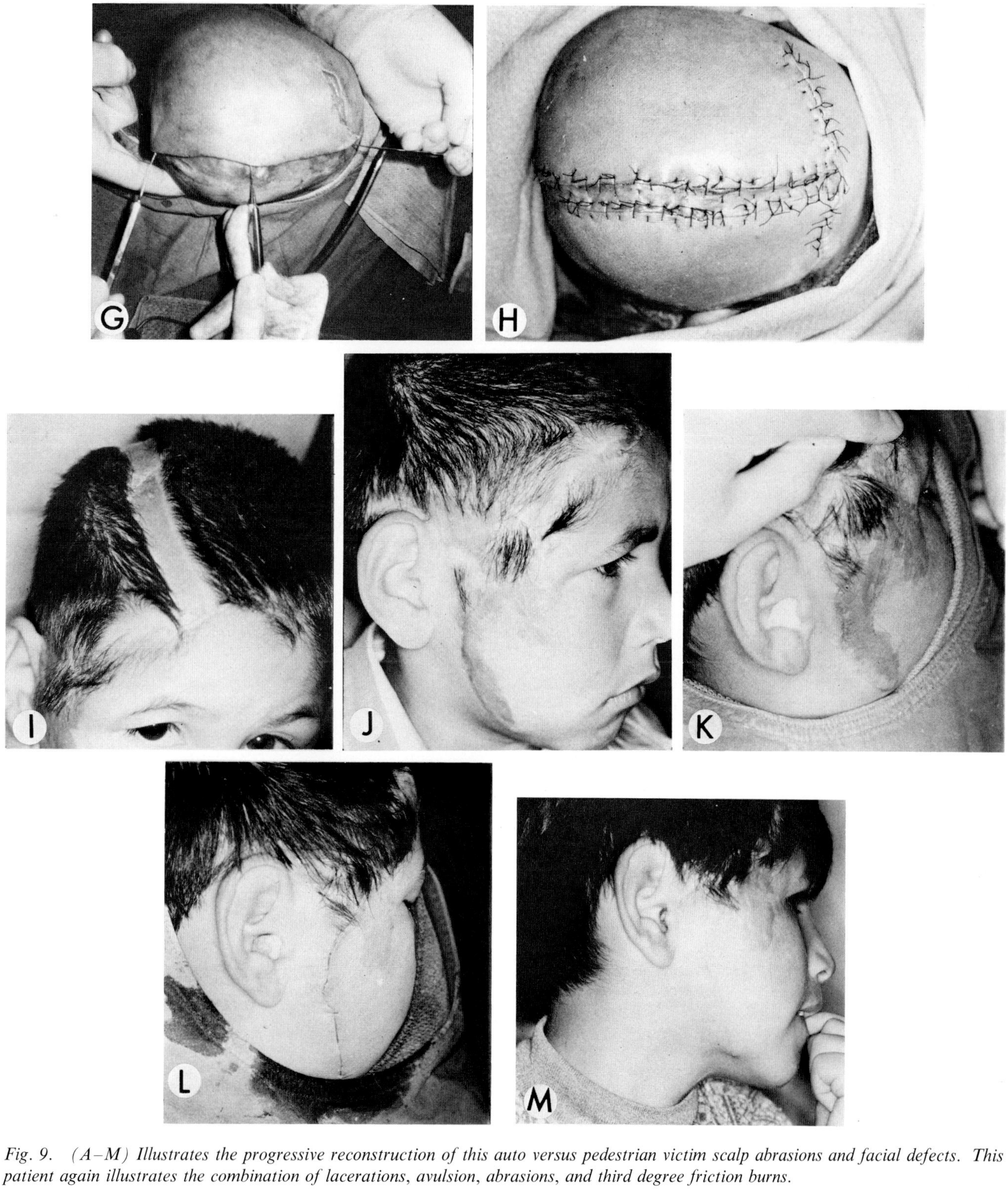

Fig. 9. (A–M) Illustrates the progressive reconstruction of this auto versus pedestrian victim scalp abrasions and facial defects. This patient again illustrates the combination of lacerations, avulsion, abrasions, and third degree friction burns.

of time. Simple gauze dressings held in place with "Surgifix" replace larger, bulkier dressings as soon as possible. The patient's dressing is periodically checked to make sure that it is not inhibiting the circulation in the area. The patient is positioned in bed so that they are not lying on the base circulation to the newly reconstructed area of scalp.

It has been our purpose to discuss basic reconstructive principles of the scalp with some of our cases. If these principles are followed the results can be rewarding for the surgeon dedicated to the reconstructive surgery of the head and neck.

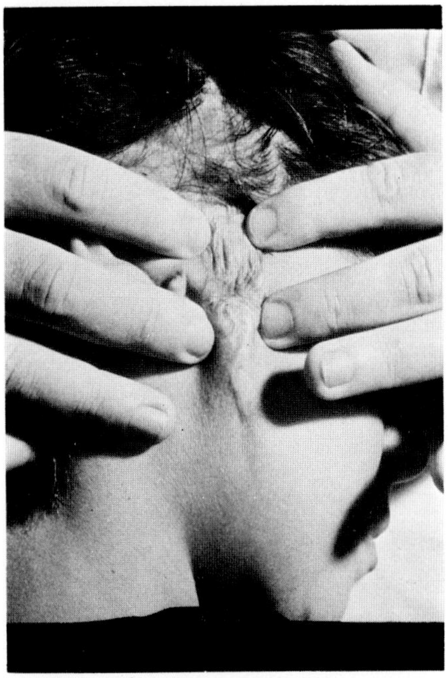

Fig. 10. When the scalp edges surrounding the temporary skin graft can be moved towards each other with ease, then a significant partial or complete closure of the defect is expected.

Index

a b c d 7 e 8 f 9 g 0 h 1 i 8 2 j